D1605131

HEALTH
POLICY
ISSUES

SIXTH EDITION

HEALTH POLICY ISSUES

AN ECONOMIC PERSPECTIVE

PAUL J. FELDSTEIN

AUPHA

Health Administration Press, Chicago, Illinois

Association of University Programs in Health Administration, Arlington, Virginia

Your board, staff, or clients may also benefit from this book's insight. For more information on quantity discounts, contact the Health Administration Press Marketing Manager at (312) 424–9470.

19   18   17   16   15   5   4   3   2   1

Library of Congress Cataloging-in-Publication Data

Feldstein, Paul J.
  Health policy issues : an economic perspective / Paul J. Feldstein.—Sixth edition.
    pages cm
  Includes bibliographical references and index.
  ISBN 978-1-56793-696-4 (alk. paper)
  1. Medical economics—United States. 2. Medical policy—Economic aspects—United States. 3. Medical care—United States—Cost control. 4. Medical care, Cost of—United States. I. Title.
  RA410.53F455 2015
  338.4'73621--`dc23

                    2014038009

The paper used in this publication meets the minimum requirements of American National Standard for Information Sciences—Permanence of Paper for Printed Library Materials, ANSI Z39.48-1984. ♾™

Acquisitions editor: Janet Davis; Project manager: Jane Calayag; Cover designer: Laurie Ingram; Layout: Virginia Byrne

Found an error or a typo? We want to know! Please e-mail it to hapbooks@ache.org, and put "Book Error" in the subject line.

For photocopying and copyright information, please contact Copyright Clearance Center at www.copyright.com or at (978) 750–8400.

Health Administration Press
A division of the Foundation of the American
    College of Healthcare Executives
One North Franklin Street, Suite 1700
Chicago, IL 60606–3529
(312) 424–2800

Association of University Programs
    in Health Administration
2000 North 14th Street
Suite 780
Arlington, VA 22201
(703) 894–0940

To Colette, Lauren, Kip, and Poppy

BRIEF CONTENTS

DETAILED CONTENTS

LIST OF EXHIBITS

PREFACE

Being an economist, I believe an economic approach is very useful, not only for understanding the forces pressing for change in healthcare but also for explaining why the health system has evolved to its current state. Even the political issues surrounding the financing and delivery of health services can be better understood when viewed through an economic perspective—that is, the economic self-interest of participants.

For these reasons, I believe an issue-oriented book containing short discussions on each subject and using an economic perspective is needed. The economic perspective used throughout is that of a "market" economist—namely one who believes markets (in which suppliers compete for customers on the basis of price and quality) are the most effective mechanisms for allocating resources. Of course, at times markets fail or lead to outcomes that are undesirable in terms of equity. Market economists generally believe that government economic interventions—no matter how well-intentioned or carefully thought out—can neither replicate the efficiency with which markets allocate resources nor fully anticipate the behavioral responses of the economic agents affected by the intervention. In cases of market failure, market economists prefer solutions that fix the underlying problem while retaining basic market incentives rather than replacing the market altogether with government planning or provision.

Healthcare reform has been an ongoing process for decades. At times, legislation and regulation have brought about major changes in the financing and delivery of medical services. At other times, competitive forces have restructured the delivery system. Both legislative and market forces will continue to influence how the public pays for and receives its medical services. Any subject affecting the lives of so many and requiring such a large portion of our country's resources will continue to be a topic of debate, legislative change, and market restructuring. I hope this book will help to clarify some of the more significant issues underlying the politics and economics of healthcare.

Changes in the Sixth Edition

For this sixth edition, both the chapters and the exhibits have been revised and updated with newer data and references. Most important, specific aspects or provisions of the Affordable Care Act (ACA) are discussed in chapters whose subject matter is directly affected by the ACA. Because the ACA has widespread implications for the entire healthcare industry, I have decided to explore this legislation throughout the book, instead of presenting only its general essence in one large chapter.

The following chapters describe, discuss, and analyze specific parts of the ACA:

Chapter 1: The Rise of Medical Expenditures

This chapter discusses whether the ACA contributed to the slowdown in rising health expenditures. Additionally, it proposes four criteria for evaluating the ACA to be considered when reading other ACA-related chapters.

Chapter 6: How Much Health Insurance Should Everyone Have?

This chapter addresses the higher individual taxes and the "Cadillac" tax (on expensive health plans) imposed by the ACA. These taxes help finance the subsidies provided to states for expanding the eligibility to state Medicaid programs and to finance those qualifying for subsidies on the health insurance exchanges.

Chapter 7: Why Are Those Who Most Need Health Insurance Least Able to Buy It?

This chapter describes many of the changes the ACA made to the health insurance market. These include establishing state and federal health insurance exchanges, providing subsidies to eligible persons buying their insurance on the exchanges, eliminating the preexisting condition exclusion, instituting an individual mandate to buy insurance, specifying the four types of health plans to be purchased on the exchanges, requiring insurers to have minimum medical loss ratios, requiring community and gender rating, adding essential benefits in health plans, and allowing adult children up to age 26 years to remain on their parent's policy. The likely consequences of these new health insurance rules on the uninsured, the newly insured, and others—as well as the response by health insurers, such as rising premiums and why insurers are using narrow provider networks—are analyzed.

Chapter 8: Medicare

This chapter highlights the ACA's changes to Medicare—including accountable care organizations, the Independent Payment Advisory Board, and the reductions in Medicare hospital payments (assumed productivity increases)—

and their implications for hospitals. The ACA's closing of the "donut hole" in Medicare Part D and the increase in Medicare payroll and income taxes to finance the ACA are also discussed.

Chapter 9: Medicaid

This chapter discusses the ACA's changes to Medicaid—particularly the expansion of eligibility to an additional 16 million low-income people. A new study presents results contrary to the ACA's expectations that emergency department visits would decline as more of the uninsured enroll in Medicaid. Factors affecting a state's decision to take advantage of ACA funding for expanding state Medicaid eligibility are explored. A reform proposal to convert Medicaid by using block grants to the states is included.

Chapter 11: The Impending Shortage of Physicians

This chapter examines how the ACA's expanded coverage (increased Medicaid eligibility and subsidies to eligible persons buying insurance on health exchanges) will cause an increase in demand for primary care services, making the shortage of physicians more severe.

Chapter 12: The Changing Practice of Medicine

This chapter analyzes the likely effects of the ACA on physician payment, the size of medical practices, and the role of the accountable care organization in the growth of hospital employment of physicians.

Chapter 16: The Future Role of Hospitals

This chapter covers the multiple effects and likely implications of the ACA on hospitals. Topics include the different approaches to reducing hospital payments—such as the Independent Payment Advisory Board, assumed hospital productivity increase, preventable hospital readmissions, and Medicare Disproportionate Share Hospital. Also discussed are new hospital payment systems—such as accountable care organizations and episode-based charges. The increase in hospital admissions as a result of Medicaid eligibility expansions and health insurance exchange subsidies is addressed.

Chapter 18: Can Price Controls Limit Medical Expenditure Increases?

This chapter presents the Independent Payment Advisory Board (IPAB) established by the ACA. The IPAB has the authority to use price controls (reduce provider payments) to decrease Medicare expenditures when they exceed the rate of growth in per capita GDP plus one percent. Also discussed are the ACA's reduced payments to Medicare Advantage plans and the likely consequences of such actions.

Chapter 19: The Evolution of Managed Care

This chapter contains a section on the effect of the ACA on managed care. Included topics are health exchanges, limited provider networks, and accountable care organizations.

Chapter 25: The High Price of Prescription Drugs

This chapter addresses ACA's reduction of the Medicare Part D "donut hole."

Chapter 31: Medical Research, Medical Education, Alcohol Consumption, and Pollution: Who Should Pay?

A footnote in this chapter describes the penalty imposed by the ACA for failure to buy health insurance under the individual mandate and the penalty's likely consequences.

Chapter 33: Employer-Mandated National Health Insurance

This chapter explains the ACA's employer mandate—how it is designed, how it is financed, and what its likely consequences are for employers and employees at different income levels. Also discussed are the health insurance exchanges, the subsidies available, age-rated premiums, and reasons that insurers use narrow provider networks on the exchanges.

Chapter 34: National Health Insurance: Which Approach and Why?

Part of this chapter spotlights the different types of taxes used to finance the ACA and their effects on efficiency and equity. An exhibit summarizes each type, including income tax, sin tax (alcohol and cigarette), sales tax (medical devices and insurers), payroll tax (employer mandate), and user tax (individual mandate). Also covered are the ACA's individual mandate, the required essential benefits to be included in health plans, and the Cadillac tax on expensive health plans.

Chapter 35: Financing Long-Term Care

This chapter describes the ACA's CLASS Act, a voluntary long-term care program that the Obama Administration determined unworkable and thus was never implemented. Congress subsequently repealed it. The problem with the CLASS Act was that it violated certain insurance principles, which are discussed.

Chapter 36: The Politics of Healthcare Reform

This chapter provides a comprehensive treatment of the political and economic interests behind the passage of the ACA. The various interest groups involved as well as their healthcare reform objectives and agendas are discussed. Also covered are how the Democratic Senate was able to achieve the necessary 60 votes to reject a Republican filibuster and pass the ACA, how the surprise election of a Republican newcomer (Senator Scott Brown) changed the legislative process and affected the outcome of the legislation, and what problems plagued the ACA implementation.

The policies and implications of the ACA, as well as other content, are repeated (although not verbatim) in related chapters. The reason for this is twofold. First, instructors are not likely to assign all 36 chapters to their students, given that not all topics in the book will be covered in class; thus, to ensure that students do not miss out on the discussion, the relevant materials appear in a few chapters that address similar issues. Second, some chapters would be considered incomplete if a particular aspect or impact of the ACA, or some other vital topic, is not included. For example, the ACA made changes to how Medicare pays hospitals; these changes and their likely consequences are discussed in both the chapter on Medicare and the chapter on the future of hospitals—as the changes affect not only Medicare patients' access to care but also hospitals' financial sustainability. Finally, an Appendix provides a brief summary of the ACA.

For the book as whole, note that some overlap between chapters occurs because of the large number of chapters (not all of which will be assigned or read) and the interrelated nature of the topics covered. To help the reader focus on the important points discussed, a list of discussion questions appears at the end of each chapter. A list of exhibits and a glossary are also included.

Teaching Tools

For instructors, a test bank, an Instructor's Manual, and PowerPoint slides are available. The Instructor's Manual includes a brief overview of each chapter and a list of the key topics covered. Also included are discussion points related to the Discussion Questions that appear at the end of each chapter. Additional questions and answers have been provided for instructor use. The test bank, Instructor's Manual, and PowerPoints reside in a secure area on the Health Administration Press website and are available only to adopters of this book. For access information, e-mail hapbooks@ache.org.

Acknowledgments

I thank Glenn Melnick, Thomas Wickizer, Jerry German, Jeff Hoch, and several anonymous reviewers for their comments. For this sixth edition, I also thank Elzbieta Kozlowski for all her assistance, particularly the collection of data and construction of the exhibits.

Paul J. Feldstein
Irvine, California

1

THE RISE OF MEDICAL EXPENDITURES

T he rapid growth of medical expenditures since 1965 is as familiar as the increasing percentage of US gross domestic product (GDP) devoted to medical care. Less known are the reasons for this continual increase. The purpose of this introductory chapter is threefold: (1) to provide a historical perspective on the medical sector; (2) to explain the rise of medical expenditures in an economic context; and (3) to set forth criteria for evaluating the Patient Protection and Affordable Care Act (ACA), which is likely to have a significant impact on the medical sector in coming years.

Before Medicare and Medicaid

Until 1965, spending in the medical sector was predominantly private—80 percent of all expenditures were paid by individuals out of pocket or by private health insurance on their behalf. The remaining expenditures (20 percent) were paid by the federal government (8 percent) and the states (12 percent) (see Exhibit 1.1). Personal medical expenditures totaled $35 billion

Source of Funds	1965		2012	
	$ (Billions)	%	$ (Billions)	%
Total	34.7	100.0	2,360.4	100.0
Private	27.6	79.5	1,244.1	52.7
Out-of-pocket	18.2	52.4	328.2	13.9
Insurance benefits	8.7	25.1	807.0	34.2
All other	0.7	2.0	108.9	4.6
Public	7.1	20.5	1,116.4	47.3
Federal	2.8	8.1	869.0	36.8
State and local	4.3	12.4	247.4	10.5

EXHIBIT 1.1
Personal Health Expenditures by Source of Funds, 1965 and 2012

SOURCE: Data from CMS (2014).

and accounted for approximately 6 percent of GDP—that is, six cents of every dollar spent went to medical services.

Two important trends have been the increasing role of government in financing medical services and the declining portion of expenditures paid out of pocket by the public. As shown in Exhibit 1.1, 47.3 percent of total medical expenditures in 2012 were paid by the government; the federal share was 36.8 percent and the states contributed 10.5 percent. Meanwhile, the private share dropped to 53 percent (from 80 percent in 1965); of that amount, 14 percent was paid out of pocket (from 52 percent in 1965).

The Greater Role of Government in Healthcare

Medicare and Medicaid were enacted in 1965, dramatically expanding the role of government in financing medical care. Medicare, which covers the aged, initially consisted of two of its current four parts—Part A and Part B. Part A is for hospital care and is financed by a separate (Medicare) payroll tax on the working population. Part B covers physicians' services and is financed by federal taxes (currently 75 percent) and by a premium paid by the aged (25 percent). Medicare Part C and Part D have since been added. Part C is a managed care option, and Part D is a prescription drug benefit—financed 75 percent by the federal government and 25 percent by the aged. Parts B, C, and D are all voluntary programs. Medicaid is for the categorically or medically needy, including the indigent aged and families with dependent children who receive cash assistance. Each state administers its own program, and the federal government pays, on average, more than half of the costs.

The rapid increase in total national health expenditure (NHE) is illustrated in Exhibit 1.2, which shows spending on the different components of medical services over time. Since 2000, NHE per capita has risen from $4,884 billion to $8,925 billion. During this time frame, hospital care and physician and clinical services—the two largest components of medical expenditures—have surged from $416 billion to $882 billion and $291 billion to $565 billion, respectively. These data indicate the enormous amount of US resources flowing into healthcare.

In the United States, $2.793 trillion (or 17.2 percent of GDP) was spent on medical care in 2012.[1] From 2000 to 2012, these expenditures climbed by about 9 percent per year. Since peaking in the early part of the decade, the annual rate of increase in NHE has been declining, although it remains above the rate of inflation. These expenditures continue to rise as a percentage of GDP.

	1965	1970	1980	1990	2000	2012
Total national health expenditures	$42.0	$74.9	$255.8	$724.3	$1,377.2	$2,793.4
Health services and supplies	37.2	67.1	235.7	675.6	1,289.6	2,633.4
Personal healthcare	34.7	63.1	217.2	616.8	1,165.4	2,360.4
Hospital care	13.5	27.2	100.5	250.4	415.5	882.3
Physician and clinical services	8.6	14.3	47.7	158.9	290.9	565.0
Dental services	2.8	4.7	13.4	31.7	62.3	111.0
Other professional care	0.5	0.7	3.5	17.4	37.0	76.4
Home health care	0.1	0.2	2.4	12.6	32.4	77.8
Nursing home care	1.4	4.0	15.3	44.9	85.1	151.5
Drugs, medical nondurables	5.9	8.8	21.8	62.7	152.5	317.0
Durable medical equipment	1.1	1.7	4.1	13.8	25.2	41.3
Other personal healthcare	0.7	1.3	8.5	24.3	64.5	138.2
Program administration and net cost of private health insurance	1.8	2.6	12.0	38.8	81.2	197.9
Government public health activities	0.6	1.4	6.4	20.0	43.0	75.0
Research and construction	4.7	7.8	20.1	48.7	87.6	160.0
Research	1.5	2.0	5.4	12.7	25.5	48.1
Construction	3.2	5.8	14.7	36.0	62.1	111.9
National health expenditures per capita	$210	$356	$1,112	$2,851	$4,884	$8,925

EXHIBIT 1.2
National Health Expenditures, Selected Calendar Years, 1965–2012 (in Billions of Dollars)

SOURCE: Data from CMS (2014).

Relationship Between NHE and GDP

The growth in medical expenditures over time can be illustrated by comparing the rate of increase in NHE per capita to the rate of change in GDP per capita. (To show the relationship between the two series more clearly, a five-year moving average of the rates of change is used.) If NHE per capita is rising faster than GDP per capita, then the former is becoming a larger share of GDP. If the two series are moving together, then changes in the economy and health spending are closely related. Exhibit 1.3 shows the relationship between the two series from 1965 to 2012.

The only major divergence between NHE per capita and GDP per capita occurred starting in the mid-1990s. Medical expenditures increased at a slower rate because of the growth of managed care (which emphasized utilization management) and price competition among providers participating in managed care provider networks. By the end of the 1990s, managed care's cost-containment approaches lost support because of public dissatisfaction with managed care, lawsuits against managed care organizations (MCOs) for denial of care, government legislation, and a tight labor market that led employers to offer their employees more health plan choices. As a result, medical expenditures rose at a more rapid rate.

The decline in the annual NHE rate increase in the past ten years (Exhibit 1.3) can be attributed to the Great Recession, slow economic recovery, high unemployment levels, large number of uninsured, decrease in the number of employers paying for employee health insurance, and rapid spread of high-deductible health plans (Fuchs 2013).[2]

EXHIBIT 1.3
Changes in National Health Expenditures and Gross Domestic Product per Capita, 1965– 2012

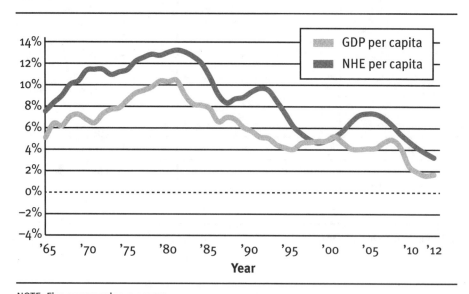

NOTE: Five-year moving averages
SOURCES: Data from CMS (2014); BEA (2014).

NHE is likely to rise at a slightly faster rate in the coming years as the economy continues to recover, more baby boomers become eligible for Medicare, new technology and specialty drugs that improve quality of life (but are higher in cost) are developed, and as the ACA is fully implemented (the expansion of Medicaid eligibility and subsidies for low-income enrollees on state health exchanges took effect in 2014). By 2022, federal, state, and local governments are expected to further increase their share of total NHE, which is expected to reach $5 trillion (almost doubling from $2.7 trillion in 2011) and to consume an even greater portion of GDP (19.9 percent) (Cuckler et al. 2013).

Exhibit 1.4 shows where healthcare dollars come from and how they are distributed among different types of healthcare providers.

Changing Patient and Provider Incentives

Medical expenditures equal the prices of services provided multiplied by the quantity of services provided. The rise of expenditures can be explained by looking at the factors that prompt medical prices and quantities to change. In a market system, the prices and output of goods and services are determined by the interaction of buyers (the demand side) and sellers (the supply side). We can analyze price and output changes by examining how various interventions change the behavior of buyers and sellers. One such intervention was Medicare, which lowered the out-of-pocket price the aged had to pay for medical care. The demand for hospital and physician services by

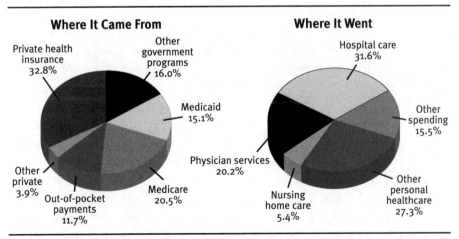

EXHIBIT 1.4
The Nation's Healthcare Dollar, 2012

Where It Came From

Private health insurance 32.8%
Other government programs 16.0%
Medicaid 15.1%
Other private 3.9%
Out-of-pocket payments 11.7%
Medicare 20.5%

Where It Went

Hospital care 31.6%
Other spending 15.5%
Physician services 20.2%
Nursing home care 5.4%
Other personal healthcare 27.3%

NOTES: "Other personal healthcare" includes dental care, vision care, home health care, drugs, medical products, and other professional services. "Other spending" includes program administration, net cost of private health insurance, government public health, and research and construction.
SOURCE: Data from CMS (2014).

the aged went up dramatically after Medicare was enacted, spurring rapid price increases. Similarly, government payments on behalf of the poor under Medicaid stimulated demand for medical services among this demographic. Greater demand for services multiplied by higher prices for those services equals greater total expenditures.

Prices also go up when the costs of providing services increase. For example, to attract more nurses to care for the higher number of aged patients, hospitals raised nurses' wages and then passed this increase to payers in the form of more expensive services. Increased demand for care multiplied by higher costs of care equals greater expenditures.

While the government was subsidizing the demands of the aged and the poor, the demand for medical services by the employed population also was increasing. The growth of private health insurance during the late 1960s and 1970s was stimulated by income growth, high marginal (federal) income tax rates (up to 70 percent), and the high inflation rate in the economy. The high inflation rate threatened to push many people into higher marginal tax brackets. If an employee were pushed into a 50 percent marginal income tax bracket, half of his salary in that bracket would go to taxes. Instead of having that additional income taxed at 50 percent, employees often chose to have the employer spend those same dollars, before tax, to buy more comprehensive health insurance. Thus, employees could receive the full value of their raise, albeit in healthcare benefits. This tax subsidy for employer-paid health insurance stimulated the demand for medical services in the private sector and further boosted medical prices.

Demand increased most rapidly for medical services covered by government and private health insurance. As of 2012, only 3.4 percent of hospital care and 9.7 percent of physician services were paid out of pocket by the patient; the remainder was paid by some third party (CMS 2014). Patients had little incentive to be concerned about the price of a service when they were not responsible for paying a significant portion of the price. As the out-of-pocket price declined, the use of services increased.

The aged—who represent almost 14 percent of the population and use more medical services than does any other age group—accounted for 36 percent of all hospital stays, as of 2011 (Pfuntner, Wier, and Elixhauser 2013, Table 2). Use of physician services by the aged (Medicare), the poor (Medicaid), and those covered by tax-exempt employer-paid insurance also increased as patients became less concerned with the cost of their care.

Advances in medical technology were yet another factor stimulating the demand for medical treatment. New methods of diagnosis and treatment were developed; those with previously untreatable diseases gained access to technology that offered hope of recovery. New medical devices (such as imaging equipment) were introduced, and new treatments (such as organ transplants) became available. New diseases (such as AIDS) also increased demand on the medical system. Reduced out-of-pocket costs and increased third-party payments (both public and private)—in addition to an aging population, new technologies, and new diseases—drove up both the prices and quantity of medical services provided.

Providers (hospitals and physicians) responded to the increased demand for care, but the way they responded unnecessarily increased the cost of providing medical services. After Medicare was enacted, hospitals had few incentives to be efficient because the program reimbursed hospitals their costs plus 2 percent for serving Medicare patients. Hospitals, predominantly not-for-profit, consequently expanded their capacity, invested in the latest technology, and duplicated facilities and services offered in nearby hospitals. Hospital prices rose faster than the prices of any other medical service. Similarly, physicians had little cause for concern over hospital costs. Physicians, who were paid fee-for-service, wanted their hospitals to have the latest equipment so that they would not have to refer their patients elsewhere (and possibly lose them). They would hospitalize patients for diagnostic workups and keep them in the hospital longer because it was less costly for patients covered by hospital insurance and physicians would be sure to receive reimbursement; outpatient services, which were less costly than hospital care, initially were not covered by third-party payers.

In addition to the lack of incentives for patients to be concerned with the cost of their care and the similar lack of incentives for providers to supply that care efficiently, the government imposed restrictions on the delivery of services that increased enrollees' medical costs. Under Medicare and Medicaid, the government ruled that insurers must give enrollees free choice of provider. Insurers such as health maintenance organizations (HMOs) that preclude their enrollees from choosing any physician in the community were violating the free choice of provider rule and were thus ineligible to receive capitation payments from the government; HMOs were instead paid fee-for-service, reducing their incentive to reduce the total costs of treating a patient. Numerous state restrictions on HMOs, such as prohibiting HMOs from advertising, requiring HMOs to be not-for-profit (thereby limiting their access to capital), and requiring HMOs to be controlled by physicians, further inhibited their development. By imposing these restrictions on alternative delivery systems, however, the government reduced competition for Medicare and Medicaid patients, forgoing an opportunity to reduce government payments for Medicare and Medicaid.

The effects of higher demand, limited patient and provider incentives to search for lower-cost approaches, and restrictions on the delivery of medical services were escalating prices, increased use of services, and greater medical expenditures.

Government Response to Rising Costs

As expenditures under Medicare and Medicaid increased, the federal government faced limited options: (1) raise the Medicare payroll tax and income taxes on the non-aged to continue funding these programs; (2) require the aged to pay higher premiums for Medicare, and increase their deductibles and copayments; or (3) reduce payments to hospitals and physicians. Each of these approaches would cost the administration and Congress political support from some constituents, such as employees, the aged, and healthcare providers. The least politically costly options appeared to be number 1 (increase taxes on the non-aged) and number 3 (pay hospitals and physicians less).

Federal and state governments used additional regulatory approaches to control these rapidly rising expenditures. Medicare utilization review programs were instituted, and controls were placed on hospital investment in new facilities and equipment. These government controls proved ineffective as hospital expenditures continued to escalate through the 1970s. The government then limited physician fee increases under Medicare and Medicaid; as a consequence, many physicians refused to participate in these programs, reducing access to care for the aged and the poor. As a result of their refusal to participate in Medicare, many Medicare patients had to pay higher out-of-pocket fees to be seen by physicians.

In 1979, President Carter's highest domestic priority was to enact expenditure limits on Medicare hospital cost increases; a Congress controlled by his own political party defeated him.

The 1980s

By the beginning of the 1980s, political consensus on what should be done to control Medicare hospital and physician expenditures was lacking, and private health expenditures continued to go up. By the mid-1980s, however, legislative changes and other events imposed heavy cost-containment pressures on Medicare, Medicaid, and the private sector.

Legislative and Government Changes

Several events in the early 1980s brought major changes to the medical sector. The HMO legislation enacted in 1973 began to have an effect in this decade. In 1974, President Nixon wanted a health program that would not increase federal expenditures. The result was the HMO Act of 1973, which legitimized HMOs and removed restrictive state laws impeding the development of federally approved HMOs. However, many HMOs decided not to seek federal qualification because imposed restrictions, such as having to offer more costly benefits, would have caused their premiums to be too high to be price competitive with traditional health insurers' premiums. These restrictions were removed by the late 1970s, and the growth of HMOs began in the early 1980s.

To achieve savings in Medicaid, in 1981 the Reagan Administration removed the free choice of provider rule, enabling states to enroll their Medicaid populations in closed provider panels. As a result, states were permitted to negotiate capitation payments with HMOs for care of their Medicaid patients. The free choice rule continued for the aged; however, in the mid-1980s they were permitted to voluntarily join HMOs. The federal government agreed to pay HMOs a capitated amount for enrolling Medicare patients, but less than 10 percent of the aged voluntarily participated. (As of 2012, 28 percent of the 42 million aged were enrolled in Medicare HMOs, referred to as Medicare Advantage plans [CMS 2013, Table 2.1].[3])

Federal subsidies were provided to medical schools in 1964 to increase the number of students they could accommodate, and the supply of physicians went up. The number of active physicians grew from 146 per 100,000 civilian population in 1965 to 195 per 100,000 in 1980; it reached 229 per 100,000 by 1990 and 283 per 100,000 in 2011 (AMA 1991, 2013). The greater supply created excess capacity among physicians, dampened their fee hikes, and made attracting physicians—and therefore expanding—easier for HMOs.

A new Medicare hospital payment system was phased in during 1983. Hospitals were no longer to be paid according to their costs. Fixed prices were established for each diagnostic admission (referred to as diagnosis-related groups [DRGs]), and each year Congress set an annual limit on the amount by which these fixed prices per admission could increase. DRG prices changed hospitals' incentives. Because hospitals could keep the difference if the costs they incurred from an admission were less than the fixed DRG payment they received for that admission, they were motivated to reduce the cost of caring for Medicare patients and to discharge them earlier. Length of stay per admission fell, and occupancy rates declined. Hospitals also became concerned with inefficient physician practice behaviors that increased the hospitals' costs of care.

In addition, in 1992 the federal government changed its method of paying physicians under Medicare. A national fee schedule (referred to as resource-based relative value system [RBRVS]) was implemented, and volume expenditure limits were established to limit the total rate of increase in physician Medicare payments. Today, the imposition of price controls and expenditure limits on payments to hospitals and physicians for services provided to Medicare patients continues to be the approach used by the federal government to contain Medicare expenditures. The RBRVS also prohibited physicians from charging their higher-income patients a higher fee and accepting the Medicare fee only for lower-income patients; they had to accept the fee for all their Medicare patients or none. Medicare patients represent such a significant portion of a physician's practice that few physicians decided not to participate; consequently, they accepted Medicare fees for all patients.

Private Sector Changes

In addition to the government policy changes of the early 1980s, important events were occurring in the private sector. The new decade started with a recession. To survive the recession and remain competitive internationally, the business sector looked to reduce labor costs. Because employer-paid health insurance was the fastest-growing labor expense, businesses pressured health insurers to better control the use and cost of medical services. Competitive pressures forced insurers to increase the efficiency of their benefit packages by including lower-cost substitutes for inpatient care, such as outpatient surgery. They raised deductibles and copayments, intensifying patients' price sensitivity. Further, patients had to receive prior authorization from their insurer before being admitted to a hospital, and insurers reviewed patients' length of stay while patients were in the hospital. These actions greatly reduced hospital admission rates and lengths of stay. The number of admissions in community hospitals in 1975 was 155 per 1,000 population. By 1990 it had fallen to 125 per 1,000 and continued to decline thereafter, dropping to 110 in 2012. The number of inpatient days per 1,000 population fell even more dramatically—from 1,302 in 1977 to 982 in 1990 to 591 in 2012 (AHA 2014).

Because of the implementation of the DRG payment system, the changes to private programs, and a shift to the outpatient sector facilitated by technological change (both anesthetic and surgical techniques), hospital occupancy rates decreased from 76 percent in 1980 to 63.3 percent in 2012 (AHA 2014).

Antitrust Laws

The preconditions for price competition were in place: Hospitals and physicians had excess capacity, and employers wanted to pay less for employee health insurance. The last necessary condition for price competition was set in 1982, when the US Supreme Court upheld the applicability of the antitrust laws to the medical sector. Successful antitrust cases were brought against the American Medical Association for its restrictions on advertising, against a medical society that threatened to boycott an insurer over physician fee increases, against a dental organization that boycotted an insurer's cost-containment program, against medical staffs that denied hospital privileges to physicians because they belonged to an HMO, and against hospitals whose mergers threatened to reduce price competition in their communities.

The applicability of the antitrust laws, excess capacity among providers, and employer and insurer interest in lowering medical costs brought about profound changes in the medical marketplace. Traditional insurance plans lost market share as managed care plans—which controlled utilization and limited access to hospitals and physicians—grew. Preferred provider organizations (PPOs) were formed and included only physicians and hospitals that were willing to discount their prices. Employees and their families were offered price incentives in the form of lower out-of-pocket payments to use these less expensive providers. Large employers and health insurers began to select PPOs on the basis of their prices, use of services, and outcomes of their treatment.

Consequences of the 1980s Changes

The 1980s disrupted the traditional physician–patient relationship. Insurers and HMOs used utilization review to control patient demand, emphasize outcomes and appropriateness of care, and limit patients' access to higher-priced physicians and hospitals by not including them in their provider networks. They also used case management for catastrophic illnesses, substituted less expensive settings for more costly inpatient care, and affected patients' choice of drugs through the use of formularies.

The use of cost-containment programs and the shift to outpatient care lowered hospital occupancy rates. The increasing supply of physicians—particularly specialists—created excess capacity. Hospitals in financial trouble closed, and others merged. Hospital consolidation increased. Hospitals' excess capacity was not reduced until years later, when the demand for care began to exceed the available supply of hospitals and physicians. Until then, hospitals and physicians continued to be subject to intense competitive pressures.

Employees' incentive to reduce their insurance premiums also stimulated competition among HMOs and insurers. Employers required employees to pay the additional cost of more expensive health plans, so many employees chose the lowest-priced plan. Health insurance companies competed for enrollees primarily by offering lower premiums and provider networks with better reputations.

The 1990s

As managed care spread throughout the United States during the 1990s, the rate of increase of medical expenditures declined (see Exhibit 1.3). Hospital use decreased dramatically, and hospitals and physicians agreed to large price discounts to be included in an insurer's provider panel. These cost-containment approaches contributed to the lower annual rate of increase. However, although price competition reduced medical costs, patients were dissatisfied. The public wanted greater access to care—particularly, less restriction on referrals to specialists. Public backlash against HMOs emerged. HMOs lost several lawsuits for denying access to experimental treatments, and Congress and the states imposed restrictions on MCOs, such as mandating minimum lengths of stay in the hospital for normal deliveries. Cost-containment restrictions weakened as a result of these events, and increases in prices, use of services, and medical expenditures reaccelerated.

The 2000s

The excess capacity that weakened hospitals in their negotiations with insurers dried up during this decade. Financially weak hospitals closed. Because consolidation reduces the number of competitors in an area, the number of hospital mergers—which enhance bargaining power—increased. As hospital prices went up, so did insurance premiums. Past approaches—decreased hospital use and price discounts—could no longer achieve large cost reductions. Instead, insurers tried to develop more innovative, less costly ways of managing patient care.

Newer approaches to cost containment included high-deductible health plans, evidence-based medicine, and disease management. Insurers' method of shifting a larger share of medical costs to consumers is referred to as consumer-driven healthcare (CDHC). In return for lower health insurance premiums, consumers pay higher deductibles and copayments. Consumers are then presumed to evaluate the costs and benefits of spending their own funds on healthcare. Instead of relying on consumer incentives to reduce medical costs, some health insurers use evidence-based medicine, which relies on the analysis of large data sets to determine the effect of different physician practice patterns on costs and medical outcomes. Other insurers employ disease management to provide chronically ill patients, who incur the most medical expenditures, with preventive and continuous care, which not only improves the quality of care but also reduces costly hospitalizations.

Another development was pay-for-performance (P4P) programs. Insurers pay physicians and other healthcare practitioners more if they provide high-quality care, which is usually defined on the basis of process measures developed by medical experts. Insurers also make report cards available to their enrollees. Report cards evaluate hospitals and medical groups in the insurer's provider network according to medical outcomes, preventive services, and patient satisfaction scores to enable enrollees to make informed choices about the providers they use.

In the latter half of the decade, rising premiums and increased unemployment (as a result of the Great Recession) prompted people to drop their insurance or switch to new types of insurance that charge lower premiums, such as high-deductible plans. Many Americans became concerned that premiums would continue increasing, making insurance even less affordable. The recession, a decrease in the number of insured, and the switch to high-deductible health plans slowed the rising health expenditures (see Exhibit 1.3).

The Affordable Care Act

The most significant health policy event of the 2010s was the enactment and implementation of the ACA. Although the 2014 implementation was fraught with website and enrollment problems, the legislation will lead to major changes in the financing and delivery of medical services. As such, it should be judged according to three criteria.

The first criterion is whether it reduced the number of uninsured, presumably the major goal of the legislation. Before it was passed, about 50 million Americans were uninsured. The ACA expanded Medicaid eligibility from 100 to 133 percent of the federal poverty level (FPL), estimating that doing so would decrease the number of uninsured by 16 million. An additional 16 million (from 133 to 400 percent of the FPL) would become eligible for government subsidies when they bought insurance on state and federal health exchanges. (The legislation included an individual mandate that requires everyone to either buy insurance or pay a penalty.) Thus, 32 million were expected to gain insurance, leaving nearly 20 million uninsured.[4] It is still uncertain how many states will increase their Medicaid eligibility levels to 133 percent of the FPL and whether the individual mandate and the subsidies, premiums, and benefits offered on the exchanges will induce many of the uninsured to seek coverage. Thus, by the end of this decade, the first criterion for judging the success of the ACA is, how many of the uninsured will have received coverage, and what will have been the cost per newly insured enrollee? Will the decrease in the number of uninsured be worth the more than trillion dollars spent to achieve it? Could another approach have achieved the same goal at a lower cost?

The second criterion relates to cost. The ACA expects to increase the demand for health insurance and, consequently, the demand for medical services without raising the costs of care. Will the ACA be able to "bend the cost curve down," "decrease premiums by $2,500 for a family of four," and "not add a dime to the deficit"? All of these were promises made by President Obama in promoting the legislation's benefits to the middle class. The cost was initially calculated over a ten-year period and was estimated by the Congressional Budget Office to be budget neutral for the first ten years by increasing taxes for the entire ten-year period but delaying the spending for several years. Whether the ACA is able to reduce the rate of increase in medical expenditures, reduce family premiums, and be budget neutral at the end of the decade will determine whether it was able to meet its second objective.[5]

The third criterion is whether people who already had insurance could keep the coverage they had, as President Obama promised. He stated numerous times, "if you like your health plan, you can keep it" and "if you like your doctor, you can keep your doctor." If the first objective of the ACA was to reduce the number of uninsured, then why was it necessary to require changes in the insurance choices of those already insured by mandating greater benefits and, consequently, higher premiums? In 2013, about half of the almost 10 million people enrolled in the individual insurance market (consisting of 5 percent of those privately insured) received cancellation notices from their insurers; their coverage no longer met the ACA's mandated benefit standards. To continue being insured, those receiving cancellation notices were forced to buy more expensive insurance on the new exchanges, which had very limited (low cost) provider networks. Many were very angry they could no longer retain their previous coverage or their physician.

The major concern regarding "keeping your coverage" relates to the remaining 170 million privately insured who receive employer-based coverage. Will employers continue to provide insurance for their employees, or will many employers pay a penalty (the employer mandate) and shift their employees to the exchanges? In a competitive labor market, employers will likely continue to offer insurance for their high-wage employees, who prefer employer coverage rather than the very limited provider networks offered by insurers on the health exchanges.[6] However, employers with low-wage employees may have a different incentive and act differently. A major disruption in the public's coverage would occur if 30 to 50 million employees lose their employer coverage, are shifted to the exchanges, end up with a limited choice of providers, and believe they are worse off and consequently feel dissatisfied. The ACA will then have failed in its promise to enable people to keep the coverage they had.

Finally, any evaluation of the ACA should be based on a comparison—not with the previous healthcare system but with other healthcare reform approaches in achieving the same objectives. Chapter 34 discusses several of these approaches, including the refundable tax credit.

Summary

The forces increasing demand and the costs of providing care have not changed. The population is aging (the first of the baby boomers retired in

2011), technological advances enable early diagnosis, and new methods of treatment are emerging—all of which stimulate increased demand for medical services. Of these three developments, new technology is believed to be the most important force behind rising expenditures. For example, the number of people receiving organ transplants has grown dramatically, as have the diffusion of new equipment and the use of imaging tests. The cost of providing medical services is also rising as more highly trained medical personnel are needed to handle advanced technology and as wage rates increase to attract more nurses and technicians to the medical sector.

The ACA will further increase the demand for care. More people will become eligible for Medicaid, and many previously uninsured individuals buying insurance on the exchanges will receive government subsidies. Everyone is required to have insurance under the legislation's individual mandate, and under the employer mandate, employers are required to provide insurance for their employees or pay a fine. However, the ACA makes no changes to patient or provider incentives to encourage them to be more efficient in their use of medical services.

The developing shortage of physicians is becoming a concern. The demand for physician services is increasing faster than the supply of physicians. Will access to care decline, indicated by increased waiting times for a physician appointment?

As the cost of financing these expansions of Medicaid eligibility and new exchange subsidies increase, the already large federal deficit is likely to grow even faster than it is growing today. The federal government will be under great pressure to reduce the rising deficit and the burden of increasing premiums faced by the middle class. Will the government rely more on regulatory (provider price controls) or competitive approaches to reduce medical expenditures and premium increases?

Innovative approaches to reducing healthcare costs are more likely to be taken in a system that has price incentives to do so (enrollees have a financial incentive to choose less costly health plans, and health insurers compete on premiums, access, and quality for enrollees) than in a regulated system. Any regulatory approach that arbitrarily seeks to reduce the rate of increase in medical expenditures will result in reduced access to both medical care and new technology.

Although the United States spends more on healthcare than does any other country, a scarcity of funds to provide for all of our medical needs and population groups—such as the uninsured and those on Medicaid—still exists. Therefore, choices must be made.

The first choice is to determine how much we as a society should spend on medical care. What approach should we use to make this choice? Should individuals decide how much they want to spend on healthcare, or should the government decide the percentage of GDP that goes to healthcare? The second choice is to identify the best way to provide medical services. Would competition among health plans or government regulation and price controls bring about greater efficiency in providing medical services?

The third choice is to establish how rapidly medical innovation should be introduced. Should regulatory agencies evaluate each medical advance and determine whether its benefits exceed its costs, or should the evaluation of those costs and benefits be left to the separate health plans competing for enrollees? The fourth choice is to specify how much should be spent on those who are medically indigent and how their care should be provided. Should the medically indigent be enrolled in a separate medical system (such as Medicaid), or should they be provided with vouchers to enroll in competing health plans?

These choices can be better understood when we are more aware of the consequences of each approach (such as which groups benefit and which groups bear the costs). Economics clarifies the implications of different approaches to these decisions.

Discussion Questions

1. What are some of the reasons for the increased demand for medical services since 1965?
2. Why has employer-paid health insurance been an important stimulant of demand for health insurance?
3. How did hospital payment methods in the 1960s and 1970s affect hospitals' investment policies and incentives to improve efficiency?
4. Why were HMOs and managed care not more prevalent in the 1960s and 1970s?
5. What choices has the federal government had to reduce greater-than-projected Medicare expenditures?
6. What events during the 1980s in both the public and private sectors made the delivery of medical services price competitive?
7. What are three criteria that have been proposed for evaluating the success of the ACA?

Notes

1. GDP represents the total value of all goods and services produced in a given year. GDP is also equal to the total income received by the resources—employees, management, and capital—that produced those goods and services.

2. Proponents of the ACA claim that part of the slowdown in medical expenditure increases was a result of the legislation. However, Chandra, Holmes, and Skinner (2013) state that the decline started several years before the ACA was enacted (as shown by Exhibit 1.3) and that most of the ACA's cost-control measures did not begin until several years after it was passed in 2010. In addition, Ryu and colleagues (2013) discuss the reasons for the decline in medical expenditure increases.

3. Medicare does not have a limit on total out-of-pocket expenses incurred by a Medicare patient. Medicare Advantage plans provide its enrollees additional benefits and limit out-of-pocket expenses.

4. Among the remaining uninsured are undocumented immigrants, who are excluded from government coverage or subsidies.

5. As shown in Exhibit 1.3, the slowdown in medical expenditures started before the ACA was enacted and should not be attributed to the legislation.

6. The narrow, low-cost networks offered on the exchanges should not be confused with the limited networks an employer (such as Walmart) or an insurer constructs to provide enrollees with a choice of centers of excellence located across the United States. These centers are carefully chosen on the basis of their high quality and low costs.

References

American Hospital Association (AHA). 2014. *Hospital Statistics*. Chicago: AHA.

American Medical Association (AMA). 2013. *Physician Characteristics and Distribution in the United States*. Chicago: AMA.

———. 1991. *Physician Characteristics and Distribution in the United States*. Chicago: AMA.

Bureau of Economic Analysis (BEA). 2014. "National Income and Product Accounts Tables." Accessed February. www.bea.gov.

Chandra, A., J. Holmes, and J. Skinner. 2013. "Is This Time Different? The Slowdown in Healthcare Spending." *NBER Working Paper* No. 19700. Boston: National Bureau of Economic Research. http://papers.nber .org/papers/W19700?utm_campaign=ntw&utm_medium=email&utm_ source=ntw.

Centers for Medicare & Medicaid Services (CMS). 2014. "Historical." Last modified January. www.cms.gov/Research-Statistics-Data-and- Systems/Statistics-Trends-and-Reports/NationalHealthExpendData/ NationalHealthAccountsHistorical.html.

———. 2013. *Medicare & Medicaid Statistical Supplement, 2013 Edition*. Last modified January. www.cms.gov/Research-Statistics-Data-and-Systems/Statistics-Trends-and-Reports/MedicareMedicaidStatSupp/2013.html.

Cuckler, G., A. Sisko, S. Keehan, S. Smith, A. Madison, J. Poisal, C. Wolfe, J. Lizonitz, and D. Stone. 2013. "National Health Expenditure Projections, 2012–22: Slow Growth Until Coverage Expands and Economy Improves." *Health Affairs* 32 (10): 1820–31.

Fuchs, V. 2013. "The Gross Domestic Product and Health Care Spending." *New England Journal of Medicine* 369: 107–09. www.nejm.org/doi/full/10.1056/NEJMp1305298?query=health-policy-and-reform.

Pfuntner, A., L. M. Wier, and A. Elixhauser. 2013. "Overview of Hospital Stays in the United States, 2011." *Statistical Brief* No. 166, November. http://hcup-us.ahrq.gov/reports/statbriefs/sb166.pdf.

Ryu, A., T. Gibson, M. McKellar, and M. Chernew. 2013. "The Slowdown in Health Care Spending in 2009–11 Reflected Factors Other Than the Weak Economy and Thus May Persist." *Health Affairs* 32 (5): 835–40.

HOW MUCH SHOULD WE SPEND ON MEDICAL CARE?

The United States spends more on medical care than does any other country—17.2 percent of its gross domestic product (in 2012)—and this percentage is expected to continue to grow. Can we afford to spend that much of our resources on medical care? Why do we view the growth of expenditures in other areas (such as the automotive industry) more favorably than the growth of expenditures in healthcare? Increased medical expenditures create new healthcare jobs, do not pollute the air, save rather than destroy lives, and alleviate pain and suffering. Why should society not be pleased that more resources are flowing into a sector that cares for the aged, the poor, and the sick? Medical care would seem to be a more appropriate use of a society's resources than cars, electronics, or other consumer products, yet increased expenditures on these goods do not prompt the concern that growth in healthcare spending causes.

Are we concerned about rising medical costs because we believe we are not receiving value for our money—that more medical services and technologies are not worth their costs when compared to other potential uses of those resources? Or is there a fundamental difference of opinion regarding the rate at which medical expenditures should increase?

To answer these questions, we must define what we consider an appropriate or "right" amount of expenditure—only then can we evaluate whether we are spending too much on medical care. If we determine that we are spending too much, how does public policy have to change to achieve the right expenditure level?

Consumer Sovereignty

The appropriate amount of health expenditure is based on a set of values and on the concept of economic efficiency. Resources are limited, so they should be used for what consumers believe to deliver the most value. Consumers decide how much to purchase on the basis of their perception of the value they expect to receive and the price they have to pay, knowing that buying one good or service means forgoing other goods and services. Consumers differ greatly in what value they place on medical care and what they are willing to forgo. In a competitive market, consumers receive the full benefits of their purchases and in turn pay the full costs of those benefits. If the benefits received from the last unit used (e.g., the last visit to the doctor) equal the cost of that unit, the quantity consumed is said to be optimal. If more or fewer services were consumed, the benefits received are said to be either less or greater than the cost of that service.

Consumer sovereignty is most easily achieved in a competitive market system. Consumers differ in the medical services they value and in their willingness to pay for a given service. Through their purchases, consumers communicate what goods and services they value. In response, producers use their resources to produce the goods and services consumers desire. If producers are to survive and profit in competitive markets, they must use their resources efficiently and produce the goods and services consumers are willing to pay for; otherwise, they will be replaced by producers that are more efficient and in tune with what consumers want.

Some people believe that consumer sovereignty should not determine how much we as a society spend on medical care. Patients lack information and have limited ability to judge their needs for medical treatment, more so than in other areas. Other concerns are the quality of care patients receive and the quantity of care that is appropriate.

Consumer sovereignty may be imperfect, but the alternatives are equally imperfect. If medical care were free to all and physicians (paid on a fee-for-service basis or salaried) decided the quantity of medical care to provide, the result would be the provision of "too much" care. Physicians are likely to prescribe services as long as they perceive the services will benefit their patients—even if only slightly—because the physicians are not responsible for the cost of that care.

The inevitable consequence of a free medical system is a government-imposed expenditure limit to halt the provision of too much care. Although physicians still would be responsible for determining who receives services and for which diagnoses, "too little" care likely would be provided—as is sometimes the case in government-controlled health systems such as those in Canada and Great Britain. Queues would be established to ration available medical care, and waiting times and age would become criteria for allocating medical resources.

No government that funds healthcare spends sufficient resources to provide all the care demanded at the going price. As does an individual making purchases, the government makes trade-offs between the benefits received from additional health expenditures and the cost of those expenditures. However, the benefits and costs to the government are different from those consumers consider in their decision-making processes. To the government, *benefit* means the political support it gains by increasing health expenditures;

cost means the political support it loses when it raises taxes or shifts resources from politically popular programs to fund additional expenditures.

Let us, therefore, assume that consumer sovereignty will continue to guide the amount we spend on medical care. Having consumer sovereignty as a guide, however, does not mean that the United States is spending the right amount on medical services. This judgment is influenced by another factor: economic efficiency.

Economic Efficiency

Efficiency in the Provision of Medical Services

If medical services were produced in an inefficient manner, medical expenditures would be excessive. For example, rather than treating a patient for ten days in the hospital, a physician might be able to achieve the same outcome and same level of patient satisfaction by treating the patient in the hospital over a fewer number of days, sending the patient home, and having a visiting nurse finish the treatment. Similarly, the patient might be able to be treated in an outpatient setting rather than in the hospital. Physicians' practice patterns vary greatly across the country, causing medical expenditures to vary widely with no apparent difference in outcomes. Unless providers have appropriate incentives to be efficient, economic efficiency in providing medical services is unlikely to be achieved.

When hospitals were paid on a cost-plus basis, they had an incentive to raise their costs. Subsequent events changed those incentives, and since the early 1980s, both the government and the private sector have been pressing for better efficiency of the delivery system. Cost-based payment to hospitals under Medicare gave way to fixed payment based on diagnosis-related groups. Price competition has escalated not just among hospitals and physicians but also among insurance companies, as they are themselves competing on the basis of premiums in the sale of group health insurance. PPOs (preferred provider organizations), HMOs, and managed care systems have expanded their market share at the expense of traditional insurers. Hospitalization rates have declined as utilization review mechanisms have increased, and the trend toward implementing case management for catastrophic illness and monitoring providers for appropriateness of care and medical outcomes has grown.

Few would contend that the provision of medical services is as efficient as it could be. Waste exists in the health system, and it is difficult to define (Brook 2011; *Health Affairs* 2012). Is it any medical intervention that provides no medical benefit, or is it a medical intervention in which the potential for a negative outcome exceeds the potential for the patient to benefit (Fuchs 2009)? Economic waste occurs when the expected benefits of an intervention are less than the expected costs. Remember that waste is also a provider's income.

The current movement by managed care plans, Medicare Advantage, and accountable care organizations away from fee-for-service and toward episode-based payment and capitation is changing provider incentives. Providers now have a financial incentive to become concerned with coordination of care and management of chronic diseases, resulting in less use of costly inpatient settings, greater use of physician extenders, and better outcomes at lower cost. It will take a number of years, however, for these new payment schemes and outcomes to become widespread throughout the medical care system.

However difficult it is to define and reduce waste, the emphasis on cost containment and the growth of managed care are efforts to decrease inefficient use and delivery of medical services. Even if administrative costs for private health plans were reduced by 50 percent (which would have saved almost $100 billion in 2012), the profits of the pharmaceutical drug companies dropped by 50 percent (saving $55 billion), and all physician incomes decreased by 25 percent (saving $40 billion), the combined savings of $195 billion represent less than two years' annual percentage increase in total medical expenditures.

Inefficiency, although important, is not the main cause for concern about the rise of medical expenditures.

Efficiency in the Use of Medical Services

Inefficiencies in the use of medical services result when individuals do not have to pay the full cost of their choices; they consume too much medical care because their use of services is based on the out-of-pocket price they pay, and that price is less than the cost of providing the service. Consequently, the cost of providing the service exceeds the benefit the patient receives from consuming additional units of the service. The resources devoted to providing these additional services could be better used for other services, such as education, that would provide greater benefits.

The effect of paying less than the full price of a service is easy to understand when the concept is applied to some other consumer product, such as automobiles. If the price of automobiles were greatly lowered for consumers, they would purchase more automobiles (and more expensive ones). To produce these additional automobiles, manufacturers would use resources that could have been used to produce other goods. Similarly, if the price people have to pay for services is decreased, people would use more services. Studies have shown that patients who pay less out of pocket have more hospital admissions, visit physicians more often, and use more outpatient services than patients who pay higher prices (Feldstein 2011). This relationship between price and use of services also holds for patients classified by health status.

Inefficient use is an important concept in healthcare because the price of medical services has been artificially lowered for many consumers. The government subsidizes medical care for the poor and the aged under Medicaid and Medicare. Those eligible for these programs use more services than they would if they had to pay the full price. Although the purpose of these programs is to increase the use of medical services by the poor and the aged, the artificially low prices also promote inefficient use—for example, when a patient uses the more expensive emergency department rather than a physician's office in a non-emergent situation.

A greater concern is that the working population contributes to use inefficiency. An employer-purchased health plan is not considered taxable income for employees. If an employer gave the same amount of funds to an employee in the form of higher wages, the employee would have to pay federal and state income taxes as well as Social Security tax on that additional income. Because employer-purchased health insurance is not subject to these taxes, in effect the government subsidizes the purchase of health insurance and—when the employee uses that insurance—the purchase of medical services. Employees do not pay the full cost of health insurance; it is bought with before-tax dollars, as opposed to all other purchases, which are made with after-tax dollars.

The greatest beneficiaries of this tax subsidy are employees in higher income tax brackets. As discussed in Chapter 1, rather than receive additional income as cash, which is then subject to high taxes (in the 1970s, the highest federal income tax bracket was 70 percent), these employees choose to receive more of their additional wages in the form of more health insurance coverage. Instead of spending after-tax dollars on vision and dental services, they can purchase these services more cheaply with before-tax dollars. The price of insurance is reduced by employees' tax bracket; as a result, they purchase more coverage than they otherwise would because they did not have to pay the full cost of coverage, and the additional coverage is worth less to employees than its full cost.

With the purchase of additional coverage, the out-of-pocket price paid for medical services declined, prompting the increased use of all medical services covered by health insurance. As employees and their families became less concerned with the real cost of medical services, few constraints limited the growth in medical expenditures. Had the inefficient use of medical services (resulting from the tax subsidy for the purchase of health insurance) been less prevalent, medical expenditures would have risen more slowly.

Inefficiencies in the provision and use of medical services are legitimate reasons for concern about how much is spent on medical care. Public policy should attempt to eliminate these government-caused inefficiencies. However, other, less valid reasons for concern exist.

Government and Employer Concerns over Rising Medical Expenditures

As payers of medical expenditures, federal and state governments and employers are concerned about growing medical costs. State governments pay half the costs of caring for the medically indigent in their state, while the federal government pays the remaining half. Medicaid expenditures have gone up more rapidly than any other state expenditure and have caused states to reduce funding for other politically popular programs so that they do not have to raise taxes. At the federal level, the government is also responsible for Medicare (acute medical services for the aged). The hospital portion of Medicare (Part A) is financed by a specific payroll tax that has been raised numerous times, and the physician and prescription drug portions (Parts B and D) are financed with general income taxes. Medicare expenditures have also risen rapidly. As a result of the Affordable Care Act (ACA), starting in 2014 government subsidies will greatly increase to pay for expanded Medicaid eligibility and for those whose income is between 133 percent to 400 percent of the federal poverty level and who buy health insurance on state healthcare exchanges.

As shown in Exhibit 2.1, federal health spending as a proportion of total federal spending is skyrocketing—from 12 percent in 1985 to 20 percent in 1995 to 26 percent in 2012 and to a projected 30 percent in 2018. The oldest of the baby boomers started to retire in 2011 and became eligible for Medicare, which will dramatically boost Medicare expenditures over the coming years. Unless the federal government can reform Medicare and reduce its growth rate, the Medicare payroll tax on the working population will be sharply raised to prevent the Medicare trust fund from going bankrupt. Funding Part B, Part D, and the subsidies under the ACA will require raising income taxes, adding to an already large federal deficit, or reducing funding for other federal programs.

Thus, even if inefficiencies did not exist in the use or provision of medical services, large increases in Medicare and Medicaid enrollments and expenses—together with the additional costs to finance the subsidies included in the ACA—will lead to federal expenditures that exceed the government's ability to finance. The consumer products comparison presented earlier can be applied here as well: If the government were the purchaser of 50 percent of all automobiles, it would become concerned with the price and use of automobiles and the associated expenditures. The pressure to continue

	1965	1975	1985	1995	2005	2012	2018*
Total federal spending	118.2	332.3	946.3	1,515.7	2,472.0	3,537.1	4,449.2
Federal health spending	3.1	29.5	117.1	307.1	614.0	922.6	1,328.4
Medicare	n/a	12.9	65.8	159.9	298.7	471.8	614.8
Medicaid	0.3	6.8	22.7	89.1	181.7	250.5	390.6
Veterans Administration	1.3	3.7	9.5	16.4	28.8	50.6	60.3
Other	1.5	6.1	19.1	41.7	105.0	149.7	262.8
Federal health spending as a percentage of total federal spending	2.6%	8.9%	12.4%	20.3%	24.8%	26.1%	29.9%

EXHIBIT 2.1
Federal Spending on Health, Fiscal Years 1965–2018 (in Billions of Dollars)

* Projected data; n/a: not applicable
SOURCE: Data from Office of Management and Budget (2014), tables 1.1 and 16.1.

funding Medicaid, Medicare, and the new healthcare entitlements through higher taxes or greater budget deficits is driving the federal government to seek ways to limit medical spending increases.

Similarly, unions and employers are concerned with the rise in employee medical expenditures for reasons other than the inefficiencies in the provision or use of services. The business sector's spending on health insurance premiums has gone up over time, both as a percentage of total employee compensation and as a percentage of business profits. Health insurance, when offered, is part of an employee's total compensation. Employers are interested only in the total cost (income) of an employee, not in the form the employee takes that income (i.e., wages or health benefits). Thus, the employee bears the cost of rising health insurance premiums because higher premiums mean lower cash wages. Large unions, whose members receive generous health benefits, want to slow the rate of growth of medical expenditures because they have seen more of their compensation gains spent on health insurance than paid out as wages.

Large employers were seriously affected by the Financial Accounting Standards Board ruling: Starting in 1993, employers that promised medical benefits to their retirees are required to list these unfunded liabilities on their balance sheets. Employers previously paid their retirees' medical expenses only as they occurred and did not set aside funds (as is done with pensions). By having to acknowledge these liabilities on their balance sheets, many large corporations, such as automobile companies, have seen their net worth decline by billions of dollars. Furthermore, because these companies have to expense a portion of these future liabilities each year (not only for their present but also future retirees), they have to report lower earnings per share. If employers were to reduce the rate of increase in their employees' medical expenditures, the net worth of companies with large unfunded retiree liabilities would rise, as would their earnings per share.

These differing reasons for concern over rising medical expenditures are important to recognize. Which concern should drive public policy—the government's desire not to raise revenues to fund its share of medical services, unions' and employers' interest in lowering employee and retiree medical expenses, or society's desire to achieve the appropriate rate of increase in medical expenditures? The interests of government, unions, and large employers have little to do with achieving an appropriate rate of growth. Instead, their particular political and economic burdens drive their proposals for limiting increases in medical expenditures.

Approaches to Limiting Increases in Medical Expenditures

The United States should strive to reduce inefficiencies in both the provision and the use of medical services. Inefficiencies in provision, however, are decreasing as managed care plans are forced to compete for enrollees on the basis of price. The large variations that exist in physicians' treatment patterns should decrease as more information on outcomes becomes available through the analysis of large insurer data sets. Vigilant application of the antitrust laws is needed to ensure that healthcare markets remain competitive and that providers, such as hospitals, do not monopolize their markets. Inefficiencies in use are also declining as managed care plans control use of services through utilization management and patient cost sharing. As these inefficiencies are reduced, the growth rate of medical expenditures will approximate the "correct" rate of increase.

Naturally, the public would like to pay lower insurance premiums and out-of-pocket costs and still have unlimited access to healthcare and to the latest medical technology. As in other sectors of the economy, however, choices must be made.

Medical expenditures have consistently grown faster than inflation, sometimes several times faster and sometimes by just several percentage points. Exhibit 2.2 shows the annual percentage change in national health expenditures and the consumer price index since 1965. During the mid-1990s, expenditures moderated as managed care enrollment rose. By the late 1990s, however, they increased more rapidly as a result of the backlash against managed care and the consequent relaxation of managed care's cost-containment methods. In the past decade, they have moderated as the

EXHIBIT 2.2

Annual Percentage Changes in National Health Expenditures and the Consumer Price Index, 1965–2012

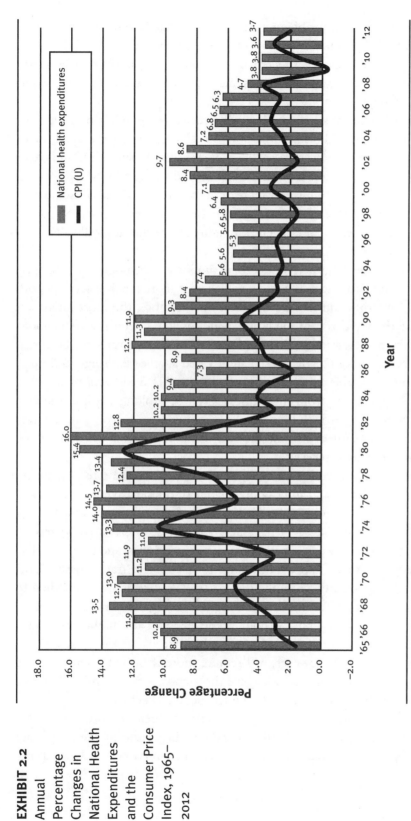

CPI (U): consumer price index for all urban consumers
SOURCES: Data from BLS (2014); CMS (2014).

economy experienced problems (such as the Great Recession) and unemployment and the number of uninsured surged. In the foreseeable future, medical expenditures are expected to continue rising faster than inflation and will be driven by higher incomes, medical advances, and a greater number of aged population.

Some politicians believe they will receive the public's political support by proposing additional discounts on drug prices for the aged, managed care regulations that give enrollees freer access to specialists and other healthcare providers, and arbitrary limits on the amount by which medical expenditures and premiums may increase. What would be the consequences of limiting expenditure and premium increases to a rate lower than what we would otherwise see in an efficient but aging and technologically advanced healthcare system?

The United States is undergoing important demographic changes. The population is aging and as such will require more medical services both to relieve suffering and to cure illnesses. Furthermore, the most important reason for the rapid rise in medical expenditures has been the tremendous advances in medical science. Previously incurable diseases can now be cured, and other illnesses can be diagnosed and treated at an earlier stage. Although no cure is yet available for some diseases (such as AIDS and various cancers), life for those suffering from these diseases can be prolonged with expensive drugs. Limiting the growth of medical expenditures to an arbitrarily low rate will decrease investment in new medical technologies and will restrict the availability of medical services.

Proposed cost-containment methods can reduce the rate of increase. Insurers and payers could impose higher out-of-pocket payments; managed care organizations could require physicians to follow evidence-based medicine guidelines and disease management protocols; or plans could restrict enrollees to using only participating physicians, specialists, and hospitals. The middle class, however, appears unwilling to make these trade-offs; it wants both lower expenditures and unlimited access. (Politicians are responding to these concerns by indicating their willingness to regulate broader access to providers and services—but without acknowledging the higher premiums that would result.) Significantly lowering the rate of increase and funding universal access to all, however, will require more than implementing these cost-containment measures. To achieve these ends, services and technology will have to be made less available to many people (Fuchs 1993).

Some politicians have led the public to believe these trade-offs are not necessary; they claim that by eliminating waste in the healthcare system, universal coverage can be achieved and everyone can have all the medical care they need at a lower cost. Such rhetoric merely postpones the time when the public realizes it must make the unpleasant choice between spending and access.

Summary

Who should decide how much is to be spent on medical care? All countries face this basic question, and each country has made a different choice. In some countries, the government determines the allocation of resources among the medical sectors and controls medical prices. When the government makes these decisions, the trade-offs between cost and access are likely to be different from those that consumers will make.

In the United States, consumer sovereignty has been the guiding principle in allocating resources; consumers (except for those enrolled in Medicare and Medicaid) determine the amount of their income to be spent on medical services. Yet, consumers have not always received value for their money. Inefficiencies in the medical sector, inappropriate provider incentives, and certain government regulations have made medical services more costly. Furthermore, subsidies for the purchase of health insurance (tax-exempt, employer-paid health insurance) have resulted in greater use of services. Thus, the debate over the appropriate amount to be spent on medical services is likely to be clarified once these two issues—consumer sovereignty and efficiency of the current system—are separated.

Discussion Questions

1. How does a competitive market determine the types of goods and services to produce, the costs to produce those goods and services, and who receives them?
2. Why do economists believe the value of additional employer-paid health insurance is worth less than its full cost?
3. Why do rising medical expenditures cause concern?
4. Why do inefficiencies exist in the use and provision of medical services?
5. Why are large employers and government concerned about rising medical expenditures?

References

Brook, R. H. 2011. "The Role of Physicians in Controlling Medical Care Costs and Reducing Waste." Commentary. *JAMA* 306 (6): 650–51. http://jama .jamanetwork.com/article.aspx?articleid=1104194.

Bureau of Labor Statistics (BLS). 2014. "Databases, Tables, and Calculators, by Subject." Accessed January. http://data.bls.gov.

Centers for Medicare & Medicaid Services (CMS). 2014. Accessed January. http://cms.gov.

Feldstein, P. J. 2011. "The Demand for Medical Care." In *Health Care Economics,* 7th ed. Albany, NY: Delmar.

Fuchs, V. R. 2009. "Eliminating Waste in Health Care." *JAMA* 302 (22): 2481–82.

———. 1993. "No Pain, No Gain—Perspectives on Cost Containment." *JAMA* 269 (5): 631–33.

Health Affairs. 2012. "Reducing Waste in Health Care." *Health Policy Brief.* Published December 13. www.healthaffairs.org/healthpolicybriefs/brief .php?brief_id=82.

Office of Management and Budget, The White House. 2014. "Fiscal Year 2014 Historical Tables. Budget of the U.S. Government." Accessed February. www.whitehouse.gov/omb/budget/historicals.

DO MORE MEDICAL EXPENDITURES PRODUCE BETTER HEALTH?

The United States spends more per capita on medical services and devotes a larger percentage of its gross domestic product to medical care than do other countries, yet our health status is not proportionately better. In fact, many countries that have lower per capita medical expenditures than the United States also have lower infant mortality rates and higher life expectancies. Is our medical system less efficient at producing good health than these other countries, or are medical expenditures less important than other factors that affect health status?

Medical Services Versus Health

Medical services are often mistakenly considered synonymous with health. When policymakers talk of "health" reform, they mean reform of the financing and delivery of medical services. Medical services consist of not only the diagnosis and treatment of illness, which can lead to improved health, but also the amelioration of pain and discomfort, reassurance of well but worried people, and heroic treatments for the terminally ill. One indication that the primary objective of government's medical spending is to treat illness—and not, more broadly, to improve the nation's health status—is that 22 percent of all medical expenditures ($278 billion in 2010) are spent on just 1 percent of the population.[1] Furthermore, 40 percent of those in that top 1 percent are older than age 65. Increased medical expenditures, therefore, may have relatively little effect on a nation's health status.

Generally, the United States is acknowledged to have a technically superior medical system for treating acute illness. (For a brief but excellent discussion of criteria used to evaluate a country's health system, see Fuchs [1992].) Financing and payment incentives have all been directed toward this goal, and physician training has emphasized treatment rather than prevention of illness. Public policy debates regarding medical services have been concerned with two issues: (1) equity—namely, whether everyone has access to medical services and how those services should be financed, and (2) efficiency—namely, whether medical services are efficiently produced. Knowing how to provide a medical treatment efficiently, however, is not the same as knowing how to produce health efficiently.

In contrast to policy regarding medical services, health policy has been less well defined. The goal of health policy presumably should be to improve the population's health status or increase its life expectancy, in which case we should be concerned with the most efficient ways to improve that status. Assuming policymakers recognize this goal, they should understand that devoting more resources to medical care is just one way to improve health and is unlikely to be the most efficient way to do so.

The more accurate the definition of health, the more difficult it is to measure. Health is a state of physical, mental, and social well-being. More simply, it is the absence of disease or injury. Empirically, it is defined by negative measures, such as mortality rates, days lost to sickness, or life expectancy. Measures of health can be broad (such as age-adjusted mortality rates) or disease specific (such as neonatal infant mortality rates within the first 27 days of birth and age-adjusted death rates from heart disease). The advantage of using such crude measures is that they are readily available and are probably correlated with more comprehensive definitions of health. Unavailability of morbidity or quality-of-life measures, however, does not mean they are unimportant or should be neglected in analyses.

Health Production Function

To determine the relative importance of medical expenditures in decreasing mortality rates, economists use the concept of *health production function*. Simply stated, a health production function examines the relative contribution of each factor that affects health to determine the most cost-effective way to improve health. For example, mortality rates are affected by the use of medical services, environmental conditions (such as the amount of air and water pollution), education levels (which may indicate knowledge of disease prevention and ability to use the medical system when needed), and lifestyle behaviors (such as smoking, alcohol and substance abuse, diet, and exercise).

Each of these determinants of health has differential effects. For example, medical expenditures may initially cause mortality rates to drop significantly, as when a hospital establishes the first neonatal intensive care unit (NICU) in its community. Beds will be limited, so the first low-birth-weight infants admitted to the NICU will be those who are most critically ill and those most likely to benefit from medical care and continuous monitoring. As NICUs are added within that community, the neonatal infant mortality rate will decline by a smaller percentage. With a larger number of NICU beds, either the beds may be unused or the infants admitted to those beds will not be as critically ill or high risk. Therefore, investment in additional NICU beds will have less of an effect on infant mortality.

Exhibit 3.1 illustrates the relationship between increased medical expenditures and improvements in health status. Higher expenditures produce a curvilinear rather than a constant effect on improved health. The marginal (additional) improvement becomes smaller as more is spent. As shown in Exhibit 3.1, an initial expenditure to improve health, moving from point A to point B, has a much larger marginal benefit (effect) than subsequent investments have, such as moving from point C to point D. The increase from point H_1 to point H_2 is greater than the increase from H_3 to H_4.

This same curvilinear relationship holds for each determinant of health. Expenditures to decrease air pollution (such as installing smog-control devices on automobiles) would reduce the incidence of respiratory illness. Additional spending by automobile owners (such as having their smog-control devices tested once a year rather than every three years) would further reduce air pollution. The reduction in respiratory illness, however, would not be as great as that produced by the initial expenditure to install smog-control devices. The reduction in respiratory illness resulting from additional expenditures to control air pollution gradually declines.

Everyone probably would agree that additional lives could be saved if more infants were admitted to NICUs (or respiratory illness further decreased if smog-control inspections were conducted more frequently). More intensive monitoring might save a patient's life. However, those same

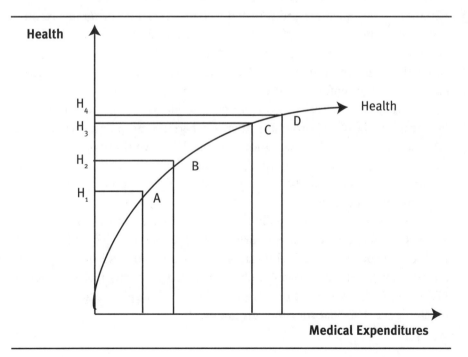

EXHIBIT 3.1
Effect of
Increased
Medical
Expenditures
on Health

funds could be spent on prenatal care programs to decrease the number of low-birth-weight infants or on education programs to prevent teen pregnancy. The true "cost" of any program to decrease mortality is the number of lives that could have been saved if those same funds had been spent on another program.

Physicians, hospitals, dentists, and other health professionals all want more government expenditures to decrease the unmet needs among their populations. However, the government cannot spend all that would be necessary to eliminate all medical, dental, mental, and other needs. To do so would mean forgoing the opportunity to eliminate other needs (such as welfare and education) because resources are limited. At some point, the forgone opportunity to save all the lives that medical science is capable of saving becomes too costly. Reallocating those same expenditures to apprehend drunk drivers or to improve highways might save even more lives.

Deciding which programs should be expanded to improve health status requires a calculation of the cost per life saved for each program that affects mortality rates. Looking at the curve in Exhibit 3.1, assume that an additional medical expenditure of $1 million results in a movement from point H_3 to point H_4, or from point C to point D, saving 20 more lives. The same $1 million spent on an education program to reduce smoking may result in a movement from H_1 to H_2, or from A to B, saving an additional 40 lives from lung cancer. The expenditure for the smoking reduction program results in a lower cost per life saved ($1 million ÷ 40 = $25,000) than if those same funds were spent on more medical services ($1 million ÷ 20 = $50,000). Continued expenditures on smoking cessation programs result in a movement along the curve. After some point, fewer lung cancer deaths will be prevented and the cost per life saved will rise. A lower cost per life saved could then be achieved by spending additional funds on other programs (such as stronger enforcement of drunk driving laws).

Crucial to the calculation of cost per life saved is knowing (1) the marginal benefit of the program—that is, where the program, such as medical treatments or smoking cessation, sits on the curve shown in Exhibit 3.1 and (2) the cost of expanding that program. The costs per life saved by each program can be compared by dividing the cost of expanding each program by its marginal benefit.

The enormous and rapidly rising medical expenditures in the United States have likely placed the return to medical services beyond point D. Further improvements in health status from continued medical expenditures are very small. The cost of expanding medical treatments has also become expensive. Consequently, the cost per life saved through medical services is much higher than that for other programs.

Improving Health Status Cost-Effectively

Numerous empirical studies have found that additional expenditures on medical services are not the most cost-effective way to improve health status. Medical programs have a much higher cost per life saved than nonmedical programs do. Researchers have concluded that changing lifestyle behavior offers the greatest promise for reducing mortality rates at a much lower cost per life saved.

The leading contributors to decreased mortality rates over the past 40 years have been the decline in neonatal infant deaths and in heart disease–related deaths.

Neonatal Infant Mortality Rate

The neonatal mortality rate represents about two-thirds (67 percent in 2011) of the overall infant mortality rate; the decline in the overall rate has been primarily attributed to the decline in the neonatal rate (Hoyert and Xu 2012). For many years, the neonatal rate had steadily dropped; however, starting in the mid-1960s the rate began to plummet more rapidly. As shown in Exhibit 3.2, the rate for whites declined from 19.4 per 1,000 live births in 1950 to 3.5 in 2011, while the rate for African Americans went from 27.8 in 1950 to 7.5 in 2011. During that period, more NICUs were established, government subsidies were provided for family planning services for low-income women, maternal and infant nutrition programs expanded, Medicaid was initiated and paid for obstetric services for those with low income, and abortion was legalized. Corman and Grossman (1985) found that higher

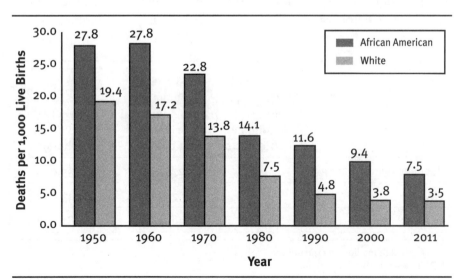

EXHIBIT 3.2
Neonatal Mortality Rates by Race, 1950–2011

SOURCES: Data from Census Bureau (2009), Table 112; Census Bureau (1985), Table 108; Hoyert and Xu (2012).

education levels and subsidized nutrition programs were the most important factors in reducing the neonatal mortality rate among whites. The availability of abortion, followed by more NICUs and higher education levels, were the most important factors among African Americans.

Simply knowing the reasons for the decline in neonatal mortality, however, is insufficient for deciding how to spend money to reduce deaths; it is important to know which programs are the most cost-effective. Joyce, Corman, and Grossman (1988) determined that, for whites, teenage family planning programs, NICUs, and prenatal care saved 0.6, 2.8, and 4.5 lives, respectively, per 1,000 additional participants. The corresponding costs of adding 1,000 participants to each of these programs (in 2013 dollars) were $274,000, $30,529,000, and $395,000, respectively. To determine the cost per life saved by expanding each of these programs, the cost of the program was divided by the number of lives saved. As shown in Exhibit 3.3, the cost per life saved was $455,000 ($274,000 ÷ 0.6) for teenage family planning; $10,713,000 for NICUs; and $87,000 for prenatal care, which is the most cost-effective. Reducing the potential number of women in high-risk pregnancies and the number of unwanted births (e.g., by providing teenage family planning programs and prenatal care) offers a greater possibility of more favorable birth outcomes than investing in additional NICUs.

Heart Disease Mortality Rate

The leading cause of death in the United States is cardiovascular disease. Between 1970 and 2011, the mortality rate from heart disease decreased faster than the death rate from any other causes—from 362 per 100,000 to 191 per 100,000 (Hoyert and Xu 2012). Improvements in medical technology (such as coronary bypass surgery, coronary care unit, angioplasty, and

EXHIBIT 3.3
Cost per Life Saved Among Three Programs to Reduce Neonatal Mortality (Whites)

	Number of Lives Saved per 1,000 Additional Participants	Cost of Each Program per 1,000 Additional Participants (in 2013 dollars)*	Cost per Life Saved (in 2013 Dollars)*
Teenage family planning	0.6	274,000	455,000
NICUs	2.8	30,529,000	10,713,000
Prenatal care	4.5	395,000	87,000

* 2013 calculations done by the author.
NICU: neonatal intensive care unit
SOURCE: Reprinted with permission as it appeared in T. Joyce, H. Corman, and M. Grossman, "A Cost-Effectiveness Analysis of Strategies to Reduce Infant Mortality," *Medical Care*, 26 (April), 1988: 348–60. © 1988 J.B. Lippincott Company.

clot-dissolving drugs) as well as changes in lifestyle (such as smoking cessation, regular exercise, and low-cholesterol diet) contributed to this decline.

One study estimated that the development and greater use of new treatment techniques over time decreased cardiovascular disease–related deaths by about one-third; the remaining two-thirds of this decline were attributed to preventive measures, such as new drugs to control hypertension, lower high cholesterol, and help with quitting smoking (Cutler and Kadiyala 2003). These lifestyle changes, however, are not seen uniformly across the population; those with more education are more likely to undertake them. Many other studies that examined heart disease deaths have reached a similar conclusion: Lifestyle changes are more important—and much less expensive—than medical interventions in improving health.

Causes of Death by Age Group

Perhaps the clearest indication that lifestyle behavior is an important determinant of mortality is the causes of death by age group. As shown in Exhibit 3.4, the top causes of death for young adults (aged 15 to 24 years) are accident (particularly automobile), suicide, and homicide. For the middle age groups (aged 25 to 44 years), the major causes are accident, cancer, heart disease, suicide, and homicide. For those in late middle age (aged 45 to 64 years), cancer and heart disease are the leading causes. After examining data by cause of death, Fuchs (1974, 46) concluded that medical services have a smaller effect on health than the way in which people live: "The greatest potential for reducing coronary disease, cancer, and the other major killers still lies in altering personal behavior."

Relationship of Medical Care to Health Over Time

The studies discussed have shown that the marginal contribution of medical care to improved health is relatively small. Improvements in health status can be achieved in a less costly manner through changing lifestyle factors. Over time, however, major technological advances have been seen in medical care, such as new drugs to lower cholesterol and blood pressure, diagnostic imaging, less invasive surgery, organ and tissue transplants, and treatment for previously untreatable diseases. Few would deny that these advances have reduced mortality rates and expanded life expectancy.

Cutler and Richardson (1999) reconcile these seemingly conflicting findings by separating medical care's effect *at a point in time* versus its technological contribution *over time*. The authors illustrate in Exhibit 3.5 the relationship between the total contribution of medical care to health and greater quantities of medical care. Comprehensive health insurance

EXHIBIT 3.4
Leading Causes
of Death by Age
Group, 2011

Age Group	Major Causes of Death	Deaths per 100,000
15–24	All causes	67.6
	Accident	27.5
	Suicide	10.7
	Homicide and legal intervention	10.3
	Cancer	3.7
	Heart disease	2.2
25–44	All causes	137.5
	Accident	35.7
	Cancer	18.5
	Heart disease	16.4
	Suicide	14.9
	Homicide and legal intervention	8.1
	Chronic liver disease/cirrhosis	3.5
45–64	All causes	610.9
	Cancer	194.6
	Heart disease	126.9
	Accident	41.8
	Pulmonary disease	23.7
	Chronic liver disease/cirrhosis	23.6
	Diabetes mellitus	22.4
	Cerebrovascular disease	20.4

SOURCE: Data from Hoyert and Xu (2012), Table 7.

and fee-for-service physician payment reduce both the patient's and the physician's incentive to be concerned with the cost of care, resulting in the healthcare system moving to point A, where the marginal contribution of medical care to health is very small. Additional medical care expenditures enhance health, but at a decreasing rate.

Eventually, however, medical advances shift the health production function upward. The level of health has improved, and the number of patients treated has risen, but the marginal contribution of medical care is still low—at point B. Too many patients whose need for treatment is doubtful are treated

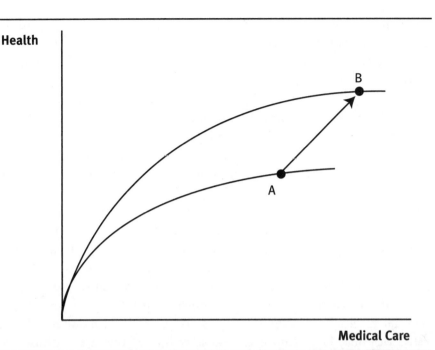

EXHIBIT 3.5
Relationship
Between
Medical Care
and Health

SOURCE: Reprinted from David Cutler and Elizabeth Richardson, "Your Money and Your Life: The Value of Health and What Affects It," in *Frontiers in Health Policy Research*, vol. 2, ed. Alan Garber (Cambridge, Mass.: MIT Press, 1999), pp. 99–132, figure 5–6.

with the new technology, or excess capacity occurs as too much of the new technology is made available. Thus, although the public believes the medical care they receive today is much more valuable than treatments offered 30 years ago, the healthcare system remains inefficient; the marginal benefit of additional medical expenditures is low (Skinner, Staiger, and Fisher 2006).

Summary

If expenditures on medical services have been shown to be less cost-effective in reducing mortality rates than are changes in lifestyle behavior, why does the United States spend a growing portion of its resources on medical care?

First, health insurance coverage has been so comprehensive—with low deductibles and small copayments—that individuals faced a very low out-of-pocket price when they went to the hospital or a specialist. Thus, patients used more medical services than if they had to pay a greater portion of the cost. The expression "the insurance will cover it" is indicative of the patients' and their providers' lack of incentive to be concerned about cost. The public also has had little incentive to compare prices among different providers, as the costs incurred in searching for less expensive providers exceed any savings on already low copayments. Given these low copayments and the incentives inherent in fee-for-service payments to providers, it is not surprising that enormous resources are spent on people in their last year of life. Rapidly rising medical expenditures and limited reductions in mortality rates are the consequences of this behavior.

Second, the primary objective of government medical expenditures has not been to improve health status and decrease mortality rates. Medicare benefits the elderly, and approximately half of Medicaid expenditures are spent for care of the elderly in nursing homes. The purpose of government medical spending is to help the aged finance their medical needs. Were the government's objective to improve the nation's health, the types of services financed would be very different—as would the age groups that would benefit the most from those expenditures. (One factor to consider is that the aged have the highest voting participation rates of any age group and perhaps have become the most politically powerful group in US society.)

Although medical expenditures have a relatively small marginal effect on health, it would be incorrect to conclude that the government should limit all medical expenditure increases. To an individual, additional medical services may be worth the extra cost even when they are not subsidized. As incomes go up, people are more willing to purchase medical services to relieve anxiety and pain—services that are not lifesaving but are entirely appropriate personal expenditures. From society's perspective, financing medical services for those with low income is also appropriate. As society becomes wealthier, its individuals and government become more willing to spend on non-lifesaving medical treatments. These "consumption" versus "investment" types of medical expenditures are appropriate as long as everyone involved recognizes them for what they are.

When government attempts to improve the health of its low-income populations (using the concept of health production function), expenditures are directed toward the most cost-effective programs—that is, those that result in the lowest cost per life saved. Allocating funds in this manner achieves a greater reduction in mortality rates for a given total expenditure than is possible with any other allocation method. The health production function is used more by employers and health plans that face financial pressures to reduce their medical costs.[2] Employers' use of health-risk appraisal questionnaires recognizes that employees' health can be improved less expensively by changes in lifestyle behavior. Incentives given to employees who stop smoking, lose weight, and exercise enable employers to retain a skilled workforce longer while reducing medical expenditures. The emphasis by health plans on reducing per capita medical costs has led them to identify high-risk groups that can benefit from measures to prevent illness and costly medical treatments.

The recognition by the government, employers, health plans, and individuals that resources are scarce and that their objective should be to improve health status rather than use additional medical services will lead to new approaches to enhance health. The health production function should clarify the trade-offs between different programs and improve the allocation of expenditures.

Discussion Questions

1. How can the health production function allocate funds to improve health status?
2. Why does the United States spend an ever-growing portion of its resources on medical services, although they are less cost-effective than other methods in improving health status?
3. How can employers use the health production function to decrease their employees' medical expenditures?
4. Describe the health production function for decreasing deaths from coronary heart disease.
5. Describe the health production function for decreasing deaths among young adults.

Notes

1. In 2010, 50 percent of total medical expenditures were spent on 5 percent of the population. The elderly represented 38 percent of those on whom a great amount of money was spent (Cohen and Uberoi 2013; Soni 2013).
2. See Chapter 21 of this book for further discussion of cost-effectiveness applied to quality-adjusted life years.

References

Cohen, S., and N. Uberoi. 2013. "Differentials in the Concentration in the Level of Health Expenditures Across Population Subgroups in the U.S., 2010." *Statistical Brief* No. 421. http://meps.ahrq.gov/mepsweb/data_files/publications/st421/stat421.pdf.

Corman, H., and M. Grossman. 1985. "Determinants of Neonatal Mortality Rates in the US: A Reduced Form Model." *Journal of Health Economics* 4 (3): 213–36.

Cutler, D. M., and S. Kadiyala. 2003. "The Return to Biomedical Research: Treatment and Behavioral Effects." In *Measuring the Gains from Medical Research: An Economic Approach,* edited by K. M. Murphy and R. H. Topel, 110–62. Chicago: University of Chicago Press.

Cutler, D. M., and E. Richardson. 1999. "Your Money and Your Life: The Value of Health and What Affects It." In *Frontiers in Health Policy Research,* vol. 2, edited by A. Garber, 99–132. Cambridge, MA: MIT Press.

Fuchs, V. R. 1992. "The Best Health Care System in the World?" *JAMA* 268 (19): 916–17.

———. 1974. *Who Shall Live?* New York: Basic Books.

Hoyert, D., and J. Xu. 2012. "Deaths: Preliminary Data for 2011." *National Vital Statistics Report* 61 (6). www.cdc.gov/nchs/data/nvsr/nvsr61/nvsr61_06.pdf.

Joyce, T., H. Corman, and M. Grossman. 1988. "A Cost-Effectiveness Analysis of Strategies to Reduce Infant Mortality." *Medical Care* 26 (4): 348–60.

Skinner, J., D. Staiger, and E. Fisher. 2006. "Is Technological Change In Medicine Always Worth It? The Case of Acute Myocardial Infarction." *Health Affairs* (web exclusive): W-34–W-47. http://content.healthaffairs.org/cgi/content/abstract/25/2/w34.

Soni, A. 2013. Personal correspondence with the author, September 25.

US Census Bureau. 2009. *The 2010 Statistical Abstract, 129th ed.* www.census.gov/compendia/statab/2010/tables/10s0112.pdf.

———. 1985. *Statistical Abstract of the United States, 1985, 105th ed.* www2.census.gov/prod2/statcomp/documents/1985-01.pdf.

IN WHOSE INTEREST DOES THE PHYSICIAN ACT?

4

P
hysicians have always played a crucial role in the delivery of medical services. Although only 24 percent of personal medical expenditures are for physician services, physicians control the use of a much larger portion of total medical resources (CMS 2014). In addition to their own services, physicians determine admissions to the hospital; lengths of stay; the use of ancillary services and prescription drugs; referrals to specialists; and even the necessity for services in nonhospital settings, such as home care. Any public policies that affect the financing and delivery of medical services must consider physicians' responses to those policies. Their knowledge and motivation will affect the efficiency with which medical services are delivered.

The role of the physician has been shaped by two important characteristics of the healthcare system. First, only physicians are legally permitted to provide certain services. Second, both patients and insurers lack the necessary information to make many medically related decisions. The patient depends on the physician for diagnosis and treatment and has limited information on the physician's qualifications or those of the specialist to whom the patient is referred. This lack of information places the patient in a unique relationship with the physician: The physician becomes the patient's agent (McGuire 2000).

The Perfect Agent

The agency relationship gives rise to a major controversy in the medical economics literature. In whose best interest does the physician act? If the physician were a *perfect agent* for the patient, he would prescribe the mix of institutional settings and the amount of care provided in each based on the patient's medical needs, ability to pay for medical services, and preferences. The physician and the patient would behave as if the patient were as well informed as the physician. Traditional insurance—once the prevalent form of health plan coverage—reimbursed the physician on a fee-for-service basis; neither the physician nor the patient was fiscally responsible or at risk for using the hospital and medical services.

Before the 1980s, Blue Cross predominantly covered hospital care; all inpatient services were covered without any patient cost sharing. Although hospital stays are more costly than outpatient care in terms of resources used, patients paid less to receive a diagnostic workup in the hospital than in an outpatient setting. While this was an inefficient use of resources, the physician acted in the patient's interest and not the insurer's. Similarly, if a woman wanted to stay a few extra days in the hospital after giving birth, the physician would not discharge her before she was ready to return home.

As the patient's agent, the quantity and type of services the physician prescribed would be based on the value to the patient of that additional care and the patient's cost for that care. As long as the value exceeded the cost, the physician would prescribe it. By considering only the services' costs and benefits to the patient, the physician neglected the costs to society and the insurance company.

Insurance and the role of the physician as the patient's agent led the physician to practice what Victor Fuchs (1968) referred to as the *technologic imperative*. Regardless of how small the benefit to the patient or how costly to the insurer, the physician would prescribe the best medical care technically possible. As a consequence, heroic measures were provided to patients in the last few months of their lives, and inpatient hospital costs rose rapidly. Prescribing "low-benefit" care was a rational economic decision because it still exceeded the patient's cost, which was virtually zero with comprehensive insurance.

Supplier-Induced Demand or the Imperfect Agent

The view of the physician as the patient's agent, however, neglects the economic self-interest of the physician. As shown in Exhibit 4.1, large increases in the total number of physicians and the number of physicians relative to population have occurred since the 1970s. The number of physicians has almost tripled since 1970, and the physician-to-population ratio has almost doubled. The standard economic model, which assumes the physician is a perfect agent for the patient, predicts that growth in supply—other things (such as higher consumer income) being equal—would result in a decline in physician fees and, consequently, in physician income.

Increases in the physician-to-population ratio, however, did not lead to decreases in physician income. This observation led to the development of an alternative theory of physician behavior. Physicians are believed to behave differently when their own income is adversely affected. In addition to being patients' agents, physicians are suppliers of a service. Their income depends on how much of that service they supply. Do physicians use their

EXHIBIT 4.1
Number
of Active
Physicians and
Physician-to-
Population
Ratio, 1950–
2011

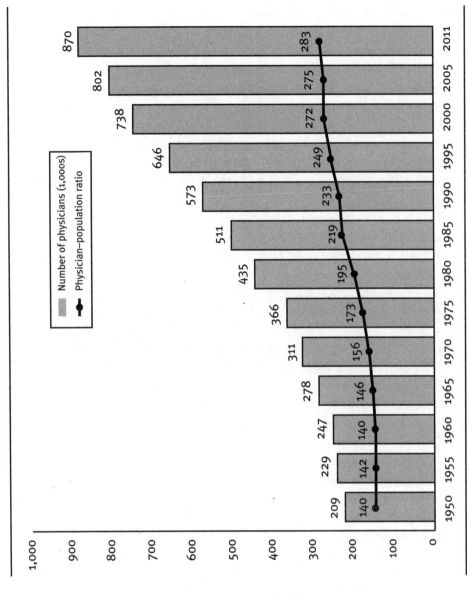

NOTE: Physician–population ratio is for active physicians and noninstitutionalized civilian population. Active physicians are federal and nonfederal physicians who are involved in patient care or non-patient care (teaching, research administration, or other professional activities) for more than 20 hours a week. Active physicians also include unclassified physicians—that is, those whose activity status or present employment setting is not known.
SOURCES: Data from AMA (1982, 2013); Census Bureau (2012).

information advantage over patients and insurers to benefit themselves? This model of physician behavior is referred to as *supplier-induced demand*.

The supplier-induced demand theory assumes that if the physician's income falls, the physician will use her role as the patient's agent to prescribe additional services. The physician provides the patient with misinformation to influence the patient to demand more services, thereby adding to the physician's income. In other words, the physician becomes an *imperfect agent*.

Physicians who are imperfect agents might rationalize some demand inducement by arguing that additional services or tests would be beneficial to the patient. However, as the physician prescribes more and more services, he must choose between the extra income he receives and the psychological cost of knowing that those services are not really necessary. At some point, the former is not worth the latter. The physician must make a trade-off between increased revenue and the dissatisfaction of deliberately providing too many services.

Thus, one might envisage a spectrum of demand inducement depending on the psychological cost to the physician. At one end of the spectrum are those physicians who act solely in their patients' interests; they do not induce demand to inflate or even maintain their income. At the other end of the spectrum are those physicians who attempt to earn as much money as possible by inducing demand; these physicians presumably incur little psychological cost. In the middle of the spectrum are those physicians who induce demand to achieve or maintain some target level of income (this is referred to as the *target income theory*).

The extent to which the physician is willing and able to generate additional demand for medical services is controversial. Few would believe that the majority of physicians do so solely to maximize their income. Similarly, few would disagree that physicians are able to induce demand. Thus, the choice is between the idea of physicians as perfect agents for their patients and physicians as imperfect agents who induce demand according to the target income theory. The issue is how much demand physicians can induce.

Demand inducement is limited to some extent by the patient's recognition that the additional medical benefits are not worth the time or cost of returning to the physician. The patient's evaluation of these benefits, however, varies according to the treatment prescribed. Patients may easily determine that monthly office visits are not worth their time and the cost of returning; however, they may have more difficulty evaluating the benefits of certain surgical services. Presumably, demand inducement is more likely to occur for services about which the patient knows the least; consequently, patients are more concern about inducement in such cases.

Many studies have attempted to determine the extent of demand inducement (see, for example, Feldstein [2011, 97–99, 234–41]), but the issue is still unresolved. Evidence shows that geographic areas (cities and counties) that have a large number of physicians (in relation to the population) also have high per capita use of physician services. This relationship, however, may merely indicate that physicians establish their practices where the population has a high rate of insurance coverage and, consequently, where demand for their services is great. One study concluded that primary care physicians are limited in the amount of demand they can induce, although how much demand they may already have induced remains unknown (McCarthy 1985). The positive correlation between the number of surgeons and the number of surgeries has been used as empirical support for the supplier-induced demand theory. Furthermore, studies have found the rate of procedures such as tonsillectomies and hysterectomies is higher when physicians are paid fee-for-service than through other income incentives (such as those available to physicians in an HMO).

Increase in Physician Supply

The growth in physician supply since the 1970s illustrates the importance of knowing which model of physician behavior—perfect agent or imperfect agent (operating under supplier-induced demand)—is prevalent. As a perfect agent, the physician would consider only the patient's medical and economic interests when prescribing a treatment, regardless of the fact that her income may decline because the greater number of physicians may decrease the number of patients she sees.

On the other hand, as an imperfect agent, the physician facing a great supply of physicians would generate demand to prevent his income from falling. Total physician expenditures would also rise as more physicians, each with fewer patients, attempt to maintain their income. Thus, whether one believes in the standard economic model (perfect agent) or in the supplier-induced demand model (imperfect agent), a larger number of physicians would lead to opposite predictions of their effect on physician prices and income.

Insurers' Response to Demand Inducement

Insurers recognize that under fee-for-service payment, physicians act either as the patient's perfect agents or as imperfect agents who boost or maintain their own income. In either case, the value of the additional services a physician prescribes is lower than the insurer's cost for those services. Consequently, the premium for insurance is higher in a fee-for-service environment than for managed care plans, which theoretically attempt to relate the value of additional medical treatments to the resource costs of those services. As a result of the higher relative premium of insurance, more of the insurer's subscribers switched to managed care. Since about 2000, therefore, insurance companies have developed mechanisms to overcome the information advantage that physicians have over both the insurers and the patients.

Insurers, for example, have implemented second-opinion requirements for surgery. Once a physician recommends certain types of surgery of doubtful medical necessity (such as back surgery), a patient may be required to obtain a second opinion from a list of physicians approved by the insurance company. Another approach is the creation of preferred provider organizations (PPOs). Physicians who have lower fees, recommend fewer medical services, and are considered to be of high quality are selected. Yet another approach is utilization review. Before a hospital admission or a surgical procedure, a patient must receive the insurer's approval; otherwise, the patient is subject to a financial penalty. The length of stay in the hospital is also subject to the insurer's approval.

These cost-containment approaches are insurers' attempts to address the imbalances in physician and patient incentives under a fee-for-service system. Furthermore, they ensure that the patient receives appropriate care (when the physician acts to increase his own income) and that the resource costs of a treatment are considered along with its expected benefits.

HMO Incentives by Imperfect Agents

The growth of HMOs and capitation payment provides physicians with income-raising incentives that are opposite those of the traditional fee-for-service approach. HMOs typically reward their physicians with profit sharing or bonuses if their enrollees' medical costs are lower than their annual capitation payments. What are the likely effects of the two models of physician behavior—perfect agent and imperfect agent—on an HMO's patients?

In an HMO setting, a perfect-agent physician would continue to provide the patient with appropriate medical services. Regardless of the effect of profit sharing on her income or pressures from the HMO to reduce use of services, the perfect agent would be primarily concerned with protecting patients' interests and providing them with the best medical care, so there is little likelihood of underservice. Unlike with insurance, in an HMO the physician would not need to be concerned whether the patient's health plan covered the medical cost in different settings. HMO patients are also responsible for fewer deductibles and copayments. Thus, the settings chosen for providing the patient's treatment are likely to be less costly for both the patient and the HMO.

The concern that patients would be underserved in an HMO exists among imperfect-agent physicians—those who attempt to boost their own income. HMO physicians have an incentive to provide fewer services to their patients and to serve a large number of patients. Those HMO physicians who are concerned with the size of their income are more likely to respond to profit-sharing incentives. At times, a physician (who may even be salaried) may succumb to an HMO's pressures to reduce use of services and thereby become an imperfect agent. If HMO patients believe they are being denied timely access to the physician, specialist services, or needed technology, they are likely to switch physicians or disenroll at the next open-enrollment period. Too high a dissatisfaction rate with certain HMO physicians could indicate that their patients are underserved.

An HMO should be concerned about underservice by its physicians. Although the HMO's profitability will improve if its physicians provide too few services, an HMO that limits access to care and fails to satisfy its subscribers risks losing market share to its competitors.

The more knowledgeable subscribers are regarding access to care provided by different HMOs, the greater will be the HMO's financial incentive not to pressure its physicians to underserve its patients. Instead, it will monitor physicians to guard against underservice. Gathering information on HMOs and their physicians and how well their enrollees are served is costly (in terms of time and money) for individuals. It is less costly for employers to gather this information, make the information available to their employees, and even limit the HMOs from which their employees can choose.

Informed Purchasers

Informed purchasers are necessary if the market is to discipline imperfect agents. An HMO's reputation is an expensive asset that can be reduced by imperfect agents underserving their patients. Performance information and competition among HMOs for informed purchasers should prevent these organizations from underserving their enrollees. The financial, reputation, and legal costs of underservice should mitigate the financial incentives to underprescribe in an HMO.

Both insurers and HMOs lack information on a patient's diagnosis and appropriate treatment needs. Thus, the insurer's or HMO's profitability depends on the physician's knowledge and treatment recommendations. Depending on the type of health plan and the incentives physicians face, a potential inefficiency exists in the provision of medical services. Physicians may prescribe too many or too few services. When they prescribe too many services, the value to the patient of those additional services may not be worth the costs of producing them. Prescribing too few services is also inefficient in that patients may not realize that the value of the services and technology they did not receive (and for which they were willing to pay) was greater than their physician led them to believe. To decrease the inefficiencies, insurers who pay physicians on a fee-for-service basis have instituted cost-containment methods.

Medicare—a fee-for-service insurer for physician services for the aged—has not yet undertaken similar cost-containment methods to limit supplier-induced demand. Until Medicare is able to institute such mechanisms, imperfect agents will be able to manipulate the information they provide to their aged patients, change the visit coding to receive higher payment, and decrease the time spent per visit with these aged patients.

Monitoring of physician behavior within HMOs and other managed care insurers has increased. Physicians who were previously in fee-for-service and who boosted their income by prescribing too many services are being reviewed to ensure that they understand the change in incentives. Once they are aware of the new incentives, these imperfect agents must be monitored to ensure that they do not underserve their HMO patients.

The market for medical services is changing. Insurers and large employers are attempting to overcome physicians' information advantage by profiling physicians according to their prices, the use and appropriateness of their services, and their treatment outcomes. These profiles allow imperfect agents less opportunity to benefit at the expense of the insurer. Information on physician performance is available on the Internet, and states (such as New York) publish data on physician and hospital performance (such as risk-adjusted mortality rates for different types of surgery).[1] Demand inducement, to the extent that it exists, will diminish. One hopes that with improved monitoring systems and better measures of patient outcomes, physicians will behave as perfect agents, providing the appropriate quantity and quality of medical services, where the costs of additional treatment as well as the benefits are considered.

Insurers serving millions of enrollees have very large data sets, and information technology allows insurers to use these data sets to analyze different treatment methods and physician practice patterns. These data will enable insurers to determine which physicians deviate from accepted medical norms.

Not all insurers or employers, however, are engaged in these informational and cost-containment activities. Those who are not are at an informational disadvantage to the physician and the HMO. Insurers and employers who are less knowledgeable regarding the services provided to their enrollees and employees pay for overuse of services and demand-inducing behavior by fee-for-service providers and for underservice by HMO physicians. Medicare and Medicaid, whose payment methods are primarily fee-for-service, are also limited in cost-containment activities to reduce demand inducement. At some point, such purchasers will realize that investing in more information will lower their medical expenditures and improve the quality of care provided.

Summary

Under fee-for-service payment, the inability of patients and their insurers to distinguish between imperfect agents and perfect agents led to the growth of cost-containment methods. The changes occurring in the private sector and in government physician payment systems must take into account the different types of physicians and the fact that, unless physicians are appropriately monitored, the response by imperfect agents will make achieving the intended objectives difficult.

Discussion Questions

1. Why do physicians play such a crucial role in the delivery of medical services?
2. How might a decrease in physician income, possibly as a result of an increase in the number of physicians, affect the physician's role as the patient's agent?
3. What are some ways in which insurers seek to compensate for physicians' information advantage?
4. What forces currently limit supplier-induced demand?
5. How do fee-for-service and capitation payment systems affect the physician's role as the patient's agent?

Note

1. Information on websites and reports on physician and hospital performance come from www.consumerhealthratings.com/index .php?action=showSubCats&cat_id=30. That website includes links to different state reports, such as the following:

- Massachusetts: Heart Bypass Surgery Hospital Ratings, 2011— www.massdac.org
- New Jersey: Cardiac Surgery Hospital and Surgeon Ratings, 2008—www.state.nj.us/health/healthcarequality/cardiacsurgery .shtml#CSR
- New York: Cardiac Surgery Ratings (hospitals and surgeons, statewide)—www.health.ny.gov/press/ releases/2012/2012-10-15_cardiac_reports_released.htm

Additional Reading

Mitchell, J. M. 2008. "Do Financial Incentives Linked to Ownership of Specialty Hospitals Affect Physicians' Practice Patterns?" *Medical Care* 46 (7): 732–37.

References

American Medical Association (AMA). 2013. *Physician Characteristics and Distribution in the United States, 2013 edition*. Chicago: AMA.

———. 1982. *Physician Characteristics and Distribution in the United States, 1981 edition*. Chicago: AMA.

Centers for Medicare & Medicaid Services (CMS). 2014. "National Health Expenditure Data." Last modified May. http://cms.gov/ Research-Statistics-Data-and-Systems/Statistics-Trends-and-Reports/ NationalHealthExpendData/index.html.

Feldstein, P. J. 2011. *Health Care Economics*, 7th ed. Albany, NY: Delmar.

Fuchs, V. R. 1968. "The Growing Demand for Medical Care." *New England Journal of Medicine* 279 (4): 190–95.

McCarthy, T. 1985. "The Competitive Nature of the Primary Care Physician Services Market." *Journal of Health Economics* 4 (2): 93–117.

McGuire, T. G. 2000. "Physician Agency." In *Handbook of Health Economics*, vol. 1A, edited by A. J. Culyer and J. P. Newhouse, 461–536. New York: North-Holland Press.

US Census Bureau. 2012. *Statistical Abstract of the United States*. Various editions. www.census.gov/compendia/statab/.

RATIONING MEDICAL SERVICES

No country can afford to provide unlimited medical services to everyone. Although few would disagree that waste exists in the current system, all of the medical needs in the United States could not be fulfilled even if that waste were eliminated and those resources redirected. A large, one-time savings would result from eliminating inefficiencies, but—driven by population growth, an aging population, and advances in medical technology—medical expenditures would continue to increase faster than inflation. As new experimental treatments (such as Avastin, a tumor-starving drug therapy used for cancer treatment) are developed—no matter how uncertain or small their effect—making them routinely available to all those who might benefit would be costly. The resources needed to eliminate all our medical needs—including prescription drugs, mental health services, long-term care, dental care, and vision care as well as acute, chronic, and preventive services—would be enormous.

The cost of eliminating all medical needs, no matter how small, means forgoing the benefits of spending those resources to meet other needs, such as food, clothing, housing, and education. Forgoing these other needs is the real cost of fulfilling all our medical needs. Because no country can afford to spend unlimited resources on medical services, each must choose some mechanism to ration or limit access to medical services.

Rationing is done by one of two methods: (1) government nonprice rationing and (2) rationing by market-determined price.

Government Rationing

The first and most frequently used method is non-price rationing, whereby the government limits access to goods and services. During World War II, for example, food, gasoline, and other goods were rationed; their prices were kept artificially low, but people could not buy all they wanted at the prevailing price. Similarly, in the 1970s, a gasoline shortage developed when the government kept the price of gasoline below its market price. The available supply was effectively "rationed" because people had to wait long hours at gasoline stations. Although they were willing to pay higher prices, they were not permitted to do so because gas prices were set by the government.

This type of rationing is also used to allocate medical services in countries such as Great Britain. The British government sets low prices for medical services and limits expenditures on those services. Because there is a shortage of services at their prevailing prices, these scarce services are explicitly allocated according to a person's age (such as when denying kidney transplants to those over a certain age) or by setting a value on a human life to determine whether costly treatments should be provided (Cox 2012; Harris 2008). In Canada, rationing is implicit according to a queue, in which a person may wait months or up to a year for certain surgical procedures, such as hip replacements (Barua and Esmail 2012).

In the United States, only Oregon has proposed such an explicit system of rationing medical services. In contrast to other states, which provide unlimited medical services to a small portion of the poor, the Oregon legislature decided to limit Medicaid recipients' access to expensive procedures (such as organ transplants) and to increase Medicaid eligibility for more low-income persons. The state ranked all medical services according to the outcomes that could be expected from treatment (e.g., "prevents death with full recovery") and according to their effect on quality of life. Because the state budget is unlikely to ever be sufficient to fund all medical procedures to all of its poor, those procedures at the lower end of the rankings would not be funded.

Rationing by Ability to Pay the Market-Determined Price

Among the general population in the United States, medical services are not rationed so explicitly. Instead, a different method of rationing is used: Everyone who can afford to pay the market-determined price has access to the goods and services. There are no shortages of services for those who are willing to pay (either out of pocket or through insurance). Those who are unable or unwilling to pay the market-determined price (such as those with low income and without health insurance) receive fewer medical services than those who have higher income.

Medical services involve a great deal of discretionary use. Empirical studies show that a 10 percent increase in income leads to an approximate 10 percent increase in medical expenditures (Congressional Budget Office 2008). As income increases, the amount spent on medical services increases proportionately. This relationship between income and medical spending exists not only in this country but also across all countries. As shown in Exhibit 5.1, the higher the country's income, the greater its medical expenditures.

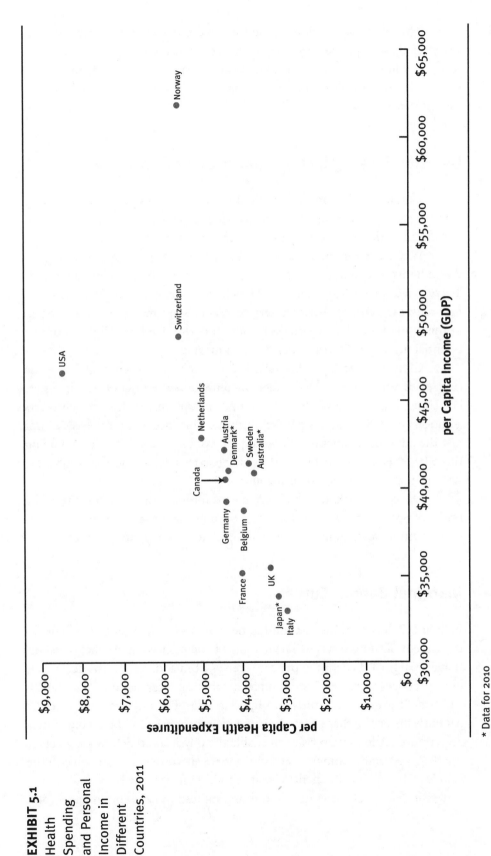

EXHIBIT 5.1
Health Spending and Personal Income in Different Countries, 2011

* Data for 2010
GDP: gross domestic product
NOTE: All values are in US dollars measured in GDP purchasing power parities.
SOURCE: Data from OECD (2013).

This observed relationship between income and medical expenditures suggests that as people become wealthier, they prefer to spend more to receive additional medical and higher-quality care. In addition, they make greater use of specialists and are willing to pay to avoid waiting to receive those services.

Decision Making by Consumers of Medical Services

Understanding why people use medical services requires more than knowing whether they are ill. Also important to understand are their attitudes toward seeking care, the prices they must pay for such care, and their income.

Whether rationing is based on ability to pay or on government expenditure limits, patients are faced with prices they must pay for medical services. These prices may be artificially low (such as in Great Britain or Canada) or may reflect the cost of providing services (such as in a market-oriented system in the United States). Regardless of how they are determined, prices are an essential ingredient in consumer decision making.

Consumers spend (allocate) their money on the basis of the value they place on different needs, their income, and the prices of their different choices. They are faced with an array of options, each of which offers additional benefits and has a different price. They decide on the basis of not just the additional benefits they would receive but also the cost of obtaining those benefits. In this manner, prices enable consumers to decide as to which services they will allocate their income.

Of course, making one choice means forgoing others. Similarly, as the prices of options increase or decrease, consumers are likely to reallocate their money. An increase in income allows consumers to buy more of everything.

Marginal Benefit Curve

Exhibit 5.2 illustrates the relationship between use of services and the cost to the patient of those services. The marginal benefit curve shows that the additional (marginal) benefit the patient receives from additional visits declines as use of services increases. For example, a patient concerned about her health will benefit greatly from the first physician visit. The physician will take the patient's history, perhaps perform some diagnostic tests, and possibly write a prescription. A follow-up visit will enable the physician to determine whether the diagnosis and treatment were appropriate and provide reassurance to the patient. The marginal benefit of that second visit will not be as high as the first visit. More return visits without any indication of a continuing health

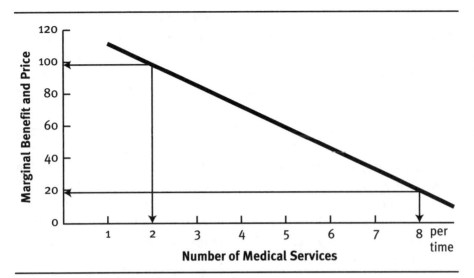

EXHIBIT 5.2
Relationship
Among Prices,
Visits, and
Marginal
Benefit of an
Additional Visit

problem will provide further reassurance, but the value to the patient of those additional visits will be much lower than the initial visits.

How rapidly the marginal benefit curve declines depends on the patient's attitude toward seeking care and the value he places on that additional care. Not all patients place the same value on medical services. For some, the marginal benefit curve will decline quickly after the initial treatment; for others, the decline will be more gradual.

The actual number of patient visits is determined by the cost to the patient for each visit. Given the patient's marginal benefit curve and a price per visit of $100, as shown in Exhibit 5.2, the marginal benefit to the patient of the first visit exceeds the cost of $100. The patient will demand a total of two visits because the marginal benefit of that second visit equals the cost of that visit. If the patient makes more than two visits, the value the patient receives from the third visit would be less than its cost.

Thus, the demand for medical services is determined by the value to the patient (either real or imagined) of those visits and the patient's cost for each visit. When the cost is greater than the value of an additional visit, the patient will not return for the additional visit; the patient could receive greater value for his money by spending it on other goods and services.

Health insurance reduces the patient's costs for medical care. Although the insurer pays the physician (or hospital) the full price, the patient pays a reduced out-of-pocket price. For example, if the charge for a physician's office visit is $100 and health insurance pays 80 percent of the charge, the "real" price to the patient is the out-of-pocket price—only $20. As the patient's cost for an office visit declines from $100 to $20, the patient will increase the number of visits. The patient will make additional visits until the value received from the last visit is worth only $20.

The patient's decision to use medical services is based solely on a calculation of her own costs (copayment) and the perceived value of those additional visits. Although the real cost of each visit is $100, the patient's cost for additional visits is only $20. The consequence is too much medical care; the value to the patient of additional visits is worth less than the full cost of those visits.

In using medical services, the patient usually incurs travel and waiting costs. The importance of these costs differs among patients. Typically, retired persons have low waiting costs, whereas working mothers have high waiting costs. To predict use of services, travel and waiting costs (as well as out-of-pocket payments) must be weighed against the marginal benefit of another visit. A medical system that has high out-of-pocket payments and low waiting costs will affect usage patterns differently than a system that relies on low prices but high waiting costs.

An important empirical question is this: How rapid is the decline in value of additional services to the patient? If the first visit is worth more than $100 to the patient and the second visit is only worth $10, little if any over-use of medical services will occur. If, however, a second visit is worth $100 and the value of subsequent visits declines slowly, the patient will make many visits before the value of a visit falls below $20.

Price Sensitivity

Research on the relationship between the out-of-pocket price paid by the patient and use of medical services indicates that for some medical services, the decline in value of additional services is gradual. In general, a 10 percent increase in price of medical services leads to about a 2 percent reduction in use of services (Morrisey 2005). Price sensitivity varies according to type of medical service. Mental health services are quite price sensitive; a 10 percent reduction in price leads to a 10 percent increase in use of services. Hospital services are the least price sensitive; hospital admissions would rise by about 1.5 percent with a 10 percent decrease in price. Lowering the price of physician services by 10 percent boosts use by about 2 percent. Higher-income groups are generally less price sensitive than lower-income groups. Nursing home services are price sensitive; reducing prices by 10 percent leads to about a 10 percent hike in use (Morrisey 2005). This finding suggests that including long-term care as part of national health insurance will result in large increases in nursing home use and expenditures.

The Medicare drug benefit is administered by private prescription drug plans (PDP), which use copayments when enrollees require prescription drugs. These copayments serve two purposes. First, by requiring a lower copayment for generic drugs, Medicare enrollees are more likely to switch to generics from brand name drugs, thereby lowering drug expenditures and reducing the cost of the private drug plan. Every 10 percent increase in the use of generic, rather than brand name, statins would reduce Medicare costs by about $1 billion annually, according to estimates by Hoadley and colleagues (2012). Second, the authors found that setting a low copayment for generic statin drugs—and even eliminating the copayment altogether—had a very large effect on encouraging Medicare enrollees to use the generic statin to control their high cholesterol, thereby minimizing costly hospital stays.

Medicare beneficiaries' price sensitivity when choosing among competing private PDPs is such that a 10 percent increase in a PDP's premium would lead to a 14.5 percent decrease in that plan's enrollment (Frakt and Pizer 2010). An important reason for such a high degree of price sensitivity is that beneficiaries can select a PDP without disrupting their doctor–patient relationship. When Medicare beneficiaries choose among competing health plans, which might require a change in the doctor–patient relationship, an increase of $10 in a plan's monthly premium decreases a plan's market share by between 2 and 3 percentage points (Buchmueller et al. 2013).

The price sensitivity faced by individual physicians, hospitals, and other providers is much greater than the overall market because each provider is a possible substitute for other providers. For example, although a 10 percent overall price decrease leads to a 2 percent increase in overall use of physician services, if an *individual* physician raises (or lowers) his price by 10 percent, and other physicians do not change their prices, the individual physician will lose (or gain) a large number of patients—approximately 30 percent. Similarly, greater price sensitivity exists toward any single health plan than toward health insurance in general. When employees have a choice of health plans and have to pay an out-of-pocket premium (copremium) for these plans, their choice of health plan is very price sensitive. One study found that a difference in HMO copremiums of as little as $5 to $10 a month would cause about 25 percent of the HMO's enrollees to switch to the less-costly HMO (Strombom, Buchmueller, and Feldstein 2002).

Moral Hazard

The behavior of patients who use more medical services because their insurance lowers the out-of-pocket cost of those services is called by the insurance industry as *moral hazard*. This term means that having insurance changes a person's behavior, and the cost of medical services to the insurance company goes up. Those with insurance (or more comprehensive insurance) use more services, see more specialists, and incur higher medical costs than those who do not have insurance (or less comprehensive insurance), and the value patients and their physicians place on many of these additional services is lower than their full costs.

Indemnity insurance also places an annual limit—referred to as a *stop loss*—on a patient's responsibility for out-of-pocket payments. If a patient has a serious illness, that out-of-pocket maximum (e.g., $5,000) is reached fairly early in the treatment process. After that point, the patient and her physician (assuming under fee-for-service payment) have an incentive to try all types of treatments that may provide some benefit to the patient, no matter how small that benefit. The expression "flat-of-the-curve medicine" indicates the use of all medical technology, even when the benefit to the patient is extremely small. The only cost to the patient is nonfinancial—the discomfort and risk associated with the treatment. Not surprisingly, medical expenditures for those who are seriously ill are, therefore, extraordinarily high. Patients in such circumstances have everything available to them that modern medicine can provide.

The problem of moral hazard has long plagued health insurers, as it results in excessive use, increased cost of medical care, and higher insurance premiums. Until the 1980s, insurers primarily controlled moral hazard by requiring patients to pay a deductible and, once the deductible was exceeded, to cover part of the cost with a copayment. In the 1980s, insurers began to use more aggressive methods to control overuse of medical services, such as prior authorization for hospital admissions, utilization review once the patient was hospitalized, and second surgical opinions. Unless prior authorization was received, the patient was liable for part of the hospitalization cost (and often the patient's physician had to justify the procedure to the insurer). Requirements to obtain a second surgical opinion were an attempt to provide the patient and the insurer with more information as to the value of the recommended surgical procedure.

These cost-containment or rationing techniques are often referred to as *managed care*. Managed care methods also include case management (which minimizes the medical cost of catastrophic medical cases) and preferred physician panels (which exclude physicians who overuse medical services). These provider panels are marketed to employer groups as less costly, thereby offering enrollees lower out-of-pocket payments and insurance premiums if they restrict their choice of physician to members of the panel.

In addition to changing patient incentives and relying on managed care techniques, moral hazard can also be controlled by changing physicians' incentives. HMOs are paid an annual fee for providing medical services to their enrolled populations. The out-of-pocket price to the enrollee for use of services in an HMO is low; consequently, usage rates are expected to be high. Because the HMO bears the risk that its enrollees' medical services will exceed their annual payments, the HMO has an incentive not to provide excessive amounts of medical services. An HMO patient must instead be concerned with receiving too little care. HMO physicians ration care on the basis of the physicians' perception of the benefits to their patients and the full costs to the HMO of further treatment. Because HMO enrollees have low copayments, the onus (and incentives) for decreasing moral hazard—hence rationing care—is placed on the HMO's physicians.

These approaches by insurers and HMOs to minimize moral hazard attempt to match the additional benefit of medical services to their full cost. Copayments and financial penalties for not receiving prior authorization are incentives to change the patient's behavior. In an HMO, the HMO's physicians are responsible for controlling moral hazard.

Summary

Important differences exist between government rationing of services and the rationing by market-determined price that occurs in a competitive market. In a price-competitive system, consumers differ in the value they place on additional medical services; however, those who place a higher value on additional services can always purchase more. As their income increases, consumers may prefer to spend more of their income on medical care than on other goods and services. If an HMO is too slow to adopt new technology or too restrictive on access to medical services provided to its enrollees, those enrollees could switch to another HMO or to indemnity insurance, pay higher premiums, and receive more services. Under government rationing, even if a patient places a higher value on additional medical services than does the government and is willing to pay the full cost of those services, the patient will still be unable to purchase them.

Medical services must be rationed because society cannot afford to provide all the medical services that would be demanded at zero prices. Which rationing mechanism should be used? Having people pay for additional services and voluntarily join an HMO or a managed care plan, or allowing the government to decide on the availability of medical resources? The first, or market, approach permits subscribers to match their costs to the value they place on additional services. Only when the government decides on the costs and benefits of medical services, and does not permit individuals to buy services beyond that level, will availability be lower than desired by those who value medical services more highly. Choice of rationing technique, relying on the private sector versus the government, is essential for determining how much medical care will be provided, to whom, and at what cost.

Regardless of which rationing approach is taken, knowledge of price sensitivity is important for public policy and for attaining efficiency. If the government wants to increase the use of preventive services—such as pre-natal care, mammograms, and dental checkups—for underserved popula-tions, would lowering the price (and waiting cost) of such services achieve that goal? If insurers raise the out-of-pocket price for some visits, would that decrease the use of care that is of low value? If stimulating competition among health plans is the goal, how great a difference in premiums would cause large numbers of employees to switch plans? If consumers are to be able to match the benefits and costs of use of medical services, and face the costs of their decisions, they will be more discriminating in their choice of health plan and use of services.

Discussion Questions

1. What determines how many physician services an individual demands?
2. What is moral hazard, and how does its existence increase the cost of medical care?
3. In what ways can moral hazard be limited?
4. Assume that medical services are free to everyone but that the gov-ernment restricts the supply of services so that physician office visits are rationed by waiting time. Which population groups would fare better?
5. How would you use information on price sensitivity of medical ser-vices for policy purposes—for example, to increase the use of mam-mograms?
6. Discuss: The high price sensitivity of insurance copremiums indicates that if employees had to pay out of pocket the difference between the lowest-cost health plan and any other insurance, market competition among health plans would be stimulated.

References

Barua, B., and N. Esmail. 2012. *Waiting Your Turn: Wait Times for Health Care in Canada, 2012 Report.* Fraser Institute. Published December. www.fraserinstitute.org/uploadedFiles/fraser-ca/Content/research-news/research/publications/waiting-your-turn-2012.pdf.

Buchmueller, T., K. Grazier, R. Hirth, and E. Okeke. 2013. "The Price Sensitivity of Medicare Beneficiaries: A Regression Discontinuity Approach." *Health Economics* 22 (1): 35–51.

Congressional Budget Office. 2008. *Technological Change and the Growth of Health Care Spending*. Published January 31. www.cbo.gov/ftpdocs/89xx/doc8947/MainText.3.1.shtml.

Cox, P. 2012. "United Kingdom: Rationing by Cost." PRI's *The World*. Accessed November 2013. http://rationinghealth.org/united-kingdom-rationing-by-cost/uprint.

Frakt, A., and S. Pizer. 2010. "Beneficiary Price Sensitivity in the Medicare Prescription Drug Plan Market." *Health Economics* 19 (1): 88–100.

Harris, G. 2008. "British Balance Benefit Versus Cost of New Drugs." *New York Times*, December 3, p. A1. www.nytimes.com/2008/12/03/health/03nice.html?pagewanted=all&_r=0.

Hoadley, J., K. Merrell, E. Hargrave, and L. Summer. 2012. "In Medicare Part D Plans, Low or Zero Copays and Other Features to Encourage the Use of Generic Statins Work, Could Save Billions." *Health Affairs* 31 (10): 2266–75.

Morrisey, M. 2005. *Price Sensitivity in Health Care: Implications for Health Care Policy*. Washington, DC: National Federation of Independent Business.

Organisation for Economic Co-operation and Development (OECD). 2013. *OECD Health Data, 2013*. Paris: OECD.

Strombom, B., T. Buchmueller, and P. Feldstein. 2002. "Switching Costs, Price Sensitivity, and Health Plan Choice." *Journal of Health Economics* 21 (1): 89–116.

HOW MUCH HEALTH INSURANCE SHOULD EVERYONE HAVE?

Why do some people have health insurance that covers almost all their medical expenditures, including dental and vision care, while others do not? Why does the government subsidize the purchase of private health insurance for those with high income? Has health insurance stimulated the growth in medical expenditures, or has it served as protection against the rapid rise in medical expenses? The answers to these questions are important in explaining the rapid increase in medical expenditures and understanding healthcare reform issues.

The purpose of health insurance is to enable people to eliminate uncertainty and the possibility of incurring a large medical expense. Buying health insurance converts the possibility of a large loss into a certain but small loss. Insurance spreads risk among a large number of people; when each person pays a premium, the aggregate amount of the premiums covers the large losses of relatively few people.

Definitions of Insurance Terms

Before this discussion continues, a number of terms should be defined. *Indemnity insurance* reimburses either the health provider or the patient a fixed amount (or a percentage of the bill), requiring the patient to pay any balance of the cost for medical treatment. When the insured patient has a *service benefit* policy, he receives all the services needed at no additional cost—regardless of the amount the insurer pays the provider. Current health insurance policies typically contain indemnity and service benefit features. Physician services and out-of-hospital services are usually treated with indemnity insurance features, whereas hospital admissions are usually paid for as a service benefit.

The difference between the provider's charge and the insurance payment is made up by deductibles and copayments. A *deductible* is a given dollar amount that the patient will have to spend before the insurer will pay any medical expenses. Typically, indemnity policies require an insured family to spend between $250 and $500 of their own money before the insurer will start paying part of their medical bills. A deductible lowers the insurance premium because it eliminates the many small medical expenses most families have each year. The insurer is also able to lower its administrative costs by eliminating the claims processing for a large number of small claims.

The effect of a deductible on an insurance premium is illustrated in Exhibit 6.1. As shown, a large percentage of families have relatively small medical expenses, while a small percentage of families have a very large (referred to as *catastrophic*) expense. Eliminating the area designated as a deductible would reduce the overall amount spent on medical care, thereby reducing the insurance premium.

When a patient pays a percentage of the physician's bill (for example, 20 percent), this is referred to as *cost sharing* or *coinsurance*. (The term *copayment* has been used to indicate a specific dollar amount, such as $20, payable by the patient.) Coinsurance provides the patient with an incentive to be sensitive to physicians' charges, perhaps by shopping around, as the patient will have to pay part of the bill. The patient will also have an incentive to use fewer services because he will have to balance the value of an additional visit against its cost (coinsurance). Coinsurance also reduces the insurer's share of medical expenses, as shown in Exhibit 6.1. Indemnity policies are typically 80/20 plans, meaning that the insurer pays 80 percent of the bill and the patient pays 20 percent. These policies also contain a *stop loss,* which places an overall limit on the patient's out-of-pocket expenses. For example, once a patient has paid a deductible and copayments that add up to, say, $2,000, the insurer pays 100 percent of all remaining expenses during that year. Without a stop loss, unlimited coinsurance or copayments could become a financial hardship. Coinsurance typically applies to out-of-hospital services considered discretionary.

Only a small percentage of families incur catastrophic claims (see Exhibit 6.1). The definition of a catastrophic expense depends on the patient's family income, as a $2,000 expense may be catastrophic to some families but not to others, but few policies define catastrophic expense this way. Insurance policies that cover only catastrophic medical expenses are referred to as *high-deductible insurance plans.*

The amount of medical expenditures paid out by the insurance company is called the *pure premium*. The pure premium for a group of people with the same risk level (age and sex) represents their expected medical cost—that is, the probability that they will need medical services multiplied by the cost of those services. For example, assuming that the probability of Person A needing surgery (given her age and sex) is 5 percent and the cost of the surgery (if needed) is $50,000, she (and others in her risk group) would have to pay a pure premium of $2,500 a year—$50,000 × 0.05. If she chooses not to buy insurance, theoretically she would have to put aside $50,000 to pay for that possible medical expense. However, she may not be

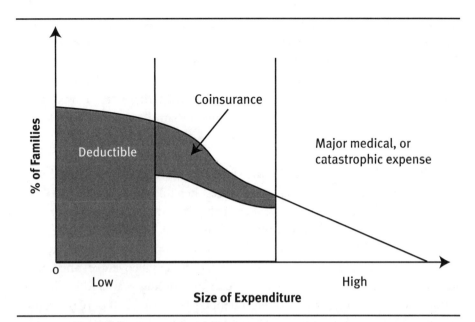

EXHIBIT 6.1
Deductibles,
Coinsurance,
and
Catastrophic
Expenses

able to put aside such a large amount—or even larger amounts (for example, the amount needed for an organ transplant)—or she may not want to tie up her funds in that way. Insurance offers Person A an alternative: It permits her to pay a premium that is equivalent to budgeting for an uncertain medical expense. She can eliminate the uncertainty of a large medical expense by paying an annual premium.

When everyone in a particular group has the same chance of becoming ill and incurring a medical expense, each person is considered to be in the same risk class and is charged the same pure premium. The *actual premium* charged, however, is always greater than the pure premium because the insurer has to recover its administrative and marketing costs and earn a profit. This difference between the pure and actual premium is referred to as the *loading charge*. (Another way to indicate the size of the loading charge is to use the *medical loss ratio*, which is the percentage of the collected premiums an insurance company pays out for medical expenses—typically 85 percent. The remaining 15 percent is the loading charge.)

Insurance-Purchase Decision Making

The size of the loading charge often explains why people buy insurance for some medical expenses but not for others. If people could buy insurance at the pure premium, they would buy insurance for almost everything because its price would reflect, on average, what they would likely spend anyway. However, when people are charged more than the pure premium, they must decide whether they want to buy insurance or self-insure—that is, bear the risk themselves. The higher the loading charge relative to the pure premium, the less insurance people will buy. For example, part of the loading charge is related to the administrative cost of processing a claim, which is not too different for small and large claims. Small claims, therefore, have higher loading costs (relative to their pure premium) than do large claims. People are more willing to pay a high administrative cost for a large claim than for a small claim.

In the Person A example in which the pure premium is $2,500 a year, even if the insurance company charged her $2,600 a year ($100 more than the pure premium), she would probably buy the insurance rather than bear the risk herself. However, her decision would be different if she were required to pay the same loading charge with a smaller expected medical expense. For example, let's say she is considering dental coverage. She knows her family will probably need dental care in the coming year, and it will cost $200. The insurance company offers a dental policy for $200 pure premium, plus the $100 administrative cost. Buying insurance for dental care is like prepaying the same amount she would otherwise spend, plus a 50 percent loading charge. In the second case, she would rather bear the small risk herself than buy insurance.

This discussion suggests that people are more likely to buy insurance for large, unexpected medical expenses than for small medical expenses (for a more complete discussion of the factors affecting the demand for health insurance, see Feldstein [2011]). This is the pattern typically observed in the purchase of health insurance. A hospital admission and the physician expenses connected with it, such as the surgeon's and anesthesiologist's fees, are more completely covered by insurance than are expenses for a physician office visit. Thus, an important characteristic of good insurance is that it covers large catastrophic expenses. People are less able to afford the catastrophic costs of a major illness or accident than they are front-end or first-dollar coverage, which is typically small expenses with relatively high loading charges.

Tax-Free, Employer-Paid Health Insurance

Surprisingly, however, many people have insurance against small claims such as dental visits, physician office visits, and vision services. How can we explain this?

Advantages

The predominant source of health insurance coverage for those under age 65 years is through the workplace, where (as of 2012) 90 percent of all private health insurance is purchased by the employer on behalf of the employee (Census Bureau 2013, Table HI01). This occurs because the federal tax code does not consider employer-paid health insurance as part of the employee's taxable income; it is exempt from federal, state, and Social Security taxes.

Until the early 1980s, marginal tax rates for federal income taxes were as high as 70 percent. Throughout the late 1960s and 1970s, inflation increased, pushing employees into higher marginal tax brackets. Social Security taxes have also risen steadily; as of 2014, the employer and employee each pay 6.2 percent of the employee's wage up to a maximum wage of $117,000 (Social Security Administration 2013). In addition, the employee and employer each pay a Medicare tax of 1.45 percent on all earned income, for a combined total of 7.65 percent on the employee and employer. Starting in 2013, the Medicare payroll tax was increased to 2.35 percent (only for the employee part) on individuals earning more than $200,000 and families earning more than $250,000. These high-income individuals and families will have to pay an additional 3.8 percent Medicare tax on all unearned income, such as investment income, dividends, and capital gains.

Marginal federal tax rates, which had declined since the 1980s, have risen again. Effective 2013, the highest federal marginal tax rate was increased to 39.6 percent for individuals earning more than $400,000 and families earning more than $450,000. Thus, the marginal tax rate on investment income for those with high income is now 43.4 percent (39.6 + 3.8 = 43.4).

Employees and their employers have a financial incentive for additional compensation in the form of health insurance benefits rather than cash income. The employer saves its share of Social Security taxes, and employees do not have to pay federal, state, or Social Security taxes on additional health insurance benefits. For example, assume Employee B is in a 30 percent tax bracket, has to pay 5 percent state income tax and 7 percent Social Security tax, already has basic hospital and medical coverage, and is due to receive a $1,000 raise. Employee B would be left with only $580 (0.30 + 0.05 + 0.07 = 0.42 subtracted from 100 percent = 0.58 × $1,000) after taxes to purchase for his family dental care and other medical services not covered by insurance. Alternately, the employer could use the entire $1,000 to purchase additional health insurance, and no taxes would be paid on it. This additional insurance would likely cover Employee B's dental care and other previously uncovered medical expenses, which could easily add up to more than the $580 he would receive if he is simply given a $1,000 raise.

As employees move into higher tax brackets, the higher loading charge on small claims is more than offset by using before-tax income to buy health insurance for those small claims. Using the example of dental care, the choice is between spending $200 of after-tax income on dental care or buying dental insurance for $300 ($200 dental expense plus $100 loading charge).

Employee B spending $200 on his family's dental care would require him to earn $350 in before-tax income (30 percent federal tax, 5 percent state tax, and 7 percent Social Security tax). However, if his employer uses that same $350 to purchase dental benefits for him, the premium—including the $100 loading charge—would be more than covered, leaving him $50 to buy even more insurance. *Tax-free, employer-purchased health insurance provides a financial incentive to purchase health insurance for small claims.*

Another way to view the tax subsidy for health insurance is to consider that if an employee saves 40 percent when buying health insurance, the price of insurance to that employee has been cut by 40 percent. Studies indicate that the purchase of insurance has an approximate proportional relationship to changes in its price (Cutler and Reber 1998). Thus, a 40 percent price reduction would be expected to increase the quantity of insurance purchased by 40 percent.

The advantages of tax-free, employer-purchased health insurance stimulate the demand for comprehensive health insurance coverage, particularly among higher-income employees. More services not traditionally thought of as insurable—such as a dental visit, an eye exam, and all small routine expenditures—have become part of the employee's health insurance.

Consequences

Employer-paid health insurance became tax exempt during World War II, when the government agreed not to consider employer-paid health insurance as an increase in an employee's income. This move came in response to wage and price controls and to prevent a West Coast shipbuilder's union from striking for higher wages. The growth in employer-paid health insurance increased rapidly in the late 1960s when inflation rose and more employees were pushed into higher marginal tax brackets. The greater comprehensiveness of tax-exempt, employer-purchased health insurance has had important consequences.

First, too many services were covered by health insurance. Administrative costs increased as insurers had to process many small claims that a deductible would have excluded. A $20 prescription drug claim and a much larger medical expense cost the same to process. Second, as insurance became more comprehensive, patients' concern with the prices charged for medical services decreased. Physicians, hospitals, and other health providers could more easily raise their charges because the patients were covered by insurance—that is, someone else was paying. Similarly, as the amount patients had to pay out of pocket for medical expenses declined, they increased their use of those services, sought more referrals to specialists, and underwent more extensive medical imaging and testing.

The growth of health insurance and medical technology was intertwined. Expensive technology, which increases the cost of a medical service, causes people to buy health insurance to protect themselves from those large, unexpected medical expenses. At the same time, the availability of insurance to pay for expensive technology stimulates its development. When comprehensive insurance removes any concern insured persons may have about the cost of their care, they (and physicians acting on their behalf) want access to the latest technology as long as it offers some additional benefit, no matter how small. The benefits of that technology to patients outweigh their out-of-pocket costs for using it. Because insurance was available to pay the costs of expensive technology, such as transplants, financial incentives existed to develop benefit-producing technology. Thus, medical technology was stimulated by, and in turn stimulated, the purchase of health insurance.

Conversely, cost-reducing technology generated little interest because employers could pass on higher insurance costs to employees in the form of reduced wages or to consumers in the form of higher prices. Furthermore, the after-tax value of savings to employees from stringent cost-containment measures was small. If, for example, insurance premiums could be reduced by $300 by limiting employees' choice of physician, the inconvenience to the employee and his family associated with changing physicians would probably not be worth the after-tax savings of $150.

The lack of concern over the price of medical services and greater use of those services caused medical expenditures to sharply increase, which in turn caused health insurance premiums to rapidly rise. Higher insurance premiums meant smaller wage increases, but this was not obvious to employees because the employer was paying the insurance premium.

Hundreds of billions of dollars in tax revenues have been lost because of employer-paid health insurance. The value of this tax subsidy was forecast to be $248 billion in 2013 in forgone federal, Social Security, and state taxes simply because employer-paid health insurance is not considered part of the employee's taxable income (Congressional Budget Office 2013a). These lost tax revenues primarily benefit high-income employees because they are in higher tax brackets. As shown in Exhibit 6.2, the higher an employee's income, the greater the value of the exclusion from income of employer-purchased health insurance. This $248 billion in lost tax revenues is equivalent to a huge subsidy for the purchase of health insurance to those who can most easily afford it. In comparison, in 2013 the federal government spent $265 billion on Medicaid, a means-tested program for the poor (Congressional Budget Office 2013b).

Exhibit 6.3 shows how the value of the exclusion from income of employer-purchased health insurance is distributed. Families with an income

EXHIBIT 6.2
Value of Tax
Exclusion for
Employer-
Paid Health
Insurance, by
Income Level,
2008

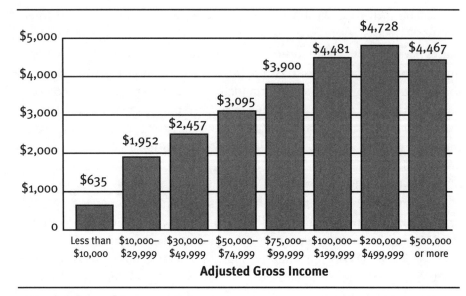

Adjusted Gross Income

SOURCE: Data from Appleby (2009), based on Joint Committee on Taxation calculations of Medical Expenditure Panel Survey data.

of $100,000 or greater in 2010 (26 percent of all families) received 40.6 percent of the federal portion of this tax subsidy for the purchase of health insurance.

Finally, tax-free, employer-paid health insurance reduced employees' incentive to choose lower-cost health plans. Many employers paid the entire premium of any plan the employee selected (or contributed more than the premium of the lowest-cost plan offered); as there was no visible cost to

EXHIBIT 6.3
Distribution
of Employer-
Paid Health
Insurance Tax
Exclusion, by
Income, 2010

Income Level	Tax Exclusion (Billion Dollars)	Percentage of Total
Less than $20,000	8.1	3.0
$20,000–$29,999	11.3	4.2
$30,000–$39,999	16.7	6.2
$40,000–$49,999	20.8	7.8
$50,000–$74,999	49.3	18.3
$75,000–$99,999	54.0	20.0
$100,000–$149,999	60.0	22.3
$150,000 or more	49.2	18.3
Total	269.6	100.0

SOURCE: Data from Sheils (2009), Figure 1.

the employee, the employee's incentive was to choose the most comprehensive plan with the easiest access to physicians and specialists.

Limitation of Tax-Free Status

To encourage competition among health plans on the basis of access to services, quality, and premiums, employers would have to require that employees pay out of pocket the additional cost of a more expensive health plan. The employee would then evaluate whether the additional benefits of that plan are worth its additional costs. Unless a limit is placed on the tax-free employer contribution, many employees will continue to select health plans on the basis of their benefits without regard to their premiums. Competition among health plans based on premiums, reputation, and access to services will not occur until employees have a greater financial stake in these decisions.

Not surprisingly, economists favor eliminating—or at least setting a maximum on—the tax-exempt status of employer-paid health insurance. Those with higher income would no longer receive a subsidy for their purchase of health insurance. Instead, increased tax revenues would come from those who have benefited most—namely those with higher income (Clemans-Cope, Zuckerman, and Resnick 2013). These funds then could be used to subsidize health insurance for those with lower income. Employees using after-tax dollars would be more cost conscious in their use of services and choice of health plans.

The Affordable Care Act (ACA) imposes a 40 percent tax on "Cadillac" health insurance (amounts greater than $27,500 a year for a family and $10,200 for an individual) starting in 2018. Unions who had negotiated comprehensive health benefits with their employers, however, opposed this provision of the legislation and were able to delay the imposition of the tax until 2018. (Starting in 2020, the value of a Cadillac health plan—set at $27,500 a year for a family—will be adjusted for inflation.) While the ACA tax on Cadillac plans was designed to raise revenue so that subsidies could be provided for other parts of the ACA, an unintended consequence is that it will likely reduce rising medical costs. If healthcare spending continues to increase faster than inflation, the percent of employer-sponsored health plans subject to the Cadillac tax is estimated to skyrocket from 15 percent in 2018 to 75 percent by 2029 (Frist 2014).

Employer-sponsored health plans will undergo changes to avoid the Cadillac tax. It will not be possible to lower premiums by decreasing covered benefits because the ACA has mandated a broad set of benefits. Instead, the likely approach for avoiding the tax will be threefold.

First, high-deductible health plans will become more prevalent. Deductibles will become much greater and the number of small claims paid by insurers will decrease, thereby decreasing administrative costs and insurance premiums. Out-of-pocket expenses will increase and become a greater financial burden on older employees and those who are chronically ill, many of whom will find that the deductibles and out-of-pocket expenses will exceed their ability to pay. As employees become more price sensitive, they will have a greater incentive (lower premiums and copayments) to use a restricted provider panel and join tightly managed care plans, such as health maintenance organizations (HMOs), in which the decision on use of services is made by the provider rather than the patient.

Second, insurers will seek to lower their premiums by using narrow (limited) provider networks. These networks rely on hospitals and physicians who are willing to discount their fees in return for a greater number of patients. Enrollees' choice of providers will be greatly reduced.

Third, several large employers are currently using *reference pricing* to reduce their employees' treatment costs and to improve treatment outcomes. An employer (or insurer) determines the maximum price it will pay the provider for an employee's medical treatment, such as a hip replacement. The reference price is usually based on the treatment price at high-quality hospitals. If the employee goes to other hospitals for their treatment, the employee pays the difference between the reference price and the hospital's price. As more employers use reference pricing, employee price sensitivity and provider competition will reduce treatment prices.

The Cadillac tax, by making patients bear more out-of-pocket expense for their care, will make patients more price sensitive. Employees may choose to join HMOs to lower their out-of-pocket expenses and thereby delegate the decision to restrict use of services to their managed care plan; in either case, use of services and medical spending will likely decline.[1] The basis for making treatment decisions will change. Employees (and physicians in managed care plans) will have to consider the costs of their treatment choices.

Summary

Health insurers play a valuable role in society. Assume a person is at risk for an operation costing $100,000. How many people would be able to pay that amount? Insurers pool risks; thus, a person can pay an insurance premium and eliminate the uncertainty that arises from whether she will incur a large expenditure if she becomes ill. Insurance reduces a person's risk of a large financial loss.[2]

However, health insurance also provides protection against relatively small losses, such as physician office visits and dental care. People buy insurance against such small losses because health insurance is subsidized; employer-paid health insurance is tax exempt. Employees purchase more comprehensive health insurance because of this tax subsidy. The primary beneficiaries of this tax subsidy are those with higher income because they are in a higher marginal tax bracket.

Tax-exempt employer-purchased health insurance has distorted consumers' choices in healthcare and diminished consumer incentives to be concerned with the cost of medical services. Reducing or limiting this tax subsidy may not only provide more funds to assist those with lower income but also make consumers more price sensitive in their choice of health plans and use of medical services.

Discussion Questions

1. How is a pure premium calculated?
2. What does the loading charge consist of?
3. How does the size of the loading charge affect the type of health insurance purchased?
4. Why does employer-purchased health insurance result in more comprehensive health insurance coverage?
5. What are the arguments in favor of eliminating (or placing a cap on) the tax-exempt status of employer-purchased health insurance?
6. How has health insurance affected the development of medical technology, and how has medical technology affected the growth of health insurance?

Notes

1. Insurers use copayments to make patients price sensitive and to discourage the use of medical services that provide little medical benefit. Patients then have to consider the costs and benefits of the additional services. For some medical services, however, copayments may increase medical costs and worsen a patient's health. For high-valued drugs, for example, a copayment may discourage a patient at risk for heart disease and stroke from taking his prescribed medications. In these circumstances, not only is it appropriate to waive the copayment but also it is in the interest of the insurer (as well as the patient) to monitor that the patient is taking his medications. Total medical costs for the patient will be lower than if a copayment were imposed on such high-valued medical services. For more on the subject of value-based insurance design, see Fendrick and Chernew (2006).

2. In addition to pooling risks, insurers can decrease their premiums by performing two additional tasks. First, to decrease the probability of a large loss occurring, insurers can encourage preventive measures among its insured population. Second, if an expensive procedure is needed, insurers can lower the cost of that procedure by selecting physicians and hospitals that are higher quality and less costly.

References

Appleby, J. 2009. "How Congress Might Tax Your Health Benefits." Kaiser Health News. Posted June 8. www.kaiserhealthnews.org/Stories/2009/June/08/taxes.aspx.

Clemans-Cope, L., S. Zuckerman, and D. Resnick. 2013. "Limiting the Tax Exclusion of Employer-Sponsored Health Insurance Premiums: Revenue Potential and Distributional Consequences." *Timely Analysis of Immediate Health Policy Issues.* Washington, DC: Urban Institute. www.urban.org/UploadedPDF/412816-Limiting-the-Tax-Exclusion-of-Employer-Sponsored-Health Insurance-Premiums.pdf.

Congressional Budget Office. 2013a. *The Distribution of Major Tax Expenditures in the Individual Income Tax System.* Accessed November. www.cbo.gov/sites/default/files/cbofiles/attachments/43768_DistributionTaxExpenditures.pdf.

———. 2013b. "Medicaid—May 2013 Baseline." Accessed November. www.cbo.gov/sites/default/files/cbofiles/attachments/44204_Medicaid.pdf.

Cutler, D., and S. Reber. 1998. "Paying for Health Insurance: The Trade-Off Between Competition and Adverse Selection." *Quarterly Journal of Economics* 113 (2): 433–66.

Feldstein, P. 2011. "The Demand for Health Insurance." In *Health Care Economics,* 7th ed., 139–69. Albany, NY: Delmar.

Fendrick, M., and M. Chernew. 2006. "Value-Based Insurance Design: Aligning Incentives to Bridge the Divide Between Quality Improvement and Cost Containment." *American Journal of Managed Care* 12 (Special Issue): SP5–SP10. www.sph.umich.edu/vbidcenter/registry/pdfs/AJMC_06speclFendrick6p.pdf.

Frist, W. 2014. "Obamacare's 'Cadillac Tax' Could Help Reduce the Cost of Health Care." *Forbes.* Posted February 28. www.forbes.com/sites/theapothecary/2014/02/26/obamacares-cadillac-tax-could-help-reduce-the-cost-of-health-care/.

Sheils, J. 2009. *Ideas for Financing Health Reform: Revenue Measures That Also Reduce Health Spending.* Statement for the Senate Committee on Finance, May 12. http://finance.senate.gov/imo/media/doc/John%20Sheils.pdf.

US Census Bureau. 2013. "Health Insurance Coverage Status and Type of Coverage by Selected Characteristics: 2012." CPS 2013 Annual Social and Economic Supplement. Last revised September. www.census.gov/hhes/www/cpstables/032013/health/toc.htm.

US Social Security Administration. 2013. "Social Security Taxable Earnings and Tax Rates for 2014." Posted November 6. http://socialsecurityinfo.areavoices.com/2013/11/06/social-security-taxable-earnings-and-tax-rates-for-2014/.

WHY ARE THOSE WHO MOST NEED HEALTH INSURANCE LEAST ABLE TO BUY IT?

We have all heard stories of individuals who are sick and need, for example, open-heart surgery, but no insurance company would sell them health insurance. Until the Affordable Care Act (ACA) required insurers to sell health insurance to anyone willing to buy it, health insurance seemed to be available only for those who did not need it. Why did health insurance companies deny insurance coverage to those who were sick and needed it most? To understand these issues and consider what should be appropriate public policy, one must understand how insurance premiums are determined and how health insurance markets work.

The Different Private Health Insurance Markets

Most private health insurance for nonelderly Americans—66 percent in 2012 (down from 77 percent in 2000)—is purchased through the workplace. While private non-group coverage has remained relatively stable at about 7 percent, employer coverage has declined from 69 percent in 2000 to 59 percent in 2012 (Fronstin 2013, Figure 1)—see Exhibit 7.1. As previously discussed in Chapter 6, employees receive important tax advantages by having their employer purchase health insurance on their behalf. Insurance purchased

Market Segment	Population (Millions)	Percentage of Total
Employment-based	156.0	58.5
Individual	19.4	7.3
Medicaid	47.3	17.7
Medicare	8.8	3.3
Tricare/CHAMPVA	9.0	3.4
Uninsured	47.3	17.7

EXHIBIT 7.1
Sources of Health Insurance Coverage of US Nonelderly (Under Age 65 Years) Population in 2012

NOTE: Numbers may not add to totals because individuals may receive coverage from more than one source.
SOURCE: Data from Fronstin (2013), Figure 1.

with before-tax dollars is equivalent to a reduction in the price of insurance compared to buying insurance with after-tax dollars. This tax subsidy is not available to those buying insurance in the individual insurance market.

Those purchasing insurance in the individual market tend to be self-employed, students, retirees not yet eligible for Medicare, unemployed, individuals between jobs, and individuals who are employed but are not offered insurance through their employer (or choose not to accept it). Individual insurance was typically purchased through a broker, directly from a health plan, or on the Internet. As part of the ACA, health insurance exchanges were established in many states to primarily serve those in the individual insurance market. Exchanges are new organizations that will offer a choice of different health plans, certify plans that participate, and provide information to help consumers better understand their options. Federal subsidies are offered to those on the exchange whose income is between 133 percent and 400 percent of the federal poverty level.

Determinants of Private Health Insurance Premiums

The insurance premium paid by an individual or an employer on behalf of its employees consists of (1) the loading charge, which represents approximately 15 percent of the premium, and (2) the claims experience of the employee group, which makes up the remaining 85 percent of the premium (see Exhibit 7.2). The loading charge reflects the insurance company's marketing costs, the administrative costs of handling the insurance claims, and profit. The claims experience of an employee group is the number of claims submitted by members of that group multiplied by the average cost per claim; this is also the medical expenditure portion of the premium, referred to as the *medical loss ratio* (medical claims expense divided by the total premium). Differences in premiums among employee groups, and the difference in annual premium increases, result primarily from differences in claims experience. An experience-rated premium is based on the claims experience of the particular group.

When a new group applies for health insurance, the insurer attempts to estimate the likely claims experience of the group. As shown in Exhibit 7.2, the insurer will consider factors that affect the group's medical expenditures, such as the following:

- Types of medical and other benefits provided to the employees and their dependents
- Types of mandates the state requires to be included in the insurance policy (e.g., hair transplants or in vitro fertilization)

Health Insurance Premiums

| Claims Experience (85 percent) | Loading Charge (15 percent) |

Determinants of Claims Experience
Benefit coverage
State mandates
Demographic characteristics of
    the insured population (age,
    sex, and family status)
Industry
Region
Medical inflation rate
Cost-containment policies
  • copayment
  • deductible
  • benefit design
  • utilization review
  • case management
  • preferred provider organization

Determinants of Loading Charge
Administrative costs
Marketing costs
Reserves
Profits

EXHIBIT 7.2
Determinants
of Health
Insurance
Premiums

- Average age of the group (older employees have higher medical expenditures than younger employees)
- Proportion of females (females have higher medical expenditures than do males)
- Industry in which the firm competes (e.g., physicians, nurses, accountants, and lawyers tend to be heavier users of healthcare than, say, bank tellers),
- Region of the country in which the employees are located (hospital costs and physician fees are higher on the West Coast than in the South)
- Estimate of the growth rate of medical inflation

Once an insurer has insured a group long enough to have a history of that group's claims experience, the insurance company will project that claims experience and multiply it by an estimate of the medical inflation rate.

Various approaches can be taken to reduce a group's claims experience. For example, increasing the deductible and the coinsurance rate will decrease employees' use of services; expanding insurance benefits to include lower-cost substitutes to inpatient admissions will reduce treatment costs; and requiring utilization review of hospital admissions, case management of catastrophic cases, and use of preferred provider organizations will lower use rates and provider charges. Thus, the claims experience of a group is related to the characteristics of that group, the medical benefits covered, and the cost-containment methods included in the insurance policy.

The insurer bears the risk of incorrectly estimating the group's medical experience. If the premium charged to that group is too low, the insurer will lose money. In the past, Blue Cross and other insurance companies have lost a great deal of money by underestimating claims experience and the medical inflation rate. An insurer cannot merely increase the premiums of the group in the following period to recover its losses because the insurance market is very price competitive. If an insurer says to an employer, "We need to increase our profit this coming year because we lost money on your employees last year," the employer may switch to a competitor, switch to a health maintenance organization (HMO), or self-insure. (The employer bears the risk and uses an insurer to administer and process claims.)

Even if the claims experience of two employee groups is similar, one group may have a lower insurance premium because it has a lower loading charge. Large groups have small loading charges because the administrative and marketing costs (which are generally fixed) are spread over a great number of employees. Furthermore, insurers earn a lower profit when they insure large groups because they fear that, if their profit is too high, the groups will decide to self-insure by bearing the risk themselves. Small groups, on the other hand, are less likely to be able to bear the risk of self-insurance. If a huge claim were to occur in one year, the financial burden could be too much for a small group to bear. In a large group, large claims are likely to be offset by premiums from employees making only small or no claims in a given year. In addition to charging small groups a higher rate, an insurer is likely to maintain a high reserve in case a large claim is made, further increasing the loading charge for small groups. However, the amount of profit the insurer is able to make from a small group is still limited by competition from other insurers and HMOs.

How Health Insurance Markets Work

This brief description of how insurance premiums are determined serves as background to examine why those who are ill have found buying insurance difficult.

Adverse Selection

Assume that Person B is without health insurance and requires a heart transplant; he wants to purchase health insurance. If the insurer does not know that he needs expensive medical treatment, his premium will be based on the claims experience of persons in a similar age (risk) group. This difference in health status information between Person B and the insurer can lead to adverse selection—that is, the insurer enrolls people whose risk level is much higher than the risk level on which their premium is based. This occurs because a person in ill health will attempt to conceal that information so that the insurer will not know of the higher risk.

For example, if 100 people were in a risk group, each with a 1 percent chance of needing a medical treatment costing $100,000, the pure premium for each (without the loading charge) would be $1,000 (0.01 × $100,000). Each year, one member of the group would require a $100,000 treatment. Now, if a person who needs that particular treatment (whose risk is 100 percent) is permitted to join that group at a premium of $1,000 (based on a mistaken risk level of 0.01), that high-risk person receives a subsidy of $99,000, as her premium should have been $100,000 because of her risk level. Because the $1,000 premium was based on a risk level of 1 percent, the insurer collects insufficient premiums to pay for the second $100,000 expense and loses $99,000. This example does not differ from one in which a man learns that he has a terminal illness and (without revealing his condition to the insurer) decides to purchase a $10 million life insurance policy to provide for his wife and children, or one in which a woman whose home is on fire quickly decides to buy fire insurance. Insurance enables an individual to protect against uncertainty. Once uncertainty no longer exists, however, the person is not insurable for that particular treatment or situation.

If the insurance company knew that Person B wanted health insurance to cover the costs of a heart transplant, it would charge a premium that reflected his expected claims experience—that is, Person B's premium would be equal to the cost of the heart transplant plus a loading charge.

We all favor subsidizing those who cannot afford but need an expensive treatment. Similarly, we favor subsidies to poor families. However, is it not more appropriate for the government, rather than the insurer, to provide those subsidies? When insurers are made to bear such losses, they will eventually be forced out of business unless they can protect themselves from people who withhold information and claim to be in lower-risk groups.

To protect themselves against adverse selection (insuring high-risk persons for premiums mistakenly based on those with low risks), the insurer could raise its enrollees' premiums, but then many low-risk subscribers—who would be willing to pay $1,000 but not $2,000 for a 1 percent risk—would drop their insurance. As more low-risk subscribers drop out, premiums for remaining subscribers would increase further, causing still more low-risk enrollees to drop out. Eventually, large numbers of low-risk people would be uninsured, although they would be willing to pay an actuarially fair premium based on their (low) risk group.

Instead, an insurer will attempt to learn as much about the individual's health status. Examining and testing the person who wants to buy health insurance is a means of equalizing the information between the two parties. Another way insurers protect themselves against adverse selection is by stating that the person's insurance coverage will not apply to preexisting conditions—medical conditions known by the patient to exist and to require treatment. Similarly, an insurer might use a delay-of-benefits clause or a waiting period; for example, obstetric benefits may not be covered until a policy has been in effect for ten months. Large deductibles will also discourage high-risk people because they will realize that they have to pay a large amount of their expenses themselves.

Insurers are less concerned about adverse selection when selling insurance to large groups with low employee turnover. In such groups, health insurance is provided by the employer as a tax-free benefit (subsidized by the government); the total group includes all the low-risk persons as well. Typically, people join large companies more for the other attributes of the job than for health insurance coverage. Once in the employer group, employees cannot just drop the group insurance when well and buy it when ill. Thus, for insurance companies adverse selection is more of a concern when individuals or small groups (with typically higher turnover) want to buy insurance. For example, an insurer might be concerned that the owner of a small firm might hire an ill family member just so she could receive insurance benefits. Thus, employees with preexisting medical conditions will be denied coverage.

Some state and local governments have attempted to assist people with preexisting conditions by prohibiting insurers from using tests to determine, for example, whether someone is HIV positive. Rather than subsidize care for such individuals themselves, governments have tried to shift the medical costs to the insurer and its other subscribers. This is an inequitable way of subsidizing care for those with preexisting conditions. Government use of an income-related tax to provide the subsidy would be fairer. Another consequence of government regulations that shift the cost of those who are ill to insurers and their subscribers is that insurers have relied on other types of restrictions not covered by the regulations, such as delay of benefits and exclusion of certain occupations, industries, or geographic areas to protect themselves.

Healthy people may not have had health insurance for several reasons. An insurance premium that is much higher than the expected claims experience of an individual will make that insurance too expensive. For example, if an employee was not part of a large insured group, he was charged a higher insurance premium because the insurer suspected he was a higher risk. When individuals and those who are self-employed buy insurance they must do so with after-tax dollars because tax-exempt employer-paid health insurance only applies when an employer purchases the coverage for the employee. The loading charge is also higher for the self-employed and those in small groups because the insurer's administration and marketing costs are spread over fewer employees, leading to a higher premium. Furthermore, state insurance mandates that require expensive benefits or more practitioners to be included in all insurance sold in that state result in higher insurance premiums; consequently, fewer people are willing to buy such insurance. (Large firms that self-insure are exempt from costly state mandates.) Many individuals and members of small groups also lack insurance coverage because premiums are too high relative to their income. Such persons would rather rely on Medicaid if they become ill. Others can afford to purchase insurance but choose not to; if they become ill, they become a burden on taxpayers because they cannot be refused treatment in emergency departments or by hospitals.

Medicare was concerned that adverse selection would occur in two of its voluntary programs—Part B (physician and outpatient services) and Part D (prescription drugs). Because the programs are voluntary (and 75 percent are subsidized by the government), the government was concerned that people would wait until they needed the services and then join the program; the programs would have a smaller risk pool of predominately sicker people, resulting in adverse selection to the government. To encourage all newly eligible Medicare beneficiaries to enroll in these programs, thereby increasing the risk pool, the monthly premiums were increased the longer an eligible beneficiary delayed enrolling in those programs.

The ACA decrees that the preexisting-condition exclusion could no longer be used by health insurers to deny health insurance to those willing to buy insurance. To eliminate the problem of adverse selection—namely people would buy insurance only when they became sick—the ACA requires everyone to have health insurance (an "individual mandate") or pay a penalty. Subsidies to purchase insurance are to be provided to those with low income. Requiring an individual mandate and removing the preexisting-condition exclusion also eliminates "job lock"; employees could change jobs without fear of losing their health insurance or being denied insurance because of a preexisting condition.

Preferred-Risk Selection

Because insurers want to protect themselves against bad risks, they clearly prefer to insure individuals who are better-than-average risks. Although their risks vary, as long as different groups and individuals pay the same premium, insurers have an incentive to engage in preferred-risk selection—that is, seek out those who have lower-than-average risks.

As shown in Exhibit 7.3, in 2010, 1 percent of the population incurred 22 percent of total health expenditures (40 percent of those in the top 1 percent are aged 65 years or older). In 1963, 1 percent of the population incurred only 17 percent of total expenditures, which demonstrates the effect medical technology has had on increasing medical expenditures. Five percent of the population incurred 50 percent of total expenditures in 2010. Given this high concentration of expenditures among a small percentage of the population, an insurer could greatly increase its profits and avoid losses by trying to avoid the most costly patients. An insurer able to select enrollees from among the 50 percent of the population that incur only 3 percent of total expenditures will greatly profit. The only way to provide insurers with an incentive to take the high-risk (hence costly) patients is to provide insurers with risk-adjusted premiums. For example, premiums for persons in older age groups should be higher than premiums for those in younger age groups. Insurers would then have an incentive to enroll these patients and manage their care to minimize their treatment cost rather than search for low-risk enrollees.

When the premium is the same for all risks, insurers attempt to enroll persons with better-than-average risks in several ways. For example, if everyone enrolling with a particular health insurer pays the same annual premium, the HMO would prefer those who have lower-than-average claims experience, are in low-risk industries, and are younger-than-average employees. To encourage younger subscribers, the HMO might emphasize services used by younger couples, such as prenatal and well-baby care. Emphasizing wellness and sports medicine programs is also likely to draw a healthier population. Similarly, de-emphasizing tertiary care facilities for heart disease and cancer

EXHIBIT 7.3
Distribution of Health Expenditures for the US Population, by Magnitude of Expenditures, Selected Years, 1928–2010

Percent of US Population Ranked by Expenditures	1928	1963	1970	1977	1980	1987	1996	2007	2010
Top 1 percent	—	17	26	27	29	28	27	23	22
Top 2 percent	—	—	35	38	39	39	38	33	32
Top 5 percent	52	43	50	55	55	56	55	50	50
Top 10 percent	—	59	66	70	70	70	69	65	66
Top 30 percent	93	—	88	90	90	90	90	89	90
Top 50 percent	—	95	96	97	96	97	97	97	97
Bottom 50 percent	—	5	4	3	4	3	3	3	3

SOURCES: Adapted with permission from "The Concentration of Health Care Expenditures, Revisited, Exhibit 1," by M. L. Berk and A. C. Monheit, *Health Affairs*, 20(2), 2001, March/April: 12. Copyright © 2001 Project HOPE—The People-to-People Health Foundation, Inc., All Rights Reserved; 2007 and 2010 data from Yu (2010); Soni (2013); Cohen and Uberoi (2013).

treatment sends a message to those who are older and at higher risk for those illnesses. Placing clinics and physicians in areas where lower-risk populations reside also results in a favorably biased selection of subscribers.

Medicare beneficiaries can voluntarily decide to join an HMO (Medicare Advantage plan). In the past, if an elderly person decided to change her mind, she could leave the HMO with only one month's notice. (This one-month notice, which was permitted for the aged but not for those in Medicaid HMOs, reflected the greater political power of the elderly.) When some HMOs determined that a Medicare patient required high-cost treatment, they were able to encourage patients to disenroll by suggesting that they might benefit from more suitable treatment for the condition outside the HMO. By eliminating these high-cost subscribers, an HMO could save a great deal of money. To discourage some HMOs from using this approach to maintain only the most favorable Medicare risks, the one-month notice by the elderly was repealed in 2003; the elderly can change health plans only once a year during open enrollment.[1]

Pricing Health Insurance: Community Versus Experience Rating

In a price-competitive health insurance market, insurers will establish their premiums based on *experience rating*. Premiums will reflect the individual's or group's risk level and will be determined as shown in Exhibit 7.2. Under experience rating, no incentive exists for insurers to engage in preferred-risk selection; insurers have an incentive to enroll and manage the care for high-risk groups, because their higher premiums will be based on their expected medical expenses. Those who have low income and cannot afford health insurance should be provided with government subsidies to buy insurance; it is not the role of insurers or their enrollees to provide subsidies to others.

An alternative approach for pricing health insurance is to require all insurers to *community rate* their subscribers—that is, charge all subscribers the same premium regardless of health status or other risk factors, such as age. The cost of high-risk individuals is spread among all subscribers. For community rating to exist, it must be mandated by the government; it cannot survive in a price-competitive insurance market. When Blue Cross started in the late 1930s, it used community rating. When commercial health insurers entered the market, it used experience rating. Because Blue Cross charged low-risk groups a premium based on the average community rate, low-risk groups moved to commercial insurers that offered them a lower experience-rated premium. As more low-risk groups switched insurers, Blue Cross's premium kept increasing and the insurer had to stop using community rating.

Community rating has serious efficiency and equity issues. It provides insurers with strong profit incentives to select preferred risks (low-risk persons) while receiving a premium based on the average for all risk groups.

Furthermore, with uniform premiums, regardless of risk status, insurers and employers no longer have an incentive to encourage risk-reducing behavior among their subscribers and employees—for example, by providing smoking cessation and wellness programs. Premiums for employee groups could not be decreased relative to other groups who do not invest in such cost-reducing behavior. Skydivers, motorcyclists, and others who engage in risky behavior are subsidized by those who attempt to lower their risks. Experience rating—with higher premiums for those who engage in high-risk activities—would provide them with an incentive to reduce such behavior and bear the full cost of their activities. Higher, community-rated premiums result in low-risk individuals dropping their coverage. The result is an increase in the number of uninsured.

When a choice exists of community-rated health plans, those who are low risk will select less costly but more restrictive plans that are less attractive to high-risk individuals. As low-risk individuals leave these more costly plans for less costly but more restrictive coverage, the more generous plans will include a greater number of high-risk individuals; this appears to have happened in New Jersey (Monheit et al. 2004). Consequently, the premiums in these more costly plans will increase, likely leading to their demise.

Community rating also has serious equity effects. A community-rated system benefits those who are high users of medical services or at high risk and penalizes those who are low users or at low risk. Low users and those at low risk pay higher premiums and those at high risk pay lower premiums than they would under an experience-rated system. Those at high risk are, in effect, subsidized by a tax on those who are low risk. Low users/low risk individuals are young and have lower income than do older, high users. Because these subsidies and taxes are based on risk rather than income, low-risk individuals who have low income end up subsidizing some high-risk, high-income people. (Not all high-risk persons are poor, and not all low-risk persons are wealthy).

The ACA's Changes to the Individual Health Insurance Market

The two approaches used in the ACA for expanding health insurance coverage to an estimated 30 million uninsured are expanding eligibility for Medicaid and providing subsidies to those who buy insurance on *state health insurance exchanges*. Although the individual health insurance market is quite small relative to the large group market, the ACA has made a number of significant changes affecting the financing and delivery of health insurance. The more significant of these changes are analyzed using previously discussed insurance concepts to determine their likely effects.

State Health Insurance Exchanges

The ACA expects each state to establish a health insurance exchange. (A federal exchange was created for those states that decided not to set up a state exchange.) These state exchanges are intended initially to serve individuals and small employer groups (up to 100 employees), but after 2017 businesses with more than 100 employees will also have access to them. The exchanges are expected to represent a market where individuals will be able to compare benefits and prices from competing insurers. Four government-standard types of health plans are to be available on the exchange, ranked from the lowest to the highest premium (Bronze, Silver, Gold, and Platinum). The Bronze plan covers 60 percent of medical expenses, while the Platinum plan covers 90 percent. Each plan limits its enrollees' out-of-pocket expenses.

Persons whose income is between 133 percent and 400 percent of the federal poverty level ($31,721 to $95,400 for a family of four in 2014) are eligible to receive a federal subsidy to purchase insurance (declining with higher income).

Elimination of Preexisting-Condition Exclusion

The ACA eliminated any preexisting-condition exclusions in the sale of health insurance. Insurers are required to sell health insurance to any person regardless of his health status. To ensure that adverse selection would not occur—that is, people buying health insurance just when they become ill—the ACA included an individual mandate. Those not buying insurance are penalized by having to pay a tax.

The elimination of the preexisting-condition exclusion was expected to bring into the insurance market high-cost people who were previously excluded from the market. However, as long as the individual mandate was required, insurers expected an increase in the demand for insurance by healthy individuals whose lower cost would more than offset the higher costs of those with preexisting conditions. Insurers, however, were strongly opposed to the individual mandate's penalty for not buying insurance (which is $95 for an individual in 2014 but increasing to $695 in 2016) versus the cost of individual insurance (which could be $3,000 to $5,000 per year). Many young, healthy people likely will opt to pay the penalty and buy insurance only if they become sick. Once they are treated and no longer need medical services, however, they will drop their coverage.

Eliminating the preexisting-conditions exclusion and imposing a penalty for not buying insurance will result in adverse selection for insurers. If insurers raise their rates to cover these high costs, more of their enrollees will drop their coverage. A private health insurance system cannot survive under these conditions.[2]

An example of how eliminating the preexisting-condition exclusion affected the health insurance market is the ACA rule (which took effect in 2010) prohibiting insurers from excluding children under age 19 years who were diagnosed with a preexisting condition. Many parents purchased child-only plans because their small employers' health insurance policies did not cover children. Concerned that they would experience adverse selection by enrolling large numbers of children with preexisting conditions (and the associated high costs), many insurers stopped selling child-only coverage while other insurers exited the market. Parents who previously enrolled their children faced much higher premiums and many disenrolled, while other parents were unable to buy child-only plans (Shaffer 2010).

Medical Loss Ratios

Health plan critics claim that insurers' profits are too high and that too little of the premium dollar goes to pay for medical expenses. These critics point to an insurance company's medical loss ratio (MLR) as an indicator of its efficiency and even the quality of care. The higher the ratio, the more of the premium dollar is paid out for medical services and the lower the administrative expenses. However, the use of the ratio as an evaluative measure is misleading. High administrative expenses (hence a low MLR) can result from a health plan (1) enrolling a great mix of small groups, which have higher marketing and administrative costs than large groups; (2) having a small enrollment base and therefore having to spread fixed administrative costs over fewer enrollees; and (3) having more insurance products, which are more costly to administer than a single product.

Additional factors are the method used to pay hospitals and physicians (by capitating providers, the administrative and claims processing expense is shifted to the provider, compared with the fee-for-service approach, in which the insurer retains those functions) and the number of cost-containment and quality review activities the insurer undertakes. For example, a health plan that merely pays out a large percentage of its premiums (high MLR) with minimal review of its claims is likely to be inefficient and lower in quality than a health plan that has a high administrative expense ratio because it reviews the accuracy of claims submitted by providers, assesses the quality of care provided, and undertakes patient satisfaction surveys.[3]

In a price-competitive health insurance market, a health plan cannot afford to be inefficient in its administrative functions. If it is inefficient and simply pays all claims submitted, its premiums would be higher and it would lose market share. An insurer must undertake a cost–benefit analysis to determine whether each of the administrative functions it performs either saves money (lower claims cost) or increases purchaser satisfaction (as shown by enrollee satisfaction surveys). To do otherwise places the plan at a competitive disadvantage.[4]

The ACA established limits on MLR rather than waiting for insurer competition to determine the size of those ratios. Health plans were required to have no less than an 80 percent ratio in the individual and small group markets and a minimum ratio of 85 percent in the large group market; otherwise, the insurer must refund the difference to their enrollees. For example, if an insurer has a ratio of 70 percent in the individual market, it is required to provide the difference between 70 percent and 80 percent back to the insured individual (Kaiser Family Foundation 2013).

A regulatory limit on MLR will result in several unintended consequences. MLRs in the individual market have generally been lower (60 percent to 70 percent) than the required 80 percent ratio because of higher enrollment, marketing, and administrative costs. Many small insurers, unable to increase their loss ratios to the higher ratio, have exited these markets, leading to less insurer competition.

Crucial to whether an insurer can meet the 80 percent MLR in the individual market is the definition of a medical or an administrative expense. Medical expenses include payment of medical claims and quality improvement programs, such as quality reporting and chronic disease management. Administrative expenses include cost-containment programs, such as fraud-and-abuse prevention activities (including medical review and provider auditing). Limiting the funds insurers spend on detecting, recovering, and litigating fraud to increase their MLR to 80 percent will result in higher—not lower—premiums. The elimination of these programs to achieve the prescribed ratios would be an unintended consequence of the ACA. Instead of requiring minimum MLR, it would be preferable to instill greater competition among insurers to keep their profits and administrative expenses down.

Community Rating

The ACA sets rules governing how health insurers are permitted to vary their premiums. Insurers are required to use a modified form of community rating. For each type of health plan, premiums are allowed to vary by family status, geography within a state, smoking status, and age. On average, the medical costs of people in their 60s differ—compared to those in their 20s—by about 6:1. However, the ACA requires that premium differences be no greater than 3:1, much less than their actual cost differences. The effect of the ACA's community rating is the redistribution of insurance costs from the old to the young.[5] (This age-rating rule was supported by AARP because it would lower premiums for older enrollees.)

Many of the uninsured are young. They have low income, are healthy, and don't see the need for expensive health insurance. Increasing their premiums through community rating, together with a weak penalty for being uninsured, will incentivize more of the young to remain uninsured.

Gender Rating of Premiums

Women generally use more healthcare services than do men of the same age. They visit the physician more often and take more prescription drugs. Because of their higher healthcare costs, a young woman's premium in the individual health insurance market would be 50 percent greater than for a young man. The ACA prohibits using gender rating for individuals (and employers with fewer than 100 employees). (The ACA further requires that contraception and maternity benefits be considered essential health benefits to be included in all health plans, even for single men and women past child-bearing age.)

Eliminating gender rating, when costs differ, is similar to community rating. Men subsidize women, regardless of their respective income. (In the price-competitive auto insurance industry, gender rating is not prohibited by the government; young men who have more accidents and incur higher costs pay larger premiums than do young women). The effect of the ACA's prohibition of gender rating increases the premiums for men, leading some to forgo buying insurance.

Expanded Health Insurance Benefits

The ACA requires insurers to cover a broad range of mandated "essential" benefits, the scope of which is greater than typical individual policies previously sold. For example, preventive services with no copayments must be included. (However, Russell [2009] notes that 80 percent of preventive services increase rather than decrease costs.) Insurers are required to permit parents to include their children (up to age 26 years) on their insurance policies and not be charged any more than for coverage of younger children. Also mandated to be included are behavioral health services, contraceptives, maternity care, outpatient prescription drugs, and pediatric dental and vision care; annual lifetime limits on health benefits are prohibited. The more comprehensive and generous the insurance, the more expensive it is.

The Effect of the ACA's Rules on Premiums in the Individual Market

Many young, healthy individuals are likely not to buy insurance. The many mandated essential benefits to be included—together with the community-rated and gender-rated premiums and the elimination of preexisting-conditions exclusion—will increase premiums. In addition, taxes were increased on insurers, pharmaceutical firms, and medical device companies to help fund the ACA. These taxes will be passed on to the enrollee in the form of higher premiums. Many young people will decide not to buy insurance because of the higher premiums. They would rather pay a penalty tax and then buy insurance if they become sick. Being uninsured will be a rational choice for many young people. (Proponents of these regulations minimize these concerns by claiming that many people will receive a subsidy when buying insurance on the state insurance exchanges. To the extent this occurs, the cost of these regulations would then be borne by taxpayers.)

Insurers are anticipating that adverse selection will occur. The insured risk pool will be biased toward those who are older and have higher risks, because many young individuals are not expected to buy insurance. To control utilization and to lower their costs, health plans are using *narrow* provider networks and high coinsurance to discourage enrollees from using out-of-network providers, which are likely to be more expensive.

Premiums on the state exchanges are higher than proponents of the ACA claimed they would be. The promise of the ACA to "bend the cost curve" is unlikely to be fulfilled.

Summary

The individual health insurance market, representing a small percentage of the overall number of the privately insured, has been the cause of much concern. Tax-exempt employer-paid health insurance is unavailable to individuals buying their own coverage, and insurers are concerned with adverse selection when individuals want to buy coverage. As a result, individual premiums are higher than those in the group insurance market and the demand for insurance is lower.

The ACA made a number of changes affecting the insurance market, particularly the individual market. State health insurance exchanges were established, four types of health plans are available on the exchanges, federal subsidies are provided to those with low income, the preexisting-condition exclusion was eliminated, and an individual mandate was imposed (which should expand the insurance pool and minimize the risk to insurers of adverse selection). Employees will be able to switch jobs without fear that they will be denied insurance.

Critics of the ACA's insurance regulations claim that imposing a penalty for not buying insurance will increase adverse selection, as many young people will wait until they are sick to buy insurance. Unless young people join the risk pool, premiums will sharply rise for those remaining in the individual market. Requiring a modified form of community rating, mandated expanded benefits, and new taxes on insurers will raise premiums for the young. These increased premiums will reduce the demand for insurance by those who believe that paying the penalty tax is less expensive than being insured. To protect themselves from likely adverse selection resulting from fewer young people joining the exchange risk pool, insurers are offering narrow provider networks, using less costly hospitals, and imposing large coinsurance rate for using non-network providers.

Mandated minimum MLRs, as an approach for limiting insurers' profits, will have unintended consequences, such as reducing competition by having fewer insurers.

The full effects of the ACA's regulations will not be known for several years because many provisions did not become effective until 2014. Although several insurance provisions of the ACA should have beneficial effects on consumers, others will have unintended consequences on the insurance markets and on some of the insured. It remains to be seen how the private health insurance market will evolve as a result of these provisions.

Discussion Questions

1. What are the different components of a health insurance premium? If an employer wanted to reduce its employees' premiums, which components could be changed?
2. What is adverse selection, and how do insurance companies protect themselves from it? If the government prohibited insurers from protecting themselves against adverse selection, how would it affect insurance premiums?
3. Why do insurers and HMOs have an incentive to engage in preferred-risk selection?
4. What are some methods by which insurers and HMOs try to achieve preferred-risk selection?
5. What is the difference between experience rating and community rating, and what are some consequences of using community rating?
6. What are some reasons the ACA is likely to cause premiums in the individual health insurance market to be higher than in the past?
7. What are unintended consequences of requiring insurers to have minimum MLRs?
8. Why have insurers developed narrow provider networks on the state and federal insurance exchanges?

Notes

1. This change was a result of the Balanced Budget Act of 1997, which sought to decrease Medicare expenditures. To compensate the aged for no longer being able to change their insurer with a 30-day notice, the aged were provided with additional preventive benefits.

2. Adverse selection is also likely to occur with the exchange's Platinum health plan, which covers 90 percent of an enrollee's medical costs. Those who are more likely to have high medical expenses will enroll in the plan that requires low copayments, while those who have low health risks will be more likely to join the cheaper Bronze plan, covering only 60 percent of their medical costs. As the Platinum plan enrolls more costly enrollees, the plan's medical costs and premiums will increase, leading those who have less costly needs to switch to plans with lower premiums, such as Silver and Bronze. This process could continue until the Platinum plan becomes too expensive and is no longer offered.

3. Robinson (1997) discusses many of these interpretive problems (and more) with MLRs and demonstrates how these ratios vary greatly within nonprofit and for-profit health plans as well as for the same health plan located in different states.

4. Expense ratios for private insurers are much larger than for Medicare. Rather than being an indication of differences in efficiency, some of the reasons for higher expense ratios among private insurers are as follows:

    *   Medicare's per capita claim costs are much higher, so their administrative expenses are a smaller proportion of total costs.
    *   The Center for Medicare & Medicaid Services, which performs administrative services for Medicare, is generally excluded from the calculation of Medicare's administrative costs.
    *   Additional costs necessary for the operation of Medicare, such as enrollment and billing, are included in the Social Security Administration's costs. The collection of Medicare payroll taxes by the IRS is not attributed to Medicare.
    *   Medicare also has lower costs because it relies on price controls and thus does not negotiate with providers or undertake cost-containment and quality improvement functions (such as medical management) or it spends too little to reduce fraud and abuse.
    *   Medicare is exempt from paying state premium taxes or incurring regulatory and compliance costs that affect insurance companies.

5. Proponents of the ACA provision that overcharges the young to subsidize those who are older claim that, over time, it evens out as today's 25-year-old becomes tomorrow's 55-year-old. This argument has several problems. First, having young people overpay for their insurance (same as an excise tax) encourages more of them to remain uninsured. Second, it is inequitable to have a 25-year-old with student debts subsidize an older person with greater income and wealth. Third, considering the time value of money, on a present value basis, the young still end up incurring greater costs than if all age groups paid experience-rated premiums. Fourth, having each generation pay for the previous generation is based on the hope that succeeding generations will honor their commitment, which—as shown by Social Security and Medicare—is unlikely to occur. Few young workers believe the benefits their taxes support today will be there for them when they retire.

Additional Readings

Feldstein, P. 2011. "The Demand for Health Insurance." In *Health Care Economics,* 7th ed. Albany, NY: Delmar.

Morrisey, M. 2008. *Health Insurance.* Chicago: Health Administration Press.

References

Berk, M. L., and A. C. Monheit. 2001. "The Concentration of Health Care Expenditures, Revisited." *Health Affairs* 20 (2): 12.

Cohen, S., and N. Uberoi. 2013. "Differentials in the Concentration in the Level of Health Expenditures Across Population Subgroups in the U.S., 2010." *Statistical Brief* No. 421, August. http://meps.ahrq.gov/mepsweb/data_files/publications/st421/stat421.pdf.

Fronstin, P. 2013. "Sources of Health Insurance and Characteristics of the Uninsured: Analysis of the March 2013 Current Population Survey." Employee Benefit Research Institute. *Issue Brief* No. 390, September. www.ebri.org/pdf/briefspdf/EBRI_IB_09-13.No390.Sources.pdf.

Kaiser Family Foundation. 2013. "Summary of the Affordable Care Act." Last modified April 23. http://kaiserfamilyfoundation.files.wordpress.com/2011/04/8061-021.pdf.

Monheit, A., J. Cantor, M. Koller, and K. Fox. 2004. "Community Rating and Sustainable Individual Health Insurance Markets in New Jersey." *Health Affairs* 23 (4): 167–75.

Robinson, J. C. 1997. "Use and Abuse of the Medical Loss Ratio to Measure Health Plan Performance." *Health Affairs* 16 (4): 164–87.

Russell, L. 2009. "Preventing Chronic Disease: An Important Investment But Don't Count on Cost Savings." *Health Affairs* 28 (1): 42–45.

Shaffer, M. 2010. "Child-Only Left Behind." *National Review.* Posted September 29. www.nationalreview.com/articles/248105/child-only-left-behind-matthew-shaffer.

Soni, A. 2013. Personal correspondence with the author, September 25.

Yu, W. W. 2010. Personal correspondence with the author, August 3.

MEDICARE

I n 1965, Congress enacted two different financing programs to cover two separate population groups: Medicare for the aged and Medicaid for the poor. As a result, the government's (particularly the federal government's) role in financing personal medical services increased dramatically. Federal and state expenditures represent about 52 percent of total medical expenditures.

Medicare and Medicaid have serious problems. Medicare's financial deficits mean that the program will require substantial changes to survive in the future. Medicaid must be improved if it is to serve more than half of those classified as poor, and it faces huge financial liabilities as an aging population requires long-term care. Medicaid is discussed in Chapter 9.

The Current State of Medicare

Medicare is a federal program that primarily serves the aged. In addition, those younger than age 65 years who receive Social Security cash payments because they are disabled become eligible for the program after a two-year waiting period. People requiring kidney dialysis and kidney transplants, regardless of age, were added to Medicare in the early 1970s. As shown in Exhibit 8.1, in 2013 Medicare covered 43.5 million aged and 8.8 million disabled beneficiaries, for a total of 52.3 million beneficiaries (CMS 2013a, Table I.1 and I.16.); the elderly population is expected to double over the next three decades.

Medicare has four parts, each of which offers different benefits and uses different financing mechanisms. Part A provides hospital insurance (HI), Part B provides supplemental medical insurance (SMI), Part C offers program beneficiaries a greater variety of health plan choices (Medicare Advantage plans), and Part D is prescription drug coverage.

Part A (HI)

All seniors are automatically enrolled in Part A when they retire at age 65. Part A covers acute hospital care (up to 90 days for each episode of care),

EXHIBIT 8.1
Number of
Medicare
Beneficiaries,
Fiscal Years
1970–2030

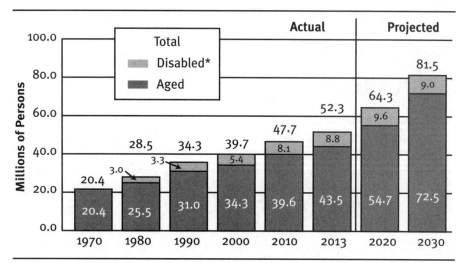

* Includes beneficiaries whose eligibility is based solely on end-stage disease.
NOTE: The disabled became eligible for Medicare in 1973; therefore, no values are included
here for the disabled prior to 1974.
SOURCES: Data from CMS (2013a); CMS (2013b), Table IV.B4.

skilled nursing home care after hospitalization (up to 100 days), and hospice care for the terminally ill. If a Medicare patient requires hospitalization, she must pay a deductible that is indexed to increase with health costs each year ($1,184 for 1 to 60 days of hospital stay as of 2013) (Kaiser Family Foundation 2010). Part A is financed by an earmarked HI payroll tax, which is set aside in the Medicare Hospital Trust Fund. In 1966, this tax was a combined 0.35 percent (0.175 percent each on the employer and the employee) on wages up to $6,600.

As Part A expenditures continually exceeded projections, the HI tax and the wage base to which the tax applied were raised. By 1994, the total HI tax grew to a combined 2.9 percent on all earned income. The Affordable Care Act (ACA) further increased the Medicare payroll tax to a combined 3.8 percent on individuals earning more than $200,000 and families earning more than $250,000. In addition, a 3.8 percent Medicare tax was imposed on all unearned income—such as investment income, dividends, royalties, and capital gains—for the same income groups; these income limits are not adjusted for inflation (IRS 2013).

The Trust Fund is a "pay-as-you-go" fund; current Medicare expenditures are financed by current employee and employer contributions. The HI taxes from current Medicare beneficiaries were never set aside for their own future expenses; instead, they were used to pay for those who were eligible at the time the funds were collected. This is in contrast to a pension fund, in which a person sets aside funds to pay for his own retirement. When Medicare actuaries have estimated that the Trust Fund will become insolvent (that is, when current HI taxes are insufficient to pay current Medicare expenditures), HI taxes on employees and employers have been increased.

In 2013, the federal government spent $278 billion on Part A; this amount is estimated to rise to $462 billion by 2023. Medicare's expenditures by type of service are shown in Exhibit 8.2.

Part B (SMI)

Part B (SMI) pays for physician services, outpatient diagnostic tests, certain medical supplies and equipment, and (since 1998) home health care (previously included in Part A). Medicare beneficiaries are not automatically enrolled in SMI—a voluntary, income-related program—but 95 percent of the elderly pay the premium. In 2013, new Part B beneficiaries pay $104.90 a month. Single individuals whose income is greater than $85,000 or married couples with a combined income of greater than $170,000 pay an additional amount. Beneficiary premiums represent only 25 percent of the

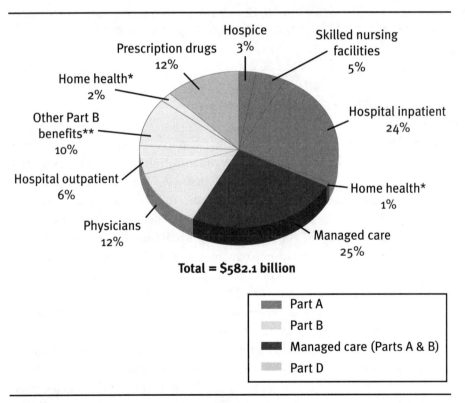

EXHIBIT 8.2
Estimated Medicare Benefit Payments, by Type of Service, Fiscal Year 2013

* "Home health" services are covered by Part A and Part B.
** "Other Part B benefits" include durable medical equipment, other carrier, other intermediary, and laboratory
SOURCE: Data from CMS (2013a).

program's costs ($63.8 billion in premiums in 2013 out of $248 billion in expenditures). The remaining 75 percent of Part B expenditures are subsidized from federal tax revenues. The aged are also responsible for an annual $147 deductible (in 2013) and a 20 percent copayment for their use of Part B services (Medicare.gov n.d.).

In 2007, against much opposition, the Part B premium became income related; seniors earning $80,000 to $100,000 receive a 65 percent premium subsidy, and those earning more than $200,000 receive only a 20 percent premium subsidy. When premiums became income related, only 3 percent of Part B enrollees were affected by the reduced premium subsidies; by 2012, 4 percent of enrollees were affected (Davis 2014). Over time, Medicare has become more of an income-related program.

When Part B expenditures exceed projections, there is no concern with insolvency (unlike in the case of the Trust Fund). The federal subsidy simply becomes larger than expected; Part B expenditures increase the size of the federal deficit. In 2012, the federal subsidy for Part B expenditures exceeded $174 billion; this is estimated to rise to $210 billion by 2018 (CBO 2013a). By way of comparison, Medicare's share of the federal budget was 15.6 percent ($551 billion) in 2012 and is expected to increase to 16.1 percent ($722 billion) of all federal expenditures in 2018 (CBO 2013b, tables 1 and 2).

Part C: Medicare Advantage Plans

Since the 1980s, the aged have been able to voluntarily enroll in a managed care plan—such as a health maintenance organization (HMO) or a preferred provider organization—referred to as *Medicare Advantage* (MA). The MA plan receives a capitation payment from Medicare based on the total Part A, Part B, and Part D expenditures for a Medicare beneficiary in that particular geographic area (adjusted for age, sex, and Medicaid and institutional status).[1] In return for this capitation payment, the MA plan provides more comprehensive benefits, such as lower out-of-pocket payments and additional services not covered by Part B. The MA plan, which is at risk for providing all the promised benefits in return for the capitation payment, limits the enrollees' choice of physicians and hospitals to those in the plan's provider network. Thus, the MA plan has a financial incentive to reduce inappropriate care and manage the elderly's care in a cost-effective manner.

About 13 million—or more than 27 percent of the aged—were enrolled in MA plans in 2012; the remainder were in traditional Medicare, where the hospitals and physicians are paid on a fee-for-service (FFS) basis and the government regulates prices. Since 2003, the elderly have to remain in a given health plan for a minimum of one year, whereas previously they were able to switch health plans with one month's notice.

Part D: Prescription Drug Coverage

In 2003, the Medicare Modernization Act was enacted, which was the largest and most significant change to Medicare since its inception. This legislation provided the aged with a new standalone outpatient prescription drug benefit starting in 2006. Part D is a voluntary program, and its cost is heavily subsidized (75 percent) by federal tax revenues. Seniors use more outpatient prescription drugs than does any other age group, and the out-of-pocket financial burden of these drugs was often of greater concern than the costs of hospital and physician services, most of which were covered by Medicare.

At the time of its enactment, the Medicare Trustees estimated that Medicare beneficiaries would pay a monthly premium of $60 a month by 2013. Instead, the monthly premium in 2013 was only $31 a month, on average, not much different than when the program started. The reason for the relatively constant Part D premium compared to the Part B premium, which increased from an average of $89 in 2006 to $105 in 2013, is that the drug benefit is provided by private, risk-bearing plans. Beneficiaries are offered a choice of competing plans at different monthly premiums. The result of offering the aged a financial incentive and a choice among competing private plans resulted in the Part D cost to the government being much less than projected, a rarity among government programs.

The design of the new prescription drug benefit was affected by an overall budgetary limit and legislators' desire that all seniors receive some benefit—not limited to just those with very large drug expenses. As shown in Exhibit 8.3, after meeting a $325 deductible, the aged must then pay 25 percent of their drug expenses between $325 and $2,970 (so that almost all of the aged would receive some benefit). Then, to remain within the budget limit for this new benefit, the elderly must pay 100 percent of their drug expenses—between $2,970 and $4,700—before the government picks up 95 percent of their remaining drug expenses. As part of the ACA, the size of the "donut hole" is reduced.

EXHIBIT 8.3
Medicare
Prescription
Drug Benefit

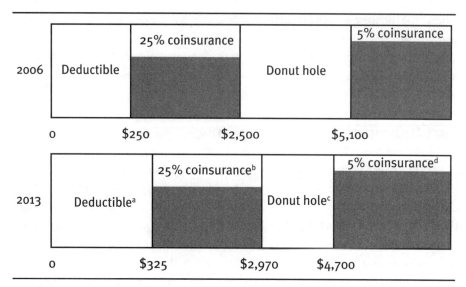

^a Some drug plans do not have a deductible.
^b Some drug plans may have a $10 copay.
^c In the donut hole, the patient pays 47.5% for brand name and 21% for generic drugs.
^d Patients pay some portion (either copays or coinsurance), but the percentage or dollar amount differs by plan.
SOURCE: 2013 data from CMS (2013c).

Medigap Supplementary Insurance

As of 2009, about 21 percent of the aged (mostly middle and high income) also purchase private Medigap insurance to cover the HI and SMI out-of-pocket costs not covered by Medicare. Twelve percent are covered by Medicaid, 31 percent have additional coverage through their previous employers, 27 percent have their out-of-pocket costs covered through their MA plan, and the remaining 20 percent have no supplementary coverage (MedPAC 2013, Chart 5.1). These out-of-pocket expenses—the HI and SMI deductibles and the 20 percent SMI copayment—can be a substantial financial burden, as *Medicare does not have any stop-loss limit for out-of-pocket expenses.* (When their out-of-pocket expenses become too great a financial burden, the low-income aged must fall back on Medicaid.) Medigap policies provide the aged with nearly first-dollar coverage, eliminating patients' financial incentives to limit their use of services or join managed care plans.

The ACA's Changes to Medicare

The ACA relies on two approaches to reduce Medicare spending.
    The first approach is funding several types of demonstration projects that rely on different payment systems that shift the financial risk of providing

care from Medicare to providers. Bundled episode-based payments are a single lump sum payment to cover all the providers involved in the patient's episode of care, such as a hip replacement or heart surgery. Accountable care organizations (ACOs)—the most important of these demonstration projects—are networks of hospitals, physicians, and other providers receiving payment incentives from Medicare for coordinating care for a defined group of Medicare patients. Providers must meet quality and performance targets in return for shared savings for the cost of delivering patient care.

The second approach is reducing Medicare provider prices. This includes lower provider payment updates based on assumed productivity increases and mandatory decreases in provider payments if Medicare spending rises faster than the gross domestic product (GDP) plus 0.5 percent annually.

ACOs

A large number of hospitals, physicians, and insurers have formed ACOs, and it is uncertain how well ACOs will be able to improve care coordination and cut down Medicare spending. ACOs differ from MA plans in several important ways that are likely to affect the ACO's performance. The designers of the ACO concept believed that traditional FFS Medicare is not as efficient as capitated MA plans and thus wanted to include more Medicare beneficiaries into a different payment system, closer to an HMO. The enrollees whose care the ACO is responsible for managing do not have to agree to become part of an ACO; they were not to be informed that they were being assigned to an ACO (based on their use of physician services), because they would likely be upset. Thus, the enrollees are still free to go to any provider without a referral or authorization from the ACO; they are not restricted to a closed provider network. However, the ACO is responsible for all of the medical expenditures of their assigned enrollees, including expenses incurred outside the ACO's provider network (Epstein et al. 2014).

The ACO is a very weak form of an HMO. The ACO concept prevents real competition. Patients are not provided with a choice of plans and a financial incentive to choose on the basis of cost, access, and quality. The ACO-assigned enrollee does not benefit if the ACO reduces its cost of caring for the patient as would occur in an HMO. Any cost savings are not passed on to the patient in the form of lower premiums or more benefits.

ACO providers continue to receive FFS payments from Medicare. The difference between ACO payment and traditional Medicare is that, at the end of the year, the ACO is evaluated on the total amount spent on its assigned enrollees and the amount that would have been spent on them in a non-ACO system. The ACO may then receive some bonuses or incur penalties. It takes years before physicians, hospitals, and other providers are able to work together in an integrated care environment; before practice patterns are changed; and before care coordination occurs.

Critics believe the ACO concept is flawed because of the lack of financial incentives among patients and providers. If, over time, ACO delivery systems are able to achieve the desired integration of services, then changes in enrollee incentives (where the enrollees would share in the cost savings) and provider payment (capitation) are more likely to be instituted and ACOs may evolve into a competitive model, as described in "premium support."

Reductions in Regulated Provider Prices

The Independent Payment Advisory Board

The Independent Payment Advisory Board (IPAB) consists of 15 appointed members whose task is to recommend policies to reduce Medicare spending if the rate of growth in Medicare spending exceeds the annual percent increase in per capita GDP plus 0.5 percent. Except for a few years, Medicare spending has historically exceeded this target goal. The IPAB is prohibited from recommending changes that would inflate beneficiaries' premiums, reducing benefits, or increasing beneficiary cost sharing. The IPAB's recommendations are to be implemented unless Congress can enact policies to achieve the same spending reductions. Given the IPAB's policy constraints, the IPAB will likely be restricted to reducing provider payments. Without changing patient or provider incentives, just reducing provider payments will not improve efficiency or care coordination.

Orszag and Emanuel (2010), two architects of the ACA, claim that the IPAB was the most important institutional change in the ACA and would result in large decreases in Medicare spending growth. However, little was said regarding its effects on providers and patient access to care.

Assumed Provider Productivity Increases

Medicare payment rates under the ACA will increase about 1.1 percent more slowly than provider input prices, which include market-based wages and energy and utility costs that are generally outside providers' control. Unless providers can increase their efficiency and productivity, the gap between costs and payments will become larger over time. Providers will find it more difficult to provide the same quality and access to care.

In his analysis of the various Medicare payment reductions, Foster (2010, 9–10) stated that as payments grow slower than costs, many providers will become unprofitable and patients' access to care will be jeopardized.

Concerns About the Current Medicare System

Three basic concerns with Medicare are (1) whether its redistributive system is fair; (2) whether it promotes efficiency; and (3) whether its rising expenditures can be reduced given that its deficit is already $34 trillion dollars, which in turn questions not only if it will be available for future generations but also who will bear the burden of funding this huge deficit.

Redistributive Aspects of Medicare

Does Medicare promote equity in terms of who receives and who finances its subsidies? When a person pays the full cost of the benefits she receives, no redistribution occurs. However, when a person pays less than the full costs of his benefits, he receives a subsidy and other population groups must bear the financial burden of that subsidy. Because Medicare is a pay-as-you-go system, on average, its beneficiaries contributed into it much less than the benefits they receive from it.

Redistribution is based on a societal value judgment that subsidies should be provided to particular groups. Typically, subsidies are expected to go to those with low income and be financed by those with high income. Medicare's redistributive system raises two concerns.

First, Medicare benefits have been the same for all of its beneficiaries regardless of income. Almost all of the elderly—96 percent—pay the same Part B premium and therefore receive the same subsidy. Medicare has relatively high deductibles and no limit on out-of-pocket expenditures. (An insurance plan should always offer protection against catastrophic expenses.) Nonacute services, such as long-term care, are not covered. Furthermore, typically, those aged requiring home care or nursing home services unrelated to an illness episode must rely on their own funds to cover such expenses. Thus, on average, out-of-pocket payments for excluded benefits as a percentage of income exceed 20 percent for the low-income elderly but are less than 6 percent for the high-income aged. Consequently, many low-income seniors find the out-of-pocket expenses a financial hardship, and 14 percent must rely on Medicaid (CMS 2013a, Table I.1 and I.16).

How equitable is the financing of Medicare? Medicare beneficiaries do not pay the full costs of the medical services they receive; the aged are subsidized by those who pay state and federal taxes and HI taxes. The subsidy to Medicaid recipients is acknowledged to be welfare, as recipients receive benefits in excess of any taxes they may have paid. As a welfare program, Medicaid is appropriately financed through the income tax system, whereby those with high income contribute more in absolute and proportionate payments in relation to their income. This is the fairest way to finance a welfare program.

Second, Medicare enrollees currently receive a very large intergenerational transfer of wealth (subsidy) from those currently in the labor force, which is no different from a conventional form of welfare. Several studies have estimated the difference between the Medicare payroll tax contributions made and the average value of the benefits received; the difference is the size of the intergenerational subsidy. As more aged became eligible over the years, they made some payroll contributions into the Trust Fund. In addition to the Part A subsidy is the 75 percent federal subsidy for Part B premiums (which exceeded $186 billion in 2013) and the 75 percent federal subsidy for Part D (which cost $53 billion in 2013) (CMS 2013b).

As shown in Exhibit 8.4, a couple who turned 65 years old in 1960 and began receiving Medicare benefits in 1966 receives a $41,000 subsidy over their lifetime. A couple who earned an average wage and turned 65 years old in 2010 receives a subsidy of $265,000 ($387,000 – $122,000). Yet another couple with average income who will turn 65 years old in 2030 is estimated to receive a subsidy of $484,000 ($664,000 – $180,000). In contrast, a couple who earned a high wage and will turn 65 years old in 2030 is estimated to receive a subsidy of $430,000.

Because the Part B and Part D subsidies are financed from general income taxes, those with high income provide relatively more of the intergenerational subsidy to the aged. With Part A, on the other hand, the subsidy to the aged is financed by a payroll tax on all employees. Thus, an inequitable situation arises. Low-income employees are taxed to subsidize the medical expenses of high-income Medicare beneficiaries.

Payroll taxes are not a desirable method of financing a welfare program. Although the employer and the employee each pay half of the HI tax,

EXHIBIT 8.4
Two-Earner Couple, Average Wage ($44,600 Each in 2012 Dollars[a])

Year Cohort Turns Age 65 Years	Lifetime Medicare Benefits[b]	Lifetime Medicare Taxes[c]	Lifetime Medicare Subsidy
1960	$41,000	0	$41,000
1980	$151,000	$17,000	$134,000
2010	$387,000	$122,000	$265,000
2020	$499,000	$153,000	$346,000
2030	$664,000	$180,000	$484,000

[a] All amounts are presented in constant 2012 dollars.
[b] Lifetime Medicare benefits represent the amount needed in an account, earning a 2% real interest rate—that is, 2% plus inflation—to pay for those benefits.
[c] Lifetime Medicare taxes are based on the value of accumulated taxes, as if those taxes were put into an account that earned a 2% real rate of interest.
SOURCE: Data from Steuerle and Quakenbush (2012).

studies confirm that employees end up paying most of the employer's share of the payroll tax as well (Brittain 1971; Gruber 1994; Summers 1989). When an employer decides how many people to hire and what wage to pay them, it considers all of the costs for each employee. Imposing any tax or regulatory cost on the employer on the basis of its number of employees is the same as requiring the employer to pay higher wages to its employees. Whether the cost of that employee is in the form of wages, fringe benefits, or taxes does not matter to the employer; each is considered a cost of labor. An increase in the employer's HI tax raises the cost of labor.

When the cost of an employee is so high that it exceeds her value to the employer, the employer will discharge the employee—unless it can reduce the employee's wage to the point where the cost is about equal to the value. Typically, when payroll taxes are increased, wages are eventually renegotiated. Raises are less than they would otherwise have been because of higher payroll taxes imposed on the employer. Most of these taxes are shifted to the employees in the form of lower wages.

A tax per employee imposed on the employer rarely stays with the employer. The part of the tax not passed on to the employee (decreasing wages) is shifted forward to customers (increasing prices of goods and services). For example, most industries are competitive and do not earn excessive profits; otherwise, new firms would enter the industry and compete away those profits. When the HI tax is increased on the employee and the employer, employment contracts cannot be immediately renegotiated. Rather than being forced to reduce its profits and potentially leave the industry, the employer will shift the tax expense to the consumer by raising prices, which is a greater proportionate burden on low-income consumers.

Why is half of the Medicare payroll tax imposed on the employer and half on the employee, even though the employer does not bear any burden of the tax? The reason is related more to a tax's visibility than to who ends up paying it. Politicians would prefer to make employees believe their share of the tax is much smaller than it actually is. Whether the tax is shifted back to the employee or forward to the consumer, the tax is regressive; those with low income pay a greater portion of their income in Social Security taxes than do high-income people. In 1994, the HI payroll tax became proportional to income, and the ACA made the tax progressive. Those with high earnings pay a greater percentage of their income on the tax, as well as paying an additional Medicare tax on unearned income. (These additional Medicare taxes, however, are *not* used to support Medicare; they are used to offset the increased expenditures under the ACA to expand Medicaid and provide subsidies for those under age 65 years who buy insurance on the new state health insurance exchanges.)

If society makes the value judgment that it wants to help the poor by providing a welfare benefit, the most equitable way to do so would be to finance those benefits by taxing the rich. The burden of financing Part A, however, has fallen more heavily on those with low earnings. Many aged who receive Part A benefits have higher income and assets than those who are provided subsidies. An income tax, which takes proportionately more from those with high income (including the aged), would be a more equitable way to finance benefits to those with low income. Although the investment and retirement income of affluent seniors are not subject to payroll taxes, they are subject to income taxes.

Efficiency Incentives in Medicare

Traditional Medicare was designed to provide limited efficiency incentives to beneficiaries or providers of medical services. The elderly had no incentives to choose less costly hospitals, as the deductible was the same for all hospitals (and hospitals were precluded from competing for the aged by decreasing the deductible) and there were no copayments for inpatient admissions or lengths of stay. To protect themselves from copayments and deductibles, many aged buy Medicare supplementary insurance, lessening any incentive they may have to be concerned with higher prices or fewer services.

Physicians under FFS have an incentive to provide more of those services whose regulated fees greatly exceed their costs and few of those whose regulated fees are less than their costs or not paid for under FFS. Chronic conditions are the costliest forms of care for Medicare patients. For example, diabetes management requires frequent checking of the patient's physical condition and blood sugar level, training the patient in self-management of their disease, discussing lifestyle changes, and ensuring the patient is taking his medications. Many of the tasks required to manage chronic conditions—such as symptom monitoring, lifestyle changes, and monitoring and adjusting medications—do not require an office visit or even a physician. However, Medicare's FFS system does not pay for many of these services, unless the patient goes to the office to be checked by the physician. Other forms of patient–physician communication, such as phone calls and e-mails, are not covered by Medicare FFS. Instead, patients with questions must schedule and travel to a doctor's appointment.

Hospitals were initially paid according to their costs for caring for an elderly patient. In 1984, Medicare changed hospital payment to a fixed price per admission, but neither hospitals nor physicians have a financial incentive to manage the overall costs of an episode of care for an aged patient or provide preventive services that lead to lower acute medical costs. (Only MA plans—such as HMOs, paid on a capitation basis—have such incentives.)

Medicare can best be thought of as a state-of-the-art 1960s health insurance plan, and its design has not changed much since then. Congress modeled Part A after Blue Cross (which paid for hospitalization) and Part B after Blue Shield (which covered physician services). To secure the support of the medical profession, Congress acceded to the profession's demand that physician payment should be FFS and that patients should have free choice of physician—namely, Medicare beneficiaries should not be required to enroll in HMOs, which would restrict their choice of out-of-network physicians. Cost containment and utilization management methods used extensively in the private insurance market are virtually nonexistent in Medicare.

The lack of financial incentives for providers to coordinate care and minimize the cost of that care led to rapid increases in the cost of Medicare over time. In 2013, Medicare spent $582 billion (compared with $1.8 billion in 1966). As Medicare expenditures exceeded government projections, every administration—regardless of political party—increased the HI payroll tax and reduced the rate of increase in hospital payments for treating Medicare patients.

As shown in Exhibit 8.5, when the Medicare hospital diagnosis-related group (DRG) pricing system was introduced in the mid-1980s and an annual limit was placed on raising the DRG price, the rate of increase in Medicare hospital expenditures declined. However, between the late 1980s and 1990s, expenditures for skilled nursing homes (particularly home health care, which were included in Part A) grew rapidly, causing total Part A expenditures to rise sharply during that period.

In 1997, concerned by the rate of increase in Part A expenditures, Congress enacted several changes intended to keep the Trust Fund solvent. Home health care expenditures, which were growing rapidly, were simply moved from Part A to Part B. This change shifted the financing of home health care from the payroll tax to the income tax. Congress also lowered payments to hospitals and to Medicare HMOs, which caused many HMOs to reduce their enrollment of Medicare beneficiaries. (Both changes decreased Part A expenditures, as shown in Exhibit 8.5.) To limit the rise of Part B expenditures, in 1997 Congress changed the method by which physicians' fees would be updated annually. Medicare physician fee increases were to be based in part on the percentage increase in real GDP per capita, which is unrelated to the supply and demand for physician services by Medicare beneficiaries. This is referred to as the *sustainable growth rate* (SGR). The consequences of the SGR were not to be felt for several years. While Congress was limiting provider payment increases, seniors were receiving additional benefits through the expansion of Medicare coverage for preventive services such as mammograms, Pap smears, and prostate and colorectal screening tests.

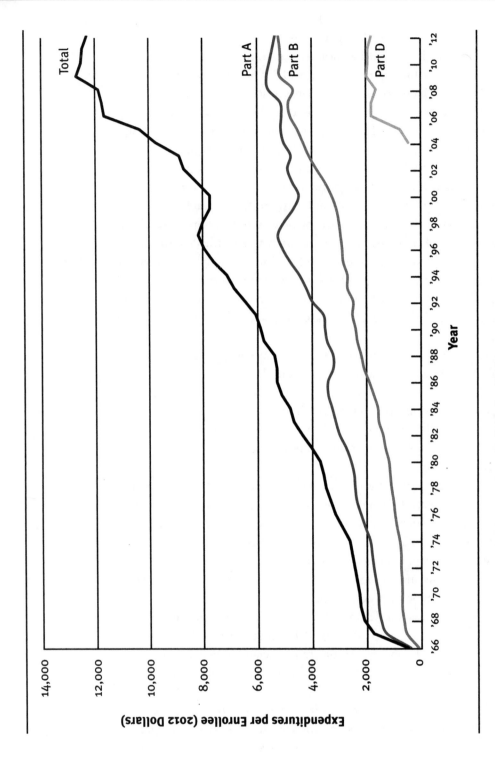

EXHIBIT 8.5
Growth in
Real Medicare
Expenditures
per Enrollee,
Part A, Part
B, and Part D,
1966–2012

Expenditures per Enrollee (2012 Dollars)

Total

Part A

Part B

Part D

Year

NOTES: Values adjusted for inflation using the consumer price index for all urban consumers.
Part A and Part B expenditures exclude patient deductible.
In 1997, home health care was moved from Part A to Part B. As a result, Part A expenditures per enrollee dropped.
SOURCES: Data from HHS and SSA (2000); 2000–2012 data from CMS (2013b), Tables III.B4, III.C4; III.D3, and V.B4.

Perhaps the clearest indication of Medicare's inefficient design is the wide variation in Medicare expenditures per beneficiary with chronic illness across states, without any difference in life expectancy or patient satisfaction.[2] For example, in 2005 Medicare spent, on average, $39,810 per beneficiary in New Jersey, compared with an average of $23,697 per beneficiary in other states. Patients with chronic illness in New Jersey had an average of 41.5 physician visits during the last six months of their lives, compared with an average of 17 visits for similar patients in Utah. Hospital days during the last six months of their lives varied from 32.1 per beneficiary at one medical center in New York to 12.9 at another medical center in Minnesota. During the last two years, Medicare spent an average of $79,280 per year at one academic medical center, compared with $37,271 at another academic center (Dartmouth Atlas Project 2006). Medicare pays for quantity, not quality.

The Unsustainable Rise in Medicare Expenditures

The current Medicare program, without improvements, is ill suited to serve future generations of seniors and eligible disabled Americans nor is it sustainable given its huge and increasing financial deficit.

Medicare's future includes a series of challenges. The numbers of aged are increasing both in absolute and percentage terms. People are living longer. Medical care costs continue to rise, and technology is driving those costs even higher. Maintaining the solvency of Part A by imposing higher payroll taxes on the working population is politically infeasible and inequitable for those with low income. Part B and Part D expenditures will require substantial increases over time in both general revenue financing and premium charges to the elderly. As the reserves in the Trust Fund are drawn down and as Parts B and D (and Medicaid) general revenue financing requirements continue to grow, the pressure on the federal budget will intensify; require politically unpopular payroll and income tax hikes; and necessitate reductions in other federal programs, such as the military, welfare, education, and the environment.

Medicare expenditures for Parts A, B, and D are expected to increase from 3.7 percent of GDP in 2013 to 4.1 percent by 2023. As a percentage of the federal budget, total Medicare expenditures are estimated to increase from 16.9 percent to 18.2 percent by 2023, based on the more likely pessimistic projections (CBO 2013b, tables 1 and 2).

In coming years, the aging of the population will place great pressures on the Trust Fund. The first of the 77 million baby boomers (those born between 1946 and 1964) started to retire in 2011. In 1960, just 9.2 percent of the population were older than age 65 years. In 2013, almost 14 percent of the population were aged 65 years or older. By 2050, the number of Medicare recipients will double from 44 million in 2013 to 87 million in

2050 (up from 70 million when the last of the baby boomers retire in 2030) (see Exhibit 8.6). In 2050, one in five Americans (21 percent) will be older than age 65 years.

People older than age 65 years have five to six times the medical costs of younger Americans. Large numbers of retirees, combined with increased longevity and more expensive and advanced medical technology, will generate huge increases in Medicare spending. The magnitude of this projected shortfall in the Trust Fund is shown in Exhibit 8.7.

The Trust Fund currently (2014) has negative cash flows, and annual cash flow deficits are expected to grow rapidly as more baby boomers retire. The growing deficits will exhaust the Trust Fund reserves by 2024.[3] (The current cash deficit is financed by previous payroll taxes in excess of outlays. The federal government gave the Trust Fund an IOU and spent the excess payroll taxes as part of general federal expenditures. Now the federal government is using general tax revenues to repay those IOUs, which contribute to the federal deficit.)

The employee base supporting Medicare is eroding. Per elderly person, the number of workers paying taxes and financing the program has steadily declined, increasing the tax burden on each employee. In 1960, there were 5.1 workers per beneficiary, in 1970 that decreased to 3.7 per beneficiary; currently, it is 3.3 per beneficiary. By 2030, the number will fall to 2.3 per beneficiary (CMS 2013b). Intermediate projections indicate that the HI tax will have to be increased from 2.9 percent to 6.21 percent (CBO 2010). However, as actual experience has been much closer to pessimistic (high-cost) assumptions, the HI tax rate will likely have to be increased to 10.86 percent by 2030.[4] These higher tax rates are only for Part A. In 2012, annual federal expenditures were $261 billion for Part A, $232 billion for Part B, and $55 billion for Part D—a total of $548 billion. Projected federal subsidies (expenditures minus premiums) in 2023 for each part of Medicare, in constant dollars, are $462 billion for Part A, $431 billion for Part B, and $169 billion for Part D—a total of $1.062 trillion (CBO 2013a).

Political support for Medicare is likely to decline as the costs to the non-aged go up, with a consequent increase in intergenerational political conflict. The US political system cannot wait until more of the baby boomers retire to resolve an issue that involves such a large redistribution of wealth among different groups in society. Those who will become eligible for Medicare in the coming decade have certain expectations about what they will receive from Medicare. Politicians cannot change Medicare's benefits at the last moment. No presidential candidate will campaign on decreasing Medicare benefits. Any changes will have to be agreed upon in nonelection years and gradually phased in. Yet the longer Congress waits, the higher the payroll tax will be.

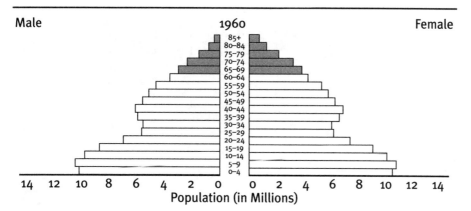

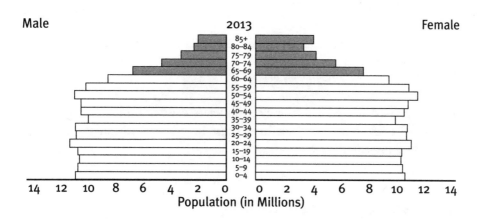

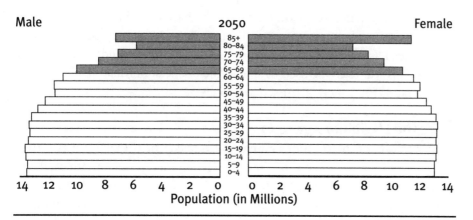

EXHIBIT 8.6
Population
Pyramid, United
States, 1960,
2013, and 2050

SOURCE: Data from Census Bureau (2013).

Enacting legislation to decrease Medicare benefits or eligibility in a presidential or congressional election year will be difficult, as Medicare has such widespread political support among the elderly, the near elderly, and their children (who might be faced with an increased financial burden of paying their parents' medical expenses). Given that a new Medicare system

EXHIBIT 8.7
Cash Deficit of the Medicare Hospital Insurance Trust Fund, 2012–2022

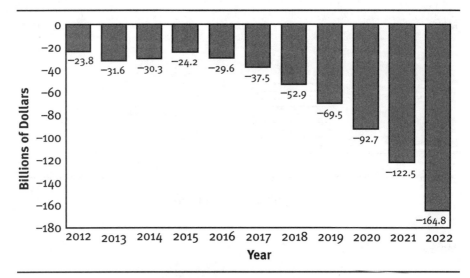

NOTE: Data based on high-cost assumption.
SOURCE: Data from CMS (2013b), Table III.B5.

must be phased in and few nonelection years exist in which to enact such controversial legislation, any changes must be enacted within the first two years after a presidential election.

Proposals for Medicare Reform

Proposals to restructure Medicare should be based on three criteria: equity, efficiency, and reduction in the rate of increase in Medicare spending. Many approaches have been proposed for reforming Medicare, and a combination of proposals will likely be used to spread the financial burden.[5] The following are several of the widely discussed proposals.

Raise the Eligibility Age to 67

Similar to one of the solutions employed to make the Social Security system more solvent, raising the age of eligibility to 67 years by one month each year would make the eligibility age for Social Security and Medicare the same. With increased life expectancy, people could work longer and maintain their employment-based health insurance.

Reduce the Rate of Increase in Medicare Provider Payments

This approach has been used previously and is likely to be part of any long-term solution. However, decreasing provider payments will ultimately reduce provider participation and access to care by Medicare beneficiaries.

Increase the HI Tax

This approach, which has also been used previously, is likely to be part of any proposed solution. Raising the HI tax would increase the financial burden on low-wage workers. In addition, the HI tax could be made more progressive.

Increase the Part B and Part D Premiums and Make Them Income Related

Most elderly people currently pay a premium that covers only 25 percent of Part B and Part C expenditures. Premiums could be increased over time to cover a higher percentage of these expenditures. With this approach, the hardship on the low-income aged would be minimized by a greater use of income-related premiums. Equity would be achieved and the deficit reduced if subsidies to high-income aged were eventually completely phased out.

Rely on Competition Between Medicare Health Plans

One proposal to increase competition among Medicare health plans is referred to as *premium support*. MA plans would compete directly with the government-administered Medicare FFS on a regional basis, and the beneficiaries would select their coverage from the competing options. Government payment to health plans, including FFS plans, would be based on the competing plans' premiums. The government contribution would be based perhaps on the second lowest plan's (risk-adjusted) bid, which would become the new benchmark premium. Thus, a beneficiary would always have a plan that requires no additional premium. Beneficiaries choosing a plan whose bid is above the benchmark would have to pay the difference between the benchmark and the more costly plan's premium. If a beneficiary chooses a relatively expensive coverage option, the additional premium would be paid entirely by the Medicare enrollee, not the government. If traditional Medicare FFS is not the cheaper plan or the benchmark, then beneficiaries would have to pay an additional premium to remain in traditional Medicare.

Competition among Medicare plans, with different premiums and different additional benefits, would provide a powerful incentive for beneficiaries to seek out high-value, low-cost plans and for plans to compete on premiums, benefits, patient access and satisfaction, and quality. Premium support changes Medicare from a defined (and continually expanding) benefit program—which is an open-ended commitment by the government to pay for the promised benefits regardless of their costs—to a defined contribution program, with the government paying on behalf of the aged a predetermined amount of money (including Parts A, B, and D) similar to a voucher to a health plan. (Older and sicker beneficiaries would receive higher amounts so that health plans would have an incentive to enroll them.) The financial risk of caring for the aged is shifted from the government to the health plan. (This approach is similar to the Federal Employees Health Benefits plan.) Proponents of competition in Medicare claim that a defined conttribution program will force competing Medicare plans to be efficient and will reduce Medicare expenditures.

Currently, MA plans could be much cheaper. However, they have less incentive to reduce their costs, rather than lower their premium or give enrollees a rebate, because the government requires them to provide more generous benefits. With more generous benefits, enrollees use more services and the plan's costs increase.

Proponents of premium support claim that health plan competition would reduce Medicare costs. Jacobson and colleagues (2012) found that the best-performing MA HMOs can offer the Medicare benefit package at premiums that are below the cost of FFS in most parts of the United States. MA plans have a greater incentive to innovate to lower costs than FFS providers, which would get paid less. Part D (a defined contribution program) provides evidence on the effect of Medicare plan competition. Medicare beneficiaries choose among competing private drug plans; as a result, premiums from these plans have stayed relatively constant over time. Plans have to cover at least one drug in each specified drug class, but the plans can vary according to what else they cover, copays, and premiums. The private drug plans have encouraged generic substitution for branded drugs by reducing copays for generics. The costs of the drug program are 40 percent less than the Medicare Actuary's projection.

A study by Baicker, Chernew, and Robbins (2013) found that greater Medicare managed care penetration (MA) in a market decreased hospital utilization (length of stay) and hospital costs for all seniors, including those in traditional Medicare, and for non-Medicare insured persons. The "spillover" effects of competition had positive effects on all sectors of the medical care system.

Allowing them to compete is the best way to judge whether traditional Medicare FFS or MA plans are more efficient. To ensure that enrollees have adequate information to choose plans, data must become available on each plan's premiums, out-of-pocket payments, quality, waiting times for access to primary care physicians and specialists, and patient satisfaction.

Critics of changing Medicare to a defined contribution program claim that many enrollees will have to pay an additional premium if they want to remain in traditional Medicare and it isn't one of the cheaper plans. Many Medicare beneficiaries would have to make a trade-off between higher premiums and restrictions on provider choice. Critics are also concerned about the ability of the elderly to make such choices and the difficulty of understanding the differences between competing health plans.

Change Medicare to an Income-Related Program

The defined contribution program could be used to change Medicare to an income-related program. Each recipient would receive premium support, but its value would be determined by the recipient's income. The subsidy would equal the entire premium required to provide a uniform set of benefits for low-income aged, but wealthy aged would receive proportionately smaller premium support vouchers. The income-related voucher would be phased in for future elderly population.

An income-related subsidy would reduce the cost of Medicare and the huge intergenerational subsidies from low-income workers to high-income aged. Income-related benefits would also help the low-income aged, who cannot afford the deductibles, cost sharing, and Part B and D premiums and thus must rely on Medicaid for these payments.

Politics of Medicare Reform

The popularity of Medicare among the aged (who have the highest voting participation rates) and their children (who are relieved of the financial responsibility of their parent's medical expenses) means that politicians who attempt to change it without the endorsement of both political parties are at great political risk. Any political party proposing decreased Medicare benefits, higher beneficiary cost sharing or premiums, or the removal of seniors' free choice of provider would lose the votes of the aged and their children. Previously, imposing financial burdens on providers by paying them less and raising payroll taxes was easier than increasing the financial burden on the elderly.

Unfortunately, the longer it takes to phase in a system that is equitable and efficient, the greater the political problems will be. Current workers will have to pay higher payroll taxes, intergenerational transfers from low-income workers will increase, beneficiaries will have less access to providers as provider fees are reduced, and the financial hardship on low-income aged who cannot afford high out-of-pocket expenditures and rising Part B and D premiums will occur. The sooner the financial burden is shared among the different groups in an equitable manner, the smaller future tax increases will be.

Summary

To make Medicare an equitable and efficient redistribution system, the "entitlement" myth of Medicare must be recognized and its large welfare component acknowledged. Government subsidies should be used primarily to help the low-income elderly. Health plans, including traditional Medicare, should be able to compete for beneficiaries on the basis of price, quality, outcomes, and enrollee satisfaction. Health plans will then have incentives to be efficient and responsive to beneficiary preferences.

The potential cost of suggesting dramatic solutions to the problems of Medicare is high to any one political party. Whatever the combination of approaches selected, a vast redistribution of wealth will result. A bipartisan commission whose recommendations are adopted by Congress has, in the past, resolved such highly visible redistributive problems. The National Bipartisan Commission on the Future of Medicare (created by Congress as part of the 1997 Balanced Budget Act) was unable to reach agreement (by just one vote) on reforming Medicare in 1999. Whether and when a commission approach will again be used for reforming Medicare remains to be seen.

Discussion Questions

1. Which population groups are served by Medicare, what are the different parts of Medicare, and how is Medicare financed?
2. Discuss how Medicare's patient and provider incentives affect efficient use of services.
3. How equitable are the methods used to finance Medicare?
4. How does the Medicare Hospital Trust Fund differ from a pension fund?
5. Why is it necessary to reform Medicare?
6. Why is it politically difficult to reform Medicare?
7. How would patient and provider incentives differ between ACOs and proposals for transforming Medicare into a premium support model?

Notes

1. The MA plans submit a premium bid for insuring Medicare beneficiaries. The government establishes a benchmark premium for deciding how much to pay MA plans. The benchmark is the average FFS expenditure for a Medicare beneficiary in that geographic area, adjusted for risk factors. If the MA plan bid exceeds the benchmark premium, then the plan receives the benchmark premium. If the plan's bid is below the benchmark, then the government pays the plan its bid and gives a rebate of 75 percent of the difference between the plan's bid and the benchmark premium. The 75 percent rebate must be returned to its enrollees in the form of additional benefits and services. About 90 percent of MA plans receive some rebate.

2. The Dartmouth Atlas Project (2006) online report, *The Care of Patients with Severe Chronic Illness*, examined differences in the management of Medicare patients "with one or more of twelve chronic illnesses that account for more than 75 percent of all US healthcare expenditures. Among people who died between 1999 and 2003, per capita spending varied by a factor of six between hospitals across the country. Spending was not correlated with rates of illness in different parts of the country; rather, it reflected how intensively certain resources—acute care hospital beds, specialist physician visits, tests and other services—were used in the management of people who were very ill but could not be cured. Since other research has demonstrated that, for these chronically ill Americans, receiving more services does not result in improved outcomes, and since most Americans say they prefer to avoid a very 'high-tech' death, the report concludes that Medicare spending for the care of the chronically ill could be reduced by as much as 30%—*while improving quality, patient satisfaction, and outcomes.*"

3. The high-cost estimates assume that the ACA payment reductions will not be implemented in all future years. Medicare actuaries claim that, under current law, Medicare's payments for health services would fall increasingly below providers' costs. "Providers could not sustain continuing negative margins and would have to withdraw from serving Medicare beneficiaries…. Under such circumstances, lawmakers might feel substantial pressure to override the productivity adjustments, much as they have done to prevent reductions in physician payment rates. In view of these issues, it is important to note that the actual future costs for Medicare are likely to exceed those shown by the current-law projections in this report, possibly by substantial amounts" (CMS 2013b, 207).

4. The rate of growth in real wages (because HI is a payroll tax) and life expectancy at retirement are important components of these projections. Pessimistic projections assume a rate of growth in real wages similar to the growth rate in the past 25 years, which is half as large as that used in the intermediate assumption. Advances in medicine, genetics, and biotechnology are also projected to result in a more rapid increase in life expectancy at retirement than the intermediate projections that assume the same rate as for the past 50 years.

5. The May 2013 issue of *Health Affairs* has many articles devoted to reducing Medicare's spending growth rate. Also see Kaiser Family Foundation (2013), which includes more than 150 options and the pros and cons for each.

References

Baicker, K., M. Chernew, and J. Robbins. 2013. "The Spillover Effects of Medicare Managed Care: Medicare Advantage and Hospital Utilization." *NBER Working Paper* No. 19070. Published May. www.nber.org/papers/w19070 .pdf.

Brittain, J. A. 1971. "The Incidence of Social Security Payroll Taxes." *American Economic Review* 61 (1): 110–25.

Centers for Medicare & Medicaid Services (CMS). 2013a. "CMS Statistics." Last modified September 12. www.cms.gov/Research-Statistics-Data-and-Systems/Research/ResearchGenInfo/CMSStatistics.html.

———. 2013b. *2013 Annual Report of the Boards of Trustees of the Federal Hospital Insurance and Federal Supplementary Medical Insurance Trust Funds.* Published May 31. www.cms.gov/Research-Statistics-Data-and-Systems/ Statistics-Trends-and-Reports/ReportsTrustFunds/Downloads/ TR2013.pdf.

———. 2013c. "Costs in the Coverage Gap." Accessed October. www.medicare .gov/part-d/costs/coverage-gap/part-d-coverage-gap.html.

Congressional Budget Office (CBO). 2013a. "CBO's May 2013 Medicare Baseline." www.cbo.gov/sites/default/files/cbofiles/attachments/44205-2013-05-Medicare.pdf.

———. 2013b. "Updated Budget Projections: Fiscal Years 2013 to 2023." Published May. www.cbo.gov/sites/default/files/cbofiles/ attachments/44172-Baseline2.pdf.

———. 2010. "The Long Term Budget Outlook." Published June 30. www.cbo .gov/ftpdocs/115xx/doc11579/06-30-LTBO.pdf.

Dartmouth Atlas Project. 2006. *The Care of Patients with Severe Chronic Illness: An Online Report on the Medicare Program.* Lebanon, NH: Dartmouth Medical School. www.dartmouthatlas.org/downloads/atlases/2006_Chronic_Care_ Atlas.pdf.

Davis, P. A. 2014. *Medicare: Part B Premiums.* Congressional Research Services. Published March 12. www.fas.org/sgp/crs/misc/R40082.pdf.

Epstein, A., A. K. Jha, E. J. Orav, D. L. Liebman, A-M. J. Audet, M. A. Zezza, and S. Guterman. 2014. "Analysis of Early Accountable Care Organizations Defines Patient, Structural, Cost, and Quality-of-Care Characteristics." *Health Affairs* 33 (1): 95–102.

Gruber, J. 1994. "The Incidence of Mandated Maternity Benefits." *American Economic Review* 84 (3): 622–41.

Internal Revenue Service (IRS). 2013. "Affordable Care Act Tax Provisions." www.irs.gov/uac/Affordable-Care-Act-Tax-Provisions.

Jacobson, G., T. Neuman, A. Damico, and the Kaiser Family Foundation. 2012. *Transforming Medicare into a Premium Support System: Implications for Beneficiary Premiums*. Published October. http://kaiserfamilyfoundation.files.wordpress.com/2013/01/8373.pdf.

Kaiser Family Foundation. 2013. *Policy Options to Sustain Medicare for the Future*. Published January. http://kaiserfamilyfoundation.files.wordpress.com/2013/02/8402.pdf.

———. 2010. "Medicare Spending and Financing Fact Sheet." Posted November 14. www.kff.org/medicare/upload/7305-05.pdf.

Medicare.gov. n.d. "Part B Costs." Accessed October 2013. www.medicare.gov/your-medicare-costs/part-b-costs/part-b-costs.html.

MedPAC. 2013. *A Data Book: Health Care Spending and the Medicare Program*. Published June. www.medpac.gov/documents/Jun13DataBookEntireReport.pdf.

Orszag, P., and E. Emanuel. 2010. "Health Care Reform and Cost Control." *New England Journal of Medicine* 363: 601–03.

Steuerle, C. E., and C. Quakenbush. 2012. "Social Security and Medicare Taxes and Benefits Over a Lifetime." Urban Institute. Published October. www.urban.org/UploadedPDF/412660-Social-Security-and-Medicare-Taxes-and-Benefits-Over-a-Lifetime.pdf.

Summers, L. 1989. "Some Simple Economics of Mandated Benefits." *American Economic Review* 79 (2): 177–83.

US Census Bureau. 2013. "International Data Base." Last updated December. www.census.gov/population/international/data/idb.

US Department of Human and Health Services (HHS) and Social Security Administration (SSA). 2000. *Social Security Bulletin, Annual Statistical Supplement*. Washington, DC: HHS.

MEDICAID

Medicaid is a means-tested welfare program for the poor, providing medical and long-term care to more than 22 percent of the population. In 1985, the program covered 22 million people, the federal government spent $23 billion on the program, and it represented 2.4 percent of the federal budget. By 2012, it covered 71 million people, a greater number than those enrolled in Medicare, total federal expenditures reached $251 billion, and the program increased its share of the federal budget to 9.2 percent (CBO 2013). These rapidly increasing Medicaid expenditures, which represent a growing financial burden on federal and state budgets, continue to provide insufficient access to care for program beneficiaries.

Medicaid is in the midst of a major enrollment expansion as a result of the Affordable Care Act (ACA). An estimated 17 million additional people—mostly low-income adults—are expected to become eligible for the program. It faces serious challenges in ensuring its enrollees have appropriate access to medical services while controlling rising medical costs.

Medicaid is administered by each state, but policy is shared by the federal government, which pays, on average, 59 percent matching funds (the range is 50 percent to 73 percent) based on each state's financial capacity (per capita income). These federal dollars make Medicaid a less expensive approach (than other state programs such as General Assistance) for the states to use in expanding access to medical care by those with low income. Each state Medicaid program must cover certain federally mandated population groups to qualify for federal matching funds.

The first and largest federally mandated population group is composed of those receiving cash welfare assistance (including single-parent families) who were previously eligible for Aid to Families with Dependent Children (AFDC) as well as those low-income aged, blind, and disabled persons who qualify for Supplemental Security Income. The second group comprises low-income pregnant women and children who do not qualify for cash assistance. The third group includes those considered to be "medically needy"—persons who do not qualify for welfare programs but have high medical or long-term-care expenses. The fourth and final group consists of low-income Medicare beneficiaries who cannot afford the deductibles, cost sharing, premiums for Medicare Parts B and D, or cost of services not covered by Medicare.

States may expand eligibility and enroll additional groups (and add services beyond those for groups mandated by the federal government). Thus, wide variations in coverage and eligibility exist among the states. Groups typically added at the state's option include medically needy groups beyond those that are federally mandated, such as the elderly and people with disabilities; children and pregnant women at a high percentage (e.g., 200 percent) above the federal poverty level (FPL); and all uninsured persons with income below a certain level. However, the percentage of the Medicaid-covered population considered poor (less than 100 percent of the FPL) varies greatly by state—from 32 percent to 67 percent. Just being poor is insufficient to qualify for Medicaid. On average, in 2012, only 47 percent of those classified as poor were enrolled in Medicaid. The percentage of near-poor—100 percent to 199 percent of the FPL—enrolled by states varies from 20 percent to 57 percent, with an average of 35 percent in 2012 (Census Bureau 2013).

In 1996, Temporary Assistance to Needy Families (TANF) was enacted to replace AFDC. TANF retains the same eligibility rules as AFDC. Before welfare reform, many poor children qualified automatically for Medicaid because their families were receiving AFDC, the national cash benefits program for poor children. Welfare reform ended that link by abolishing AFDC. Because Congress did not want anyone to lose Medicaid eligibility as a result of welfare reform, it decreed that states should continue using their old AFDC rules for determining Medicaid eligibility, such as covering pregnant women, the medically needy, and children (if their parents would have qualified for AFDC). The children of women who leave welfare for work are still eligible for Medicaid if their family income remains low enough.

An Illustration of Medicaid Eligibility

Within federal guidelines, states may set their own income-and-asset eligibility criteria for Medicaid. Following is an illustration of how the medically needy qualify for Medi-Cal (Medicaid in California). A person cannot have more than $2,000 in assets ($3,000 if there is a family member older than age 60 years), excluding a house, car, and furniture. One's financial assets can be reduced in many legitimate ways to qualify for Medicaid. Money could be spent fixing up one's house, purchasing a new car, or taking a vacation, or it could be put in a special burial account. Selling one's house and giving the cash to one's children will make one ineligible for Medicaid for months. The penalty period for doing so is determined by dividing the amount transferred by the average private pay cost of a nursing home in the state. For example, if a person gave away property to his children worth $100,000 and the monthly cost of nursing home care in California in 2013 was $6,900 (for a semi-private room; a private room was $8,040), the person would be ineligible for Medicaid benefits for 16 months (Genworth Financial Inc. 2013, 25).

When a couple is involved, special spousal financial protections exist. If a husband enters a nursing home, the wife can remain in their home and is entitled to have about $2,931 a month in income and $117,240 in financial assets (excluding primary residence and a car). If the wife's Social Security payments are below $2,931, the husband's Social Security can be used to bring her monthly income to $2,931 (as of 2014) (DHCS 2013). Retirement accounts and other assets can be partially shielded from the government by counting the income from those retirement accounts toward the $2,931 monthly income. For example, if a person has $100,000 in an investment account and takes out $500 a month, the $500 counts toward his monthly income, but the $100,000 does not count as an asset. A number of states have begun to crack down on various schemes used by some wealthy aged to shield their assets to become Medicaid eligible, such as setting up annuities, trusts, and life contracts.[1] In general, many middle-class elderly become distraught when they find they must spend down their hard-earned assets for a spouse to become Medicaid eligible.

State Children's Health Insurance Program (SCHIP)

A major expansion of Medicaid eligibility occurred in 1997. As part of the 1997 Balanced Budget Act, Congress enacted the State Children's Health Insurance Program (SCHIP). SCHIP was enacted to provide coverage for low-income children whose family income was too high to qualify for Medicaid. Politically, children are considered a vulnerable and more deserving group than other uninsured groups; consequently, this program expansion received bipartisan support. (Medical benefits for children are considered relatively inexpensive when compared with benefits for uninsured adults.) Furthermore, providing coverage to older children was viewed as an expansion of existing Medicaid policies, extending to infants, younger children, and pregnant women in the late 1980s. This program provided the states with federal matching funds to initiate and expand healthcare assistance for uninsured low-income children up to age 19 years with family income as high as 400 percent of the FPL. Federal matching funds may be as high as 83 percent (Kaiser Family Foundation 2014).

The number of children eligible for public coverage increased dramatically, as did participation rates in SCHIP. The percentage of uninsured children whose family income is between 100 percent and 200 percent of the FPL (as well as those whose family income was less than 100 percent of the FPL) has declined since 1997. In each of these groups, the percentage of children with public coverage climbed, while the percentage of children with private insurance fell over this same period. Not all of the increase in public coverage for poor and low-income children was the result of uninsured children being enrolled in SCHIP. Significant growth in public coverage also resulted from a movement from private insurance to free or low-cost public coverage (referred to as *crowd-out* because public insurance "crowds out" private insurance). It has been estimated that as many as 60 percent of those newly enrolled in public insurance programs, such as SCHIP, were formerly in private insurance plans (Gruber and Simon 2008).

Bipartisan support for SCHIP was achieved as a result of an ideological compromise on how SCHIP services would be delivered to eligible children. States may either purchase health insurance coverage for eligible children in the private market or include them in the state's Medicaid program.

The SCHIP, now called Children's Health Insurance Program (CHIP), was renewed in 2010. A concern with CHIP was that it was originally intended for children of low-income families but has now been extended to include more children from middle-income families. CHIP eligibility in some states is as high as $94,200 for a family of four (e.g., New York in 2014) (CMS 2013a); further, a number of states use CHIP funds to cover adults other than expectant mothers.

The ACA requires any child whose parents earn between 100 percent and 133 percent of the FPL to switch from CHIP to Medicaid. Many children previously enrolled in CHIP and in private health plans, such as Blue Cross, will be required to receive their care from Medicaid networks, whose access to and coordination of care is less than that provided by private health plans.

Medicaid Beneficiaries and Medicaid Expenditures

Broadened eligibility requirements for Medicaid have caused the number of recipients to sharply rise from 22 million in 1975 to 71 million in 2012 to an estimated 91 million by 2023. Most of the past enrollment growth resulted from federal and state expansions in coverage of low-income children and pregnant women. As of 2011, the major beneficiary groups consist of low-income children (49.7 percent); nondisabled low-income adults (pregnant women and adults in families with children receiving cash assistance, 24.1 percent); aged persons receiving Medicare who need Medicaid ("dual eligibles") to pay for their deductibles, cost sharing, premiums for Medicare

Parts B and D, and other services not covered by Medicare (8.8 percent); and blind and disabled persons receiving acute medical and long-term care services (17.2 percent).

As shown in Exhibit 9.1, the distribution of Medicaid expenditures does not match the distribution of Medicaid enrollees. Although about 74 percent of Medicaid recipients are low-income parents and children, they account for only about 35 percent of Medicaid expenditures. By comparison, about 65 percent of Medicaid expenditures are for medical services and institutional care for the aged, people with disabilities, and people with mental handicap (26 percent of Medicaid recipients).

Although the number of Medicaid beneficiaries has increased over time, from about 22 million in the 1970s and 1980s, to about 35 million in the 1990s, to more than 70 million in 2012, the distribution of beneficiary groups has stayed roughly constant over this period. State and federal Medicaid expenditures have rapidly increased and are expected to continue to rise sharply over the next decade. Medicaid represents one of the largest items

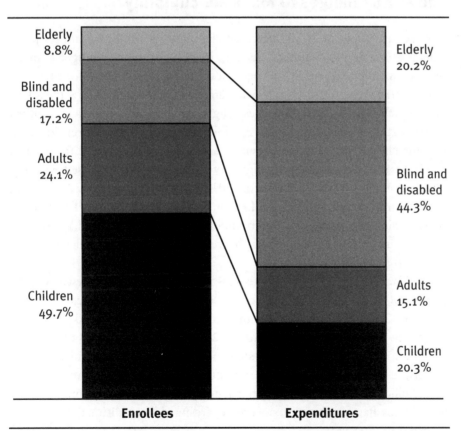

EXHIBIT 9.1
Percentage Distribution of Medicaid Enrollees and Benefit Payments, by Eligibility Status, Fiscal Year 2011

NOTE: Totals exclude disproportionate share hospital expenditures, territorial enrollees and expenditures, and adjustments.
SOURCE: Data from CMS (2013b), Table 2.

in state budgets, along with elementary and secondary education expenditures. Federal and state Medicaid expenditures were $55.1 billion in 1988; spending rose to an estimated $409 billion in 2012 and is expected to reach $839 billion by 2022. During this same period, the number of beneficiaries is expected to grow by 29 percent (see Exhibit 9.2).

Exhibit 9.3 shows the distribution of Medicaid expenditures by type of service. The largest share of Medicaid expenditures is for acute care (66 percent), which is made up of fee-for-service payments (50 percent), managed care (45 percent), and Medicare premiums (5 percent). Long-term care (which includes nursing home care and home health care) represents the second-largest category (30 percent). Because Medicaid pays providers relatively low rates, payments to disproportionate-share hospitals (4 percent) compensate those hospitals that serve proportionately more Medicaid beneficiaries and low-income people.

The ACA's Changes to Medicaid Eligibility

The ACA, enacted in 2010, increased eligibility for Medicaid and projected federal Medicaid expenditures. Starting in 2014, all those younger than age 65 years with income up to 133 percent of the FPL are eligible for Medicaid. (As of 2014, this meant $16,105 for an individual and $32,913 for a family of four). For the first time, these eligibility standards, which are uniform for all states, will include childless adults. As parents of children in CHIP become eligible for Medicaid, their children will be transferred from CHIP to Medicaid. These changes in eligibility are expected to increase total Medicaid enrollment from 71 million in 2012 to 91 million by 2023, assuming all states implement the Medicaid expansion under the ACA. (The estimate of 91 million represents the total number of individuals enrolled in Medicaid at any point during the fiscal year; however, average enrollment for 2023 is projected to be 70 million.)

The ACA provides full federal financing of those newly eligible (from 100 percent up to 133 percent of the FPL) for the years 2014 to 2016. In 2017, the federal matching rate will decline from 100 percent for these new eligibles to 90 percent by 2020 and thereafter (Kaiser Family Foundation 2013). If all of the states implement the Medicaid expansion under the ACA, the federal government is expected to spend an additional $952 billion on Medicaid while the states will spend an additional $76 billion. States have expressed concern regarding their additional costs to be incurred in later years.

Given the large expected increase in Medicaid enrollment starting 2014, the government was concerned that the Medicaid population would

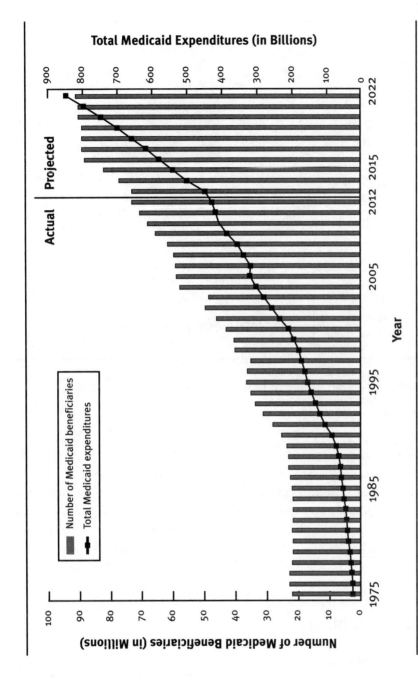

EXHIBIT 9.2
Number of
Medicaid
Beneficiaries
and Total
Medicaid
Expenditures,
Actual and
Projected,
1975–2022

Total Medicaid Expenditures (in Billions)

Number of Medicaid beneficiaries
Total Medicaid expenditures

Year

Number of Medicaid Beneficiaries (in Millions)

Actual Projected

SOURCES: Data on the "Number of Medicaid beneficiaries" from CMS (2013c); projected data from CBO (2013); data on the "Total Medicaid expenditures" from CMS (2014a).

EXHIBIT 9.3
Medicaid
Expenditures,
by Service,
2012

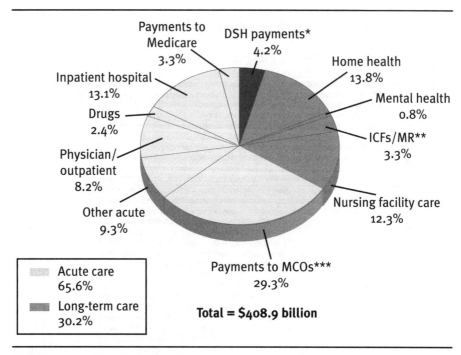

* DSH: Disproportionate share hospital
** ICFs/MR: Intermediate care facilities for the mentally retarded
*** MCOs: Managed care organizations
SOURCE: Data from CMS (2014b).

have limited access to primary care physicians, particularly given that Medicaid pays physicians lower fees than any other payer. Thus, for just the years 2013 and 2014 (covering the congressional midterm elections), the ACA requires the federal government to pay the additional cost of making Medicaid fees to primary care physicians equal to Medicare fees. After 2014, Medicaid fees will be determined by the states and will return to their previous lower levels, with a consequent sharp drop in physician availability.

Medicaid Problems

Medicaid Coverage

Although Medicaid is the government's major healthcare financing system for the poor—including low-income families, children, childless adults, elderly, and those requiring long-term care—it is generally perceived to be highly inadequate. The program does not cover a large portion of those with low income. On average, only 47 percent of people below 100 percent of the FPL were covered and only 35 percent of those who are considered poor and near-poor (below 200 percent of the FPL) were covered in 2012.

The likelihood of a poor person being eligible for Medicaid varies greatly by state. States with higher per capita income were more likely to cover a higher percentage of their poor population and provide more generous Medicaid benefits. The variation among states of the percentage of poor eligible for Medicaid varied from 32 percent to 67 percent in 2012. (In 2014, 100 percent of the FPL was $23,850 for a family of four, $15,730 for a couple, and $11,670 for a single person [Census Bureau 2013; HHS 2014].)

Expanding Medicaid coverage to a greater portion of those with low income involves maintaining incentives for working low-income persons who have health insurance to maintain their private insurance. Working low-income people with insurance have an incentive to drop their private insurance and accept the free public insurance. Medicaid is considered less valuable than private insurance (because of the stigma cost and more restricted access to physicians because of low Medicaid reimbursement), but as the cost of private insurance increases, Medicaid becomes a more desirable substitute. Expanded public coverage in some states has displaced existing private coverage with little additional overall gain in coverage. (Part of the private coverage replaced by public coverage may have had relatively limited benefits.)

Because income is one criterion for Medicaid eligibility, those on the program lose their eligibility once their incomes rise above their state's cut-off level, which could still be below the FPL. The potential loss of their medical benefits is a disincentive for Medicaid recipients to accept low-paying jobs. A Medicaid-eligible person must make a trade-off between earning a higher income versus losing all their benefits (this is referred to as the *notch effect*). Program eligibility would be increased if, as people's wages go up, they would lose only a portion of their Medicaid benefits. Graduating benefits according to income would provide an incentive for those who want to keep their benefits to work more hours and seek higher-paying jobs.

Medicaid Effectiveness

Medicaid is a fragmented, fee-for-service system in which care is not coordinated and accountability for outcomes is nonexistent; poor care often results in greater reimbursement for the provider. The traditional program has been shown to be ineffective in improving its beneficiaries' health, compared to those who are uninsured. In 2008, Oregon enrolled an additional 10,000 low-income individuals, chosen by lottery, to its Medicaid system. Baicker and colleagues (2013) compared the health status of those who were with those who were not selected by lottery to be enrolled in Medicaid. The researchers found that Medicaid coverage had no significant effect on the prevalence or diagnosis of hypertension or high cholesterol levels or on the use of medication for those conditions, and no improvement in individuals' diabetes was observed. Medicaid recipients, however, had reduced out-of-pocket expenses, decreased rates of depression, and increased use of preventive services and doctors' services.

In a further analysis of the Oregon data, Taubman and colleagues (2014) found that Medicaid coverage significantly increased emergency department (ED) visits by 40 percent per person, compared to ED use by those not selected for Medicaid. The higher numbers of ED visits were for broad types of visits and conditions, including conditions readily treatable in primary care settings. These findings are contrary to the expectations of the ACA that as more of the uninsured are enrolled in Medicaid and treated in physician offices, costly ED visits would decline and money would be saved.

The ACA is expanding Medicaid eligibility to many millions of people at a cost of hundreds of billions of dollars. If the program merely expands eligibility, significant changes in participants' health status will not occur. Unless the delivery of Medicaid services is radically transformed, a great deal of money will have been spent with little effectiveness in improving the health of its beneficiaries.

State Funding

Rising Medicaid expenditures have become a great financial burden to the states and the federal government. Continuing to spend an increasing portion of state budgets on Medicaid would require a tax hike or a reduction of expenditures on politically popular programs, such as education and prisons. Each option is politically costly. Instead, to reduce rising Medicaid expenditures, many states have resorted to reducing Medicaid eligibility and setting low fee-for-service provider-payment rates.[2] The consequences of reduced provider fees are low provider participation rates, limited access to care, less willingness of a physician to spend much time with a Medicaid patient, a shift away from physician offices to hospital EDs, and a lack of care coordination (Decker 2009; Zuckerman, Williams, and Stockley 2009).

Conflict exists between Medicaid's goals of expanding eligibility, improving access to care, providing coordinated and effective care, and slowing the rate of increase in Medicaid expenditures. Federal financing of Medicaid expansion (and subsidies for the state health insurance exchanges) started in 2014. The federal government, however, currently faces a huge deficit, which will get bigger as a result of the ACA. Unless the federal government is able to reduce current and future Medicaid (and Medicare) expenditures, it will be unable to reduce its ever-growing deficit.

States' Decision to Expand Medicaid Eligibility

Many states have not decided whether they will expand Medicaid eligibility from 100 to 133 percent of the FPL as proposed (but not mandated) by the ACA. The federal government will pay 100 percent of the costs of expanding Medicaid for the newly eligible population—childless adults—up to 133 percent of the FPL, for the first three years and declining to a 90 percent Federal Medical Assistance Percentage (FMAP) thereafter. In 2013, the FMAP varied by state from 50 percent to 72 percent.

Each state must consider the trade-off of receiving a high FMAP for those newly eligible against the burden of higher state Medicaid expenditures. Hospitals and healthcare providers—important political constituencies—have lobbied their states to expand Medicaid eligibility. Financial considerations making many states hesitant to do so include the following:

- The aging population will place an increasing burden on Medicaid long-term care budgets.
- States face substantial Medicaid expenditures for currently eligible populations, separate from the coverage expansion.
- States are concerned that many who are currently eligible for Medicaid (below 100 percent of the FPL) but not enrolled may decide to enroll, increasing state Medicaid expenditures. A recent study indicates this effect could be substantial. The federal matching rate does not increase for anyone newly enrolling in Medicaid if they were previously eligible (Sonier, Boudreaux, and Blewett 2013).
- Even the 10 percent matching rate for the newly eligible population will add billions over time to many state budgets—funds that states can ill afford to spend without raising taxes or reducing other programs.
- Is the federal government a reliable business partner? The growth in federal Medicaid spending is currently believed by many to be unsustainable and must be cut. There is no guarantee that Congress would not reduce that 90 percent matching rate in the future to control federal spending. Should this occur, the state would be faced with a huge increase in its Medicaid budget, likely leading to sharply decreased provider payments for all those eligible, or the state will have to drop eligibility for many currently eligible.

Many states will delay making a long-term commitment on expanded Medicaid eligibility to see how federal policy and funding evolves. A few states are considering enrolling the newly eligible population in state health insurance exchanges (if the state has such an exchange) where enrollees would qualify for federal subsidies, thereby shifting the financial risk to the federal government. Individuals would likely have greater access to care on the exchange than in fee-for-service Medicaid.

Medicaid Reforms

Medicaid Managed Care

Managed care offers Medicaid programs a way to reduce rising Medicaid expenditures and provide coordinated care to its enrollees. By paying managed care plans, such as HMOs, a fixed fee per person per month (i.e., a capitation fee), states are able to shift their risk for higher expenditures to a managed care plan. In addition, states should be able to monitor how well the managed care plan achieved specific goals, such as immunization rates, preventive care, reduced use of hospital EDs, and so on. Medicaid managed care has become an important approach to providing Medicaid services.

The largest change in the distribution of Medicaid expenditures has been the growth in Medicaid managed care. Almost all states rely on some form of managed care for their Medicaid populations. About 74 percent (as of 2011) of beneficiaries are enrolled in some form of managed care program. The types of managed care plans states use vary. Initially, many states used primary care case management, whereby beneficiaries are enrolled with a primary care gatekeeper, who does not assume financial risk but receives a monthly fee of about $2 to $3 per enrollee per month and is responsible for coordinating the enrollee's care. Under the primary care case management concept, providers themselves are paid fee-for-service. In the mid-1990s, many states moved toward contracting with HMOs and paying them a capitated amount for each enrolled Medicaid beneficiary. Under full-risk capitation, the HMO provides a comprehensive range of required benefits that includes preventive and acute care services.

States contract with managed care plans for two reasons. First, it reduces the rate of increase in Medicaid expenditures. Managed care produced substantial savings in the private sector. Similar savings have not occurred in fee-for-service Medicaid programs, where providers do not have similar incentives to decrease inpatient utilization, use less costly outpatient settings, and minimize unnecessary use of the ED.

Second, it expands Medicaid enrollees' access to care. To save money, Medicaid programs have reduced payments to hospitals and physicians (well below rates paid by other insurers) so that many providers refuse to serve Medicaid patients. Enrollees have typically had to rely on EDs and clinics that predominantly serve large numbers of Medicaid patients. By contracting with managed care plans, the states expect their enrollees to have greater access to primary care providers, receive coordinated care, and spend fewer dollars than previously. The percentage of Medicaid beneficiaries enrolled in managed care plans has increased rapidly—from 4.5 percent in 1991 to 74 percent in 2011.

Medicaid managed care programs have a great deal of experience caring for relatively young demographic groups, such as children and working-age adults, similar to their commercial businesses. However, these population groups—children and nondisabled, low-income adults (who make up about 74 percent of Medicaid beneficiaries)—account for a relatively small share of Medicaid spending (about 35 percent of Medicaid expenditures). Managed care plans have had less experience in caring for chronically ill and disabled populations, a more difficult group for which to provide managed care but for whom the potential savings of coordinated care is much greater. The aged, blind, and disabled as well as those in nursing homes (about 26 percent of beneficiaries) account for most Medicaid expenditures (about 65 percent). Until managed care plans enroll and manage care for the chronically ill, those with severe mental illness, and the institutionalized aged who require long-term care, Medicaid managed care savings will not be very large (CMS 2013b).

If managed care plans are to enroll these more costly Medicaid beneficiaries, states must provide these plans with appropriate financial incentives. State capitation payments should reflect the costs of caring for different types of beneficiaries (risk-adjusted payments). If the payment rate is set too low, managed care plans will be unwilling to enroll high-cost groups. To date, it has been difficult to develop capitation rates that adequately reflect the costs of caring for elderly and chronically ill population groups.

In addition, it is necessary for state Medicaid programs to monitor the care provided and the access to care by beneficiaries in any delivery system, whether it is managed care or traditional fee-for-service. Unfortunately, many states' performance in monitoring the quality of care their Medicaid populations receive has been notoriously inadequate. For budgetary reasons, some states are unwilling to monitor and punish low-performing providers. Nursing home scandals continue to surface, and many Medicaid programs' quality of care and accessibility are inadequate. Private insurers use various monitoring mechanisms and financial incentives, such as pay for performance, to reward providers who practice high-quality care. It remains to be seen how well state agencies will use the quality information they receive to similarly reward or penalize Medicaid providers.

Block-Granting Medicaid

Federal law restricts the ability of states to change Medicaid benefits. To make such changes, a state must apply for a federal waiver, which is a time-consuming process. Having the federal government provide to the states block grants based on a fixed amount per Medicaid beneficiary, which would increase by an inflation index, has been proposed as a means of limiting the open-ended financing commitment by federal and state governments. Currently, the federal government matches (by 50 percent to 73 percent) what states spend on Medicaid.

Many state governors would prefer receiving federal block grants in return for greater state flexibility in the design of Medicaid benefits and administration. Fewer restrictions on how states spend Medicaid dollars would enable them to be more innovative in providing care to their Medicaid population; improving access to care; and reducing their Medicaid budgets, which are crowding out state expenditures on education and public safety. Block grants would also improve equity among the states because wealthier states that can afford to spend more receive a greater amount of federal Medicaid funds. The Medicaid benefits received by the poor vary greatly depending on where they live.

Several states have experimented with federal Medicaid waivers, and not all have had favorable outcomes. An important reason for the success of waivers in Rhode Island and Washington has been careful planning and engaging important interest groups, such as the medical societies. Too rapid an implementation causes confusion among providers and recipients. Low payment rates, failure to adequately adjust risk-based payments, and adverse selection negatively affected the implementation of Tennessee's reforms (Beaulier and Pizzola 2012). Rhode Island, for example, was able to reduce Medicaid costs while increasing patient's access and reducing the use of EDs for routine visits. Reduced admissions to nursing homes by better case management programs for Medicaid patients with asthma, diabetes, and heart problems as well as home care subsidies to provide long-term care patients services in the home and in a community-based facility all saved money for Rhode Island (Lewin Group 2011).

States could mine utilization data to determine patients at high risk and offer preventive services to minimize costly hospital admissions. States could fund nonmedical services, such as supportive housing for the mentally ill; allow Medicare/Medicaid patients to use Medicaid funds for services, such as caregivers, that enable them to remain in their residence rather than enter a nursing home; and permit Medicaid patients to get care from nurse practitioners in a retail medical clinic rather than doctors in the ED. Care management techniques can reduce ED use and improve health outcomes for adults with chronic diseases. Increasing home and community-based services would decrease the number of nursing home users.

Block grants would have to be adjusted by type of Medicaid recipient—child, young adult, person with an addiction-related illness, or patient in a nursing home; otherwise, states could game the system by enrolling more low-cost people, such as children. The federal government's ongoing monitoring of the health outcomes of state programs that receive block grants would alleviate the concern that the poor would be harmed by states not providing necessary services and access to care. Medicaid block grants (per capita) also would be counter-cyclical economic policy. In an economic downturn, as more people qualify for Medicaid, the total block grant would increase—as compared to the current situation in which the state receives less tax revenues and cutbacks are made when instead there should be an increase (Cassidy 2013).

Many state governors have requested waivers providing fewer Medicaid funds in exchange for greater flexibility in how they spend those dollars. Allowing states to receive block grants with fewer rules and mandates would encourage greater experimentation with approaches to care for the poor, disabled, and elderly populations that are more satisfactory but less expensive. Other states would be able to copy those approaches that improve health outcomes and better meet the needs of their Medicaid populations.

Income-Related Vouchers

Another Medicaid reform proposal is to do away with sharp eligibility levels and instead include all those with low income through an income-related voucher. The size of the subsidy would decline as income grows, and the person would be able to use his voucher to choose among competing managed care plans. Because those receiving a subsidy would lose only a portion of their subsidized voucher as their incomes rose, they would no longer have a disincentive to accept a low-paying job. An income-related voucher would eliminate the large differences among states in the percentage of their populations eligible for Medicaid.[3]

The ACA provides income-related subsidies only to those whose income is between 133 percent and 400 percent of the FPL and who buy private insurance through the state insurance exchanges. It would be preferable to treat everyone, including those on Medicaid, in the same way and permit them to also buy private insurance on the state exchanges.

An income-related subsidy would improve efficiency (and equity) while reinforcing the movement toward Medicaid managed care, with its emphasis on coordinated care, better access to primary care physicians, and incentives to provide care in less costly settings.

To be effective in having health plans compete for Medicaid enrollees, the income-related voucher should be risk adjusted; specifically, chronically ill enrollees should receive more valuable vouchers than those who are younger and in better health. Risk-adjusted premiums will induce health plans to compete for chronically ill enrollees and to develop disease management programs to better care for them.

When Medicaid beneficiaries have a choice among managed care plans, managed care firms have an incentive to compete for Medicaid patients. States, however, need to provide the Medicaid population with relevant information on their plan choices. To the extent that beneficiaries do not choose and are assigned to a managed care plan, the role of choice in disciplining plan performance is negated. To reduce Medicaid expenditures, attention must be focused on those groups consuming the largest portion of Medicaid expenditures—namely the chronically ill and people with disabilities. (These groups are also the fastest-growing segment of the Medicaid population.) The challenge for the states in the coming years is to include these vulnerable population groups in managed care, pay managed care plans appropriately for their care, and vigorously monitor the care they receive.

Medicaid's movement to managed care has made survival difficult for many "safety-net" providers, such as public and not-for-profit hospitals and community clinics that have traditionally served large Medicaid and uninsured populations. These providers rely on disproportionate-share hospital payments and need Medicaid patients if they are to survive. As managed care firms seek less expensive hospital settings and cut down inpatient use, these safety-net providers must become part of a network that competes for Medicaid capitation contracts. Unless they are able to do so, their financial stability is threatened. The loss of safety-net providers would be unfortunate, as an income-related voucher will not likely be enacted in the near future. Until then, those without private insurance or Medicaid coverage will need access to medical care, which is likely to be delivered primarily by safety-net providers.

Summary

Medicaid is a means-tested program that pays for the medical care provided to those with low income. Although state Medicaid programs are federally required to serve designated population groups, states have discretion to include additional medical services and population groups in their programs. Medicaid does not cover all those with low income or all of the uninsured. In contrast to Medicare, Medicaid recipients and their supporters are not able to provide legislators with political support. For these reasons, the generosity of Medicaid programs (eligibility levels and included services) varies across states, and Congress does not mandate the level of funding as it does with Medicare.

(Medicare is a defined-benefit program to specific population groups, which requires the federal government to fund those benefits.) In times of budget difficulties, many states attempt to reduce their deficits by cutting Medicaid eligibility and benefits.

In 2014, the ACA expanded Medicaid eligibility. A major problem is that the higher number of newly and previously eligible beneficiaries greatly increased the demand for physician services. Unless Medicaid raises physician fees, beneficiaries will not have more access to coordinated care but instead will have to rely on hospital EDs.

Several approaches have been proposed to increase Medicaid's effectiveness. Providing beneficiaries with the option to use managed care plans will increase their access to care because plans will be able to lower the costs of caring for Medicaid patients by providing coordinated care and boosting physician productivity. Instituting a federal income-related subsidy to all those eligible for Medicaid would improve equity among those with low income who live in different states and give them an incentive to earn more without the fear of completely losing their Medicaid eligibility. Block-granting Medicaid to the states in return for fewer federal regulations will permit each state to innovate in how medical services are provided, which in turn provides greater patient satisfaction at lower cost.

An important challenge facing Medicaid reform are the most costly Medicaid beneficiaries—people with disabilities and long-term care patients in nursing homes. The current Medicaid system has not performed adequately in this arena, and managed care plans have to demonstrate their ability to care for such patients.

Importantly, the federal government has a huge debt and large annual deficits. The ACA will further increase federal expenditures and the deficit. The financial markets will soon place great pressure on the federal government to reduce its deficits. Medicaid is an important contributor to federal deficit spending, and its recipients are less politically powerful than Medicare and Social Security beneficiaries. Thus, changes in Medicaid's financing and eligibility are likely to occur.

Discussion Questions

1. Describe the Medicaid program. What are the differences between Medicare and Medicaid?
2. How well does Medicaid achieve its objectives?
3. Why would it be difficult to enroll all of the Medicaid population in HMOs?
4. What are some approaches to reforming Medicaid?

5. What are the arguments for and against having one government pro-
    gram instead of both Medicare and Medicaid?
6. What does the ACA do with respect to the Medicaid program?

Notes

1. As part of deficit-reduction legislation in 2005, Congress included
    limits on the ability of people with homes and assets to get Medicaid
    to pay their nursing home costs. The legislation toughened rules that
    prevent individuals seeking to become Medicaid eligible from trans-
    ferring assets—usually to their children. Examples of these changes
    include lengthening the time period in which states can examine
    the inappropriate transfer of assets to five years and excluding from
    Medicaid coverage those people whose home equity is in excess of
    $500,000 (previously, a home equity limit did not exist).
2. States have used various financing schemes to inappropriately increase
    federal Medicaid payments. For example, a state may impose a $100
    million tax on its hospitals and then return those funds to the hos-
    pitals in the form of Medicaid expenditures. The state then receives
    federal Medicaid matching funds of $100 million to $200 million,
    depending on its matching formula. Once the state receives the fed-
    eral matching payments, it can substitute those funds for its share
    of future Medicaid spending or even for non-Medicaid purposes (if
    the state does not return the full amount of the tax payments to the
    hospitals). Because all states, except Alaska, game the system by using
    these "provider taxes" to raise federal Medicaid spending, Congress
    has been reluctant to close this loophole.
3. To provide income-related subsidies, Medicaid would have to be fed-
    eralized. States would continue to spend what they currently spend,
    and the federal government would have to pay for the difference
    between what is currently spent and what is required for an equal
    income-related subsidy across all states.

References

Baicker, K., S. Taubman, H. Allen, M. Bernstein, J. H. Gruber, J. P. Newhouse, E.
    C. Schneider, B. J. Wright, A. M. Zaslavsky, and A. N. Finkelstein. 2013.
    "The Oregon Experiment—Effects of Medicaid on Clinical Outcomes."
    New England Journal of Medicine 368 (18): 1713–22. www.nejm.org/doi/
    pdf/10.1056/NEJMsa1212321.

Beaulier, S., and B. Pizzola. 2012. "The Political Economy of Medicaid Reform: Evidence from Five Reforming States." *Mercatus on Policy* No. 107, April. Fairfax, VA: Mercatus Center, George Mason University.

California Department of Health Care Services (DHCS). 2013. *California Partnership for Long-Term Care,* Issue 21. Published November. www.dhcs .ca.gov/services/ltc/Documents/IB2014.pdf.

Cassidy, A. 2013. "Per Capita Caps in Medicaid." *Health Affairs/RWJF Health Policy Briefs* 32 (4). www.rwjf.org/en/research-publications/find-rwjf-research/2013/04/per-capita-caps-in-medicaid.html.

Centers for Medicare & Medicaid Services (CMS). 2014a. "Projected." Last modified November. http://cms.gov/Research-Statistics-Data-and-Systems/Statistics-Trends-and-Reports/NationalHealthExpendData/NationalHealthAccountsProjected.html.

———. 2014b. "CMS-64 Quarterly Expense Report." Medicaid Budget and Expenditures System (MBES), FY2012 Net Expenditures. Accessed January. http://medicaid.gov/Medicaid-CHIP-Program-Information/By-Topics/Data-and-Systems/MBES/CMS-64-Quarterly-Expense-Report.html.

———. 2013a. "State Medicaid and CHIP Income Eligibility Standards Effective January 1, 2014." Table. Accessed March 2014. www.medicaid.gov/AffordableCareAct/Medicaid-Moving-Forward-2014/Downloads/Medicaid-and-CHIP-Eligibility-Levels-Table_HHsize4.pdf.

———. 2013b. *2012 Actuarial Report on the Financial Outlook for Medicaid.* Accessed March 2014. http://medicaid.gov/Medicaid-CHIP-Program-Information/By-Topics/Financing-and-Reimbursement/Downloads/medicaid-actuarial-report-2012.pdf.

———. 2013c. *CMS Statistics Reference Booklet.* Various editions. Tables on Medicaid and CHIP enrollments. www.cms.gov/Research-Statistics-Data-and-Systems/Statistics-Trends-and-Reports/CMS-Statistics-Reference-Booklet/2013.html.

Congressional Budget Office (CBO). 2013. *Medicaid Spending and Enrollment Detail for CBO's May Baseline, 2013.* Accessed March 2014. www.cbo.gov/sites/default/files/cbofiles/attachments/44204-2013-05-Medicaid.pdf.

Decker, S. 2009. "Changes in Medicaid Physician Fees and Patterns of Ambulatory Care." *Inquiry* 46: 291–304.

Genworth Financial Inc. 2013. *Genworth 2013: Cost of Care Survey,* 10th ed. Accessed March 2014. www.genworth.com/dam/Americas/US/PDFs/Consumer/corporate/130568_032213_Cost%20of%20Care_Final_nonsecure.pdf.

Gruber, J., and K. Simon. 2008. "Crowd-Out Ten Years Later: Have Recent Expansions of Public Insurance Crowded Out Private Health Insurance?" *Journal of Health Economics* 27 (2): 201–17.

Kaiser Family Foundation. 2014. "Table 1: Medicaid and CHIP Income Eligibility Limits for Children as a Percent of the Federal Poverty Level as of January 2014." Accessed March. http://kaiserfamilyfoundation.files.wordpress .com/2014/01/7993-04-tables-where-are-states-today-medicaid-and-chip-eligibility-levels.pdf.

———. 2013. "Medicaid: A Primer—Key Information on the Nation's Health Coverage Program for Low-Income People." Published March. www.kff .org/medicaid/7334.cfm.

Lewin Group. 2011. *An Independent Evaluation of Rhode Island's Global Waiver.* Published December. www.ohhs.ri.gov/documents/documents11/Lewin_ report_12_6_11.pdf.

Sonier, J., M. Boudreaux, and L. Blewett. 2013. "Medicaid 'Welcome-Mat' Effect of Affordable Care Act Implementation Could Be Substantial." *Health Affairs* 32 (7): 1319–25.

Taubman, S. L., H. Allen, B. Wright, K. Baicker, and A. Finkelstein. 2014. "Medicaid Increases Emergency-Department Use: Evidence from Oregon's Health Insurance Experiment." *Science* 343 (6168): 263–68.

US Census Bureau. 2013. "Current Population Survey." Accessed March 2014. www.census.gov/cps/data/cpstablecreator.html.

US Department of Health and Human Services (HHS). 2014. "2014 Poverty Guidelines." Accessed January. http://aspe.hhs.gov/poverty/ 14poverty.cfm.

Zuckerman, S., A. Williams, and K. Stockley. 2009. "Trends in Medicaid Physician Fees, 2003–2008." *Health Affairs* 28 (3): w510–w519.

HOW DOES MEDICARE PAY PHYSICIANS?   **10**

I n 2012, fee-for-service Medicare spent more than $68 billion on physician services (CBO 2013a). Medicare represents, on average, more than 20 percent of total physician revenues (about 23 percent in 2011), although for many physicians and specialties it represents a sizable portion of revenues. As such, understanding how Medicare pays physicians is important. In 1992, a new payment system was instituted for physician services under Medicare. Why was it necessary to change the system? How does the new payment system compare with the previous one? What are the effects of this new payment system on access to care by Medicare patients, on physician fees paid by the nonaged working population, and on physicians' income? And what are the likely changes to Medicare payment for physician services?

Previous Medicare Physician Payment System

When Medicare Part A (which pays for hospital care) was enacted in 1965, Part B (which pays for physician and out-of-hospital services) was included. (Part B is a voluntary benefit for which the aged pay a monthly premium that covers only 25 percent of the total cost of that program.) Physicians were paid on a fee-for-service basis and given the choice to participate (including for some medical claims but not others). When physicians participated, they agreed to accept the Medicare fee for that service, and the patient was responsible for only 20 percent of that fee after she paid the annual deductible.

If a physician was not a participant, the patient would have to pay the physician's entire charge (which was higher than the Medicare fee) and apply for reimbursement from Medicare. When the government reimbursed the patient, it would pay the patient only 80 percent of the Medicare-approved fee for that service. Thus, a patient who visited a nonparticipating physician would have to pay 20 percent of the physician's Medicare-approved fee plus the difference between the approved fee and the actual charges. This difference is referred to as *balance billing*. Medicare patients who saw nonparticipating physicians were also burdened by the paperwork involved with sending their bills to Medicare for reimbursement.

Physicians' fees and Medicare expenditures rapidly increased, and in 1972 the government placed a limit—referred to as the Medicare Economic Index—on physicians' Medicare fee increases. Physicians' fees, however, continued to rise sharply in the private sector, and as the difference between private-physician charges and the Medicare-approved fees became larger, fewer physicians chose to participate in Medicare. Consequently, more of the aged were balance billed for the difference between their physician's fee and the Medicare-approved fee.

Another consequence of limiting increases on participating physicians' charge was the possibility that physicians would encourage more visits and engage in more testing to raise their Medicare billings (called *induced demand*). Even with limits on physicians' fees, Part B expenditures continued to increase rapidly, as shown in Exhibit 8.5.

Reasons for Adopting the New Payment System

The new Medicare physician payment system was adopted for three reasons.

The first and most important reason was the federal government's desire to limit the increase in the federal budget deficit, an issue of great political concern in the early 1990s. In 1992, physicians received 75 percent of all Part B payments (this has decreased to 30 percent as of 2009); the remaining expenditures were for other nonhospital services (this portion was growing rapidly at approximately 10 percent per year). Part B expenditures rose from $777 million in 1967 to more than $50 billion by 1992 and were expected to continue to climb. In 2012, Part B expenditures reached $232 billion; they are expected to be $431 billion by 2023 (CBO 2013a). As Medicare physician payments continued to increase, the government's portion of the cost of the program—75 percent of the total (again, the aged paid a monthly premium that covered only 25 percent of Part B expenditures)—contributed directly to the growing federal budget deficit. Both Republican and Democratic administrations believed that if the government reduced the size of the federal deficit, the growth in Part B expenditures had to be slowed. The government, however, was constrained in the approaches it could take to limit Part B expenditures. Given the political power of the elderly, the government was reluctant to ask seniors to pay higher Part B premiums or to increase their cost sharing. Furthermore, the government could not simply limit Medicare physician fees for fear that physicians would decrease their Medicare participation, which would adversely affect the aged.

Thus, the second reason Part B was changed was that members of Congress were concerned that unless they ensured that the aged had access to physicians, they would lose their political support at election time. As limits were placed on Medicare physician fee increases, fewer physicians were willing to participate (accept Medicare payment), so more seniors were either charged additional amounts by nonparticipating physicians (balance billed) or, if they could not afford the additional payments, had to face decreased access to physician services. Congress wanted to increase physician participation in Medicare.

Third, many physicians and academicians believed the previous Medicare payment system was inequitable and inefficient. A newly graduated physician establishing a fee schedule with Medicare could receive higher fees than could an older physician whose fee increases were limited by the Medicare Economic Index. Physicians who performed procedures such as diagnostic testing and surgery were paid at a much higher rate per unit of physician time than were physicians who performed cognitive services, such as office examinations. Medicare fees for the same procedure varied greatly across geographic areas and were unrelated to differences in practice costs. The fee-for-service payment system encouraged inefficiency by rewarding physicians who performed more services. These inequities and inefficiencies caused differences in physician income and affected their choice of specialty and practice location.

Components of the New Payment System

Reducing the federal deficit by limiting Part B expenditures, achieving greater Medicare fee equity among physicians, and limiting the aged's payments led to the three main parts of the physician payment reform package. The inefficiencies inherent in the fee-for-service system were not addressed by the new payment system.

Resource-Based Relative Value Scale Fee Schedule

The first, and most publicized, part of the physician payment reform package was the creation of a resource-based relative value scale (RBRVS) fee schedule. The RBRVS attempted to approximate the cost of performing each physician service. Its premise was that, in the long run, in a competitive market, the price of a service will reflect the cost of producing that service. Thus, the payment for each physician service should reflect his resource costs. However, this cost-based approach to determining relative values was complex, as it required a great deal of data; relied on interviews; was based on certain assumptions, such as the time required to perform certain tasks; and needed to be continually updated because any of the elements of cost and time could change.

Three resource components were used to construct the fee for a particular service. The first—the work component—estimated the cost of providing a particular service, including the time, intensity, skill, mental effort, and stress involved.[1] The second were the physician's practice expenses, such as salaries and rent. The third was malpractice insurance, because its cost varies across specialties. Each component was assigned a relative value that was summed to form the total relative value of the service; the greater the costs and time needed, the higher the relative value unit (RVU) was. A procedure with a value of 20 was believed to be twice as costly as one with a value of 10.

The actual fee was then determined by multiplying these RVUs by a politically determined conversion factor. For example, "transplantation of the heart" was assigned 44.13 work RVUs, 49.24 practice-expense RVUs, and 9.17 malpractice RVUs for a total of 102.54 RVUs. The 1992 conversion factor was $31, making the fee for this procedure $3,178 ($31 × 102.54). This fee was then adjusted for geographic location. (The initial conversion factor was set so that total payments under the new system would be the same as under the previous one—that is, the system was "budget neutral.") A separate conversion factor was used for surgical services, primary care, and other nonsurgical services. (In 1998, a single conversion factor was instituted for all services.) Exhibit 10.1 illustrates how the RBRVS and the conversion factor are used to calculate the fee for a visit to an office (located in the Anaheim, Santa Ana, region in California).

RBRVS reduces the variation in fees both within specialties and across geographic regions. New physicians receive 80 percent of the Medicare fee schedule in their first year, and the percentage rises to 100 percent by the fifth year. Medicare fees can still vary geographically by 12 percent less and 18 percent more than the average, but this is greatly reduced from the previous

EXHIBIT 10.1
Calculations of Physician Payment Rate Under RBRVS Office Visit (Mid-Level), Anaheim, Santa Ana (California), 2013

	Relative Value		Geographic Adjustment	Adjusted Relative Value
Physician work	0.97	×	1.04	1.01
Physician expense*	1.09	×	1.22	1.33
PLI**	0.07	×	0.68	0.05
				2.39
			Conversion factor ×	34.02
			Payment rate	$81.31

* Nonfacility practice expense
** PLI: Professional liability insurance

geographic variation. As a result, fees dropped for physicians in California, whereas fees in Mississippi increased by 11 percent.

The new payment system reflected the cost of performing 7,000 different physician services, including visits, procedures, imaging, and tests. When constructing the RBRVS fee structure, Harvard professor William Hsiao and colleagues (1988) found that physician fees were not closely related to the resource costs needed to produce those services. In general, cognitive services (such as patient evaluation, counseling, and management of services) were greatly undervalued compared with procedural services (such as surgery and testing). The RBRVS reduces the profitability of procedures while increasing payment for cognitive services. By changing the relative weights of different types of services, the system caused substantial shifts in payments—and consequently incomes—among physicians. In large metropolitan areas, for example, surgeons' fees declined by 25 percent. The "winners" and "losers" among physician specialties after the new system was introduced are shown in Exhibit 10.2.

Medicare Expenditure Limit

The RBRVS approach is still fee-for-service payment and by itself does not control volume, mix of services, or total physician expenditures. Because the government was concerned that physicians would induce demand to offset their lower Medicare fees, the second part of the new payment system limited overall physician Medicare expenditures. This limit was achieved by linking the annual update on physician fees (the conversion factor) to the

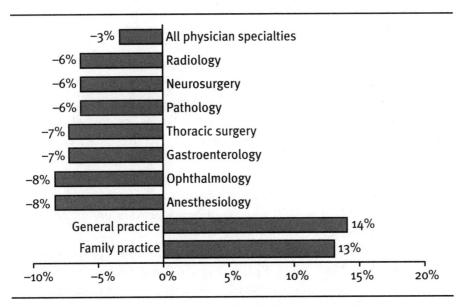

EXHIBIT 10.2
Medicare Physician Fee Schedule Effect on Fees, by Specialty, 1992

SOURCE: Data from US Senate Subcommittee on Medicare and Long-Term Care (1991).

growth in volume and mix of services. If volume grew more rapidly than a target rate based on increases in inflation, number of beneficiaries, newly covered services, and technological advances, Congress would lower the annual fee update the following year. Too rapid an increase in services would result in a smaller fee update.

As it turned out, volume and mix of services grew less rapidly than expected for surgical services. Consequently, to maintain the target rate of Medicare payments for surgical services, the conversion factor increased more rapidly. These changes in fees were unrelated to any supply or demand changes for such services.

As part of the Balanced Budget Act of 1997, the annual update method was changed. The sustainable growth rate (SGR) in Medicare physician expenditures became the new government objective. The SGR was designed to reduce physician fee updates if physician spending growth exceeded a specified target. This new system holds Medicare spending growth for physician services to that of the general economy (the gross domestic product [GDP]), adjusting for several factors. (Tying the SGR to GDP per capita represented an affordability criteria—how much the government could afford to subsidize physician Part B expenditures.)

The SGR consists of four elements:

1. The percentage increase in real GDP per capita
2. A medical inflation rate of physician fee increases
3. The annual percentage increase in Part B enrollees (other than Medicare Advantage enrollees)
4. The percentage change in spending for physicians' services resulting from changes in laws and regulations (e.g., expanded Medicare coverage for preventive services)

Under the SGR system, physician fee updates are adjusted up or down depending on whether actual spending has fallen below or has exceeded the target. Over time, fees tend to rise at least as fast as the cost of providing physician services as long as volume (number of services provided to each beneficiary) and intensity growth (complexity and costliness of those services) remain below a specified rate—about 1.5 percent per year. If volume and intensity grow faster than the specified rate, the SGR lowers fee increases or causes fees to fall. The SGR formula does not provide any incentives for *individual* physicians to control volume growth.

During the late 1990s and early 2000s, physicians received generous fee increases from Medicare (5.4 percent in 2000 and 4.5 percent in 2001). However, the government then revised upward its estimate of previous years' actual physician expenditures and lowered the spending target on the basis of revised GDP data. Physician fees dropped by 5.4 percent in 2002, a decline that was, in part, a correction for fees that had been set too high in previous years because of errors in forecasting. Physician fees were also to be decreased in subsequent years to recoup excess spending accumulated from averted cuts in previous years and partly because real spending per beneficiary (volume and intensity) on physician services increased faster than allowed under the SGR. Responding to pressure from physicians and concerned about Medicare patients' access to care after the 2002 reduction in physician fees, Congress repealed all scheduled fee reductions, which, if implemented all at once, would total almost 25 percent in 2014 (CBO 2013b).

In Exhibit 10.3, the years 2000 to 2013 describe actual physician updates. The sharp decline in physician fees for 2014 shows the accumulated required fee decreases according to the SGR formula. However, as in previous years, Congress overrode the 25 percent scheduled fee decrease and pushed them further into the future.

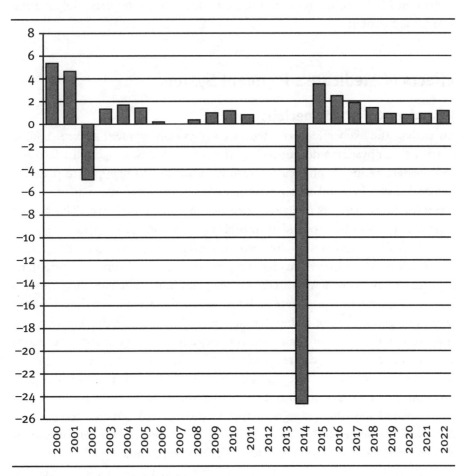

EXHIBIT 10.3
Recent and Projected Payment Updates for Physician Services

SOURCE: Data from CMS (2013), Table IV.B1.

Congress faces a dilemma. Recognizing that rapid expenditure growth in Medicare physician expenditures is not sustainable, Congress can maintain fiscal discipline by relying on an automatic mechanism, such as the SGR. By doing so, however, Congress risks having physicians limit their participation with Medicare, thereby dramatically reducing Medicare beneficiaries' access to physician services. Tying Medicare physician fees to economic growth completely ignores changes in physician supply and demand.

Balance-Billing Limit

The third part of the new payment system limits the amount physicians are able to balance bill Medicare patients. Physicians can no longer participate in Medicare for some patients but not others. Few physicians are able to forgo such a significant source of revenue. Physicians who decide not to participate in Medicare still cannot charge a Medicare patient more than 109 percent of the Medicare-approved fee. Thus, even physicians who decide not to participate in Medicare are restricted in how much they can charge for treating a Medicare patient.

Effects of Medicare's Payment System

Procedure-Oriented Specialists

To analyze the likely effects of Medicare's physician payment system, assume initially that physicians do not induce demand—that is, as specialist fees and incomes are reduced, physicians are not motivated to manipulate patients' demand. Keep in mind that physicians work in at least two markets: They serve Medicare patients and private or non-Medicare patients. (The private market could also be subdivided into HMO and non-HMO patients.)

RBRVS reduces fees for procedures and increases fees for cognitive services. With lower fees for surgery, for example, surgeons might be expected to perform fewer Medicare surgeries and reallocate their time to performing surgeries for private patients, whose fees were not reduced. However, if surgeons are not as busy as they would prefer, and the Medicare fee still exceeds the value of their time spent doing nonsurgical tasks, surgeons will not lower their Medicare surgeries. The effect of lower fees for procedures with no change in the number of procedures will decrease Medicare procedure-type expenditures and specialists' incomes.

Would specialists raise their fees to their private patients to make up for lower Medicare fees? Fees for private patients are presumably already at their highest level, which is consistent with making as much profit as possible from those patients. If specialists do not charge as much as the market will bear, they forgo income they could have earned. If private fees are increased beyond what the market will bear, the loss in revenue from lower volume would exceed the gain in revenue from those higher fees. The specialist would be worse off (see Chapter 17). A specialist might be able to increase her volume from private-pay patients by decreasing her fees to health plans to increase the number of private patients. Lowering the fee would be a more profitable strategy than raising it if the gain in revenue from higher volume more than offsets the loss in revenues from decreased fees.

Assume that before Medicare lowered specialist fees, specialists were allocating their time between private and Medicare patients so that the profit from each type of patient was the same. Once Medicare reduces its fees, the profit per hour of the specialist's time becomes greater when serving *private* patients. The specialist should serve fewer Medicare patients and more private patients. However, the only way the specialist can serve more private patients is to reduce her fees (to managed care organizations). Thus, the specialist would not likely want to or be able to cost shift to private patients.

If a specialist has excess capacity and does not attempt to induce demand, the aged would have the same access as before specialist fees were reduced. Specialists would provide the same volume of services, but their income would be reduced and overall Medicare expenditures for specialist services would decline.

Physicians who are willing to create demand to offset declines in their income would first attempt to induce demand among their private patients. A greater volume of private patients would be more profitable because the private fee has not been lowered. Only after private fees were reduced would the specialist create demand among the Medicare patients, whose fees had already been lowered. If specialists are not busy enough, they have probably already tried to induce as much demand as possible and would be unable to further induce demand. Instead, they might engage in such fraudulent practices as "code creep" as a way of increasing their Medicare fees.

Medicare expenditures and specialist incomes would still be expected to decline among physicians who are inclined to induce demand, assuming that these specialists previously had excess capacity. To the extent that demand inducers are able to engage in code creep, they will be able to offset some of the decline in their income. If specialists are fully busy, the reductions in Medicare specialist fees would result in a reallocation of specialists' time to private patients (whose fees are higher) and, consequently, less access by Medicare patients.

Given the excess capacity that existed among specialists, when Medicare introduced the RBRVS system and lowered Medicare fees to surgical specialties, the new fees likely reduced such specialists' incomes and the Medicare expenditures for such services but not Medicare patients' access to these services.

Primary Care Physicians

Under RBRVS, Medicare fees for cognitive services rose. Because the higher fees increase the profitability of Medicare patients, primary care physicians were expected to serve more Medicare patients and fewer private patients (assuming the Medicare fees are higher than private insurance fees). As physicians were expected to decrease their available time for private patients, and as demand exceeded the available physician time for private patients, fees for private patients were expected to increase. Total Medicare expenditures for cognitive services, particularly for primary care physicians, rose.

Primary care physicians who may otherwise have been willing to induce demand to raise their income might have been less inclined to do so because their income increased as a result of their higher fees. Those still inclined to induce demand would have found that it was more profitable to do so for their Medicare patients than for their private patients.

What was the RBRVS fee schedule's likely overall effect on expenditures? Assuming specialists were not busy enough, little additional demand inducement occurred, and (adjusting for the increased number of aged) Medicare Part B expenditures for specialists did not rise. Medicare expenditures for primary care physicians were expected to go up because their fees were raised; however, these increases were smaller than the decreases in specialist expenditures. Exhibit 8.5 illustrates these changes in the trend in Part B expenditures after the new physician payment system was introduced in 1992. (Part B expenditures have grown slightly more rapidly in recent years as a result of Congress shifting home health care expenditures from Part A to Part B in 1997 to solve an impending bankruptcy in the Part A Trust Fund.)

The expenditure limit that was part of the RBRVS system was meant to control demand inducement. Although specialists had excess capacity, demand inducement—hence volume of surgical services—was less than the government anticipated.

Concerns with Medicare's Physician Payment System

The SGR formula has, for a number of years, required decreases in physician fees, given that actual expenditure growth has exceeded SGR projected physician expenditures. Congress, concerned that decreasing physician fees will lessen the aged's access to care, has postponed these annual fee decreases. Under the law, the accumulated amount of these fee decreases, which will grow to 25 percent (in 2014), must be recouped by even larger fee reductions in the following year. Although Congress realizes that Medicare physician fees will not be cut by such a large amount, they are reluctant to change the SGR formula. To do so would mean that, according to budget rules, Congress would have to raise taxes, reduce other federal spending, or acknowledge a $175 billion increase in the federal deficit over the next ten years.[2] Given the political concern over increasing federal deficits, each Congress prefers to make adjustments one year at a time.

The SGR formula, by limiting increases in Medicare physician expenditures, was intended to provide physicians with an incentive to practice more efficiently, thereby not exceeding the overall expenditure limit. However, because the SGR is based on the aggregate Medicare payment for physician services, individual physicians have no incentive to limit their services. In fact, their incentive is to provide more services because the penalty of exceeding the aggregate Medicare spending limit will fall proportionately on all physicians. Those physicians who do limit their services are penalized. An overall spending limit cannot be effective unless the incentives are based on the behavior of individual physicians.

The elderly's demand for physicians continues to rise because of growth in the aged population (many baby boomers started retiring in 2011), advanced technologies, and legislated new benefits. The ACA further increased demand for physician services by expanding Medicaid eligibility (to 133 percent of the federal poverty level) and providing subsidies to those persons (whose income is between 133 percent to 400 percent of the federal poverty level) purchasing health insurance on newly formed state health insurance exchanges. With the increased demand for physician services, unless Congress allows for greater flexibility to allow for physician fee increases, shortages of primary care physicians will occur. As demand for care by Medicare, Medicaid, and private patients grows, primary care physicians will attempt to raise their fees. To the extent that Medicare fees remain less than those of private patients, physicians will find it more profitable to serve a greater number of private patients. As Congress limits Medicare fee increases to save money, the relative profitability to physicians of Medicare patients will continue to decline.

As Medicare fees fall relative to private fees, only by "raising" their Medicare fees—by such methods as reducing the time spent per Medicare visit, having the patient return more often, or performing more imaging tests (for which the physician receives payment)—would it be equally profitable for primary care physicians to continue seeing the same number of Medicare patients.

As the demand for Medicare services exceeds the amount physicians are willing to supply at Medicare's relatively lower fee, some primary care physicians have begun charging their Medicare patients an annual "concierge" fee of about $2,000. This fee is technically for services not provided under Medicare and provides a concierge patient with greater access to his physician. Because a concierge physician sees fewer patients, the shortage of primary care physicians is exacerbated for those who do not or are unable to pay such a fee. A concierge fee is an indication that the demand for physicians exceeds the supply at the fees Medicare is willing to pay.

To determine whether Medicare's physician fees are too low, thereby affecting Medicare patients' access to care, the Medicare Payment Advisory Commission (MedPAC) undertakes several types of surveys. The first is a survey of physicians' willingness to serve Medicare patients; the second is a survey of Medicare patients' access to care. Both surveys take several years to conduct and analyze before the results become available. Because of this delay, MedPAC conducts a telephone interview survey of Medicare beneficiaries and non-Medicare privately insured persons aged 50 years to 64 years to compare any differences in their access to physician services. As of 2012, these data indicate that access to care by Medicare patients was generally good, although some new Medicare patients were having difficulty finding a primary care physician[3] (MedPAC 2013, 83–90). In 2011, Medicare fees remained at about 82 percent of private insurer fees.

Unless the SGR formula is changed, projected reductions in Medicare physician fees for the next several years (under current law) will decrease Medicare patients' access to care, particularly as more baby boomers become eligible for Medicare, enrollment in Medicaid increases, and those eligible for subsidies join the state health insurance exchanges.

Given the delay in receiving information with which to evaluate the adequacy of Medicare physician fees in different parts of the country, MedPAC is unlikely to be able to bring Medicare demand and supply of physicians into equilibrium. In a normal market situation, rising doctor fees would indicate demand growing faster than supply and the need to take corrective action. But because balance billing—which acted as a market-driven indicator—is no longer allowed, no automatic mechanism exists to indicate a current shortage and hence access problems. According to a survey by the American Academy of Family Physicians, the proportion of family doctors who accepted new Medicare patients in 2012—81 percent—was down from 83 percent in 2010 (Beck 2013).

Physician fee schedules result in numerous problems. Certain services are "overvalued"—that is, their fee is too high relative to the cost or difficulty of providing the service. Overvalued services are more profitable than undervalued services (the fee is too low relative to the cost of providing the service). Thus, imaging and procedure-oriented services have increased more rapidly than services provided by primary care physicians. These differences in fees relative to their cost also affect the career choice of physicians, providing greater rewards to some specialties over others.

A single committee of the American Medical Association (AMA) decides on the time required for a physician (and different specialties) to perform various tasks, such as colonoscopies. These time requirements become part of the relative values used by Medicare for determining the fee for performing a particular medical service. However, a recent study has determined that the AMA's estimates of the time involved in many procedures are greatly overstated (Whoriskey and Keating 2013). Some of the physicians in the study performed procedures, that, according to the AMA's and Medicare's time estimates, have them working 24, 30, and even 50 hours a day.

Establishing a uniform fee schedule among physicians in the same specialty provides the wrong incentives to physicians. In a competitive market where fees vary, differences in fees for the same service will reflect differences in that service. For example, some physicians are of higher quality or spend more time listening to the patient's concerns. Although the service code may be nominally similar, the content of that service will vary. The costs of providing that service in terms of the physician's time differ. Medicare uniform fee schedules provide no incentive for physicians (other than their own integrity) to add value to their patients. Recently, Medicare initiated a Physician Quality Reporting System to encourage higher quality. However, the quality bonus is so small that it provides minimal incentive for physicians to change their behavior; the bonus is limited to only 0.5 percent of the previous year's Medicare payments to that provider. The physician's cost of collecting quality data will exceed any financial return from the program.

Patients are willing to pay more for certain physician attributes, such as their ability to relate to the patient. A uniform fee schedule provides perverse incentives by preventing a physician treating Medicare patients from charging for these extra attributes. Busy primary care physicians could provide additional visits and earn a higher income instead of spending time cultivating these attributes, which are not rewarded.

Proposed Physician Fee Changes

Various demonstration projects are being undertaken to change physicians' incentives from rewarding volume of services provided (fee-for-service) to improving quality and reducing medical costs (MedPAC 2010). One type of demonstration project is a bundled or episode-based payment—a single payment to a provider to cover all the services related to a specific disease or condition during a specific time period. The hospital, specialists, and primary care physicians involved in the patient's treatment would receive a specified amount (which they would have to share) for a patient's episode of care, such as a heart attack or a joint replacement, including follow-up care. Episode-based payment would require physicians and hospitals to more closely coordinate the patient's care. Each participant would have an incentive to be concerned with the efficiency and the coordination of care among specialists. The participants' performance outcome in providing an episode of care can be more easily evaluated in terms of quality compared to the care provided by other organizations for the same episode of illness.

Under pay for performance (P4P), physicians meeting certain quality guidelines, such as lower complication rates for knee arthroscopic surgery, receive higher payments. P4P offers incentives to physicians that are different from fee-for-service, in which quality is not rewarded. The National Commission on Physician Payment Reform also recommends that physician payment for "evaluation and management" services be raised. The current fee-for-service system provides a disincentive for physicians to spend time with patients having complex chronic conditions and to neglect illness prevention and disease management (National Commission on Physician Payment Reform 2013).

These examples of payment reform offer improved physician incentives for quality and care coordination; however, it will take a number of years before these payment systems become widespread among physicians. Until then, Medicare fee-for-service payment will continue to be the dominant method of paying for physician services (Ginsburg 2012). Nevertheless, it is important to reform Medicare fee-for-service to ensure that the relationship between fees and cost of providing services is uniform across all physician services and specialties, that payments for the same services are adjusted for differences in quality of care provided, and that greater incentives are provided for evaluation and management services.

Summary

The RBRVS national fee schedule (with expenditure controls and limits on balance billing) attempted to limit federal expenditures for Medicare physician services, improve equity among different medical specialties, and limit out-of-pocket payments and Part B premiums by the aged while increasing the aged's access to care. Medicare expenditures, however, will continue to rise as the number of eligible aged grows along with inflation, legislated new Medicare benefits, advances in technology, and increases in demand by newly insured patients.

Under the present Medicare SGR formula for paying physicians, Congress continually faces the decision between limiting Medicare physician fees and expenditures and decreasing the aged's access to care. Congress is unlikely to be able to accurately forecast the "right" rate of increase in Medicare expenditures (SGR) because it is more likely to be concerned with limiting the rise in Medicare expenditures than with properly adjusting for changes in the number of aged, inflation, and technology. The consequences to seniors of "too slow" an increase in Medicare expenditures will be a shortage of primary care services.

A uniform fee schedule cannot indicate that a shortage is developing in some geographic areas or among certain physician specialties, nor can uniform fees eliminate such shortages. Unless a national fee schedule is flexible and allows fees for some services, physicians, and geographic regions to grow more rapidly than others, shortages will arise and persist. Furthermore, delays in gathering survey data and data analysis to determine whether the elderly have physician access problems is likely to result in imbalances between physician supply and demand by Medicare patients.

Market-based fees provide information; they signal that changes have occurred in the costs of providing care, the demand for that care, or both. If the government does not want to overpay specialties and services that are in oversupply while underpaying those that are in short supply, a flexible payment mechanism is needed. Otherwise, the aged will find that they have reduced access to care, and the government will not be spending its money wisely. Movement toward episode-based payment and pay for performance offer the possibility of greater care coordination and improved efficiency, which are lacking in the fee-for-service payment system.

Discussion Questions

1. What were the reasons for developing a new Medicare physician payment system?
2. In what ways does the current physician payment system differ from the previous system?
3. What are the likely effects of Medicare's payment system on its patients' out-of-pocket expenses, Part B premiums, and access to physicians (primary care versus specialists)?
4. What, if any, are the likely effects of Medicare's payment system on patients in the non-Medicare (private) sector?
5. What are the likely effects of Medicare's physician payment system on physicians (by specialty)?
6. Contrast the likely effects of fee-for-service versus episode-based payment.

Notes

1. Two methods were used to estimate the complexity of a task: personal interviews and a modified Delphi technique in which each physician was able to compare her own estimate with the average of physicians within that specialty. Many assumptions were required; for

example, in calculating opportunity cost, it was assumed that the years required for training in a specialty were the minimum necessary. Further assumptions were made regarding the lengths of working careers across specialties, residency salaries, hours worked per week, and an interest rate to discount future earnings.

2. The recent slower growth in Medicare physician expenditures reduced the increase in the federal deficit that would be incurred by eliminating the SGR formula—from $275 billion in 2011 to $175 billion in 2013 (CBO 2013b).

3. A 2013 survey by Merritt Hawkins found an average acceptance rate by physicians of new Medicare patients of 75 percent, indicating that Medicare patients have access problems in a number of physician markets (Miller 2014). For example, the family practice physician acceptance rate for new Medicare patients was 42 percent in New York City and 55 percent in Dallas and Denver.

References

Beck, M. 2013. "More Doctors Steer Clear of Medicare." *Wall Street Journal*, July 29, page A4.

Centers for Medicare & Medicaid Services (CMS). 2013. *2013 Annual Report of the Boards of Trustees of the Federal Hospital Insurance and Federal Supplementary Medical Insurance Trust Funds.* Accessed September. www .cms.gov/Research-Statistics-Data-and-Systems/Statistics-Trends-and-Reports/ReportsTrustFunds/Downloads/TR2013.pdf.

Congressional Budget Office (CBO). 2013a. "CBO's May 2013 Medicare Baseline." Accessed September. www.cbo.gov/sites/default/files/cbofiles/ attachments/44205-2013-05-Medicare.pdf.

———. 2013b. "Cost Estimate, H.R. 2810, Medicare Patient Access and Quality Improvement Act of 2013." Published September. www.cbo.gov/sites/ default/files/cbofiles/attachments/hr2810.pdf.

Ginsburg, P. B. 2012. "Fee-for-Service will Remain a Feature of Major Payment Reforms, Requiring More Changes in Medicare Physician Payment." *Health Affairs* 31 (9): 1977–83.

Hsiao, W. C., P. Braun, D. Yntema, and E. R. Becker. 1988. "Estimating Physicians' Work for a Resource-Based Relative Value Scale." *New England Journal of Medicine* 319 (13): 835–41.

Medicare Payment Advisory Commission (MedPAC). 2013. *Report to the Congress, Medicare Payment Policy.* Published March. www.medpac.gov/documents/ Mar13_entirereport.pdf.

————. 2010. "Appendix A." In *Report to the Congress: Aligning Incentives in Medicare.* http://medpac.gov/documents/Jun10_EntireReport.pdf.

Miller, P. 2014. *2014 Survey of Physician Appointment Wait Times and Medicaid and Medicare Acceptance Rates.* Irving, TX: Merritt Hawkins. www .merritthawkins.com/uploadedFiles/MerrittHawkings/Surveys/ mha2014waitsurvPDF.pdf.

National Commission on Physician Payment Reform. 2013. *Report of the National Commission on Physician Payment Reform.* Published March. http:// physicianpaymentcommission.org/wp-content/uploads/2012/02/ physician_payment_report.pdf.

US Senate Subcommittee on Medicare and Long-Term Care. 1991. "Medicare Physician Payment Reform Regulations." Hearing before the Subcommittee on Medicare and Long-Term Care of the Committee on Finance, July 19.

Whoriskey, P., and D. Keating. 2013. "How a Secretive Panel Uses Data That Distort Doctors' Pay." *Washington Post*, July 20. www.washingtonpost.com/ business/economy/how-a-secretive-panel-uses-data-that-distorts-doctors- pay/2013/07/20/ee134e3a-eda8-11e2-9008-61e94a7ea20d_story_4 .html.

THE IMPENDING SHORTAGE OF PHYSICIANS **11**

About every 10 to 20 years, concern arises that the United States is producing either too many or too few physicians. In 1992, the Council on Graduate Medical Education (COGME), which advises the government on the size of the physician workforce and its training, warned that by 2000 a surplus of specialists would be seen—as high as 15 to 30 percent of all physicians—as well as a shortage of primary care physicians (COGME 1992). Evidence for the belief in a large physician surplus was the rapid growth occurring in the number of active physicians, which increased from 435,000 in 1980, to 573,000 in 1990, to 738,000 in 2000, to 870,000 in 2011. When adjusted for population, the number of active physicians per 100,000 population (the physician-to-population ratio) increased from 195 in 1980, to 234 in 1990, to 270 in 2000, to 283 in 2011 (see Exhibit 4.1 in Chapter 4). Some researchers, assuming that a large portion of the US population would be enrolled in HMOs, compared the relatively low physician ratio within HMOs to the national physician ratio and claimed that an overall surplus of 165,000 physicians (or 30 percent of the total number of patient care physicians) would occur by 2000. A 30 percent surplus in the number of specialists was also projected.

The projected physician surplus was expected to have adverse effects on physician income—especially specialist income—for many years. To forestall such surpluses, COGME and physician organizations recommended reducing medical school enrollments, decreasing the number of specialists and increasing the number of primary care physicians (from 30 percent to 50 percent of all physicians), and limiting the number of foreign medical school graduates entering the United States.

By 2005, COGME issued a new report warning that an overall shortfall of 85,000 to 95,000 physicians is likely by 2020 (COGME 2005). A 2012 study by the American Association of Medical Colleges (AAMC) similarly predicted a shortage of 62,900 physicians by 2015, growing to more than 90,000 by 2020 (45,000 primary care physicians and 46,000 surgeons and medical specialists) and creating a deficit of 130,000 physicians by 2025 (AAMC Center for Workforce Studies 2012). This expected shortfall is the result of several factors, one of which is the demand for physicians will sharply increase because of the 30 million newly insured under the Affordable Care

Act (ACA) and the growing number of aged (who have the highest needs for care). Though the supply of physicians has been rising, more physicians are leaving primary care because of decreased fees, fewer medical students are choosing a primary care specialty because the income is lower than in other medical specialties, and about one-third of all physicians are expected to retire by 2020. The shortage is becoming more severe and will adversely affect the most vulnerable members of the population.

What is the basis for these projections of physician surpluses and shortage? What is an economic definition of a physician surplus or shortage? What are the consequences and self-correcting mechanisms of a shortage or surplus?

Definitions of a Physician Shortage or Surplus

Physician-to-Population Ratio

Different approaches have been used to determine whether a shortage (or surplus) exists in a profession. One approach often taken in the health field is a physician-to-population ratio. This ratio often relies on a value judgment about how much care people should receive or on a professional determination of how many physician services are appropriate for the population.

In this method, generally the existing physician-to-population ratio is compared with the physician-to-population ratio likely to occur in some future period. First, the *supply ratio* is projected by estimating the future population and the likely number of medical graduates that will be added to the stock of physicians (less the expected number of deaths and retirements). Second, the *physician requirement ratio* is projected by estimating the extent of disease in the population (usually based on survey data), the physician services necessary to provide care for each illness, and the number of physician hours required to provide preventive and therapeutic services. (Some studies attempt to modify the requirements ratio by basing it on utilization rates of population subgroups—such as age, sex, location, and insurance coverage—and multiplying these utilization rates by the future population in each category.) Third, assuming a 40-hour workweek per physician, the number of hours is translated into number of physicians and into a physician-to-population ratio. The same approach is used to determine the number of physicians in each specialty. The difference between the supply ratio and the requirements ratio is the anticipated shortage or surplus. The Graduate Medical Education National Advisory Committee (the predecessor organization to COGME) also used a physician-to-population ratio methodology to determine the appropriate number of physicians.

This ratio technique has served as the basis for much of the health manpower legislation in the United States and has resulted in many billions of dollars of subsidies from federal and state governments. Nonphysician health professional associations, such as those for registered nurses, have used this approach as well in their quest for government subsidies. Using a physician-to-population ratio for judging whether a shortage (or surplus) exists has serious shortcomings.

First, the use of a ratio—whether based on health professional esti- mates of the need for services or on the current physician-to-population ratio—as a guideline for determining whether future ratios will be adequate does not consider changes in physician demand. For example, if demand for physicians is growing faster than the supply because of an aging population, an expansion of Medicaid eligibility, new medical advances that encourage the public to use medical care, or an increase in the number of privately insured on state insurance exchanges, then maintaining a particular ratio is likely to result in too few physicians.

Second, the ratio method does not include productivity changes that are likely to occur or could be attained. Adding physician services is possible without increasing the number of physicians. Technology (such as health information systems) and personnel with less training can be used to relieve physicians of many tasks; delegation of some tasks would permit the number of physician visits to grow. A smaller physician-to-population ratio would be needed if productivity growth were considered. Conversely, if the percentage of female physicians (who work fewer hours, on average, than male physi- cians do) rises or if physicians prefer an easier lifestyle, will more physicians be needed?

Third, the ratio technique does not indicate how important a surplus or shortage is—if, in fact, one exists. Is a shortage or surplus of 10,000 physicians significant, or does the number have to reach 200,000 to warrant concern? What are the consequences to physician fees, income, and patients' access to care?

Projections of shortages and surpluses using the ratio technique have been notoriously inaccurate. Many assumptions are used in calculating future ratios, and public policies based on inaccurate projections will take many years to correct, exacerbating future shortages or surpluses.

How an economic shortage of physicians can occur can be analyzed in two ways.

The Market for Physician Services

The first approach is to examine the market for physician services. A shortage exists when the demand for these services exceeds the supply of these services—at a given price. Patients are then unable to purchase all the physician services they want at the going market price. The available supply is rationed by patients, who have to wait longer to see a physician. This type of shortage may be temporary. Initially, as demand increases, physicians may be unaware that the higher demand is permanent and that they can raise their prices. As physicians conclude that demand will remain high, they can increase their fees and still retain at least the same number of patients. Some patients will demand fewer physician visits as fees rise, but overall the number of visits will likely go up.[1] Higher payments provide physicians with an incentive to supply more services. In addition to working longer hours, physicians can hire additional staff to boost their productivity. Market equilibrium is restored when patients can buy all the physician visits they want at the going market price.

A more serious type of economic shortage—referred to as a *static shortage*—occurs when physicians are unable to raise their fees in response to an increased demand for their services. When the government regulates physician fees, as occurs under Medicaid and Medicare, the government may take a long time to recognize that a shortage has occurred and determine how much the fees need to be increased to eliminate the shortage. Also, state Medicaid programs may decide not to raise physician fees because it will increase the state's deficit. In these cases, the shortage of physician services will persist, and for many Medicaid programs the shortage becomes permanent. The demand for physician services continues to exceed the supply of such services at the government's regulated physician fees.

Rate of Return on a Medical Education

The second approach is to determine the rate of return on a medical education. Medical education is viewed as an investment. The rate of return is calculated by estimating the costs of that investment and the expected higher financial returns from that investment while discounting that cash flow to the present.

If a person decides to enter medical (or any graduate) school, she is in effect making an investment in an education that offers a higher future income. The costs of that investment include tuition, books, and other expenses. Often, the largest part of this investment is the income that could have been earned had the person taken a job, which is the biggest opportunity cost of a graduate education.

The return earned on this educational investment is the higher income received. Because this income is earned in the future, and future income is valued less than current income, it must be discounted to the present. Does the discounted rate of return on a medical education exceed what the student could have earned had she invested an equivalent amount of money in a savings or bond account? If the rate of return is higher than what could have been earned by investing an equivalent sum of money, a shortage of physicians occurs. If the rate of return is lower than alternative investments or an investment in education for other professions, a surplus exists.[2]

The rate-of-return approach does not imply that every prospective student makes a rate-of-return calculation before deciding on a medical or other graduate education. Many students would become physicians even if future income prospects were low, simply because they believe medicine is a worthwhile profession. However, some students are at the margin; they may be equally excited about a career in medicine, business, or computer science. Changes in rates of return affect these students. High rates of return in medicine shift more students to medicine (eventually lowering the rate of return), whereas low rates of return shift them into other professions, eventually eliminating the physician surplus.

This approach incorporates into its calculations all the relevant economic factors, such as likely income lost if the person does not become a physician and the longer time to become a specialist (greater opportunity costs). In addition, changes in likely physician income by specialty and educational costs (such as tuition) alter the rate of return on a medical education.

Consequences of an Imbalance in the Physician Supply and Demand

What is likely to occur if demand for physicians exceeds supply? A shortage has short-term and long-term consequences. And these effects will vary depending on whether the individual demanding the service is a private-pay patient or a publicly funded patient for whom the government regulates the physician's fee.

Private Market for Physician Services

Short-Term Effects of a Physician Shortage

As discussed, a temporary shortage results in an increase in the number of patients seeking physician services. Initially, patients will find scheduling an appointment with a physician more difficult. Wait times will increase. Physicians' bargaining position with insurers will improve, and they will eventually raise their fees. They will likely add staff to increase their productivity so that they can see more patients. Physician income will rise as well.

Equilibrium will be reestablished—similar to what existed before demand increased—as a consequence of the higher physician fees. Patients will pay higher insurance premiums (or out-of-pocket payments), and some patients will not see their physicians as often as they did previously.

Long-Term Effects of a Physician Shortage

Over time, as physician income increases, so will the rate of return on a medical education. That return will exceed the return achieved by professionals with comparable training times, such as professors. The demand for medical education will increase, as will demand for residency positions in those specialties experiencing the largest growth in service demand. An important consideration is whether medical schools will accommodate the higher demand for a medical education. If medical schools expand and new medical schools open, the supply of US-trained physicians will slowly increase. If not, the applicant-to-acceptance ratio will rise, driving students who desire a medical education but cannot obtain it in the United States to seek that training overseas and then return to the United States for their residencies. Eventually, a greater supply of physicians will moderate physician fee increases and enter those specialties in which demand for services has surged. With physician supply growing faster than physician demand, the rates of return will decline to the point that they become comparable to those of other professions.

The response by patients, physicians, college graduates, and medical schools will result in the elimination of a shortage. The response will not be immediate, as it takes time for patients and physicians to realize that demand for physicians has risen; for some college graduates to decide to enter medicine; and for these medical students to graduate, complete their residencies, and practice full time.

Crucial assumptions regarding the long-term response to a shortage in the private market are (1) physician fees can increase, (2) the number of medical school spaces grow to accommodate the high demand for medical education, and (3) the number of residency positions in teaching hospitals expands to allow more medical graduates to be trained. Higher physician fees will eliminate any shortage in the physician services market. However, if medical school spaces and residency positions do not expand to meet greater demand, physicians will continue to earn higher rates of return, particularly in those specialties where the demand for residencies is greatest. Limited medical school spaces and the inability to gain a residency are entry barriers that have kept physician rates of return high, particularly in those specialties offering the highest income.

Although physician fee increases will achieve equilibrium in the private and public physician services markets, a shortage will continue to exist in the demand and supply of medical education and in more lucrative medical specialties. Expanding the number of medical school spaces will do little to alleviate the shortage unless the number of residency positions also expands.[2] Soon, increasing the number of graduates—both US- and foreign-trained graduates—to fill residency positions will be difficult (Iglehart 2013). About 30,000 positions are offered each year. Of the total number of residencies,

104,000 are at teaching hospitals, and the number of federally subsidized residencies—94,000—has been constant since 1997.

Public Market for Physician Services

Short-Term Effects of a Physician Shortage

The public and private physician services markets are interrelated. Physicians will allocate their time according to the relative profitability of serving patients in each market. (This is not meant to imply that all physicians behave similarly but that a sufficient number of physicians are willing to shift their services on the basis of the profitability of serving Medicare, Medicaid, and private-pay patients [Rice et al. 1999].) Consequently, the effects of a physician shortage on patients depend on the flexibility of physician fees in each market. Markets that permit greater flexibility in fees and entry of new physicians are more likely to resolve a shortage situation than markets that rely on government-regulated fees, which are slow to adjust to changes in demand and supply.

The main difference between the private and public markets is that the government regulates the price of physician services in public markets (Medicare and Medicaid). Governments are rarely able to accurately determine the price for physician services and for each specialty so that it can equilibrate service supply and demand for Medicare and Medicaid patients. Often, budget considerations influence how much the government will spend on physician services.

If a shortage situation occurs in the private market and insurers increase physician fees, physicians will serve fewer Medicare and Medicaid patients unless the government also raises physician fees. Physicians will shift their time to higher-paying private patients. This is currently occurring with Medicare patients and is a continual problem for Medicaid patients.

Long-Term Effects of a Physician Shortage

Unlike in the private market, a shortage may continue indefinitely in the public market if government fees are not sufficiently increased to match those in the private market. Low out-of-pocket payments by Medicare and Medicaid patients result in high demand, which will continue to exceed the supply of services physicians are willing to devote to these patients at the regulated price. The consequence is that the excess demand is rationed by increased wait times for an appointment, an important deterrent to receiving care. Some physicians are able to increase their hourly fee by reducing the time they spend with each patient, others engage in "upcoding"—for example, billing for a comprehensive visit when a brief visit was provided, and still other physicians are unwilling to see new patients.

When regulated fees are below fees in the private market, physicians have no incentive to increase the supply of their services in the regulated markets. Instead, physicians will reallocate their time to private patients, in a setting where fees are higher and where physicians can receive greater revenue per visit. Patients in the regulated public market—generally the poor and aged—will have to wait longer for an appointment. When regulated fees prevent equilibrium from occurring—such as in some Medicare markets where demand exceeds supply—physicians will be able to charge an annual "concierge" fee of $1,500 to $2,000 for better access. In addition to same-day access and more time per visit for concierge patients, the physician helps the patient negotiate the bureaucratic medical system. To provide the time for concierge patients, physicians reduce the size of their practice from about 2,500 to 600 patients, thereby forcing those unable to pay the concierge fee to search for another physician. The growth of concierge medicine will continue in our current multitiered healthcare system, whereby those with high income receive more and timelier care than those with low income.

With decreased access to physicians, patients in the public market will search for substitutes to private physician services, such as hospital emergency departments. Similarly, to have greater access, more publicly funded patients will join HMO-type organizations, which are able to attract physicians by paying them a higher rate. (More Medicare patients will enroll in Medicare Advantage plans.) These organizations, which are paid an annual amount per enrollee (known as *capitation payment*), are able to cut their costs by using more nonphysicians and providing preventive and disease management services, which reduce costly hospital care.

Economic Evidence on Trends in Physician Demand and Supply

Several measures are used to determine whether a shortage exists and, if so, whether it is temporary or permanent. A shortage in the physician services market is characterized by high fees and income, lengthy wait times, and high rates of return on a medical education. A temporary shortage is distinguished from a permanent shortage by whether the supply of physician services is increasing (which is consistent with a temporary shortage). Regulatory limits on physician fee hikes when demand goes up will result in a permanent shortage for Medicare and Medicaid patients, a shortage that will become more severe as physicians shift their time to the private sector where they can earn more per visit. A shortage for public patients is indicated by long wait times, given that Medicare and Medicaid physician fees are prevented from rising as fast as the fees in the private market.

Each of these indicators is discussed in the following sections.

Trends in Physician Fees

In the late 1980s, physician fees rose much more rapidly than did inflation (indicative of demand increasing faster than supply) and more rapidly than in the 1990s, when managed care began having an effect. Exhibit 11.1 indicates that physician fee increases have barely exceeded inflation in the previous decade but inflation actually exceeded physician fee growth in recent years.

A growing divergence in fees exists between the private and public markets for physicians, leading to a growing shortage of physician services among Medicare and Medicaid patients. While average private physician fees have been similar to the rate of inflation in the past three years, Medicare physician fees have declined when adjusted for inflation (see Exhibit 10.3). Physicians have tried to compensate for these declining Medicare fees by increasing the volume of imaging and testing services, thereby raising their Medicare revenue per patient (MedPAC 2013).

Trends in Patient Wait Times and Acceptance Rates

A 2013 physician survey examined how long new patients would have to wait for an appointment with a physician in 5 medical specialties—family practice, cardiology, dermatology, obstetrics–gynecology, and orthopedic surgery—in 15 major metropolitan markets in the United States (Miller 2014). The survey also asked physicians whether they accepted Medicare and Medicaid patients. A similar survey was conducted in 2004 and 2009.

Very large differences existed in new-patient wait times for a physician appointment between cities. Boston had the highest wait times (66 days) among other physician markets studied (the wait time in Dallas was 5 days). Boston also had the highest wait times in the 2009 and 2004 surveys. Family practice was not included in the earlier surveys so it was not possible to determine whether wait times for a new patient seeking a family physician changed over time. Average wait times to see a cardiologist and a dermatologist increased since 2009 but decreased for obstetrician/gynecologists and orthopedic surgeons.

The acceptance rates of new Medicaid patients by physicians in all 5 specialties and in all 15 markets surveyed was 45.7 percent, down from 55.4 percent in 2009. Although physician acceptance rates of new Medicare patients were not included in earlier surveys, the average acceptance rate in 2013 in all 5 specialties and in all 15 markets was 76 percent.

These data show that wait times vary widely among specialties and in different markets, indicating that physician shortages are much greater in

EXHIBIT 11.1
Annual
Percentage
Changes in
the Consumer
Price Index and
in Physicians'
Fees, 1965–
2013

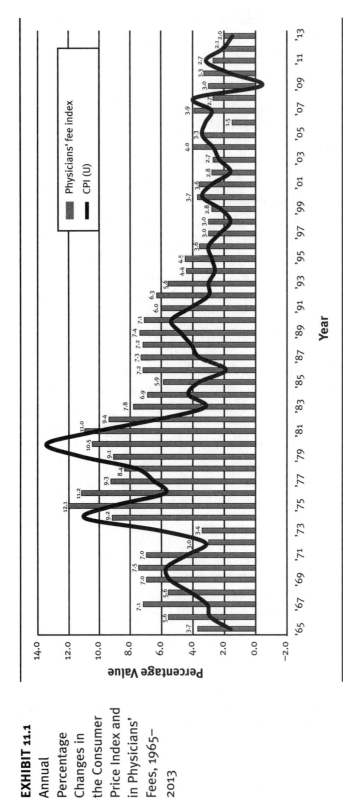

CPI (U): consumer price index for all urban consumers
SOURCES: Data from BLS (2014); CMS (2014).

some parts of the country than in others and by specialty. Medicaid patients, particularly, face a shortage that results in severe access problems. The limited number of physicians willing to serve these patients is caused by Medicaid's low physician fees. Physicians have greater financial incentive to serve other patients whose payments are higher.

Although Medicare has higher physician payment rates than Medicaid does, the average 75 percent acceptance rate for Medicare patients indicates that Medicare patients have access problems in a number of physician markets. For example, the family practice physician acceptance rate for new Medicare patients is 42 percent in New York City and 55 percent in Dallas and Denver. When demand and supply for physicians vary around the country, a single government payment system will not fully reflect these different market conditions; shortages are bound to occur in those areas where demand for physicians is increasing faster than the supply and where Medicare fees are not sufficiently flexible to reflect these differences.

Trends in Physician Income

Exhibit 11.2 shows that, over the 2002–2012 period, physician income has risen more than the inflation rate by about 1 percent to 2 percent per year. These data are also indicative of demand for physician services increasing faster than the supply.

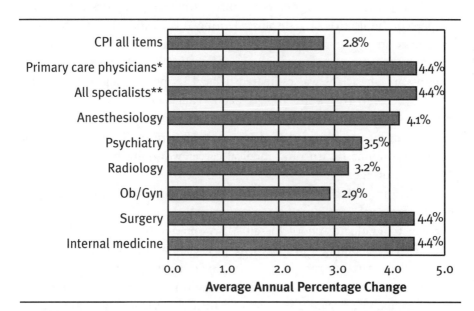

EXHIBIT 11.2
Average Annual Percentage Change in Physicians' Median Salaries from Medical Practice, by Specialty, 2002–2012

* "Primary care physicians" group includes family practice (without obstetrics), internal medicine, and pediatric/adolescent medicine. ** "All specialists" group includes anesthesiology, cardiology, dermatology, emergency medicine, gastroenterology, hematology/oncology, neurology, obstetrics/gynecology, ophthalmology, orthopedic surgery, otorhinolaryngology, psychiatry, pulmonary medicine, radiology, general surgery, and urology.
SOURCE: Data from MGMA (2008, 2009, 2013), Table A.

Trends in Rates of Return on a Medical Education

To determine whether a shortage of physicians (and by specialty) exists, examining the economic rate of return on a medical education is useful—namely, whether an investment in medical education offers higher returns than do other professional educational opportunities or working after graduating from college. High relative rates of return are indicative of a shortage. A permanent shortage is characterized by high relative rates of return and limited entry into the profession so that the high rates of return persist. (The applicant-to-acceptance ratio for medical schools is further evidence of whether prospective medical students believe the returns to a medical career are more favorable than for other professions.)

Data on rates of return on a career in medicine are intermittent and only available up to 1997.[3] These studies have been conducted by different researchers, and their methodologies may not be similar. What do they indicate? Throughout the post–World War II period, rates of return on a medical career were sufficiently high to suggest that a shortage existed. In 1962, the rate of return was estimated to be 16.6 percent. By 1970, it had risen to 22 percent. The rate of return declined slightly between 1975 and 1985, when it was estimated to be 16 percent, which indicates a shortage (Feldstein 2011).

Rates of return have varied greatly among physician specialties. In 1985, some specialties—such as anesthesiology and surgical subspecialties—earned 40 percent and 35 percent returns, whereas pediatrics earned only 1.3 percent (indicative of a surplus). During this period, the rate of return on a physician education was more than 100 percent greater than the rate of return on the education of a college professor. In 1994, the rate of return for primary care physicians was estimated to be 15.9 percent and for specialists was 20.9 percent. Weeks and Wallace (2002) calculated that in 1997 the rate of return for primary care physicians was about the same as in 1994 at 15.8 percent, but for specialists it had declined to 18 percent. These data indicate that the economic return on a medical career was quite high, indicating a physician shortage.

Vaughn and colleagues (2010) provide additional information on the economic value of a medical career by calculating the net present value of going to graduate school for an MBA (master of business administration) degree, becoming a primary care physician, and becoming a cardiologist—and compared to the net present value of an undergraduate (bachelor) degree. In contrast to a rate-of-return calculation, in which the discount rate of a future income stream is the rate of return, the calculation of net present value uses a predetermined interest rate to discount future income streams.

Because the higher income of a graduate education occurs over time, and a dollar earned in the future is worth less than a dollar earned today, those income streams are discounted by an interest rate to determine the economic value of the additional educational investment in current dollars.

Exhibit 11.3 shows the income streams for the four career paths and illustrates when the income starts for each career path and its magnitude at different ages. Based on these data, Vaughn and colleagues (2010) calculated that the net present value from college graduation to age 65 years was $5,171,407 for cardiologists, $2,475,838 for primary care physicians, $1,725,171 for those with an MBA, and $340,628 for those with only a bachelor's degree. Thus—even accounting for the many years of training, the delay in earning an income and for fewer years, and the high levels of debt incurred—a medical career (particularly one in cardiology) has a great deal of economic value.

The economic returns of an investment in medical education are sufficiently high to indicate that a physician shortage exists. (If a surplus were indicated, the net present value of a medical career would be less than that of a career of a regular college graduate.) Whether or not the investment return on a medical career has fallen in the past several decades, the rate is still sufficiently high to suggest that there are too few physicians. An increase in physician supply would lower the current high returns on medical education investment.

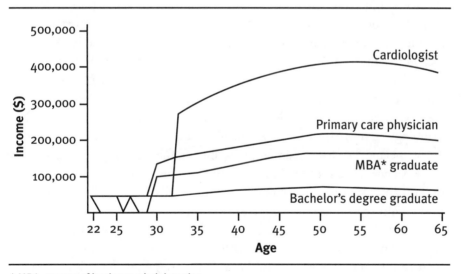

EXHIBIT 11.3
Annual Ordinary Income (Before Taxes) for Various Professions and Educational Attainment Levels, Ages 22–65 Years

* MBA: master of business administration
SOURCE: Adapted with permission from Vaughn and colleagues (2010).

Applicant-to-Acceptance Ratio in Medical Schools

Another indicator of the economic value of a medical career is the demand for medical education. The applicant-to-acceptance ratio has always been greater than one (see Exhibit 23.1 in Chapter 23). After reaching a high of 2.9:1 in 1973, the applicant-to-acceptance ratio steadily declined to 1.6:1 in 1988; rose again in the mid-1990s; and, after declining again and reaching 1.9:1 in 2002, has increased and is 2.2:1 in 2012. An excess demand for a medical education still exists.

Summary of the Evidence on a Physician Shortage

What can one conclude from the data on wait times, physician fees, rates of return, net present value, and the applicant-to-acceptance ratio? A shortage appears to exist in the physician services market, particularly in some markets. Medicare and Medicaid physician fees have not been increasing, and these patients will experience greater access problems, particularly access to primary care physicians. The ACA—which expands coverage to an additional 30 million by increasing Medicaid eligibility and providing federal subsidies to those enrolled in state and federal health insurance exchanges—together with the demographic trends resulting in a growing number of elderly will greatly raise the demand for primary care services, making the shortage (and limited access to care) even more severe.

The shortage of physicians has existed for many years. A medical career is an attractive investment. Physician income is still sufficiently large to offer a high economic return on a medical career, relative to other careers available to prospective medical students. Also indicative of a shortage is the continual excess demand for a medical education; more qualified students seek admission to medical school than are accepted. A growth in the supply of physicians would reduce these high relative rates of return, making them comparable to the rates of return on other educational investments.

Consistently high returns—particularly for medical specialties such as cardiology—are barriers that prevent many qualified students from becoming physicians and from gaining entry into highly remunerative specialties. These barriers consist of the limited number of medical school spaces, resulting in many US students going overseas to receive a medical education at a substantial expense. Limited expansion of medical residencies also prevents entry into those specialties having high rates of return. Medical students have strong financial incentives to enter the specialties, not just because of the much higher income but also because that remuneration allows them to quickly pay off their large medical school loans.

The supply of primary care physicians will likely not grow sufficiently to reduce the physician shortage. Further, under the current fee-for-service payment system, the large differences in returns between primary care physicians and many specialties will continue to exist.

Long-Term Outlook for the Physician Shortage

The demand for physicians is expected to increase sharply in coming years, thereby exacerbating the physician shortage. The ACA requires most US citizens to have health insurance, and about 32 million additional people have become eligible for Medicaid and health insurance exchange subsidies. Exhibit 11.4 shows the increasing role of government in physician payment. Unless Medicare and Medicaid increase physician fees when demand is increasing faster than supply, those with low income (Medicaid) and the aged (Medicare) will suffer a significant decrease in access to physician services.

Reducing the shortage of physician services requires two approaches: a decrease in demand and an increase in supply.

Demand Strategies for Reducing the Shortage

Three general approaches can be used to decrease the demand for physician services.

First, patient incentives can be changed by increasing the price patients pay for low-value services. For example, most people on Medicare purchase private supplementary health insurance (Medigap) policies. This coverage

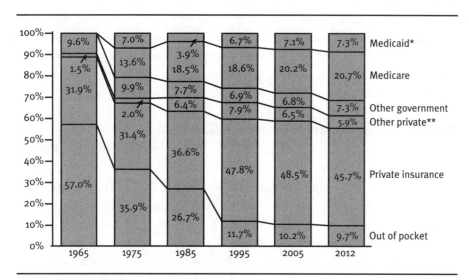

EXHIBIT 11.4
Percentage Distribution of Physician Expenditures, by Source of Funds, Selected Years, 1965–2012

* Total Medicaid (excluding Medicaid expansion).
** This category includes industrial inplant and other private revenues (such as philanthropy); other private funds in 1965 and 1975 were 1.5% and 2.1%, respectively.
SOURCE: Data from CMS (2014).

pays for their Medicare deductibles and copayments, greatly lowering the price they must pay for physician services (some Medigap policies cut the price to zero) and decreasing their price sensitivity to physician fees. With virtually complete coverage for physician services, many elderly patients excessively use physician and specialist services. Requiring a copayment for Medicare patients able to afford it will decrease the use of low-value services and make patients more aware of the cost of services.

Second, physician incentives can be changed by switching from fee-for-service to a broader payment system, such as capitation or a single fee for an episode of illness. In this way, physicians will use more innovative and less costly approaches to providing care, particularly to the chronically ill. Physicians will have an incentive to identify high-risk patients and manage their care before a costly episode occurs. For example, getting more patients to control their hypertension will decrease the number of patients suffering a stroke. Similarly, foot exams for patients with diabetes will reduce the number of amputations. All of these will decrease demand for costly medical services.

Under fee-for-service, the better a primary care physician cares for her patients, the fewer the complications that could occur, leading to fewer office visits and thus lower physician income. Under a broader payment system, physicians are rewarded for improving quality and for minimizing the use of costly services for their chronically ill patients. Further, physicians have a greater incentive to assist individuals with becoming and remaining healthy and better managing their conditions, which decrease the demand for services.

Third, a controversial approach is to rely on government guidelines for how care should be provided. Physician payment for publicly insured patients would be based—all or in part—on whether the physician used recommended protocols in treating different illnesses. (The advantages and disadvantages of treatment guidelines are discussed completely in Chapter 21).

Supply Strategies for Reducing the Shortage

The supply of physician services may be increased in several ways, and efforts to this end are currently under way.

First, new medical schools are launching, and existing schools are expanding their number of spaces. However, producing a primary care physician takes about 12 years after high school—four years of undergraduate college education, four years of medical school, and three to four years of residency training. Further, innovations will have to occur in medical education, such as reducing completion time from the current four years to three years.

However, simply increasing the number of medical school graduates to solve the physician shortage will neither be quick nor adequate. Only about 32 percent of MDs (doctor of medicine degree) are in primary care, which include internists, family physicians, pediatricians, and geriatricians. Although graduates of foreign medical schools make up about 25 percent of all physicians, they represent about 50 percent of primary care physicians. Unless more residency positions are created, the growing number of graduates of US medical schools will just replace foreign medical graduates without adding to the physician supply.

Second, in coming years, physicians will have to boost their productivity to serve more patients by using lesser-trained personnel—known as *physician extenders*—to perform certain tasks when medically appropriate. Nurse practitioners, physician assistants, and similarly prepared personnel perform some physician-type services (particularly primary care), and their numbers are likely to grow.[4] In some states, nurse practitioners and physician assistants are assuming more responsibility for delivering primary care, especially in underserved communities (Yee et al. 2013). In a national survey of physicians and nurse practitioners in primary care practice, Donelan and colleagues (2013) found that

> [n]urse practitioners were more likely than physicians to believe that they should lead medical homes, be allowed hospital admitting privileges, and be paid equally for the same clinical services. When asked whether they agreed with the statement that physicians provide a higher-quality examination and consultation than do nurse practitioners during the same type of primary care visit, 66.1% of physicians agreed and 75.3% of nurse practitioners disagreed.

Medical associations, however, are strongly opposed to physician extenders expanding their scope of practice and working without the supervision of physicians. Under fee-for-service, physicians and independent nurse practitioners are competitors. Under a broader system, physicians and nurse practitioners are in less economic competition for patients.

Third, technological advances are making the physician's office more efficient, enabling the office to increase the number of patients seen and to use the physician's time more effectively. Physicians are beginning to prescribe smart phone applications and medical devices—such as a glucose meter and blood pressure monitor—that remind patients to take their medications and manage their chronic diseases (such as heart disease, diabetes, and asthma). Clinical decision support systems, such as IBM's Watson supercomputer, are being developed that can make more accurate diagnosis and treatment recommendations. Telehealth applications provide easier access to physicians and enable them to respond to patients in a more timely manner.

Fourth, an important supply response to the shortage has been the rise of retail medical clinics. As of 2013, there were more than 1,400 retail medical clinics, twice as many as six years ago (Robeznieks 2013). When regulated fees cause a shortage, the *effective price*—the out-of-pocket payment for a visit and the value of the wait time to see a physician—to the patient increases. A higher effective price makes patients more willing to use substitutes, whose out-of-pocket price may be higher but whose wait time cost may be lower.

An example of the growth of substitutes to physician office visits and time-consuming waits at emergency departments is the rise of retail medical clinics, which are available every day of the week and some of which are open 24 hours a day. A large percentage of the population do not have a primary care physician. Walgreens and CVS Caremark, for example, have expanded their health services from providing acute episodic care (such as giving flu shots and treating sore throats) to managing chronic diseases (such as diagnosing and treating patients for asthma, diabetes, and high cholesterol). Diagnosis and treatment—areas long controlled by physicians—are now provided by nurse practitioners and physician assistants, who prescribe tests, make diagnoses, write prescriptions, and advise patients on managing their conditions at home. Retail chains have entered the potentially lucrative business of treating customers with long-term medical problems, which often require prescription drugs or other supplies that could be purchased at these stores. These convenient and low-cost substitutes will eventually take business from physicians by using physician extenders and by controlling referrals to healthcare professionals and hospitals, because whoever controls the entry point to medical services will also determine referrals to other healthcare providers.

Also driving the demand for retail clinics are high-deductible health plans offered by employers. Because more employees are choosing high-deductible health plans (which make them responsible for "first dollar" coverage), they have become more cost-conscious purchasers of medical services. In addition, insurers—once skeptical of retail medical clinics—now reimburse for vaccines and family physicals obtained from these clinics.

Medical associations, such as the American Academy of Family Physicians, are seeking state legislation that limits the scope of services retail medical clinics offer because these clinics (which use independent nurse practitioners) are providing disease management services that adversely affect physician income.

The role of the physician will have to change over time as innovations occur in the payment system; the technology used in diagnosis, treatment, and management of illness; the professions involved in providing services (i.e., physician extenders who desire to become independent practitioners); and the settings in which services are delivered.

Summary

Regulated fees prevent equilibrium from occurring when demand exceeds supply in Medicare and Medicaid physician services markets. The resulting shortage will cause Medicare and Medicaid patients to endure much longer wait times and experience decreased access to care. Continual high rates of return on medical education and an increasing applicant-to-acceptance ratio for medical schools are further signals of a physician shortage. Adding to the supply of physicians together with expanding residency positions would lower these high rates of return, making them comparable to the return on other educational investments.

Shortages and surpluses are resolved over time through the adjustment of rising or falling fees. Market imbalances are not resolved quickly, as it takes many years to train additional physicians. A particular problem with medical education is that it is highly regulated by the medical profession. It is difficult for entrepreneurs to develop new medical schools with innovative curricula, shorten the required education time for students, and achieve the same outcomes as graduates from traditional medical schools. As long as these restrictions continue—along with an excess demand for a medical education—medical schools will be unresponsive to increased demands for a medical education and to curriculum innovations.

To reduce the shortage of physician services, two approaches should be used. First, decrease the demand for physician services by providing financial incentives to patients to use fewer, less-valued services and to physicians to better manage the care of chronically ill patients. Second, increase the supply of physician services by boosting physician productivity, using more physician extenders, and using more technology that improves physician efficiency.

Whether a shortage or surplus is beneficial often depends on whether one is a patient or a physician. A small physician supply raises physician income, whereas greater competition among physicians benefits patients by improving their access to care.

Discussion Questions

1. Evaluate the use of the physician-to-population ratio as a means of determining a physician surplus or shortage.
2. Describe and evaluate how a rate of return on a medical education would determine the existence of a physician surplus or shortage.

3. What demand and supply trends in the physician services market will affect the income of surgical specialists and primary care physicians?

4. Prices change in a competitive market for two basic reasons: high operating costs and changes in physician demand. In what ways do these reasons explain physician fee increases?

5. Based on the evidence presented on physician income, physician fees, physician-to-population ratio, and applicant-to-acceptance ratio in medical schools, would you conclude that a physician shortage currently exists?

Notes

1. Typically, physicians will require higher fees from insurers, who in turn will pass these costs to their enrollees in the form of higher health insurance premiums. Insurers may also impose higher cost-sharing amounts on patients seeing a physician.

2. In the United States, a residency is a three- to seven-year long on-the-job training in a US teaching hospital that medical school graduates must complete before they can practice medicine. Each year, graduates from US medical schools compete with thousands of graduates from osteopathic schools, thousands of US-citizen graduates from international medical schools, and thousands of non–US citizen graduates from international medical schools for a limited number of new residency positions.

3. The internal rate of return is the discount rate that, when applied to the future earnings stream, will make its present value equal to the cost of entry into the profession or the present value of the expected outlay or cost stream. A normal rate of return might be similar to the rate of return on a college education or on the return the individual could have received had he or she invested a sum of money comparable to what was spent on a medical education.

4. Nurse practitioners are registered nurses who have completed a postgraduate nursing degree with a specialization in primary care, acute care, or psychiatric/mental health care and sometimes with a focus on pediatrics, adult/gerontology, or women's health. State scope-of-practice laws vary widely in the level of physician oversight required for nurse practitioners: Some states allow nurse practitioners to practice independently, while others prohibit nurse practitioners to diagnose, treat, and prescribe medications to patients without supervision. Medicare reimburses nurse practitioners 85 percent of the fee received by physicians for the same services.

References

AAMC Center for Workforce Studies. 2012. "Physician Shortages to Worsen Without Increases in Residency Training." Accessed March 2014. www.aamc.org/download/286592/data/physicianshortage.pdf.

Bureau of Labor Statistics (BLS). 2014. "Consumer Price Index." Accessed March. www.bls.gov/cpi/.

Centers for Medicare & Medicaid Services (CMS). 2014. "National Health Expenditure Data." Last modified May. http://cms.gov/Research-Statistics-Data-and-Systems/Statistics-Trends-and-Reports/NationalHealthExpendData/index.html.

Council on Graduate Medical Education (COGME). 2005. *Physician Workforce Policy Guidelines for the United States, 2000–2020. Sixteenth Report.* Published January. www.hrsa.gov/advisorycommittees/bhpradvisory/cogme/Reports/sixteenthreport.pdf.

———. 1992. *Improving Access to Health Care Through Physician Workforce Reform: Directions for the 21st Century. Third Report.* Published October. https://archive.org/details/thirdreportimpro00heal.

Donelan, K., C. DesRoches, R. Dittus, and P. Buerhaus. 2013. "Perspectives of Physicians and Nurse Practitioners on Primary Care Practice." *New England Journal of Medicine* 368 (20): 1898–906. www.nejm.org/doi/full/10.1056/NEJMsa1212938.

Feldstein, P. J. 2011. "Health Manpower Shortages and Surpluses." In *Health Care Economics*, 7th ed. Albany, NY: Delmar.

Iglehart, J. K. 2013. "The Residency Mismatch." *New England Journal of Medicine* 369 (4): 297–99. www.nejm.org/doi/full/10.1056/NEJMp1306445?query=TOC.

Medical Group Management Association (MGMA). 2013. *Physician Compensation and Production Survey: 2013 Report Based on 2012 Data.* Englewood, CO: MGMA.

———. 2009. *Physician Compensation and Production Survey: 2009 Report Based on 2008 Data.* Englewood, CO: MGMA.

———. 2008. *Physician Compensation and Production Survey: 2008 Report Based on 2007 Data.* Englewood, CO: MGMA.

Medicare Payment Advisory Commission (MedPAC). 2013. *Report to the Congress: Medicare Payment Policy.* Washington, DC: MedPAC. www.medpac.gov/documents/Mar13_entirereport.pdf.

Miller, P. 2014. *2014 Survey of Physician Appointment Wait Times and Medicaid and Medicare Acceptance Rates.* Irving, TX: Merritt Hawkins. www.merritthawkins.com/uploadedFiles/MerrittHawkings/Surveys/mha2014waitsurvPDF.pdf.

Rice, T., S. C. Stearns, D. E. Pathman, S. DesHarnais, M. Brasure, and M. Tai-Seale. 1999. "A Tale of Two Bounties: The Impact of Competing Fees on Physician Behavior." *Journal of Health Politics, Policy and Law* 24 (6): 1307–30.

Robeznieks, A. 2013. "Retail Clinics at Tipping Point: Pharmacies, Chains Answering Demand for Access and Affordability." *Modern Healthcare* 43 (18): 6–7.

Vaughn, B., S. DeVrieze, S. Reed, and K. Schulman. 2010. "Can We Close the Income and Wealth Gap Between Specialists and Primary Care Physicians?" *Health Affairs* 29 (5): 933–40.

Weeks, W., and A. Wallace. 2002. "The More Things Change: Revisiting a Comparison of Educational Costs and Incomes of Physicians and Other Professionals." *Academic Medicine* 77 (4): 312–19.

Yee, T., E. Boukus, D. Cross, and D. Samuel. 2013. "Primary Care Workforce Shortages: Nurse Practitioner Scope-of-Practice Laws and Payment Policies." *NIHCR Research Brief* No. 13, February. www.nihcr.org/PCP-Workforce-NPs.

THE CHANGING PRACTICE OF MEDICINE

The practice of medicine has changed dramatically since the mid-1980s. For many years, the predominant form of medical practice was solo practice with fee-for-service reimbursement. With the increase in medical knowledge and technological advancements, however, more physicians became specialists. Insurer payment and federal education subsidies also encouraged the growth of specialization. The development of managed care changed the practice of medicine; more physicians joined together in increasingly large medical groups.

What are the reasons for this shift away from solo and small group practice toward large medical groups? Is the consolidation of medical practices into large groups likely to continue? What impact will the Affordable Care Act (ACA) have on how physicians practice?

Types of Medical Groups

Different types of medical groups have formed to serve the varied needs and preferences of practicing physicians. Following is a description of these two basic types.

Single Specialty or Multispecialty Groups

Physicians in these groups share facilities, equipment, medical records, and support staff. Physicians may be paid according to one or more methods: salary plus a share in remaining net revenues, discounted fee-for-service with a share in remaining net revenues, or capitation. Leaving a group practice is difficult for physicians, as they cannot take their patients with them. Any contracts the group has with a health plan belong to the group and include the patients covered by those contracts.

Independent Practice Associations

Physicians who want to be associated with other physicians (on a nonexclusive basis) for the purposes of joint contracting with a health plan will form a loose organization, such as an independent practice association (IPA). These physicians continue to practice in their own offices, see their own patients, hire and pay their own staff, and do their own billing.

When the IPA contracts with a health plan, the IPA physicians are paid on a discounted fee-for-service basis. If an IPA receives a capitation contract from a health plan, the physicians may be paid a discounted fee-for-service with the possibility of receiving additional amounts if total physician billings are less than the total capitation amount at the end of the year. The IPA may also subcapitate some specialists. As IPAs competed for capitated contracts and assumed financial risk, they began to exercise more oversight of their physicians' practice patterns.

Changes in the Size and Type of Medical Groups

Data on physicians' practice settings were based on nationally representative surveys (published by the Center for Studying Health System Change) of physicians who spend at least 20 hours a week in direct patient care. These surveys were conducted over different periods, starting in 1996 to 1997, with the latest in 2008. The survey methods differed (the earlier survey was taken via telephone, while 2008 data were based on a mail survey) and were not directly comparable; however, they provide an indication of the changes that have occurred over time. Unfortunately, data based on a 2012 American Medical Association (AMA) survey were not comparable with the previous surveys.

Exhibit 12.1 shows the changing distribution of office-based physicians according to physician subspecialty and size of group for different time periods. Three types of physicians are examined: primary care physicians,

EXHIBIT 12.1
Physicians by Subspecialty and Practice Setting, 1996–1997 and 2008

	Solo–2 Physician Practice		3–5 Physician Practice		6+ Physician Practice		Other*	
	1996–1997	2008	1996–1997	2008	1996–1997	2008	1996–1997	2008
Primary care	37.5	34.6	10.3	15.7	15.1	26.0	37.1	23.7
Medical specialist	38.1	27.3	9.6	10.0	17.3	24.6	35.1	38.2
Surgical specialist	47.8	34.4	17.9	18.8	15.5	26.0	18.8	20.9

* Includes physicians employed by medical schools, health maintenance organizations, hospitals (including office-based practices), community health centers, freestanding clinics, and other settings as well as independent contractors
SOURCES: Adapted from Liebhaber and Grossman (2007); based on Boukus (2008).

medical specialists, and surgical specialists. Over the period surveyed, all three types appear to have moved toward practicing in large groups.

According to the 2012 AMA survey, single-specialty practice was the most common type of practice, reported by 45.5 percent of physicians (Kane and Emmons 2013). A greater percent of radiologists (57.3 percent), anesthesiologists (55.8 percent), and obstetricians/gynecologists (52.7 percent) belonged to single-specialty groups. Primary care physicians were less likely to be in a single-specialty group. Female physicians—who are more likely to be in primary care (52.7 percent) than men (22.3 percent)—were less likely to be in a single-specialty group. Twenty-two percent of physicians were in multispecialty groups, including 36 percent of internists and 28.3 percent of family practice physicians.

Exhibit 12.2 illustrates the changes in physician practice arrangements by type of setting. In 1996 to 1997, 40.7 percent of physicians practiced in solo- or two-physician practices, with only 2.9 percent in groups of greater than 50 physicians. Only 10.7 percent worked in a hospital setting. (The trend toward hospital-employed physicians is discussed more fully later.) In 2008, the number of physicians in solo- and two-physician practices declined to 32 percent, the largest physician group increased to 6 percent, and physicians working in hospitals increased to 13 percent. The 2012 data show a greater number of physicians have become part of physician groups with 50

EXHIBIT 12.2
Physicians by Practice Setting, 1996–2001, 2004–2005, and 2008

	1996 –1997 (%)	1998 –1999 (%)	2000– 2001 (%)	2004– 2005 (%)	2008 (%)
Solo–2 physician practice	40.7	37.4	35.2	32.5	32.0
3–5 physician practice	12.2	9.6	11.7	9.8	14.5
6–50 physician practice	13.1	14.2	15.8	17.6	19.4
>50 physician practice	2.9	3.5	2.7	4.2	6.1
Medical school	7.3	7.7	8.4	9.3	7.3
Health maintenance organization	5.0	4.6	3.8	4.5	3.5
Hospital[1]	10.7	12.6	12.0	12.0	13.1
Other[2]	8.3	10.5	10.4	10.1	4.1

1 Includes physicians employed in hospitals and office-based practices owned by hospitals. Forty percent of physicians in this category were in office-based practices in 2004–2005.
2 Includes physicians practicing in community health centers, freestanding clinics, and other settings as well as independent contractors
SOURCE: Adapted from Liebhaber and Grossman (2007); based on Boukus (2008).

or more physicians—12 percent compared with 6 percent in 2008. (The AMA data are not comparable with the earlier practice size categories.) The trend appears to be physicians becoming part of large groups and working in hospitals.

In a highly competitive managed care market, physicians in individual and small group practices were at a disadvantage. Therein lies an important explanation for the formation of large medical groups.

Medical Groups as a Competitive Response

Before managed care became dominant in the insurance marketplace, physicians were less concerned with being included in an insurer's provider panel or competing for insurance contracts. The growth in private insurance reduced the out-of-pocket price of physician services paid by private patients. As patients' out-of-pocket payments declined, they became less price sensitive to physicians' fees, and their demand increased. Patients had access to all physicians, who were paid according to their established fee schedules. Patients had similar insurance (indemnity) and limited, if any, information on physician qualifications or the fees charged.

Price competition among managed care plans for an employer's enrollees changed all that. To be price competitive, insurers had to reduce the price they paid for their inputs (physician and hospital services) and reduce the quantity of services used.

The physician services market in the 1980s consisted of a growing supply of physicians—particularly specialists—and a high proportion of them were in solo or small group practices. Physicians were eager to contract with new managed care health plans. Insurers and health maintenance organizations (HMOs) were able to form limited provider networks by selecting physicians according to whether they were willing to sharply discount their fees in return for a greater volume of patients. Physicians excluded from such networks lost patients.

The growth of managed care had two main effects on physicians. First, managed care forced physicians to deeply discount their fees in return for a greater volume of the plan's enrollees. Patients enrolled in managed care plans were required to use providers who were part of their plan's provider network; otherwise, the patient had to pay the full price charged by a non-network provider. For physicians to have access to an insurer's enrollees, the physician had to be part of the insurer's provider network. Managed care plans limited the number of physicians in their provider networks and selected physicians based on how much they were willing to discount their fees (and not overuse medical services).

Second, managed care reduced enrollee access to specialists. Managed care relied on gatekeepers—primary care physicians—to determine whether a patient would receive a referral to a specialist. The growth of managed care increased the demand for primary care physicians and decreased the demand for specialists.

The growth of medical groups was a competitive response to the greater bargaining power of insurers and HMOs. Being part of a medical group—particularly a large group—provided physicians with a competitive advantage over physicians who were not similarly organized. Large medical groups were able to bid for HMO contracts and serve as preferred provider organizations for employers and insurers. Negotiating and contracting with one large medical group is less costly than carrying out separate, time-consuming negotiations with an equivalent number of individual physicians. Tasks performed by the insurer, such as utilization management, can be delegated to the medical group. Thus, large medical groups were better able than individual physicians and small medical groups to compete for patients.

HMOs were also able to shift their insurance risk to a large medical group by paying that group on a capitation instead of a fee-for-service basis. Similarly, a large medical group can spread financial risk over a large number of capitated enrollees and physicians.

Capitation also provided medical groups with financial incentives to be innovative in the delivery of medical services and the practice of medicine, because by saving part of the capitation payment, they could increase their profits. These incentives do not exist in small group practices that are paid on a fee-for-service basis. As a consequence, several large medical groups developed expertise in managing care and in developing "best-practice" guidelines.

In the 1990s, medical groups in California (more so than medical groups in other states) sought more financial risks and rewards by accepting a greater percentage of the HMO premium (Gillies et al. 2003). These medical groups believed that by being responsible for all of the patient's medical services, they could better manage care; further, by reducing hospital admissions, lengths of stay, and payments to hospitals, they could make greater profits. Unfortunately, many of these medical groups were inexperienced in managing the financial risks associated with capitation and suffered financially. Most medical groups no longer accept capitation payments.

Increased Market Power

An employer or a health plan contracting with a large medical group has less reason to be concerned with physician quality. Large medical groups have more formalized quality control and monitoring mechanisms than do independently practicing physicians. Within a large group, physicians refer to their own specialists; thus, specialists who are not part of a group are less likely to have access to patients. These contracting, quality review, and referral mechanisms provide physicians in large medical groups with a competitive advantage over physicians who are unaffiliated with such groups.

These advantages gave large groups greater bargaining power over health plans than had by independent and small physician practices. As a result, large groups were more likely to be able to negotiate higher payments and increased market share (receiving a greater portion of the health plan's total number of enrollees).

Large medical groups also have greater leverage over hospitals. Because such groups control large numbers of enrollees, it can determine to which hospitals it will refer its patients. Hospitals, in turn, were willing to share some of their capitated revenues with these groups. When hospitals were capitated, a *risk-sharing pool* was formed from part of the hospital's capitation payments, whereby the savings from reduced hospitalization were shared between the hospital and the medical group. These risk-sharing pools enabled physicians in medical groups to increase their income compared with what they would have earned in independent or small group practices.

Economies of Scale in Group Practice

An obvious reason for moving toward large medical groups in a price-competitive environment is to take advantage of economies of scale. Large groups have lower per-unit costs than do small groups. They also are better able to spread certain fixed costs over a larger number of physicians. The administrative costs of running an office (including making appointments; billing patients, government, and insurance companies for services rendered; maintaining computerized information systems to keep track of patients; and staffing aides to assist the physician) do not rise proportionately to the increase in the number of physicians. Multispecialty groups also can more easily provide care coordination to their patients and arrange for consultations with other physicians in the group. In addition, they are able to receive volume discounts on supplies and negotiate lower rates on their leases than can the same number of physicians practicing separately or in small groups.

Informational economies of scale also provide large groups with a competitive advantage over small or independent practices. A distinguishing characteristic of the physician services market is the lack of information about the physicians, including their quality, their fees, their accessibility, and the manner in which they relate to patients. Physicians are better able than patients to evaluate other physicians. Evaluating and monitoring member physicians are less costly for the medical group than for patients. Being a member of a medical group conveys to patients information regarding quality, giving physicians in that group the equivalent of a brand name.

A new physician entering a market is at a disadvantage (compared with established physicians) because developing a reputation and building a practice take time. Joining a medical group immediately transfers the group's reputation to the new physician. The reputation of the group for specialist services that are less frequently used is more important to the patient and more difficult for the patient to evaluate. Multispecialty groups offer greater informational economies of scale than do groups made up of family practitioners.

Medical Groups and Quality of Care

Large medical groups are more likely than physicians in solo or small groups to invest in management and clinical information systems, such as electronic medical record (EMR). On average, large multispecialty medical groups have been found to deliver higher quality care and lower annual costs per patient than physicians who are in solo practice or small groups (Weeks et al. 2010). Medical groups are likely to use more recommended care management processes for patients with chronic illnesses. Large groups are able to hire professional management to deal with an increasingly burdensome regulatory environment and achieve operational efficiencies by taking advantage of economies of scale.

The growing emphasis by insurers, employers, and Medicare on monitoring systems to measure patient outcomes and satisfaction and the greater interest in pay-for-performance give large medical groups a competitive advantage in attracting patients and receiving bonuses for achieving certain quality benchmarks. Pay-for-performance revenue is likely to become a large share of physician income; thus, medical groups that invest in information technology and can demonstrate improved patient performance will receive more physician revenues.

Reversal of Fortunes of Large Multispecialty Groups

The promise of large multispecialty medical groups in managing patient care and being rewarded for accepting greater capitation risk foundered in the late 1990s, particularly in California.

Changing Market Environment

The prosperity created by the economic expansion in the United States in the late 1990s led employees to demand broader provider networks and freer access to specialists from their HMOs. Large medical groups had been using primary care gatekeepers to control specialist referrals and utilization management to control the growth in medical costs. But when the market changed, it was no longer willing to reward large capitated medical groups for strict cost-control measures.

During this time, competition among HMOs led to low premium increases, leaving large capitated groups with low capitation rates. Medical groups found themselves in financial difficulty as their costs increased and state and federal governments enacted patient protection measures. These included 48-hour hospital stays for normal deliveries, requiring HMOs to allow obstetricians/gynecologists to serve as primary care physicians and prohibiting limited lengths of stay after a mastectomy. These measures further made the medical groups' costs more expensive.

HMOs were wary of being sued for withholding appropriate treatment even when the HMO had delegated such treatment decisions to its large medical groups. As HMOs began to undertake those decisions themselves, some of the advantages of capitation payment to large groups faded.

Difficulty of Developing a Group Culture

A well-functioning medical group cannot be formed overnight; the group may not coalesce even after years. An important difference between group and nongroup physicians is the willingness of group physicians to give up some of their autonomy and abide by group decisions. Physicians may not share values or accept the same assumptions regarding their external environment, mission, and relationships with one another. This cultural difference often determines whether physicians will remain in a group. Many physicians are very independent and do not want other physicians involved with their practice, whether the issue relates to contracting with certain health plans, reviewing practice patterns, or determining compensation.

A large multispecialty group must have various committees, one of which determines physician compensation. Disputes among physicians over their compensation are an important reason such groups have dissolved. For example, when a multispecialty group is capitated for a large number of enrollees, the group must decide how the primary care physicians and each specialist will share in those capitation dollars. In the past, when specialists had excess capacity and the primary care physicians controlled specialist referrals, some groups paid the primary care physicians more than they would earn under a discounted fee-for-service environment. These funds came from paying specialists less.

Another issue in medical group compensation is how much of each physician's income should be tied to productivity. Productivity incentives decline when a physician's payment is not directly related to his clinical work. More productive physicians may decide to leave if large differences occur between productivity and compensation.

When physicians in a large group share the use of inputs—personnel and supplies—they are less concerned with those costs than they would be if they were in an independent or a small group practice, where their costs are more directly related to their earnings. This lack of efficiency incentives offsets some savings from economies of scale.

Lack of Management Expertise

As medical groups increased in size and number, many had inadequate management expertise to handle the clinical and financial responsibilities of the group. The groups did not have adequate information systems for tracking expenses and revenues, they lacked actuarial expertise for underwriting risk when they were receiving capitation payments, and they did not have sufficient management specializing in marketing, finance, and contracting. Unfortunately, many medical groups expanded more rapidly than their management ability to handle the increased risk and patient volume.

Instead of developing such management expertise themselves, many groups joined for-profit (publicly traded) physician practice management (PPM) companies. These companies promised a number of benefits to a participating medical group, such as including the group in a larger contracting network with health plans, handling its administration, and improving its efficiency. In return for these services, the PPM company received a percentage (e.g., 15 percent) of the group's revenues. However, several publicly traded PPM companies were themselves poorly managed and declared bankruptcy. A further disappointment with these companies was that the cost savings they were able to achieve in the medical group and the additional contracting revenue they were able to bring to the group were often lower than the 15 percent management fee they charged.

Lack of Capital

Medical groups typically pay out all of their net revenues to their member physicians. Thus, no funds are available to reinvest in expanding the group, such as by establishing new clinics, purchasing expensive diagnostic services, or buying costly hardware and software for information technology. Their lack of capital is an important reason expanding medical groups seek partners.

Hospitals have generally been willing to provide the capital for medical groups to expand and to develop their infrastructures. In return for such investments, hospitals hope to secure the medical group's inpatient referrals and negotiate joint contracting arrangements with a health plan. The hospital may also manage or become a part owner in a joint management company that contracts with the medical group for medical services.

The main concerns groups have with hospitals as capital partners are that the hospital will somehow gain control of the group and that it may not be the most advantageous facility to which to refer patients. Many hospitals have lost a great deal of money investing in their physician partners because the hoped-for returns have been lower than anticipated—particularly when hospitals purchased physician practices and physician productivity (separated from compensation) declined.

The Outlook for Medical Practice

The organization of medical practice is based on a number of factors, but one increasing in importance is the method of payment for medical services. Fee-for-service (FFS) payments are likely to increase more slowly under government programs. As major payers, Medicare and the ACA's accountable care organization (ACO) are likely to have a strong impact as they experiment with alternative payment strategies for medical services—away from FFS and toward episode-based care and capitation.

Physicians and hospitals will be under intense pressure to control rising healthcare costs while demonstrating to payers that the quality of the care they provide and their outcomes are measurably improved. Provider organizations will have to better coordinate care for chronic illness, manage the health of their enrolled populations, and ensure easier access to care—while doing so under more stringent payment conditions. It will be increasingly difficult for solo practitioners and small medical practices to compete in this new economic environment.

The Movement to Single-Specialty Groups

An important trend is the growth of single-specialty medical groups. Under FFS, greater profits accrue to those physicians who can provide profitable procedures and ancillary services, such as imaging and diagnostic services. Single-specialty groups are also able to take advantage of economies of scale. (Although, on average, multispecialty groups are larger, more physicians belong to single-specialty groups [Kane and Emmons 2013].)

Medical groups have become more entrepreneurial as they attempt to increase physician revenues. Because of concerns that growth in physician revenues from providing services to Medicare and Medicaid patients is limited, medical groups have become more aggressive in expanding the services they offer. Medical groups are more likely than physicians in solo practice to invest in equipment to provide ancillary services, such as imaging and laboratory testing, within their existing practices. Patients' use of such services has sharply increased. If it were not for the ancillary services, some groups would not make any money.

The emergence of new imaging and surgical technologies made it possible to provide outpatient imaging and surgical services. Specialists have an incentive to move these services out of the hospital and into their own facilities. Physicians with specialties in cardiology and orthopedics invested in freestanding specialty hospitals and ambulatory surgical centers that competed with their own community hospitals. (To eliminate competition from specialists-owned hospitals, the American Hospital Association successfully lobbied Congress, as part of the ACA, to prohibit the development of new physician-owned single-specialty hospitals.) Large groups—particularly single-specialty groups—invested in costly imaging equipment, surgical services, and information technology, all of which are usually beyond the means of small groups. By investing in these outpatient facilities, specialists are able to receive the fees for such services (which would otherwise go to the hospital) and thereby increase their income. Physicians have claimed that such "focused factories" are more convenient for patients and improve patient care.

The profit potential of performing services with a high markup over cost in their own outpatient facilities provided specialists with an incentive to form large single-specialty groups. Specialists are able to generate more profit than are primary care physicians. Specialty groups that own expensive imaging equipment (such as an MRI or magnetic resonance imaging) and facilities (such as ambulatory surgery centers) are more profitable when paid on an FFS basis than are primary care physicians that provide cognitive services. Further, single-specialty groups do not have to share their revenues or governance with primary care physicians, as occurs in a multispecialty group.

A further economic advantage of single-specialty groups is their increased leverage when bargaining with health plans and community hospitals. The consolidation of many specialists into a single group lessens competition among specialists, enabling them to increase their fees in negotiations with health plans. Health plans are reluctant to lose a large network of specialists. Physicians in solo practice and small groups are at a competitive disadvantage in dealing with health plans.

The Growth of Hospital-Employed Physicians

An important trend is the growth in hospital-employed physicians. In the 1990s period of tightly managed care, excess capacity existed among physicians, the demand for primary care physicians rose as they became gatekeepers and restricted access to specialists, and specialist fees decreased. To increase their referrals and gain market share, hospitals bought medical practices. As managed care became less restrictive and hospitals found they were losing money on their medical groups, hospitals divested the groups.

Hospitals have again started to employ physicians. Of the 685,000 physicians who were in patient care (as of 2012), the number of physicians employed by community hospitals increased by 32 percent between 2000 and 2010—from 160,000 to 212,000 (Kane and Emmons 2013, 2). This growth has been more rapid since 2007.

Hospitals have several reasons for again employing physicians: an important medical group may be considering moving its admissions to another hospital, the hospital may be trying to enter a new market, the hospital may lack specialists in some services, or the hospital may be trying to preempt competition from specialists who have started their own outpatient services. In addition to capturing the physician's referrals, employing specialists and primary care physicians is likely to increase the hospital's negotiating leverage over health plans; if the health plan does not raise the hospital's rates, it may lose both the hospital and its physicians.

Another reason hospitals employ physicians is to enlarge their Medicare payments. When a physician's practice is purchased by a hospital and the physician treats the same patients in the same location as previously, under Medicare Part A the hospital can charge more for the same service than if the physician is an independent practitioner and bills under Medicare Part B. Medicare's cost of care goes up as does the patient's copayment. For example, "...when a Medicare beneficiary receives a certain type of echocardiogram in a doctor's office, the government and the patient together pay a total of $188. They pay more than twice as much— $452—for the same test in the outpatient department of a hospital." "From 2010 to 2011, ... the number of echocardiograms provided to Medicare beneficiaries in doctors' offices declined by 6 percent, but the number in hospital outpatient clinics increased by nearly 18 percent." Medicare's financial incentives have resulted in more than tripling the number of hospital-employed cardiologists—from 11 percent in 2007 to 35 percent in 2012 (Pear 2013).

Although hospitals have sought to employ both primary care physicians and specialists, hospitals are more likely to have an ownership interest in multispecialty groups (Kane and Emmons 2013). Multispecialty groups' wider scope of practice and use of primary care physicians are the apparent reasons for hospitals' great interest in such groups. In addition to providing a strong referral base, hospitals appear to be preparing for changes in payment that shift from FFS to broader payment arrangements that make providers accountable for the cost and quality of care provided (O'Malley, Bond, and Berenson 2011).

Physicians—particularly new graduates—have become more receptive to hospital employment because it provides them with regular work hours and eliminates the paperwork, regulations, necessity to invest in EMR, and administrative responsibilities of dealing with the government and private insurers. Employment also eliminates for physicians the financial risks of operating their own medical practice. More than half of all physicians work for hospitals and other organizations rather than in private practice.[1] It is not obvious whether hospital-employed (salaried) physicians are more productive than those working in small medical groups and whether their earnings are more directly related to the FFS revenue derived from their productivity.

The Effect of Payment Changes on Medical Practices

Medicare payment changes are likely to have a major effect on the organization of physician and hospital services, decreasing the growth of single-specialty groups while increasing the number of multispecialty groups and hospital employment.

The organization of medical services has been greatly affected by the payment system. FFS encourages the provider to perform more services and shifts the open-ended financial risk of paying for all the services to the insurer or to Medicare and Medicaid. When each type of provider (such as hospital, primary care physician, specialist, nursing home, and home health agency) is paid FFS, the delivery system is likely to be fragmented. Coordination of services and the alignment of each provider's incentives are less likely to occur than under a broader payment system.

Capitation payment shifts the financial risk to the provider; the provider receives a fixed payment and has to provide all the necessary medical services, so its incentive is to perform fewer services. Under a broader payment system, however, the incentive to coordinate care by each of the participating providers is greater so as to reduce the costs of providing that treatment.

Each type of payment system requires monitoring and quality reporting. Under FFS, monitoring the quality of many different unaffiliated providers is more difficult; duplication of services is more likely to occur and costs are harder to control. Because the incentive under capitation is to provide fewer services, it is also necessary to monitor treatment outcomes, which is easier than measuring the care given by each provider, as under FFS. Controlling rising medical costs is less difficult under capitation, as the organization bears the financial risk of exceeding the overall payment per enrollee.

Over time, Medicare has recognized the difficulty in controlling utilization of services and costs under FFS and has tried to move to a broader payment system. One such example is the change from paying hospitals according to their costs to a fixed price per admission. The financial risk of the costs per admission was shifted from Medicare to hospitals. Hospitals responded by reducing lengths of stay and becoming more efficient. Medicare was better able to control rising hospital costs. However, hospitals have no incentive to be concerned with the costs of treating the patient either before or after being discharged. Thus, an even broader hospital payment system is being considered. Medicare still relies on FFS for physician payment. Although physician fees are regulated, use of physician services is not; consequently, Medicare finds it difficult to limit rising physician expenditures.

Medicare Advantage plans, which are like HMOs, are paid a risk-adjusted capitation amount for each Medicare enrollee, and the private plans compete against each other as well as with traditional Medicare FFS. Medicare Advantage enrollees are provided with increased benefits and decreased cost sharing, in return for enrollees' limiting their access to the plan's provider network. Both political parties differ on the use of private managed care plans, and as part of the ACA, payments to Medicare Advantage plans were reduced. This reduction will likely decrease enrollment in such plans as they raise fees to their Medicare enrollees.

Medicare is considering moving toward broader payment systems, such as using episode-based payment and offering financial incentives to organizations to form ACOs, thereby shifting more of the financial risk of controlling costs to providers. Under episode-based payment, the insurer pays a single fee that includes all the services involved in treating a certain procedure, such as heart surgery or hip replacement. Eventually, the goal is to use episode-based payment for more types of treatments. ACOs are meant to encourage hospitals and physicians to collaborate to manage care and limit rising costs.

These broader payment systems, if successful, are likely to transform the delivery of medical services. More multispecialty medical groups will form to be able to undertake financial risk by becoming ACOs, and hospital employment of physicians will expand to enable the hospital to become an ACO and provide episode-based care in a less costly manner. Under this scenario, single-specialty medical groups will be at a disadvantage, as will physicians who own various surgery and imaging centers and those who are not affiliated with a hospital or a multispecialty group. With broader-based payment, the financial risk of rising costs is shifted to providers, and provider incentives for coordinating care and investing in EMR will increase.

Should attempts by Medicare to institute a broader-based payment system be politically unsuccessful and FFS remains the predominant system, the current trend toward single-specialty medical groups and hospital-employed physicians will likely continue. (Hospital consolidation and their control over access to physician services enhance their bargaining power with insurers.) The financial risk of controlling Medicare costs will remain with the government, and price controls will become more likely. The consolidation of the delivery of medical services will then make it easier for government to impose regulatory controls on large organizations of hospitals and physicians than if the industry consisted of many small organizations.

Summary

The organization of medical practices is changing. Large medical groups have advantages over physicians in solo or small group practices. In addition to being able to hire professional management, achieve economies of scale, and attain greater bargaining leverage with health plans and hospitals, large medical groups—particularly single-specialty groups—are able to increase their revenues by taking into their own outpatient settings more services that were previously provided in hospitals.

As budget pressures from federal (Medicare) and state (Medicaid) governments limit physician fee increases, new sources of revenue will increase in importance for physicians. The trend by multispecialty and single-specialty medical groups to invest in technologically advanced services that can be provided in an outpatient setting will continue.

Medical groups face challenges in coming years. Employers, insurers, and Medicare are increasing emphasis on monitoring patient outcomes and satisfaction. As payers become more sophisticated and quality is rewarded, large medical groups will have an advantage because quality and outcome measures are more accurate for medical groups than for individual physicians. Medical groups will also have to become more proficient in managing chronic illness for an increasingly aged population while demonstrating improved medical outcomes and patient satisfaction. Large medical groups will be better able than small medical groups to invest in the necessary information technology to evaluate practice patterns and patient outcomes.

A broader payment system provides incentives for hospitals to expand their role in the delivery of medical services. The trend toward lower hospital utilization, greater reliance on less costly outpatient services, and movement away from FFS toward bundled payments and capitation has placed hospitals at financial risk for delivering episodes of treatment at a fixed price. To provide coordinated care across all delivery settings, hospitals have been employing more physicians and purchasing medical groups.

The opportunity exists for large medical groups to remain independent of hospitals and increase their role in the delivery of medical services. It is uncertain, however, whether medical groups will be sufficiently entrepreneurial to achieve their promise in innovating new treatment methods that decrease medical costs while demonstrating improved patient outcomes.

Discussion Questions

1. Why has the size of multispecialty medical groups increased?
2. Why do large medical groups have market power?

3. Why do medical groups occasionally break up?
4. Describe how an IPA functions.
5. What are the different types of capital partners available to medical groups? What do they expect in return for providing capital?

Note

1. Health plans are also acquiring physician groups to increase their control over physician practices, utilization, and healthcare costs. In 2011, United Health Care purchased the largest physician group in Orange County, California. To date, physicians have preferred to become part of hospitals rather than health plans. The ACA offers incentives for hospitals (as well as insurers and medical groups) to form ACOs to provide healthcare for Medicare enrollees, basing payment on a capitation or a shared-savings model. When the organization is paid on a basis other than FFS, the financial risk is shifted from the payer to the organization. The organization at risk requires physicians to provide coordinated care, reduce hospital admissions (and readmissions), and better manage chronically ill patients to reduce the costs of care.

Additional Readings

Goldsmith, J. 2010. "Analyzing Shifts in Economic Risks to Providers in Proposed Payment and Delivery System Reforms." *Health Affairs* 29 (7): 1299–304.

Welch, W. P., A. Cuellar, S. Stearns, and A. Bindman. 2013. "Proportion of Physicians in Large Group Practices Continued to Grow in 2009–11." *Health Affairs* 32 (9): 1659–66. http://content.healthaffairs.org/content/32/9/1659.full.

White, C., A. Bond, and J. Reschovsky. 2013. "High and Varying Prices for Privately Insured Patients Underscore Hospital Market Power." *HSC Research Brief* 27, September. Washington, DC: Center for Studying Health System Change. www.hschange.org/CONTENT/1375/.

References

Boukus, E. 2008. Personal correspondence with the author.

Gillies, R., S. Shortell, L. Casalino, J. Robinson, and T. Rundall. 2003. "How Different Is California? A Comparison of U.S. Physician Organizations."

Health Affairs (web exclusive): W3-492–502. http://content.healthaffairs .org/cgi/reprint/hlthaff.w3.492v1.

Kane, C., and D. W. Emmons. 2013. "New Data on Physician Practice Arrangements: Private Practice Remains Strong Despite Shifts Toward Hospital Employment." In *American Medical Association Policy Research Perspectives*. Chicago: American Medical Association. www.ama-assn.org/ resources/doc/health-policy/prp-physician-practice-arrangements.pdf.

Liebhaber, A., and J. Grossman. 2007. "Physicians Moving to Mid-Sized, Single Specialty Practices." *HSC Tracking Report* 18, August. Washington, DC: Center for Studying Health System Change.

O'Malley, A., A. Bond, and R. Berenson. 2011. "Rising Hospital Employment of Physicians: Better Quality, Higher Costs." *Issue Brief* 136, August. Washington, DC: Center for Studying Health System Change. http:// hschange.org/content/1230/1230.pdf.

Pear, R. 2013. "Medicare Panel Urges Cuts to Hospital Payments for Services Doctors Offer for Less." *New York Times*, June 14, p. A14. www.nytimes .com/2013/06/15/health/medicare-panel-urges-cuts-to-hospital- payments-for-services-doctors-offer-for-less.html?_r=0.

Weeks, W. B., D. J. Gottlieb, D. E. Nyweide, J. M. Sutherland, J. Bynum, L. P. Casalino, R. R. Gillies, S. M. Shortell, and E. S. Fisher. 2010. "Higher Health Care Quality and Bigger Savings Found at Large Multispecialty Medical Groups." *Health Affairs* 29 (5): 991–97.

RECURRENT MALPRACTICE CRISES

13

Three malpractice crises have occurred in the last 35 years. The last one began in 2002. The median annual increase in malpractice premiums was between 15 and 30 percent in most states, and some states experienced rate increases as high as 73 percent.

The first malpractice crisis occurred in the mid-1970s, when physicians' malpractice premiums rose more than 50 percent between 1974 and 1976; for some specialties, such as obstetrics/gynecology and surgery, the increases were even greater. During this first malpractice crisis, some insurers completely withdrew from the malpractice insurance market, while others increased their premiums by as much as 300 percent. Physicians threatened to strike if state legislatures did not intervene. To ensure access to malpractice insurance at the lowest possible rates, some medical societies formed their own mutual insurance companies.

By the late 1970s and early 1980s, malpractice premiums had stabilized somewhat, but they rose sharply again in the mid-1980s. This event precipitated the second malpractice crisis. Again, physicians demanded that state legislators take action to alleviate the burden of high premiums. In the late 1980s, malpractice premiums and awards started to decline and then stabilized through the mid-1990s.

The annual percentage change in malpractice premiums appears to be cyclical. After years of falling malpractice premiums, the third malpractice crisis started in 2002, as premiums again rose rapidly and premiums for some medical specialties sharply increased. With the rapid rise in premiums, medical societies once again pressured federal and state legislatures for malpractice reform—that is, tort changes that would limit malpractice awards and claims filed.

Since 2006, malpractice premiums have either been relatively stable or have declined, as price competition among malpractice insurers has increased, yet insurers continue to remain profitable; the cost of claims plus the money spent defending the claims has been less than collected premiums (Medical Liability Monitor 2013). If history is any guide, another malpractice crisis will likely arise in several years. As long as insurers remain profitable, they will try to expand their market share by competing on price until they realize their costs are exceeding their premiums; they will begin to suffer underwriting losses and then sharply raise their premiums to make up for those losses.

Explanations for the Rise in Malpractice Premiums

Insurers take several factors into account when setting malpractice premiums, such as recent payments, the anticipated cost of future payments, the expected rate of return on invested premium income, and administrative expenses. Further, because malpractice claims may take years to settle, insurers may find that previously they did not correctly predict malpractice payments and therefore have to either increase premiums to cover their losses or decrease premiums. This uncertainty in the market for medical malpractice insurance, together with changes in interest rates, contributes to the cyclical nature of this industry.

The components of malpractice premiums that receive the most attention are (1) economic costs, which include current and future medical expenses and lost wages; (2) the costs of pain and suffering, which usually cover the physical and emotional stress caused by an injury; this is the component that damage caps seek to limit; and (3) the factors affecting the malpractice insurer's profitability, including its operating loss ratio, investment returns, and legal defense costs. To understand the cyclical rise in malpractice premiums, it is important to learn how each of these components has been changing.

Insurers' malpractice payments per physician are based on economic costs and the costs of pain and suffering. These payments are based on two factors: the number of claims filed and the size of jury awards and out-of-court settlements per claim.

Claims Filed

Two reasons account for the general increase in malpractice cases over time. First, physicians are performing more procedures using complex new technologies, which carry greater risks of injury. Second, liberalized applications of tort law have created uncertainty among insurers regarding how much the awards are for pain and suffering and who is liable, which have placed some defendants (those with "deep pockets," such as health insurers and hospitals) at greater financial risk, although their contributions to injuries may be minor. Large jury awards and the ability to include more defendants increase the likelihood of a greater payoff to lawyers for bringing a malpractice case, hence increasing the number of such claims.

The number of claims per 100 physicians has risen at various times and then fallen. Since 1990, the number has been declining. Claims against obstetricians—typically the group with the highest number of claims filed—have dropped sharply since the early 1990s. The number of claims filed does not appear to explain the sharp increase in malpractice premiums in 2002, as the frequency of claims has continued to decline (CBO 2004).

Claims Payment

The second component of malpractice payments is the average payment per claim. Most claims (about 14,000 per year) are resolved by settlement with the insurer, whereas successful jury awards to the injured party number only about 400 per year.

An interesting factor in the rising costs for malpractice insurance is the difference between the average (mean) jury award and the median jury award, which represents the midpoint of all of the awards (half the awards are above and half are below the median award). Although the median jury award has risen slightly over time, the average jury award has increased sharply since the late 1990s (see Exhibit 13.1). The average jury award in any year (2012) is generally two to six times greater than the median award (e.g., more than $5 million versus $750,000, meaning juries make many small awards and a few large ones, although the latter receive the greatest publicity. Trial judgments (which account for only 4 percent of all malpractice payments) are, on average, about twice the size of settlements (which account for the remaining 96 percent), although the median settlement award also has increased—from $500,000 in 1997 to $750,000 in 2012.[1]

Large damage awards and financial settlements for patients, however, do not appear to be the driving force behind the surge in physicians' malpractice insurance premiums in 2002. One study, based on data from the National Practitioner Data Bank, found that payments to patients between 1991 and 2003 rose by 4 percent annually, a figure consistent with the increase in overall medical costs over that same period (Chandra, Nundy, and Seabury 2005). Malpractice premiums, however, grew much more rapidly.

Insurer Profitability

The third component of (and possible explanation for) malpractice payments is the changing financial condition and market structure of malpractice insurers. Profitability of insurers is determined by their loss ratio (jury awards, settlements, and defense costs as a percentage of premiums) and their investment returns, which are often used to offset high loss ratios. If the loss ratio is high, investment returns may offset those losses and the insurer may still be profitable.

As the frequency and size of physicians' malpractice claims rose in the early 1980s, several large insurers sharply increased their rates. The frequency and size of claims leveled off by the late 1980s, leaving insurers with large

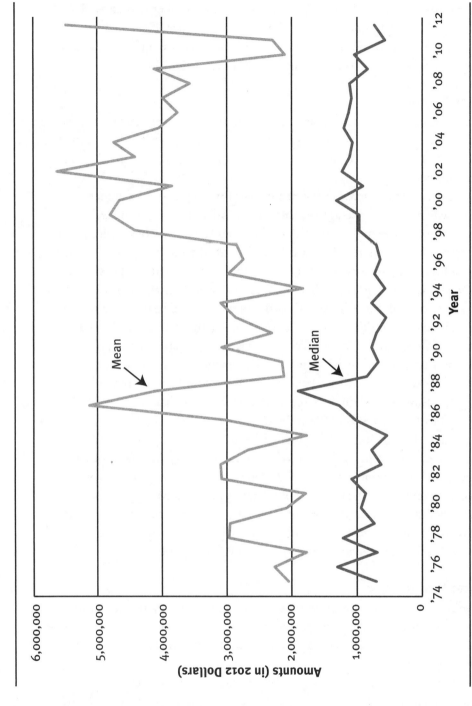

EXHIBIT 13.1
Jury Awards
for Medical
Malpractice
Cases, 1974–
2012

SOURCES: 1974–1990 data from ACS (n.d.); 1991–1992 data and 1993–2012 data from Jury Verdict Research (n.d.).

reserves that had been set aside for expected continued increases in malpractice payouts. During the early and mid-1990s, these insurers had substantial reserves against possible losses, so by releasing these reserves (changing them from expenses to income), insurers greatly increased their income. During this period also, insurers' loss ratios were favorable—at about 92 percent—and investment returns were high; insurers were profitable and malpractice premiums were generally stable.

Seemingly unaware that insurers' high profitability was based on previous years' reserves (when insurance actuaries were predicting that previous claims trends would continue to rise) and believing large profits could be had in malpractice insurance, new insurers entered the business. To attract business, these new insurers offered lower premiums, and existing insurers responded by cutting their premiums. Intense price competition among insurers led to premiums that were inadequate to cover malpractice payouts (Zimmerman and Oster 2002). As a result, the loss ratio rose as high as 98 percent of premium income by 2001 (see Exhibit 13.2). Reserves were consumed; further, investment returns fell sharply as bond yields and equities declined.[2] To improve their loss ratios and compensate for their lower investment returns, insurers increased their premiums. Another malpractice crisis occurred.

Two additional factors reinforced insurers' rate increases. First, reinsurers, who cover large malpractice insurance payouts, began to raise their reserves (and consequently their rates to malpractice insurers) as the percentage of million-dollar jury awards increased. Second, the structure of the malpractice insurance industry changed. By 2001, many insurers were losing money, became insolvent, and either exited the business or withdrew from markets in which they had been losing money. These temporary disruptions in availability of coverage in several markets led to much higher rates.[3]

By increasing their premiums, insurers became profitable by 2003. Insurer loss ratios declined, and they started to build up their reserves. As loss ratios continued to decline relative to premiums, investment income rose, profitability continued to grow, and malpractice premium increases became stable and even declined. Currently (2013), malpractice insurers continue to be profitable. With rising profitability and low loss ratios, premium competition among insurers for market share will rise and, as this occurs, loss ratios will similarly increase, leading to another malpractice crisis in several years. The cycle is likely to repeat itself.

Objectives of the Malpractice System

Tort law is the basis for medical malpractice. It entitles an injured person to compensation as a result of someone's negligence. Damages include

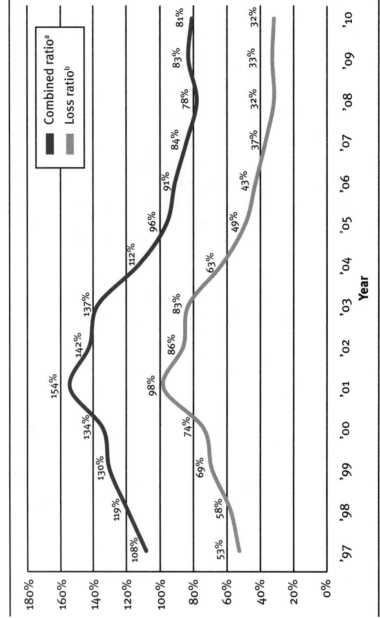

EXHIBIT 13.2
Medical
Malpractice
Industry
Financial
Ratios, 1997–
2010

[a] Awards, settlements, and defense costs plus dividends, administrative costs, and corporate income taxes as a percentage of premium
[b] Awards, settlements, and defense costs as a percentage of premium
SOURCE: Data from Lantry (2012), pp. 3 and 46.

economic losses (lost wages and medical bills) and noneconomic losses (referred to as *pain and suffering*). Thus, physicians have a financial incentive to provide good treatment and perform only those procedures for which they are competent.

The purposes of tort law are (1) to compensate the victim for negligence and (2) to deter future negligence. How well does the malpractice system fulfill these two objectives? Can legislative reforms achieve them at a lower cost than can the current system? Physician advocates maintain that too many claims have little to do with negligence (so the insurer will settle to avoid legal expenses that would exceed the settlement cost) and that juries award large sums unrelated to actual damages. Further, *defensive medicine*—additional tests and procedures prescribed by physicians to protect themselves against malpractice claims—adds billions of dollars to the nation's health expenditures.

Patient advocates counter those claims. They say physician negligence is more extensive than reflected by the number of claims filed, large jury awards are infrequent, incompetent physicians must be discouraged from practicing because physicians do not adequately monitor themselves, and defensive medicine is caused by the fee-for-service insurance system that rewards physicians for performing more services and eliminates patients' incentives to be concerned about the cost of care.

Compensation of Victims

A 1990 Harvard University study found that too few of those injured by negligence are compensated under the malpractice system (Localio et al. 1991). The authors examined hospital records from 1984 in 51 New York hospitals and determined that almost 4 percent of all patients suffered an injury while in the hospital and that one-quarter of those injuries were the result of negligence. Thus, about 1 percent of all patients discharged from New York hospitals in 1984 experienced some type of negligence. Examples of injuries occurring in hospitals are errors in diagnosis, falls, hospital-caused infections, and surgical complications.

Surprisingly, fewer than 2 percent of the patients identified as victims of negligence filed malpractice claims. However, 6 percent of injured patients who had not been victims of negligence filed claims. (Even though no negligence may have been committed by the surgeon, not all surgical procedures are successful, and the patient could be left with a disability or even die.) According to the Harvard study, half the patients who file claims eventually receive some compensation. Many patients settle within two years without receiving any compensation, and the rest may wait years for compensation. Few victims of actual negligence ever receive compensation—only about 1 percent. Of those patients injured through negligence who do not file claims

(98 percent of negligence victims), 20 percent have serious injuries—disabilities that last six months or more—and this figure includes fatalities (Localio et al. 1991).

A later study (involving cases in Colorado and Utah) also found a poor relationship between medical negligence and malpractice claims; 97 percent of those who suffered a medical negligence injury did not sue. Studdert and colleagues (2000) found that the elderly and the poor were least likely to sue for medical negligence. When physicians were sued, the claims were generally for injuries not caused by negligent care. (Also see Studdert and colleagues [2006] for an additional study on medical negligence and malpractice claims.)

Several reasons account for the low percentage of negligence claims filed. A patient may not know that negligence caused an injury. Some claims may be difficult to prove. Recoverable damages may be less than the litigation costs, particularly in the case of minor injuries.

The cost of administering the compensation system is high, and only a small portion of malpractice premiums is returned to those injured through negligence. Overhead, including legal fees, consumes the major portion of premiums. For every dollar paid into the liability system, 54 cents goes to legal fees and administrative costs (Studdert et al. 2006). Health insurance, on the other hand, returns 80 to 85 percent of the premium for medical expenses. If the sole purpose of malpractice insurance is to compensate those who are negligently injured, more efficient means at lower administrative costs exist. A different approach could compensate a greater number of victims and return a greater portion of premiums to those injured.

Deterrence of Negligence

Justification of the current malpractice system must depend, therefore, on how well the system performs its second, more important purpose: deter future negligence. Compensation tries not only to make whole the injuries suffered by victims of negligence but also to force negligent healthcare providers to exercise greater caution in future caregiving situations. Concerns exist, however, that not enough injuries are prevented by the current system to justify the high costs of practicing defensive medicine, determining fault, and prosecuting malpractice claims.

The standard of care used in determining negligence is what one would expect from a reasonably competent person who is knowledgeable about advances in medicine and who exercises care. Some cases of malpractice—such as amputating the wrong leg or leaving surgical supplies in a patient's abdomen—are easily established. With other forms of physician behavior, however, uncertainties exist in both diagnosis and outcome of medical treatment. Many medical procedures are inherently risky. Even with correct diagnosis and treatment, a patient may die because of poor health conditions, or a baby may be born with a birth defect through no fault of the obstetrician. Physicians do differ in the quality of care they provide and in their success rates, but it is difficult—hence costly—to determine whether a specific outcome is a result of physician negligence, poor communication of the risks involved, or the patient's underlying health condition.

The potential for malpractice suits increases the cost of negligent behavior to the physician. Physicians, therefore, would be expected to change their behavior and restrict their practices to forestall such costs—to stop performing procedures and tasks for which they lack competence. Prevention costs time and resources; therefore, physicians should invest their time, training, and medical testing in prevention up to the point at which the additional cost of prevention equals the additional value of injuries avoided (forgone malpractice costs). Too much prevention could occur if a great deal of time and resources (the additional costs) are used to prevent occasional minor injuries. A requirement that the injury rate be zero would be too costly for society and would discourage skilled specialists from performing procedures that involve an element of risk of injury but could benefit the patient.

How Well Does the Malpractice System Deter Negligence?

Is the value to patients of the negligence prevented greater than the costs (defensive medicine, determining liability, and litigation) of the malpractice system? Experts differ on this issue.

First, critics of the current system claim that physicians are not penalized for negligence, as only 2 to 3 percent of negligence victims file claims. Second, because less than half of malpractice insurance premiums—approximately $4.6 billion, or one-sixth of 1 percent of total healthcare spending—are returned to victims of negligence and the remainder is spent on overhead and legal fees, the system is too costly. Third, because most malpractice insurance does not experience-rate physicians within their specialties, incompetent physicians are not penalized by higher premiums; their behavior merely raises premiums for all physicians in that specialty. Fourth, not all physicians who are sued are incompetent. Although incompetent physicians may be sued more often, competent physicians may also be sued because of occasional errors or because they are specialists who treat more difficult cases; for example, board-certified physicians are sued more often than are other physicians.[4] Fifth, a characteristic of the current system is the amount of money spent on tests and services that are not medically justified but that help protect physicians from malpractice claims. Physicians overuse tests because the costs of such defensive medicine are borne by patients and insurers, whereas an injury claim could result in physician liability. Thus, physicians are able to shift the costs of their greater caution to others.

In Defense of the Malpractice System

Defenders of the malpractice system claim that the incentive to avoid malpractice suits changes physicians' behavior and makes them act more carefully. Physicians have limited their scope of practice, they are more conscientious in documenting their records, and they take the time to discuss with their patients the risks involved in a procedure. Although physician premiums are not experience-rated, lawsuits are a costly deterrent in terms of time spent defending against them and potential damage to the physician's reputation.

The Costs of Defensive Medicine

The costs of defensive medicine are probably overstated because, under a fee-for-service system, excessive testing would occur even if the threat of malpractice were eliminated. Physicians order too many tests because insured patients pay only a small portion of their price. Although the benefits of the tests are less than the costs of performing them, patients rationally want those tests because the benefit to them may be greater than their share of the costs. Physicians are reimbursed a fee-for-service benefit from prescribing extra tests, while physicians in health maintenance organizations (HMOs) have less of an incentive to perform excessive testing. Thus, physicians' use of excessive testing results in part from traditional insurance payment systems and a lack of policing of such tests by insurers, not necessarily from malpractice.

The costs imposed by defensive medicine are difficult to measure. Estimates of the extent of that practice often rely on conjectural surveys of providers, and what one provider may consider defensive medicine may be deemed prudent medicine by another. However, Mello and colleagues (2010, Exhibit 1) estimated the cost of defensive medicine in 2008 dollars to be $45.59 billion—$38.79 billion for hospital services and $6.8 billion for physician/clinical services—which is not an insignificant amount.

Physicians with malpractice insurance are not at risk for a large financial loss resulting from a malpractice case. However, a malpractice case imposes other, nonfinancial, costs on a physician. During the time it takes to resolve a malpractice claim, about five years after the incident, the physician is likely to be concerned about the damage to her reputation, the time lost from work, and the general stress of the process. These costs often weigh larger in the mind of the physician than the possible financial costs, which the physician does not bear, causing her to be defensive in the tests and treatments she prescribes.

A study by Carrier and colleagues (2013) found that physicians who were more concerned about malpractice were more likely to engage in defensive medicine—such as ordering more diagnostic tests than medically necessary, performing more procedures, requiring more visits, and being more likely to hospitalize a patient or to refer him to other physicians.

Removing the threat of malpractice leaves few alternatives for monitoring and disciplining physicians. The emphasis on quality control in organized medicine has always been on the process of becoming a physician—that is, spending many years on education, graduating from an approved medical school, and passing national examinations. However, once a physician is licensed, he is never re-examined for re-licensure. State medical licensing boards do not adequately monitor physician quality or discipline incompetent physicians. Finally, patients have little or no access to information on physicians' procedure outcomes. Until recently the medical profession actively discouraged public access to such information. What recourse, other than filing a malpractice claim, would a patient have after being injured by an incompetent physician?

Few would disagree that victims of negligence are not adequately compensated. The controversial issues are whether malpractice actually deters negligence and whether alternatives are available for monitoring and disciplining incompetent physician behavior.

Proposed Changes to the Malpractice System

Many changes have been proposed to correct perceived inadequacies in the malpractice system. Generally, proposals seek to lower malpractice premiums by limiting the size of jury awards for pain and suffering (economic costs for medical expenses and lost wages are not subject to a cap) and the number of claims filed. Both changes would reduce lawyers' incentives to accept malpractice cases.

Damage Caps

Proposals to limit the potential recovery of damages decrease the value of malpractice claims and thereby reduce the number of malpractice claims filed. One study found that malpractice premiums in states with damage caps are 17 percent lower than in states without damage caps (Thorpe 2004).[5] In 1975, California enacted a $250,000 damage cap on pain and suffering, which has not been updated for inflation. (If adjusted for inflation, the cap would be $1.083 million in 2013 dollars.) Caps such as those in California's lower the amount of malpractice awards that can be used to pay legal fees, as the remainder of the award is for lost wages and medical expenses. Zeiler and Hardcastle (2012) reviewed multiple studies that have estimated the effect of damage caps on malpractice premiums and concluded that little weight can be placed on any one study because of their methodological shortcomings.

Collateral Offset Rule

Under the collateral offset rule, the amount of an injured party's jury award or insurer's settlement is reduced because of the amounts paid by other sources, such as health insurance and worker's compensation. Proponents of this rule believe additional payments from other sources provide the injured party with much more than he is entitled to. Opponents of this rule believe that unless the injured party collects the full amount of his award, even though he is paid by other sources, the negligent defendant benefits because her liability is reduced. Proposals to reduce awards by amounts paid by other sources would have the same effect as imposing damage caps. Lawyers would have less incentive to bring suits on behalf of patients.

Limits on Attorney's Fees

Fewer malpractice cases would be brought if a limit were placed on lawyers' contingency fees (currently these can be as high as one-third to one-half of the award). Lawyers accept malpractice cases on the basis of the probability of winning and the size of the likely award. They have less financial incentive to invest their resources in cases whose awards would be small. They are in a competitive market and may represent either plaintiffs or defendants in malpractice cases. Defendants pay them an hourly rate. Fewer lawyers would choose to represent plaintiffs if contingency fees were reduced.

Joint and Several Liability

Joint and several liability occurs when an injured person sues multiple defendants and is able to collect the entire award from any of the defendants, regardless of the defendant's degree of fault. Even if a defendant is only 10 percent liable, she may end up paying most of the damages. This rule creates an incentive for the injured party to sue as many defendants as possible to make sure the damages can be paid. Some states have limited a defendant's liability to the individual degree of fault. Limiting a defendant's liability decreases the potential size of the award, which might lessen the defendant hospital's oversight of its staff physicians to avoid malpractice suits.

Special Health Courts

In a special health court, the jury is replaced with a specially trained judge (with both medical and legal training) who would be advised by neutral experts. Proponents of this approach claim that proceedings would be expedited (the case would be decided in a matter of months); that costs would be dramatically lower than those of the current system, which consumes about 60 percent of the premium for legal fees and administrative costs and takes about five years to resolve a case; and that it would provide a system of justice based on accepted medical standards, thereby reducing the need for defensive medicine.

As part of the proposal for special health courts, patient compensation for medical negligence would be decided by a separate administrative agency (which would act as a neutral fact finder) rather than by the current court system (which is adversarial, with each side having its own experts).

If special health courts were adopted, filing a claim would be less costly, a greater number of patients would be able to file claims, and more injured patients would be compensated for medical negligence. The amount of compensation for a patient negligently injured likely would be lowered given that so many more patients would receive compensation. Although special courts have been used in other areas where special expertise is needed—such as in tax courts, bankruptcy courts, and family courts—special health courts have not been used in the United States; their implementation is opposed by trial lawyers, who benefit from the current malpractice system.

Evidence-Based Guidelines

The adoption of national (as opposed to local) standards of care has been proposed for judging malpractice suits. Guidelines are written documents of what is considered the best clinical practices for a set of symptoms, type of patient, and a specific disease. Local standards of care differ greatly among various US localities, leading to wide variations in tests and procedures. Physicians who are able to demonstrate that they practiced according to well-accepted, evidence-based national guidelines would then be exempt from liability in malpractice lawsuits. The current tort-based malpractice system would not be changed if the use of national guidelines were adopted; however, the evidence of whether a physician was negligent would be based on these national rather than local standards of care.

Frakes (2013) examined geographic variations in physician practice patterns and estimated that if states were to adopt national standards for judging malpractice claims, geographic variations in use of medical services would decrease by 30 percent to 50 percent. Frakes also found no associated changes in patient health as a result of a change to national guidelines.

The adoption of national guidelines for malpractice cases is controversial. Critics claim that such guidelines are unable to account for the wide variation in patients' conditions and their health problems. (A similar criticism has been leveled against the use of comparative effectiveness research—see Chapter 21.)

No-Fault Malpractice

A no-fault system would compensate an injured patient whether or not negligence was involved. In return, patients would forfeit their right to sue. A no-fault system has two main advantages. First, litigation costs would be lower because proving who was at fault for the injury is not necessary, and these savings could be used to increase victim compensation. Second, all injured patients—most of whom could not win malpractice suits because either their claims were too small to attract a lawyer's interest or no one was at fault in causing their injuries—would receive some compensation. A no-fault system could have a payment schedule according to types of injuries, which led to loss of income and medical expenses. The schedule could include payment for pain and suffering in cases of severe injury.

A no-fault system, however, has two important problems. First, such a system has no deterrence mechanism to weed out incompetent providers or encourage physicians to exercise greater caution. Second, because all injuries would be subject to compensation, no clear line would be drawn between injuries resulting from negligence, injuries not resulting from negligence, unfavorable treatment outcomes caused by the patient's health condition and lifestyle, and outcomes of risky procedures (such as transplants and delivery of low-birth-weight infants) that are never 100 percent favorable. Compensating patients for all injuries and unfavorable outcomes could be very expensive given the large number of injuries for which no claims are filed.[6] Who should bear these costs?

Studdert, Brennan, and Thomas (2000) estimated that a no-fault compensation system for patients who are injured from all events (negligent and non-negligent) would cost more than four times as much as the current tort system.

Enterprise Liability

Deterring physician negligence continues to be difficult. Regulatory approaches—such as state licensing boards for monitoring and disciplining physicians—have performed poorly. One approach that seeks to improve on the malpractice system for deterring negligence is enterprise liability. Changing the liability laws so that liability is shifted away from the physician to a larger entity of which the physician is required to be a part—such as a hospital, medical group, or managed care plan—would place the incentive for monitoring and enforcing medical quality with that larger organization. These organizations would balance the increased costs of prevention and risk-reducing behavior against the potential for a malpractice claim.

The shift to enterprise liability is already occurring because of market trends and court rulings. The growth of managed care organizations and the fact that they are liable for physicians they employ or contract with have increased such organizations' monitoring of physician behavior. Further, the concept of joint and several liability—wherein the physician is the primary defendant but the hospital or managed care plan is also named as a defendant with potentially 100 percent liability for damages (although it may have been only 10 percent at fault)—provides hospitals and HMOs an incentive to increase their quality assurance and risk management programs. Many physicians, however, perform surgery only in outpatient settings or do not practice within a hospital. Other physicians may have multiple hospital staff appointments, and still others do not belong to large health plans. These physicians would be most affected by such a shift in liability laws because they would lose some of their autonomy as they become subject to greater supervision by larger entities.

Placing liability for malpractice on a large entity would enable insurers to experience-rate the organization.[7] As more healthcare organizations become experience-rated, they will devote more resources to monitoring their quality of care and disciplining physicians for poor performance. Many organizations—such as HMOs, preferred provider organizations, and large medical groups—have information systems in place to profile the practice patterns of their physicians. Competition on price and quality provides organizations with an incentive to develop quality-control mechanisms. These organizations, rather than regulatory bodies, have the incentives and the ability to evaluate and control physicians.

Disclosure, Apology, and Offer Programs

A relatively new approach for resolving malpractice claims that does not require new legislation is referred to as *disclosure, apology, and offer* (Sage et al. 2014). The physician and hospital voluntarily disclose any adverse events and errors, apologize for such injuries and errors, and offer compensation to the patient and family. Further, all hospital and professional fees are waived if the patient received substandard care. A number of institutions using this approach state that it has reduced the number of malpractice claims filed against them and the time to settle malpractice cases; it has also eliminated the high costs of defending a malpractice lawsuit, including attorney fees, expert witnesses, and court costs (which can be as high as $350,000). In addition, these institutions claim that defensive medicine by physicians—such as additional lab and radiology tests—has also decreased.

Disclosing medical errors, apologizing, and offering compensation is contrary to the approach used by many hospitals and physicians fearful of a malpractice case. Their approach has been (1) deny that such adverse events and errors have occurred and (2) defend themselves. But such a defensive approach often leads to the filing of a malpractice case because a patient may feel that doing so is the only way to find out what caused the injury.

An important advantage of the disclosure, apology, and offer approach is that physicians and hospitals can improve patient safety by learning how to prevent similar adverse events in the future. The major elements of this approach include reporting errors, analyzing what occurred, issuing an apology, offering compensation, improving process and performance, and educating professional and staff personnel.

The Effects of Various Tort Reforms

Many proposals have been made to improve the current tort system, which does not adequately compensate patients injured by medical negligence or act as a deterrent to negligent physicians. Exhibit 13.3, adapted from Mello and Kachalia (2010), summarizes the likely impact of selected proposals on the following outcomes of malpractice reform: frequency of malpractice claims and costs, overhead costs of the medical liability system (including legal defense costs), healthcare providers' liability costs, defensive medicine, supply of medical services (including supply of physicians and patients' health insurance premiums), and quality of care. In addition, the exhibit indicates the certainty of the evidence as to these effects. Unfortunately, for many of the proposals the level of certainty is low.

Summary

The current medical malpractice system has several important flaws. First, most patients injured by medical negligence (97 percent to 98 percent) do not sue and are not compensated for their injuries. Second, given the small percentage of injured patients who sue, physicians' negligent behavior is rarely deterred. Third, the current system is inefficient. A large percent of the malpractice premium is not used for patient compensation but for legal costs and administrative expense. Further, physicians have an incentive under fee-for-service payment (and insurance that results in low patient copayments) to engage in defensive medicine, prescribing care of doubtful value to decrease the probability of a malpractice lawsuit.

Experts do not agree on malpractice reform. Reform proposals that decrease the size of an award or make filing claims more difficult are addressing the wrong problem. These remedies are directed at reducing the number of claims, but the real problem appears to be that too few bona fide *negligence* claims are brought. Reform should be evaluated in terms of whether it deters negligent behavior and improves victim compensation. Some proposals, such as special health courts and enterprise liability, have academic

EXHIBIT 13.3
Evidence and Probable Effects of Malpractice Reform

	Claims Frequency and Costs	Overhead Costs	Liability Costs	Defensive Medicine	Supply	Quality of Care
Caps on noneconomic damages	o for frequency (M), ↓↓ for costs (M)	↑ (L)	↓ for premiums (M)	↓ (H)	↑ (M) for physician supply, o (L) for health insurance premiums	o (L)
Attorney fee limits	o (H) for frequency and costs	↓ (L)	o (H)	o (L)	o (M)	o (L)
Joint-and-several liability reform	o (L) for frequency, o (H) for costs	o (L)	o (M)	o (M)	o (M) for physician supply, ↓ (L) for health insurance premiums	o (L)
Collateral-source rule reform	o (M) for frequency, o (H) for costs	o (L)	o (M)	o (H)	o (M) for physician supply, ↓ (L) for health insurance premiums	o (M)
Administrative compensation systems or "health courts"	Medical court model: o (L) for frequency, o (L) for costs Administrative model: ↑↑ (M) for frequency, o (L) for costs	Medical court model: ↓ (L) Administrative model: ↓↓ (H)	Medical court model: o (L) Administrative model: o (L)	Medical court model: o (L) Administrative model: ↓ (L)	Medical court model: o (L) Administrative model: o (L)	Medical court model: o (L) Administrative model: ↑ (M)
Enterprise liability	o (L) for frequency, (L) for costs	↓ (L)	↓ (L)	↓ (L)	o (L)	↑ (L)

NOTES: Effects are classified as large increase (↑↑), modest increase (↑), no change (o), modest decrease (↓), or large decrease (↓↓). Evidence or certainty levels for these effects are classified as low or theoretical only (L), moderate (M), or high (H).
SOURCE: Adapted from Mello and Kachalia (2010), tables 3 and 4.

support. However, enacting reform is a difficult political problem. Proposals often reflect the interests of those who might benefit from the change. Medical societies are often pitted against the trial lawyers' associations (and their respective political parties). The battle for changes in the malpractice system is occurring in almost every state and, because of the opposition of trial lawyers, only demonstration projects were included in the Affordable Care Act. All proposals by whatever interest group should be judged by how well they achieve the two goals of the malpractice system: compensating victims injured by negligence and deterring future negligence.

Discussion Questions

1. How well does the malpractice system compensate victims of negligence?
2. How effective is the deterrence function of the malpractice system?
3. Discuss the advantages and disadvantages of no-fault insurance.
4. Do you think the costs of defensive medicine would be reduced under a no-fault system?
5. Evaluate the possible effects of the following on deterrence and victim compensation:
   a. Limiting lawyers' contingency fees
   b. Special health courts
   c. Limiting the size of malpractice awards
   d. Placing the liability for malpractice on the healthcare organization to which the physician belongs

Notes

1. Vidmar (2009) summarizes findings from various studies regarding jury decisions in malpractice cases:

   > Juries are skeptical about inflated claims. Jury verdicts on negligence are roughly similar to assessments made by medical experts and judges. Damage awards tend to correlate positively with the severity of injury. There are defensible reasons for large damage awards. Moreover, the largest awards are typically settled for much less than the verdicts.

2. A decline in investment return of 1 percent is estimated to lead to a 2 percent to 4 percent increase in malpractice premiums (Thorpe 2004, W4–23).

3. Rising malpractice premiums are not the result of collusion among insurers. Collusion would be difficult given the large number of insurers—including physician-owned insurance companies (although few companies exist from whom these insurers purchase reinsurance)—and the high level of competition among them.

4. Jena and colleagues (2011) analyzed the percentage of physicians experiencing a malpractice claim in a year by specialty, the average claim payment by specialty, and the cumulative risk of ever being sued for physicians in both high- and low-risk specialties. The authors found that by age 65, 99 percent of physicians in high-risk specialties had a malpractice claim compared to 75 percent of physicians in low-risk specialties.

5. Malpractice liability has affected physicians' participation in a market. Physicians claim that the financial burden of high malpractice premiums has led some physicians to retire early, others to stop performing high-risk procedures, and still others to move to states with lower malpractice premiums—all of which affect patients' access to medical care. For example, states that capped noneconomic damages in malpractice cases experienced a relatively modest 3.3 percent increase in physician supply compared with states without such caps (Kessler, Sage, and Becker 2005). Rural counties in states with noneconomic damage caps had 3.2 percent more physicians per capita than did rural counties in states without caps. Obstetricians and surgeons, who are considered more vulnerable to lawsuits than other physicians, were most influenced by the presence or absence of caps (Encinosa and Hellinger 2005).

6. The Institute of Medicine and others have issued reports documenting high rates of medical error causing serious harm or death in the United States. Not all of these injuries to patients, however, are believed to be the result of provider negligence. Appropriate systems are lacking to prevent human error (Kohn, Corrigan, and Donaldson 1999).

7. The reason generally given for the lack of experience-rating, except by specialty, is that malpractice suits and awards are unrelated to medical negligence or the physician's history of negligence. Instead, they are more related to the physician's bedside manner—manner of relating to the patient. Whether this is correct is debatable.

References

American College of Surgeons (ACS). n.d. *Socio-economic Factbook for Surgery.* Various editions. Chicago: ACS.

Carrier, E., J. Reschovsky, D. Katz, and M. Mello. 2013. "High Physician Concern About Malpractice Risk Predicts More Aggressive Diagnostic Testing in Office-Based Practice." *Health Affairs* 32 (8): 1383–91.

Chandra, A., S. Nundy, and S. Seabury. 2005. "The Growth of Physician Medical Malpractice Payments: Evidence from the National Practitioner Data Bank." *Health Affairs* (web exclusive): http://content.healthaffairs.org/cgi/content/abstract/hlthaff.w5.240v1.

Congressional Budget Office (CBO). 2004. "Limiting Tort Liability for medical Malpractice." Accessed October 2013. www.cbo.gov/sites/default/files/cbofiles/ftpdocs/49xx/doc4968/01-08-medicalmalpractice.pdf.

Encinosa, W., and F. Hellinger. 2005. "Have State Caps on Malpractice Awards Increased the Supply of Physicians?" *Health Affairs* (web exclusive): http://content.healthaffairs.org/cgi/content/abstract/hlthaff.w5.250v1.

Frakes, M. 2013. "The Impact of Medical Liability Standards on Regional Variations in Physician Behavior: Evidence from the Adoption of National-Standard Rules." *American Economic Review* 103 (1): 257–76.

Jena, A., S. Seabury, D. Lakdawalla, and A. Chandra. 2011. "Malpractice Risk According to Physician Specialty." *New England Journal of Medicine* 365 (7): 629–36. www.ncbi.nlm.nih.gov/pmc/articles/PMC3204310/.

Jury Verdict Research. n.d. *Current Award Trends in Personal Injury.* Various editions. Horsham, PA: LRP Publications and Thomson Reuters.

Kessler, D., W. Sage, and D. Becker. 2005. "Impact of Malpractice Reforms on the Supply of Physicians." *JAMA* 293 (21): 2618–25.

Kohn, L., J. Corrigan, and M. Donaldson (eds.). 1999. *To Err Is Human.* Washington, DC: National Academies Press.

Lantry, K. J. H. 2012. "Malpractice Loss Trends, 2012." Powerpoint presentation. Accessed March 2014. www.scha.org/files/klantry_medical_malpractice_trends_update.pdf.

Localio, A. R., A. Lawthers, T. Brennan, N. Laird, L. Hebert, L. Peterson, J. Newhouse, P. Weiler, and H. Hiatt. 1991. "Relation Between Malpractice Claims and Adverse Events Due to Negligence." *New England Journal of Medicine* 325 (4): 245–51.

Medical Liability Monitor. 2013. *Annual Rate Survey Issue* 38 (10). www.milliman.com/uploadedFiles/insight/2013/MLM-Rate-Survey.pdf.

Mello, M., and A. Kachalia. 2010. *Evaluation of Options for Medical Malpractice System Reform.* Washington, DC: Medicare Payment Advisory Commission.

Mello, M., A. Chandra, A. A. Gawande, and D. M. Studdert. 2010. "National Costs of the Medical Liability System." *Health Affairs* 29 (9): 1569–77.

Sage, W., T. Gallagher, S. Armstrong, J. Cohn, T. McDonald, J. Gale, A. Woodward, and M. Mello. 2014. "How Policy Makers Can Smooth the Way for Communication-and-Resolution Programs." *Health Affairs* 33 (1): 11–19.

Studdert, D., T. Brennan, and E. Thomas. 2000. "Beyond Dead Reckoning: Measures of Medical Injury Burden, Malpractice Litigation, and Alternative Compensation Models from Utah and Colorado." *Indiana Law Review* 33 (4): 1643–86.

Studdert, D., M. Mello, A. Gawande, T. Gandhi, A. Kachalia, C. Yoon, A. Puopolo, and T. Brennan. 2006. "Claims, Errors, and Compensation Payments in Medical Malpractice Litigation." *New England Journal of Medicine* 354 (19): 2024–33. www.nejm.org/doi/pdf/10.1056/NEJMsa054479.

Studdert, D., E. Thomas, H. Burstin, B. Zbar, E. Orav, T. Brennan, and A. Troyen. 2000. "Negligent Care and Malpractice Claiming Behavior in Utah and Colorado." *Medical Care* 38 (3): 250–60.

Thorpe, K. 2004. "The Medical Malpractice 'Crisis': Recent Trends and the Impact of State Tort Reforms." *Health Affairs* (web exclusive): http://content.healthaffairs.org/cgi/reprint/hlthaff.w4.20v1.

Vidmar, N. 2009. "Juries and Medical Malpractice Claims: Empirical Facts versus Myths." *Clinical Orthopaedics and Related Research* 467 (2): 367–75. www.ncbi.nlm.nih.gov/pmc/articles/PMC2628507/.

Zeiler, K., and L. Hardcastle. 2012. "Do Damages Caps Reduce Medical Malpractice Insurance Premiums? A Systematic Review of Estimates and the Methods Used to Produce Them." Georgetown Law and Economics Research Paper 12–042. http://scholarship.law.georgetown.edu/cgi/viewcontent.cgi?article=2140&context=facpub.

Zimmerman, R., and C. Oster. 2002. "Assigning Liability: Insurers' Missteps Helped Provoke Malpractice 'Crisis.'" *Wall Street Journal*, June 24, pp. A1 and A8.

DO NONPROFIT HOSPITALS BEHAVE DIFFERENTLY FROM FOR-PROFIT HOSPITALS?

14

Hospitals initially cared for the poor, the mentally ill, and those with contagious diseases, such as tuberculosis. Many hospitals were started by religious organizations and local communities as charitable institutions. More affluent patients were treated in their own homes. Things began to change with the development of ether in the mid-1800s, which allowed operations to be conducted under anesthesia. By the late 1800s, antiseptic procedures began to increase the chances of surviving surgery. Then the introduction of the X-ray machine around the beginning of the twentieth century enabled surgeons to become more effective by improving their ability to determine the location for the surgery, and some exploratory surgery was eliminated.

As a result of these improvements, hospitals became the physician's workshop. Similarly, the type of patients the hospital served changed. Hospitals were no longer places in which to die or be incarcerated but rather places in which paying patients could be treated and then returned to society. The development of drugs and improved living conditions reduced the demand for mental and tuberculosis hospitals, and the demand for short-term general hospitals grew.

The control of private nonprofit hospitals also changed. As more of the hospital's income came from paying patients, reliance on trustees to raise philanthropic funds declined. Physicians, who admitted and treated patients, became more important to the hospital. As they were responsible for generating the hospital's revenue, physicians' control over the hospital increased.

Most hospitals in the United States are nonprofit, either nongovernmental institutions or controlled by religious organizations. Together, these are referred to as *private nonprofit hospitals*. As Exhibit 14.1 shows, the ownership of a majority of hospitals (2,894 of the 5,010 hospitals in 2012) is voluntary, meaning private nonprofit. In 2012, 1,037 state and local government and 202 federal hospitals were in operation. Investor-owned (for-profit) institutions accounted for 1,068 of total hospitals. Together, private nonprofit and for-profit hospitals admitted 83 percent of patients (68.5 percent and 14.5 percent, respectively). The main legal distinctions between nonprofit and for-profit hospitals are that nonprofits cannot distribute profits

EXHIBIT 14.1
Selected Hospital Data, 2012

Type of Hospital	Number of Hospitals	Percentage Change			Beds	Admissions	Percent Distribution of Admissions	Occupancy Rate[a]
		75–85	85–95	95–12				
Short-term							97.7	
General[b]	5,010	–3.3	–9.8	–4.0	800,566	34,422,071	95.2	63.5
State and local government	1,037	–10.4	–16.5	–23.2	120,271	4,446,594	12.3	63.8
Not-for-profit	2,894	0.3	–8.1	–8.9	545,287	24,751,485	68.5	64.9
Investor-owned	1,068	3.9	–6.6	42.0	135,008	5,223,992	14.5	56.8
Federal	202	–10.2	–12.8	–32.4	36,342	884,609	2.4	62.7
Long-term[c]	511	–6.3	4.0	–33.7	82,737	833,766	2.3	83.8

[a] Ratio of average daily census to every 100 beds
[b] "Short-term general" includes community hospitals and hospital units of institutions. Community hospitals group consists of state and local government, nongovernment not-for-profit, and investor-owned hospitals.
[c] Includes general, psychiatric, tuberculosis and other respiratory diseases, and all others
SOURCE: Data from AHA (n.d.): 1986 edition, Text Table 2; 1995–1996 edition, Table 3A; 2014 edition, Table 2.

to shareholders and their earnings and property are exempt from federal and state taxes; they also may receive donations.

Since the mid-1980s, when managed care competition started, debate has ensued over whether nonprofit hospitals are really different from for-profit hospitals. The issues surrounding this debate center on the following questions: Do nonprofits charge lower prices than for-profits do? Do nonprofits provide a higher level of quality than for-profits do? Do nonprofits provide more charity care than for-profits do? Or, as some critics of nonprofits maintain, is there no difference between the two other than the tax-exempt status of nonprofits' surpluses? If the latter position is correct, is continuing nonprofit hospitals' tax advantages and government subsidies justified? Alternatively, if nonprofits provide more charity care and higher quality of service and charge lower prices, will eliminating for-profits enable nonprofits to better serve their communities?

Why Are Hospitals Predominantly Nonprofit?

Several hypotheses have been offered to explain the existence of nonprofit hospitals. The most obvious is that when hospitals were used predominantly as institutions to serve the poor, they were dependent on donations for their funds. However, the possibility of receiving donations does not explain why the majority of hospitals continue to be nonprofit. Donations account for a small percentage of hospital revenue. As public and private health insurance became the dominant sources of hospital revenue, the potential for profit increased, as did the number of for-profit hospitals.

Although both public and private insurance have increased, many people are still uninsured. Some believe that only nonprofit hospitals provide uncompensated care to those who are unable to pay. Nonprofit hospitals presumably are willing to use their surplus funds to subsidize both the poor and money-losing services.

Another related explanation is the issue of trust. A relationship based on trust is needed in markets in which information is lacking. Patients are not sure what services they need. They are dependent on the provider for their diagnoses and treatment recommendations, and they do not know the skill of the surgeon. The quality of medical and surgical treatments is difficult for patients to judge, and they cannot tell whether the hospital failed to provide care to save costs. In such situations, patients are more likely to rely on non-profit providers, believing that because they are not interested in profit, they will not take advantage of a patient who lacks information and is seriously ill.[1]

Another explanation for nonprofit status is that the hospital's managers and board of directors want to be part of a nonprofit hospital, where their activities would be subject to limited community oversight. The managers and board would have greater flexibility to pursue policies according to their own preferences, such as offering prestigious but money-losing services even if these services are provided by other hospitals in the community.

Still another explanation is that hospitals are nonprofit because it is in physicians' financial interest. Being associated with nonprofit organizations allows physicians to exercise greater control over the hospital's policies, services offered, and investments in facilities and equipment. In a for-profit hospital, physicians have less money available for facilities and equipment of their choosing because the surplus has to be divided with shareholders and the government through payment of dividends and taxes. The hospital's physicians also benefit from the hospital's ability to receive donations and from the trust the community has in a nonprofit hospital.

The importance of trust, the provision of community benefits, and the financial interests of physicians appear to be key reasons for the nonprofit status of hospitals.[2]

Performance of Nonprofit and For-Profit Hospitals

For-profit hospitals have a more precise organizational goal—namely profit—than nonprofit hospitals do. A concern of any organization is monitoring its managers' success in achieving the firm's goal. In a for-profit firm, the objective is straightforward, and the shareholders have an incentive to monitor the performance of its managers and replace them if their performance is lacking.

A nonprofit firm has multiple objectives, making monitoring its managers more difficult. The various stakeholders of the nonprofit hospital—medical staff, board members, managers, employees, and the community—have different and conflicting objectives as to how the hospital's surplus should be distributed. Should the profits be used to subsidize the poor, increase compensation for managers, raise wages for employees, establish prestige facilities, or provide benefits (e.g., low office rent and resources) to medical staff? Less incentive exists to monitor a nonprofit hospital, as the board of directors generally has less financial interest in the hospital's performance and must depend on the managers for information on achieving the hospital's multiple goals. Furthermore, if the nonprofit hospital is not performing efficiently, it may be able to survive on community donations.

Given the differing goals and incentive-monitoring mechanisms between for-profit and nonprofit hospitals, it is important to examine how the behavior of nonprofits differs from that of for-profits.

Pricing

For-profit hospitals attempt to set prices to maximize their profits.[3] Do non-profit hospitals set lower prices than for-profit hospitals do? Three aspects of hospital pricing shed light on how nonprofit hospitals set prices.

First, nonprofits price to earn sufficient revenues to cover their costs. The nonprofits set prices to private insurers below their profit-maximizing price but raise those prices when the government lowers the price it pays for Medicare or Medicaid patients. For cost shifting to occur, a hospital (1) must have market power—that is, be able to profitably raise its price and (2) must decide not to exploit that market power before the government reduces its price. The extent to which cost shifting occurs indicates that hospitals do not set profit-maximizing prices to private payers. (A more complete discussion of cost shifting is provided in Chapter 17.)

Evidence for cost shifting is based on data from prior to the mid-1980s, before managed care competition. With the start of intense price competition among hospitals, insurers became more sensitive to the prices charged by hospitals. Hospitals' market power declined because insurers were willing to shift their volume to hospitals offering lower prices. Any ability nonprofit hospitals may have had to shift cost disappeared with hospital competition for managed care contracts. Instead, as the government reduced the prices it paid for Medicare and Medicaid patients, hospitals experienced greater pressure to lower their prices to be included in an insurer's provider network.

Second, the pricing practices of nonprofit hospitals to uninsured patients have received a great deal of media publicity recently. Large purchasers of hospital services (such as health insurers, Medicare, and Medicaid) receive deep discounts from a hospital's billed charges—often as high as 50 percent. Uninsured patients were asked to pay 100 percent of the hospital's billed charges. Newspaper stories have described the hardship faced by many of these patients who do not have the resources to pay their hospital bills. Several lawsuits were filed on behalf of the uninsured against nonprofit hospitals because the hospitals charged those least able to pay the highest prices and hounded patients for unpaid debts. These lawsuits (several of which have been settled by hospitals) claimed that nonprofit hospitals violated their charitable mission by overcharging the uninsured and sought to have these hospitals' tax-exempt status revoked. The pricing practices of nonprofits for the uninsured appear to be no different than those of for-profits. (Under public and political pressure, both types of hospitals have modified their pricing practices to the uninsured.)

Third, do nonprofit hospitals increase prices if they merge with other nonprofit hospitals? The number of hospital mergers has grown in recent years. Consolidation of for-profit firms or hospitals in a market causes concern that competition will decline, enabling the hospitals to raise their prices. Would a merger of nonprofit hospitals similarly result in higher hospital prices, or are nonprofit hospitals different?

In previous court cases in which the merger of nonprofit hospitals was contested by federal antitrust agencies, the presiding judges ruled that nonprofit mergers are different from for-profit mergers. The judges believed that merging nonprofits were unlikely to raise their prices—even if they acquired monopoly power—because the boards of directors are themselves local citizens and would not take advantage of their neighbors. Empirical studies, however, contradict the judges' belief that nonprofit ownership limits price increases after a merger (Capps and Dranove 2004; Melnick, Keeler, and Zwanziger 1999). Researchers found that nonprofits with great market power charge significantly higher prices than do nonprofits in competitive markets. These results suggest that some nonprofit hospitals merge simply as a means to increase their market power and negotiate higher prices with managed care plans. This type of behavior is no different from the behavior expected of for-profit hospitals.

In October 2005, the Federal Trade Commission (FTC) won an antitrust suit against nonprofit Northwestern Healthcare for a previously consummated hospital merger. The FTC claimed that a hospital merger that occurred in 2000 violated federal antitrust law because the newly created three-hospital system sufficiently boosted its market power to illegally control hospital prices in its market. The FTC claimed that, as a result of the merger, Northwestern Healthcare used its post-merger market power to impose huge price increases—40 percent to 60 percent and, in one case, even 190 percent—on insurers and employers (FTC 2006). The FTC's decision was upheld on appeal, and the system hospitals were ordered to negotiate independently with insurers, rather than have Northwestern Healthcare divest itself of one hospital as the initial decision recommended. Mergers of nonprofit hospitals are no longer likely to be viewed as different from mergers of for-profit hospitals (Morse et al. 2007).

Quality of Care

Sloan (2000) reviewed several large-scale empirical studies of quality of care received by Medicare beneficiaries in nonprofit and for-profit hospitals. The studies examined various measures of quality, such as the overall care process and the extent to which medical charts showed that specific diagnostic and therapeutic procedures were performed competently. They assessed different hospital admissions (such as hip fracture, stroke, coronary heart disease, and congestive heart failure) and different outcome measures (such as survival, functional status, cognitive status, and probability of living in a nursing home). These studies found that although patients admitted to major teaching hospitals did better, no statistically significant differences were found between nonteaching private nonprofit hospitals and for-profit hospitals.

In an extensive study, McClellan and Staiger (2000) compared patient outcomes of all elderly Medicare beneficiaries hospitalized with heart disease (more than 350,000 per year) in for-profit and nonprofit hospitals between 1984 and 1994. The authors (2000, 4) found that

> [o]n average, for-profit hospitals have higher mortality among elderly patients with heart disease, and ... this difference has grown over the last decade. However, much of the difference appears to be associated with the location of for-profit hospitals. Within specific markets, for-profit ownership appears if anything to be associated with better quality care. Moreover, the small average difference in mortality between nonprofit and for-profit hospitals masks an enormous amount of variation in mortality within each of these ownership types. Overall, these results suggest that factors other than for-profit status per se may be the main determinants of quality of care in hospitals.

Charity Care

Nonprofit hospitals have a long tradition of caring for the medically indigent. They were given tax-exempt status and community donations in the belief that they would provide charity care. However, the advent of price competition in the mid-1980s has changed their ability to provide the level of charity care some believe is necessary to maintain their tax-exempt status. The extent of charity care they provide has been examined in terms of (1) hospital conversions (a nonprofit becomes a for-profit) and (2) the effect of greater competitive pressures from managed care.

Concern has arisen that once a hospital converts to for-profit status, its charity care will decline as the profit motive becomes dominant. Various studies, however, have found no difference in provision of uncompensated care once a hospital converts from nonprofit to for-profit. Norton and Staiger (1994) found that for-profit hospitals are often located in areas with a high degree of health insurance (Medicare, Medicaid, and private). However, once differences in location are accounted for—such as by examining nonprofit and for-profit hospitals in the same market—no difference was found in the volume of uninsured patients cared for by the two types of hospitals.

Price competition is expected to negatively affect a nonprofit hospital's ability to provide charity care by decreasing the "profits" or surplus available for such care. As competition reduces the prices charged to privately insured patients, profits decline and thus less funds are available for charity care. Gruber (1994) found that increased competition among hospitals in California from 1984 to 1988 led to decreased revenues from private payers, net income, and consequently provision of uncompensated care. The comptroller general David Walker (2005) stated that in four of the five states studied in 2003, state and locally owned hospitals provided an average of twice as much uncompensated care as did either nonprofit or for-profit hospitals. In Florida, Georgia, Indiana, and Texas, nonprofits delivered more uncompensated care than did for-profits, but the difference was small. In California, for-profits delivered more uncompensated care than did nonprofits. In a study of uncompensated care in five states, the US Congressional Budget Office (2006, 2) found that the cost of uncompensated care as a percentage of hospital operating expenses was much larger in government or public (13 percent) than in nonprofit (4.7 percent) or for-profit (4.2 percent) institutions. Individual nonprofit and for-profit hospitals, however, varied widely in the amount of uncompensated care they provided.

Overall, competitive pressures result in lower income available for charity care in nonprofit and for-profit hospitals, while public hospitals experience higher uncompensated care costs.

The Question of Tax-Exempt Status

Nonprofit hospitals have received tax advantages that obligate them to serve the uninsured. Nonprofits, however, vary greatly in the amount of care they provide to the uninsured. In some cases, the value of the hospital's tax exemption exceeds the value of charity care it provides. Consequently, it has been proposed that, in return for their tax-exempt status, nonprofit hospitals should be required to deliver a minimum amount of charity care.

If the tax exemption is to be tied to the value of charity care/community benefits, the measure to be used and the amount of care to be provided must be defined. The following are proposed possible measures:

- *Pure charity care:* care for which payment is not expected and patients are not billed
- *Bad debt:* value of care delivered and billed to patients believed to be able to pay but from whom the hospital is unable to collect
- *Uncompensated care:* the sum of bad debt and charity care
- *Medicaid and Medicare shortfalls:* the difference between charges and the amount Medicare and Medicaid reimburse
- *Community benefits:* the previous items plus the amount of patient education, prevention programs, medical research, and provision of money-losing services (such as burn units and trauma centers)

Deciding which definition should be used and what percentage of a nonprofit hospital's revenue should be devoted to that measure is an important public policy issue being debated by state and federal governments. For example, if the charity care definition is used, is the amount of free care measured by the hospital's full charges (which few payers actually pay) or the lower prices a health maintenance organization would pay? Further, using the broadest definition of community benefits may result in a hospital delivering no charity care but relying instead on Medicare and Medicaid shortfalls and some community prevention programs, which may also be viewed as a marketing effort by the hospital.[4] If such a broad definition were used, little difference would be found between many nonprofit and for-profit hospitals.

Many states have begun to engage in limited monitoring of the uncompensated care provided by nonprofits (see, for example, Day 2006; Reece 2011). Stringent requirements have not been imposed on hospitals to maintain their tax-exempt status. Included as part of the Affordable Care Act (ACA) is the requirement that nonprofits conduct and submit a community needs assessment, after which their progress toward meeting those needs will be measured every three years. Those nonprofits making little or no progress toward meeting their identified needs will risk losing their tax-exempt status. Nonprofits also are required to ensure that their patients are aware when free or discounted care is available. These conditions are less severe than requiring nonprofits to spend a given percentage of their surplus on charity or uncompensated care.

Summary

In examining whether the behavior of nonprofit hospitals is different from that of for-profit hospitals, one must keep in mind that wide variations in behavior exist within both types of hospitals. Although little difference is found between ownership type in pricing behavior, quality of care delivered, or even the amount of uncompensated care provided, these comparisons are based on averages.

As price competition among hospitals increases, ownership differences become less important in determining a hospital's behavior regarding pricing, quality of care, and even charity care. In a price-competitive environment, both nonprofits and for-profits must have similar behavior to survive; nonprofits will have less of a surplus to pursue other goals.

Ideally, the poor and uninsured should not have to rely on nonprofit hospitals for charity care. Expanding health insurance to the uninsured—either through private insurance vouchers or Medicaid—will more directly solve the problem of providing care to the medically indigent. According to the ACA, starting in 2014, 95 percent of the uninsured should have insurance coverage either through increased eligibility for Medicaid or through tax credits on state health insurance exchanges. As more people obtain some form of coverage, the tax-exempt status of many nonprofit hospitals is likely to be questioned. Although certain nonprofits will continue to provide care to those who remain uninsured, the majority of nonprofit hospitals will have to justify their role in society.

Discussion Questions

1. Discuss the differences and similarities among theories on why many hospitals are nonprofit.
2. Do you agree with the ruling by a federal judge that mergers of nonprofit hospitals should not be subject to the same antitrust laws as mergers of for-profit hospitals?
3. How has price competition affected the ability of nonprofit hospitals to achieve their mission?
4. What conditions should be imposed on nonprofit hospitals to retain their tax-exempt status?
5. In what ways, if any, are nonprofit hospitals different from for-profit hospitals?

Notes

1. The trust relationship between the patient and provider, however, applies more strongly to the patient–physician relationship. The physician diagnoses the illness, recommends treatment, refers the patient to specialists, and monitors the care the patient receives from different providers. Yet physicians are for-profit.
2. An additional explanation for the existence of nonprofit status is that the stochastic nature of the demand for medical services requires hospitals to maintain excess capacity for certain services. It can be very costly for patients if they cannot access hospital care when needed. For-profit hospitals, some believe, would be unwilling to bear the cost of idle hospital capacity. Further, certain hospital services (e.g.,

emergency departments; trauma centers; neonatal intensive care units; teaching, research, and care for certain groups [such as AIDS patients and drug addicts] that benefit the community) generally lose money and would otherwise not be provided.

3. Lakdawalla and Philipson (2006) claimed that the traditional for-profit analysis of a firm can be used to explain nonprofit hospitals but with a lower cost structure because of their nonprofit status. The type of services, in addition to the pricing strategy, a hospital chooses to offer will also affect its profitability. Horwitz and Nichols (2009) found that nonprofit hospitals' services vary according to the relative market share of nonprofit, for-profit, and government hospitals in a market. Nonprofits in markets with high for-profit market share were more likely to offer relatively profitable services and less likely to offer unprofitable services compared to nonprofits in markets with low for-profit penetration.

4. Young and colleagues (2013) surveyed nonprofit hospitals to determine how much they spent on IRS-defined measures of community benefit. They found that hospitals in the study spent, on average, 7.5 percent of their operating expenses on community benefits. On average, more than 85 percent of these expenditures went to patient care, and almost 50 percent of the 85 percent were used to supplement the low prices paid by government for services provided to Medicaid and other means-tested patients. Community benefit spending not related to patient care was devoted to community health improvement activities and health professions education. Only 1.9 percent of the study hospitals' operating expenditures was, on average, spent on charity care.

References

American Hospital Association (AHA). n.d. *Hospital Statistics*. Various editions. Chicago: AHA.

Capps, C., and D. Dranove. 2004. "Hospital Consolidation and Negotiated PPO Prices." *Health Affairs* 23 (2): 175–81.

Congressional Budget Office. 2006. "Nonprofit Hospitals and the Provision of Community Benefit." Published December. www.cbo.gov/sites/default/files/cbofiles/ftpdocs/76xx/doc7695/12-06-nonprofit.pdf.

Day, K. 2006. "Hospital Charity Care Is Probed." *Washington Post*, September 13. www.washingtonpost.com/wp-dyn/content/article/2006/09/12/AR2006091201409.html.

Federal Trade Commission (FTC). 2006. "In the Matter of Evanston Northwestern Healthcare Corporation." Last updated April 28, 2008. www.ftc.gov/os/adjpro/d9315/070806opinion.pdf.

Gruber, J. 1994. "The Effect of Competitive Pressure on Charity: Hospital Responses to Price Shopping in California." *Journal of Health Economics* 13 (2): 183–212.

Horwitz, J., and A. Nichols. 2009. "Hospital Ownership and Medical Services: Market Mix, Spillover Effects, and Nonprofit Objectives." *Journal of Health Economics* 28 (5): 924–37.

Lakdawalla, D., and T. Philipson. 2006. "The Nonprofit Sector and Industry Performance." *Journal of Public Economics* 90 (8–9): 1681–98.

McClellan, M., and D. Staiger. 2000. "Comparing Hospital Quality at For-Profit and Not-for-Profit Hospitals." In *The Changing Hospital Industry: Comparing Not-for-Profit and For-Profit Institutions*, edited by D. Cutler, 93–112. Chicago: University of Chicago Press.

Melnick, G., E. Keeler, and J. Zwanziger. 1999. "Market Power and Hospital Pricing: Are Nonprofits Different?" *Health Affairs* 18 (3): 167–73.

Morse, M., B. Kevin, R. McCann, and L. Bryant Jr. 2007. "Federal Trade Commission Finds Evanston Northwestern Healthcare Merger Unlawful but Orders 'Separate and Independent Negotiating Teams' Rather than Divestiture." Published August 17. www.lexology.com/library/detail.aspx?g=a1132f5c-4483-41e5-a31d-dc832f51f1ea.

Norton, E., and D. Staiger. 1994. "How Hospital Ownership Affects Access to Care for the Uninsured." *RAND Journal of Economics* 25 (1): 171–85.

Reece, M. 2011. "Bill Scrutinizes Nonprofit Property Tax Structure." Published February 7. http://flatheadbeacon.com/2011/02/07/bill-scrutinizes-nonprofit-property-tax-structure/.

Sloan, F. 2000. "Not-for-Profit Ownership and Hospital Behavior." In *Handbook of Health Economics*, vol. 1B, edited by A. J. Culyer and J. P. Newhouse, 1141–73. New York: North-Holland Press.

Walker, D. M. 2005. "Nonprofit, For-Profit and Government Hospital Uncompensated Care and Other Community Benefits." Publicly released May 26. Testimony before the Committee on Ways and Means, House of Representatives, GAO-05-743T. www.gao.gov/new.items/d05743t.pdf.

Young, G. J., C-H. Chou, J. Alexander, S-Y. D. Lee, and E. Raver. 2013. "Provision of Community Benefits by Tax-Exempt U.S. Hospitals." *New England Journal of Medicine* 368: 1519–27.

COMPETITION AMONG HOSPITALS: DOES IT RAISE OR LOWER COSTS?

C urrent federal policy (the antitrust laws) encourages competition among hospitals. Hospitals proposing a merger are scrutinized by the Federal Trade Commission (FTC) to determine whether the merger will lessen hospital competition in that market, in which case the FTC will oppose the merger. Critics of this policy believe hospitals should be permitted—in fact encouraged—to consolidate and co-operate the facilities and services they provide. They claim that the result will be greater efficiency, less duplication of costly services, and higher quality of care. Who is correct, and what is appropriate public policy for hospitals—competition or cooperation?

Important to understanding hospital performance are (1) the methods used to pay hospitals (different payment schemes offer hospitals different incentives) and (2) the consequences of having different numbers of hospitals compete with one another.

Origins of Nonprice Competition

After the introduction of Medicare and Medicaid in 1966, hospitals were paid their costs for the services they rendered to the aged and poor. Private insurance, which was widespread among the remainder of the population, reimbursed hospitals generously according to either their costs or their charges. The extensive coverage of hospital services by private and public payers removed patients' incentive to be concerned about the costs of hospital care. Patients pay less out-of-pocket costs for hospital care (3.4 percent in 2012) than for any other medical service.

Third-party payers (government and private insurance) and patients had virtually no incentive to be concerned about hospital efficiency and duplication of facilities and services. Further, most hospitals are organized as nonprofit (nongovernment) organizations that are either affiliated with religious organizations or controlled by boards of trustees selected from the community. With the introduction of extensive public and private hospital insurance after the mid-1960s, the use of nonprofit hospitals increased. Lacking a profit motive and assured of survival by the generous payment methods, nonprofit hospitals also had no incentive to be concerned about efficiency. This caused the costs of caring for patients to rise rapidly.

Exhibit 15.1 illustrates the dramatic growth in hospital expenditures from the 1960s to 2012. After Medicare and Medicaid were enacted in 1966, hospital expenditures rose by more than 16 percent per year, which was primarily attributable to sharp increases in hospital prices (as shown in Exhibit 15.2). Price increases moderated during the early 1970s, when wage and price controls were imposed, but then continued once the controls were removed in mid-1974. Hospital expenditure growth was less rapid in the mid- to late 1980s as Medicare changed its hospital payment system and price competition increased. The rate of increase in hospital expenditures and hospital prices continued to fall during the 1990s.[1] These declines, discussed later, are indicative of the changes that have occurred in the market for hospital services.

In the late 1960s, the private sector also did not encourage efficiency. Although services such as diagnostic workups could be provided less expensively in an outpatient setting, BlueCross paid for such services only if they were provided as part of a hospital admission. Small hospitals attempted to emulate medical centers by having the latest in technology, although those services were infrequently used. Because cost was of little concern to patients or purchasers of services, it did not matter whether large organizations had lower costs per unit and higher-quality outcomes than small facilities did.

The greater the number of hospitals in a community, the more intense was the competition among the nonprofit hospitals to become the most prestigious. Hospitals competed for physicians by offering all the services available at other hospitals to maximize the physicians' productivity and convenience and discourage them from referring patients to another hospital. This wasteful form of nonprice competition was characterized as a "medical arms race" and caused the rapid rise in hospital expenditures.

As the costs of nonprice competition ballooned, federal and state governments attempted to change hospitals' behavior. Regulations were enacted to control hospital capital expenditures; hospitals were required to have certificate-of-need (CON) approval from a state planning agency before they could undertake large investments. According to proponents of state planning, controlling hospital investment would eliminate unnecessary and duplicative investments. Unfortunately, no attempts were made to change hospital payment methods, which would have changed hospitals' incentives to undertake such investments. Numerous studies concluded that CON had no effect on limiting the growth in hospital investment. Instead, CON was used in an anticompetitive manner to benefit existing hospitals in the community, which ended up controlling the CON approval process. Ambulatory surgery centers (unaffiliated with hospitals) did not receive CON approval for construction because they would take away hospital patients; health maintenance organizations (HMOs), such as Kaiser, found entering a new market

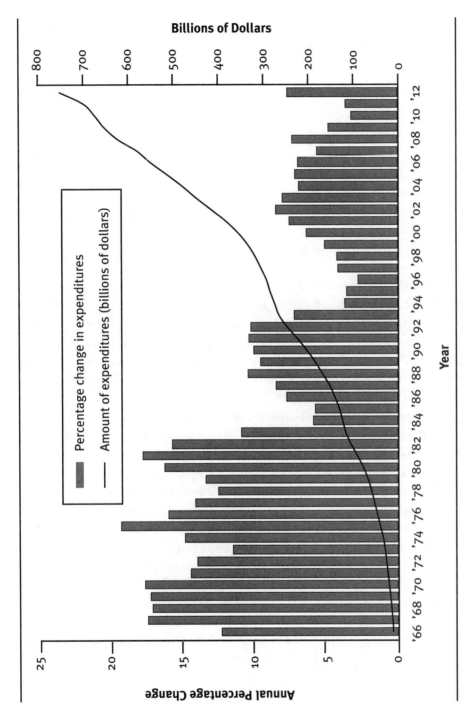

EXHIBIT 15.1
Trends in
Hospital
Expenditures,
1966–2012

NOTE: Data are for total nonfederal short-term general and other special hospitals.
SOURCE: Data from AHA (2014), Table 1.

difficult because they could not receive CON approval to build a new hospital; and the courts found that the CON process was used in an "arbitrary and capricious manner" against for-profit hospitals attempting to enter the market of an existing nonprofit hospital (Feldstein 2011).

Transition to Price Competition

Until the 1980s, hospital competition was synonymous with nonprice competition, and its effect was wasteful and rapidly rising expenditures.

During the 1980s, hospital and purchaser incentives changed. Medicare began to pay hospitals a fixed price per admission, which varied according to the type of admission. This new payment system—referred to as *diagnosis-related groups (DRGs)*—was phased in over five years starting in 1983. Faced with a fixed price, hospitals now had an incentive to reduce their costs of caring for aged patients. In addition, hospitals reduced lengths of stay for aged patients, which caused declines in hospital occupancy rates. For the first time, hospitals became concerned with their physicians' practice behavior. If physicians ordered too many tests or kept patients in the hospital longer than necessary, the hospital lost money, given the fixed DRG price.

Pressure to reduce hospital costs also came from private insurers, primarily because employers became concerned about the rising costs of insuring employees. Insurers changed their insurance benefits to encourage patients to have diagnostic tests and minor surgical procedures performed in less costly outpatient settings. Insurers instituted utilization review to monitor the appropriateness of inpatient admissions, which further reduced hospital admissions and lengths of stay. These changes in hospital and purchaser incentives reduced hospital occupancy rates from 76 percent in 1980 to 67 percent by 1990; as of 2012, the rate was about 63 percent. The decline in occupancy rates was much more severe for small hospitals, where they fell to below 50 percent (NCHS 2014, Table 107). As occupancy rates fell, hospitals became willing to negotiate price discounts with insurers and HMOs that could deliver a large number of patients to their hospitals. This initiated price competition among hospitals by the late 1980s.

Price competition does not imply that hospitals compete only on the basis of lowest price. Purchasers are also interested in characteristics of a hospital, such as reputation, location in relation to patients, facilities and services available, patient satisfaction, and treatment outcomes. In recent years, as mergers have occurred and price competition has lessened, hospitals' market power has expanded (relative to that of health insurers), and hospital prices (adjusted for inflation) have risen rapidly; see Exhibit 15.2.

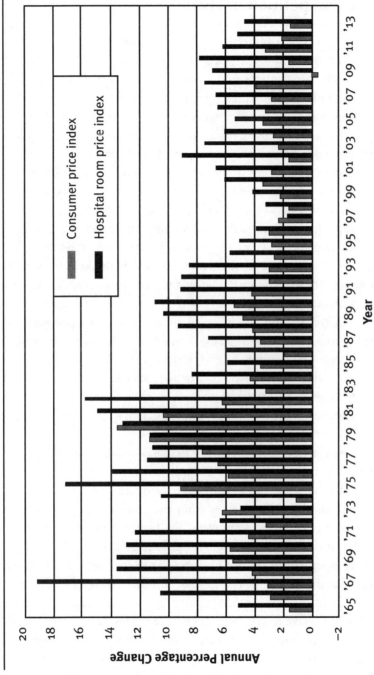

EXHIBIT 15.2
Annual
Percentage
Changes in the
Consumer Price
Index and the
Hospital Room
Price Index,
1965–2013

NOTE: Because of changes in Bureau of Labor Statistics coding, data after 1996 are for hospital services.
SOURCE: Data from BLS (2014).

Price Competition in Theory

How did hospitals respond to this new competitive environment in which purchasers demand lower prices? Let us examine two hypothetical situations.

In the first situation, only one hospital exists in an area; it has no competitors, and no substitutes for inpatient services are available. The hospital is a monopolist in providing services and has no incentive to respond to purchaser demands for lower prices, quality information, and patient satisfaction. The purchaser has no choice but to use that one hospital. If the hospital is not efficient, it can pass on the resulting higher costs to the purchaser. If the patients are dissatisfied with the services or the hospital refuses to provide outcomes information, the purchaser and patients have no choice but to use the hospital. (Obviously, at some point, it becomes worthwhile for patients to incur large travel costs to go to a distant hospital or facility.) When only one hospital serves a market, that hospital is unlikely to achieve high performance. It has little incentive to be efficient or respond to purchaser and patient demands.

In the second situation, many hospitals—perhaps ten—serve a geographic area. Now assume a large employer in the area is interested, on behalf of its employees, in not only high-quality care and high patient satisfaction but also in low hospital costs. Further, assume each of the ten hospitals is equally accessible to the employees in terms of short travel distance and staff appointments for the employees' physicians). How are hospitals likely to respond to this employer's demands?

At least several of the ten hospitals would be willing—in return for gaining many new customers from the employer—to negotiate on prices and accede to demands for information on quality and satisfaction. As long as the price the hospital receives from the employer is greater than the direct costs of caring for the employees, the hospital will make more money than if it did not accept this business. Further, unless each hospital is as efficient as its competitors, it cannot hope to obtain such a contract. A more efficient hospital is always able to charge less. Similar to competing on price is competing on willingness to provide information on treatment outcomes. As long as the hospitals have to rely on purchaser revenues to survive, they will be driven to respond to purchaser demands. If Hospital A is not responsive to these demands, other hospitals will be, and Hospital A will soon find that it has too few patients to remain in business. When hospitals compete on quality, satisfaction, price, and other purchaser demands, their performance is opposite that of a monopoly provider. In price-competitive markets, hospitals have an incentive to be efficient and respond to purchaser demands.

What if, instead of competing with one another, the ten hospitals decide to agree among themselves not to compete on price or provide purchasers with any additional information? The outcome would be similar to a monopoly situation. Prices would be higher, and hospitals would have less incentive to be efficient. Patients would be worse off because they would pay more, and patient quality and patient satisfaction would be lower because employers and other purchasers would be unable to select hospitals based on patient quality and satisfaction information.

The more competitive the market, the greater the benefits to consumers. For this reason, society seeks to achieve competitive markets through its antitrust laws. Although competitive hospitals might be harmed and driven out of business, *the evaluation of competitive markets is based on their effect on consumers rather than on any competitors in that market*. Antitrust laws are designed to prevent hospitals from acting anticompetitively. Price-fixing agreements, such as those described earlier, are illegal because they reduce competition. Barriers that prevent competitors from entering a market are also anticompetitive. If two hospitals in a market are able to restrict entry into that market (perhaps through the use of regulations such as CON approval), they will have greater monopoly power and be less price competitive and less responsive to purchaser demands. Mergers may be similarly anticompetitive. For example, if nine out of the ten hospitals merged, leaving only two organizations, the degree of competition would be less than if ten are independently operating. For this reason, the FTC examines hospital mergers to determine whether the consolidation is eliminating competition in the market.

Price Competition in Practice

The previous discussion provides a theoretical basis for price competition. To move from price competition's theoretical benefits to reality, two questions must be considered. First, does any market have enough hospitals for price competition to occur? Second, is there any evidence on the actual effects of hospital price competition?

The number of competing hospitals in a market is determined by the cost–size relationship of hospitals (economies of scale) and the size of the market (the population served). A large hospital—for example, one with 200 beds—is likely to have lower average costs per patient than a hospital with the same set of services but only 50 beds. In a large hospital, some costs can be spread over a greater number of patients. However, some costs do not change whether the hospital has 50 or 200 patients, such as costs for an administrator, an X-ray technician, and imaging equipment (which can be used more fully in a large organization). These economies of scale, however, do not continue indefinitely; at some point, the high costs of coordinating services begin to exceed the gains from being large. Studies have generally indicated that hospitals in the size range of 200 to 400 beds have the lowest average costs.

If the population in an area consists of only 100,000, only one hospital of 260 beds is likely to survive (assuming 800 patient days per year per 1,000 people and 80 percent occupancy). If more than one hospital is in the area, each has higher average costs than one large hospital has; one of the hospitals may expand, achieve lower average costs, and be able to set its prices lower than the other hospital. An area with a population of 1 million is large enough to support three to six hospitals in the 200- to 400-bed range.

Hospital services, however, are not all the same. The economies of scale associated with an obstetrics facility are quite different from those associated with organ transplant services. Patients are less willing to travel great distances for a normal delivery than for a heart transplant. The travel costs of going to another state for a transplant represent a smaller portion of the total cost of that service than the travel costs of going to another state for childbirth would represent (and the travel time is less crucial). Thus, the number of competitors in a market depends on the particular service. For some services, the relevant geographic market served may be relatively small, whereas for others the market may be the state or region.

As of 2012, approximately 84 percent of hospital beds were located in metropolitan statistical areas (MSAs). An MSA may not necessarily be indicative of the particular market in which a hospital competes. For some services, the travel time within an MSA may be too great, whereas for other services (organ transplants) the market may encompass multiple MSAs. However, the number of hospitals in an MSA provides a general indication of the number of competitors in a hospital's market. As shown in Exhibit 15.3, 192 MSAs (45 percent) have fewer than four hospitals, and 80 MSAs (19 percent) have four or five hospitals. The remaining MSAs (36 percent) have six or more hospitals; however, that 36 percent of MSAs contains 76 percent of the hospitals located in metropolitan areas. Therefore, the majority of hospitals in MSAs (76 percent) are located in MSAs with six or more hospitals. Even in an MSA with few hospitals, competition still occurs and substitutes to the hospitals' services (for example, outpatient surgery) are often available, which decrease those hospitals' monopoly power.

When few providers of specialized facilities exist in a market (because of economies of scale and the size of the market), the relevant geographic market is likely to be much larger because the highly specialized services are generally not of an emergency nature and patients are more willing to travel to access them. Insurers negotiate prices for transplants, for example, with several regional *centers of excellence*—hospitals that perform a high number of transplants and have good outcomes. Thus, price competition

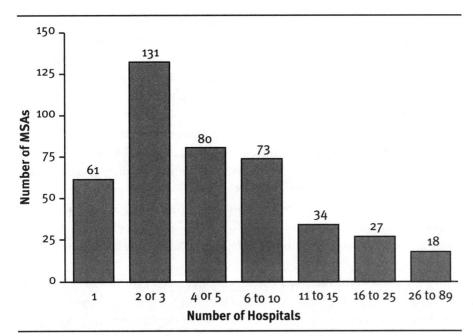

EXHIBIT 15.3
The Number of Hospitals in Metropolitan Statistical Areas, 2012

SOURCE: Data from AHA (2014), Table 8.

among hospitals appears to be feasible. As insurers and large employers have become concerned about the costs of hospital care and have become better informed on hospital prices and patient outcomes, hospitals are being forced to respond to purchaser demands and compete according to price, outcomes, and patient satisfaction. Data shown in exhibits 15.1 and 15.2 show how competition lowered the rate of increase in hospital expenditures and prices during the late 1990s. As hospitals had to compete to be included in provider panels of managed care plans, they had to become more efficient and discount their prices.

A number of studies have been published on the effects of hospital price competition. This research provides further support for traditional economic expectations regarding competitive hospital markets. The change to hospital price competition was not uniform throughout the United States. Price competition in California developed earlier and more rapidly than in other areas. Bamezai and colleagues (1999) classified hospitals within California according to whether they were in a high- or low-competition market and whether the managed care penetration was high or low. Hospitals in more competitive markets (controlling for other factors) were found to have a much lower rate of increase in the costs per discharge and per capita than were hospitals in less competitive markets. Bamezai and colleagues also found that an increase in managed care penetration reduced the rise in hospital costs (see Exhibit 15.4). The decrease in costs, however, was much greater for hospitals in more competitive markets. Also, regardless of the degree of managed care penetration, competition was important in slowing hospital cost increases. These findings imply that hospital mergers that decrease competition are likely to result in higher hospital prices. A subsequent study by Melnick, Chen, and Wu (2011) confirmed these findings, showing that greater hospital market concentration leads to higher hospital prices.[2]

Other studies have found similar results using different methods and data on specific types of hospital treatment. For example, Kessler and McClellan (2000) analyzed Medicare claims data (from 1985 to 1994) for Medicare patients admitted to the hospital with a primary diagnosis of a heart attack. They found that before 1990, hospital competition on the basis of the latest technology led to higher costs and, in some cases, lower rates of adverse health outcomes. After 1990, hospital price competition substantially reduced costs and rates of adverse outcomes. Patients had lower mortality rates in the most competitive markets.

After the consumer backlash against managed care in the late 1990s and early 2000s, health plans broadened their provider networks to give their enrollees more provider choices. As insurers included more hospitals in their networks, their bargaining power over hospitals decreased (Dranove et al. 2008). Reinforcing this shift in relative bargaining power was the decrease in the number of hospitals. Hospital closures and mergers resulted in fewer hospitals competing within a market.[3] The result was that hospital prices increased much more rapidly. Insurers' reliance on broad provider networks and the decreased number of competing hospitals enabled hospitals to maintain their relative bargaining power over insurers.

The relative bargaining power between hospitals and insurers is beginning to change as insurers—particularly those insurers competing on state and federal health insurance exchanges (established as part of the ACA)—are relying on limited provider networks. The ACA mandates a comprehensive set of benefits and a modified form of community rating. Thus, to prevent their premiums from becoming too high to those who are young, insurers are using lower-cost hospitals and limited provider networks.

EXHIBIT 15.4
Hospital Cost Growth in the United States, by Level of Managed Care Penetration and Hospital Market Competitiveness, 1986–1993

Level of Managed Care Penetration	Level of Hospital Competition		% Difference
	Low	High	
Low	65	56	16[a]
High	52	39	33[a]
% difference	25[a]	44[a]	67[b]

[a] % difference = [(High − Low)/Low]
[b] [Low/Low (65) − High/High (39)] / [High/High (39)]
SOURCE: Calculations by Glenn Melnick, Rand Corporation.

Summary

The controversy over whether hospital competition results in higher or lower costs is based on studies from two different periods. When hospitals were paid according to their costs, nonprice competition occurred and resulted in rapidly rising hospital costs. Medicare's switch to fixed-price hospital payment and managed care plans' switch to negotiated prices changed hospitals' incentives. Hospitals had incentives to be efficient and compete on price to be included in managed care plans' provider panels. Consequently, hospital costs and prices rose less rapidly in more competitive hospital markets. Public policies (such as antitrust laws) that encourage competitive hospital markets will be of greater benefit to purchasers and patients than policies that enable hospitals to increase their monopoly power.

As enrollment in managed care plans rose, the demand for hospital care fell. Hospitals developed excess capacity and were willing to discount their prices to be included in insurers' limited provider networks. Hospital prices declined. With excess capacity, some hospitals closed and many merged with financially stronger hospitals. Under public pressure to expand their provider networks, insurers were less able to offer hospitals a greater volume of patients in return for heavily discounted prices. Currently, with fewer hospital competitors in a market and insurers' willingness to contract with a larger number of hospitals, the relative bargaining positions of hospitals and insurers changed. Hospital price increases have been higher than in the 1990s, when managed care limited provider networks and hospitals had excess capacity.

Discussion Questions

1. Why did hospital expenditures rise so rapidly after Medicare and Medicaid were introduced in 1966?
2. What changes did Medicare DRGs cause in hospital behavior?
3. What is the likely response of hospitals when only one hospital is in a market, compared with their response when ten hospitals are competing for a large employer's employees?
4. What determines the number of competitors in a market? Apply your answer to obstetrics and to transplant services.
5. What are some anticompetitive hospital actions that the antitrust laws seek to prevent?

Notes

1. Starting in the mid-1980s, hospital price increases—as calculated in the consumer price index (CPI)—were greatly overstated because the CPI measured "list" prices rather than actual prices charged. The difference between the two became greater with the increase in hospital discounting (Dranove, Shanley, and White 1991). To correct this discrepancy, the Bureau of Labor Statistics, in constructing the CPI, began to use data on actual hospital prices in the early 1990s.

2. In 2006, the English government tried to introduce competition among hospitals by allowing patients to choose among different hospitals and providing patients with information on hospital quality and timeliness of care. Gaynor, Moreno-Serra, and Propper (2013) found that patients discharged from hospitals in more competitive markets were less likely to die, had shorter lengths of stay, and were no more costly than patients in less competitive markets.

3. An example of the effect of fewer competing hospitals on hospital prices is the study by Wu (2008), who analyzed hospital closures between 1993 and 1998 and found that as the number of competitors decreased, competitors located near the closed hospitals improved their bargaining position over insurers. As these hospital markets became more concentrated, hospitals were able to raise their prices more than less concentrated markets could.

References

American Hospital Association (AHA). 2014. *Hospital Statistics.* Chicago: AHA.

Bamezai, A., J. Zwanziger, G. Melnick, and J. Mann. 1999. "Price Competition and Hospital Cost Growth in the United States: 1989–1994." *Health Economics* 8 (3): 233–43.

Bureau of Labor Statistics (BLS). 2014. "Consumer Price Index Databases, All Urban Consumers (Current Series)." Accessed March. www.bls.gov/cpi/data.htm.

Dranove, D., R. Lindrooth, W. White, and J. Zwanziger. 2008. "Is the Impact of Managed Care on Hospital Prices Decreasing?" *Journal of Health Economics* 27 (2): 362–76.

Dranove, D., M. Shanley, and W. White. 1991. "How Fast Are Hospital Prices Really Rising?" *Medical Care* 29 (8): 690–96.

Feldstein, P. 2011. "The Market for Hospital Services." *Health Care Economics*, 7th ed. Clifton, NJ: Thomson Delmar Learning.

Gaynor, M., R. Moreno-Serra, and C. Propper. 2013. "Death by Market Power: Reform, Competition and Patient Outcomes in the National Health Service." *American Economic Journal: Economic Policy* 5 (4): 134–66. http://pubs.aeaweb.org/doi/pdfplus/10.1257/pol.5.4.134.

Kessler, D., and M. McClellan. 2000. "Is Hospital Competition Socially Wasteful?" *Quarterly Journal of Economics* 115 (2): 577–615.

Melnick, G., Y. Chen, and V. Wu. 2011. "The Increased Concentration of Health Plan Markets Can Benefit Consumers Through Lower Hospital Prices." *Health Affairs* 30 (9): 1728–33.

National Center for Health Statistics (NCHS). 2014. *Health United States, 2013: With Special Feature on Prescription Drugs.* Accessed May 2014. www.cdc.gov/nchs/data/hus/hus13.pdf.

Wu, V. 2008. "The Price Effect of Hospital Closures." *Inquiry* 45 (3): 280–92.

THE FUTURE ROLE OF HOSPITALS

Hospitals have traditionally been the center of the healthcare system. Before Medicare and Medicaid were implemented in 1965, hospital expenditures represented 40 percent of total health expenditures. During the late 1960s and the 1970s, the growth of Medicare, Medicaid, and private insurance stimulated the demand for hospital services. By 1975, 46 percent of health expenditures were for hospital services. Although hospital expenditures have continued to increase, hospitals' share of total health expenditures has declined, falling to 32 percent in 2012. Will the traditional role of the hospital continue to decline, or will hospitals expand their role beyond treating inpatients and become responsible for a greater portion of the spectrum of care?

From Medicare to the Present

During the post-Medicare period (1966 to early 1980s), hospitals were reimbursed for their costs, engaged in nonprice competition to attract physicians, and quickly adopted new technology. Facilities and services grew rapidly, and hospitals were the largest and fastest-increasing component of healthcare expenditures.

Starting in the mid-1980s, the financial outlook for hospitals changed. Medicare introduced diagnosis-related groups (DRGs), which changed Medicare payment from a cost basis to a fixed price per admission (by type of admission). Hospitals realized that reducing their costs and patients' lengths of stay raised their net income because they could keep the difference between the DRG price and the cost of caring for Medicare patients. Under pressure from employers, insurers introduced managed care with its cost-containment measures, such as utilization review; second surgical opinions; and lower-cost substitutes to inpatient care, including ambulatory surgery and outpatient diagnostic testing. To reduce treatment costs, managed care shifted services out of the most expensive setting—the hospital. Greater use occurred in outpatient facilities and step-down facilities, such as skilled nursing facilities, rehabilitation units, and home health care.

Hospitals experienced excess capacity as they cut Medicare patients' lengths of stay and as private cost-containment measures reduced hospital use. With excess capacity, hospitals were willing to compete on price to be included in managed care preferred provider organizations. Managed care competition, hospitals' excess capacity, and the resulting pressures on hospitals to compete on price led to bankruptcies, mergers, falling profit margins, and a distressed industry for hospitals. The DRG Medicare payment system and managed care's utilization management methods left the industry with too much excess capacity. The financial survival of many hospitals was in doubt.

Exhibit 16.1 describes the changes that occurred in the hospital industry. The number of hospitals and beds, the average length of stay, and the occupancy rates all declined during the 1980s and 1990s. With the movement to less expensive settings, outpatient visits and surgeries sharply rose. These trends have continued to the present time. Inpatient use of the hospital has continued to decline.

To increase their admissions, hospitals bought physicians' practices, thereby increasing physician referrals. However, employed physicians, with their changed incentives, became less productive, so hospitals abandoned the practice. Hospitals were not adept at managing physicians' practices, and physicians were suspicious of working too closely with hospitals. Hospital–physician relationships have been a continual concern to hospitals, especially as physician-owned outpatient surgery centers brought physicians into competition with hospitals.

Hospital profitability had gradually returned by the late 1990s. Financially troubled hospitals closed or merged with other hospitals. To survive and prosper, hospitals adopted strategies that emphasized monopolization of the market. Mergers between competing hospitals increased, and large

EXHIBIT 16.1
US Community Hospital Capacity and Utilization, 1975–2012

Year	Number of Hospitals	Number of Staffed Beds (Thousands)	Inpatient Admissions (Thousands)	Average Length of Inpatient Stay (Days)	Average Inpatient Occupancy Rate (%)	Outpatient Visits (Thousands)
1975	5,875	942	33,435	7.7	74.9	190,672
1980	5,830	988	36,143	7.6	75.6	202,310
1985	5,732	1,001	33,449	7.1	64.8	218,716
1990	5,384	927	31,181	7.2	66.8	301,329
1995	5,194	873	30,945	6.5	62.8	414,345
2000	4,915	824	33,089	5.8	63.8	521,404
2005	4,936	802	35,239	5.6	67.3	584,429
2012	4,999	801	34,422	5.4	63.3	674,971

SOURCE: Author's analysis based on data from AHA (2014a), Table 1.

multihospital systems developed. The number of hospital competitors in a market decreased. The Federal Trade Commission (FTC), concerned that mergers were creating monopoly power that enabled hospitals to raise their prices, brought several antitrust suits against mergers. The FTC, however, lost every merger case. The judges in these cases believed nonprofit hospitals were different from for-profits in that the nonprofits would not exploit their market power by raising prices.

The managed care backlash, which occurred in the late 1990s, resulted in health plans expanding their provider networks, thereby providing enrollees with more choice. With broader networks, insurers were less able to guarantee hospitals increased patient volume in return for large price discounts. The weakening of managed care's cost-containment methods further enhanced hospitals' bargaining power over insurers.

Hospital consolidation, the reduction in hospital bed capacity, and the demise of managed care's limited provider networks in the late 1990s led to higher prices for hospital services and increased hospital profitability. As shown in Exhibit 16.2, hospital profit margins reached a high in 1996 and 1997. Profit margins then declined for several years as Medicare reduced hospital payments to postpone bankruptcy of the Medicare Trust Fund. Profit margins increased throughout most of the decade, reaching a high in 2007. A deep recession, large numbers of uninsured, and bad debts reduced profit margins in 2008. Starting in 2009, hospitals' finances started to improve and by 2012 reached the highest total margins (7.8 percent) in more than 30 years.

Hospitals have gained greater market power as a result of mergers, decreased excess capacity, and insurers' reliance on broad provider networks (White, Bond, and Reschovsky 2013). These actions enabled hospitals to increase their prices and profitability. Hospitals' market power has limited insurers' ability to reduce growing hospital expenditures, one of the fastest-rising components of insurance premiums.

These changing trends, which have affected hospitals since the 1960s, are shown in Exhibit 16.3, which describes the annual rate of increase in hospital expenditures (adjusted for inflation). Medicare and Medicaid led to a large increase in spending growth rates in the late 1960s. Thereafter, annual growth rates have been on a generally downward trend. Although spending growth rates rose after the sharp drops during managed care, in recent years expenditure growth rates have continued to decrease, as the United States entered a severe recession, unemployment remained high, the percentage of employees with employer-paid health insurance declined, and more employees have chosen high-deductible health plans with lower premiums.

The future for hospitals is uncertain. The federal and state (Medicare and Medicaid) governments are major payers of hospital services, and both

EXHIBIT 16.2
Aggregate
Total Margins
and Operating
Margins for
US Hospitals,
1980–2012

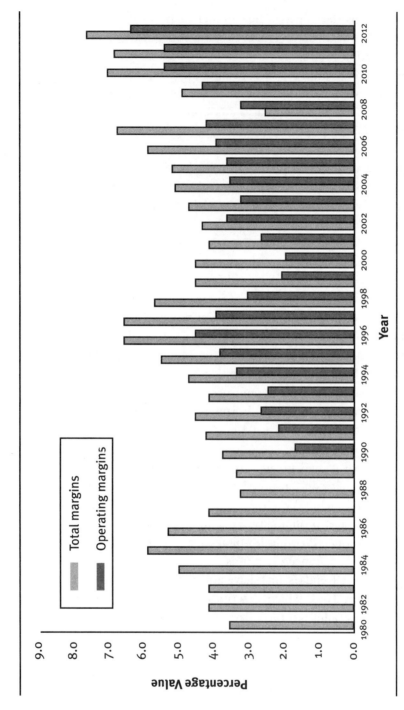

NOTE: Total margin is calculated as the difference between total net revenue and total expenses divided by total net revenue. Operating margin is calculated as the difference between operating revenue and total expenses divided by operating revenue. Data on operating margin before 1990 are not available.
SOURCES: 1980–1989 data are author's calculations from data in AHA (n.d.); 1990–2012 data from Lewin Group analysis of data in AHA (2014b), Table 4.1.

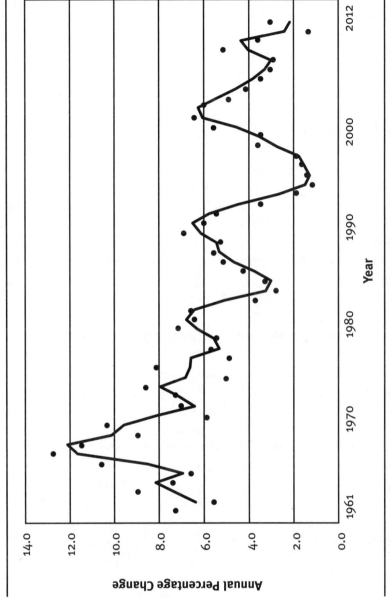

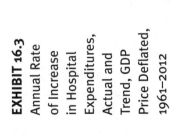

EXHIBIT 16.3
Annual Rate
of Increase
in Hospital
Expenditures,
Actual and
Trend, GDP
Price Deflated,
1961–2012

NOTE: Line represents two-year moving average.
SOURCES: Author's calculations based on data from CMS (2014a); GDP data from Office of Management and Budget (2014),
Table 10.1.

face severe financial deficits. The privately insured sector is declining, and the Affordable Care Act (ACA) is also likely to significantly affect hospital revenues and their future role. Will hospitals be able to generate sufficient funds to replace aging buildings, upgrade their facilities, purchase the latest technology, and continue to play an important role in the delivery of medical services?

The Hospital Outlook

Forecasting the industry outlook over the next five to ten years requires an analysis of trends affecting hospital costs and revenues (subdivided into hospital payment [price] and utilization). The hospital's margin (profit) is the difference between revenues and costs. Further, the actions of the two major payers of hospital care—government (Medicare and Medicaid) and private insurers—should be considered, along with the likely consequences of the ACA. Lastly, two scenarios can be envisioned: the status quo and a new role for hospitals.

Hospital Costs: The Public and Private Sectors

The greatest certainty regarding hospitals is that their costs will continue to grow faster than inflation. Two drivers warrant discussion. First is increasing labor costs. Salaries and benefits are the largest component of hospital costs, making up 53 percent of hospitals' overall expenses. The supply of and demand for registered nurses (RNs) determine their wages. Although the recession that began in 2008 caused many RNs who had left the workforce to return and although enrollments in nursing schools are up, this increase in supply of nurses (which has exceeded the demand for nurses) has limited raises in nurse wages in the past several years. As many baby boomers become eligible for Medicare and thus demand more medical services and as the number of the "old-old" elderly goes up, the demand for RNs will also grow. Although RNs are used predominantly in hospital settings, they also work in other care settings—from outpatient facilities, to home health care, to hospices. RNs represent 26 percent of hospital personnel, and their wages are likely to rise in coming years. (See Chapter 24 on the shortage of nurses for a more complete discussion of the nurse labor market.)

Economists consider new technology—including equipment, technicians, and expensive drugs—as the second most important reason for rising medical costs. In addition, hospitals are making large investments in information technology such as electronic medical records, which capture patient information related to visits with physicians and specialists, laboratory tests, prescription refills at pharmacies, and use of hospitals and outpatient facilities in the communities. Further, hospitals are investing large sums in clinical information technology to streamline clinical decision making, promote quality, and reduce medication errors. These investments, while likely to improve quality and cut costs, will require nonprofit hospitals to incur debt, which will add to their cost structure.

Caring for both public and private patients will continue to become more costly. Whether hospitals will have the revenue to cover these costs depends on future utilization and payments from the public and private sectors.

Hospital Revenues

Hospital revenues are determined simply by multiplying price by quantity—namely utilization. Several of the factors likely to affect trends in hospital utilization are considered in the following sections, followed by a discussion of likely changes in hospital payment.

Hospital Utilization

The Public Sector

Demographically, the population is aging. In 2011, the oldest of the baby boomers became eligible for Medicare. Forty million people began shifting from private insurance to Medicare. While Medicare discharges per enrollee (a measure of hospital use) have been decreasing in recent years, outpatient services per enrollee have been sharply increasing as more surgical procedures are performed in outpatient settings (CMS 2013, Table 5.1). Both trends are likely to continue.

The ACA, enacted in 2010, expands coverage for an estimated 32 million uninsured persons starting in 2014 (Kaiser Family Foundation 2013). About half of the 32 million people are eligible for Medicaid as a result of the expanded eligibility levels (to 133 percent of the federal poverty level), and the remainder (those between 133 to 400 percent of the federal poverty level) are eligible for subsidies for private coverage purchased on state health insurance exchanges.[1] Hospitals anticipated an increase in admissions as a result of the ACA's expansion of coverage and payment for previously uninsured patients. However, many hospitals are likely to be disappointed. The 16 million newly eligible for Medicaid are likely to be enrolled in Medicaid managed care plans. These managed care plans, to reduce their costs, will try to limit their enrollees' use of the hospital. The 16 million expected to purchase private insurance on state health insurance exchanges are offered a choice of health plans with narrow provider networks and high copayments for going out of network. Teaching hospitals are generally excluded from these provider networks to enable insurers to offer lower-priced insurance while protecting themselves from adverse selection; insurers fear that a higher number of less healthy than healthy enrollees will purchase insurance on the exchanges. Although the impact of the ACA's expanded coverage may be higher utilization, this increase may be less than originally expected.

The Private Sector

Hospital utilization by private, nongovernment patients is likely to decline as the baby boomers, a high-risk/user group, become eligible for Medicare. To limit increases in private insurance premiums, insurers will continue to examine approaches to decrease hospitalization—the most costly component of medical care. Hospitals will become more dependent on inpatient utilization from the expanding public sector.[2]

Hospital Payment

How hospitals are paid—and how much—has a significant effect on revenues. Individual hospitals cannot negotiate with the government over the price Medicare pays for services. Instead, hospital associations negotiate politically with legislators who determine Medicare's annual rate increases. Medicaid payment is determined at the state level. Hospital price negotiation with private insurers depends on their relative bargaining power. Thus, hospital prices are determined in both a competitive and a political marketplace.

Public Payers

Hospital payment sources have changed over time. Government now accounts for about 55 percent of hospital revenue, and this is likely to sharply increase as the ACA provisions are instituted (see Exhibit 16.4). Hospitals receive about 89 percent of their average costs of treatment for Medicaid patients and 86 percent for Medicare patients (see Exhibit 17.1). Lower government payment-to-cost ratios for Medicare and Medicaid enrollees reduce hospital profitability.

Medicaid will continue to be constrained in its payments to hospitals. States—which pay about half the costs of Medicaid on average (the remainder is paid by the federal government)—have difficulty financing rising Medicaid expenditures. Under the ACA, the federal government will pay for most of the cost of expanding the Medicaid eligible population. States, however, will bear some financial liability for this larger population. (As of 2014, many states have not decided whether they are going to expand Medicaid eligibility.) Medicaid payments have not kept up with rising hospital costs and are unlikely to do so in the future. The increasingly large number of low-income aged requiring Medicaid long-term care will place additional pressures on state Medicaid programs to limit hospital and other provider payments.

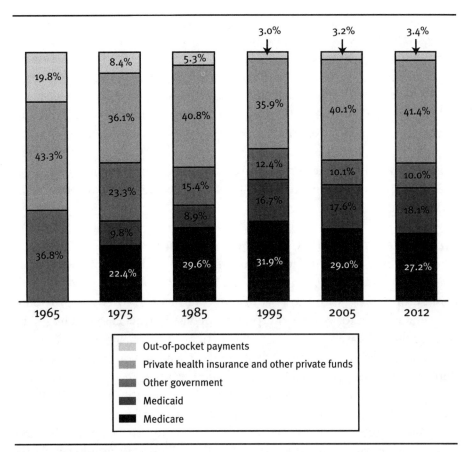

EXHIBIT 16.4
Sources of Hospital Revenues, by Payer, Selected Years, 1965– 2012

NOTE: "Medicaid" includes CHIP and Medicaid CHIP expansion. "Other government" includes workers' compensation, Department of Defense, maternal/child health, Veterans Administration, vocational rehabilitation, temporary disability, and state/local hospitals and school health.
SOURCE: Author's calculations based on data from CMS (2014b).

The Impact of the ACA on Medicare Hospital Payments

The ACA lowers Medicare hospital payments in several ways. The ACA also established an Independent Payment Advisory Board (IPAB) that must recommend payment reductions for hospitals and other Medicare providers if the per capita growth rate in Medicare spending exceeds the per capita growth rate of gross domestic product (GDP) plus one percent, which is lower than the historic average. (The IPAB's recommendations will have the force of law if Congress is unable to enact alternative measures to achieve the same spending reduction.) In addition, the ACA reduces hospital payments if a patient is readmitted for what is known as a *preventable hospital readmission*.[3] The hospital is now at financial risk for the appropriateness and quality of care received by their patients in settings other than the hospital.

An ACA change with large financial consequences for the hospital is a change to the DRG price update. Under the Medicare hospital DRG system,

Congress annually decided the percentage increase in the DRG price, which is supposed to be based on technical factors, such as hospital input price increases and productivity changes. The ACA, however, bases the DRG update on an assumed increase in hospital productivity (whether or not the productivity increase occurs). These assumed productivity improvements, which will reduce the DRG price update, will occur automatically in coming years and cannot be modified or rescinded except through new legislation.

Medicare's chief actuary has testified that the ACA's hospital payment cuts will, over time, result in Medicare hospital rates being much lower than Medicaid rates and that many hospitals will be forced into bankruptcy (Foster 2011, 7–8).

Accountable Care Organizations and Episode-Based Payment

The ACA also included several new voluntary Medicare payment models—accountable care organizations (ACOs) and bundled payments for an episode of illness—with the goal of reducing medical costs and providing coordinated care for a defined group of Medicare beneficiaries. The intent of coordinated care is to ensure that patients—especially the chronically ill—receive appropriate care when needed while avoiding unnecessary duplication of services. ACOs may include hospitals, medical groups, and other providers. Payment would vary according to the financial risk the ACO is willing to bear. Minimum financial risk involves a shared savings program whereby the ACO accepts responsibility for the overall quality and cost of caring for a defined group of Medicare fee-for-service beneficiaries and shares in any cost savings. A model including greater risk requires the ACO to share both savings and losses.

A concern with the ACO model is that Medicare fee-for-service patients are not informed that they have been assigned to an ACO and they are allowed to seek care anywhere—even outside the ACO. Medicare patients have no financial incentive to seek care just from the ACO, so they can still go to any hospital or specialist. The ACO, however, may incur penalties based on the patients' cost of care, regardless of who delivers it and where.

Episode-based (or bundled) payment pays hospitals and physicians a single price for all the services included in a particular diagnosis; the financial risk is shifted from the payer to the provider. The payment is made to an organization, such as a hospital, which then divides the payment among the participating providers. Episode-based payment changes providers' incentives so that providers have incentives to innovate, coordinate care, reduce costs, and improve quality.

Geisinger Health System (Danville, Pennsylvania) uses a bundled payment model as follows: For cardiac procedures, bundled payment includes the costs of the physician visit at which surgery was determined to be necessary, all hospital costs for the surgery and related care for 90 days after the surgery, and cardiac rehabilitation. Any associated complications and their treatment are also the provider's financial responsibility. Because of this bundled payment model, since 2006 Geisinger has seen surgery complications decrease by 21 percent, readmissions by 44 percent, and average length of stay by half a day (Paulus, Davis, and Steele 2008). Geisinger has expanded this model beyond cardiac procedures; it is now applied to hip replacement procedures, cataract surgery, obesity surgery, prenatal care, and cardiac catheterization.

Expanding episode-based payment to many more diagnoses is difficult. Patients are frequently treated for multiple chronic conditions, and bundled payment—which has a single-condition focus—may not be best for these patients. Changes in government payment policy, such as the move away from Medicare's DRG system and toward a broader system, occur slowly. Until such changes occur (if they do occur), hospital's incentives continue to be to increase admissions.

Private Payers

Hospital prices are referred to as *charges*. However, few purchasers of hospital services pay full (100 percent) charges.[4] Almost all payers receive discounts on charges. Hospitals may discount their charges by up to 50 percent. Most insured patients are insensitive to the prices hospitals charge because they typically do not pay any out-of-pocket costs when they are admitted to the hospital. (Only about 3.4 percent of hospital revenue is paid out of pocket by patients, which is lower than any other insured service.) The insurer negotiates a prearranged price with the hospital, which has separate contracts with many different health plans.

Insurers attempt to include in their network those providers whom their enrollees prefer and who are willing to give large price discounts in return for a greater volume of the insurers' enrollees. The insurer's ability to shift patients to competing hospitals determines its hospital discount. Its ability to shift patients is limited by the degree of hospital competition in a market. In markets with only one hospital, the hospital is a monopolist and can exercise its market power by charging more than hospitals charge in markets where multiple similar hospitals exist.[5] In competitive markets, insurers can shift their enrollees to lower-cost (but equal-quality) hospitals. The greater the number of hospitals competing on price, the lower the hospital's price markup and the greater the hospital discount (Ho 2009).

As a large percentage of the population is included in Medicare and Medicaid, hospitals will try to serve more privately insured patients, whose payment rates are higher (see Exhibit 17.1). However, private insurers are under competitive pressure to reduce rising premiums. Hospitals with little market power will face difficult price negotiations with insurers and will be pressured to limit their price increases and move to episode-based payment, potentially causing conflict with their medical staff. Thus, in the private sector, hospitals integrated with their physicians are likely to fare better than those hospitals that continue to rely on fee-for-service. Only those hospitals with strong market power will be able to receive high private fee-for-service payments—from a shrinking private sector, however.

The Current Hospital Outlook

Hospital Consolidation

A great deal of hospital consolidation has been occurring over the past two decades. Increased hospital spending in recent years is the result of higher hospital prices charged to commercial insurers, not because patients are using hospitals more (see Exhibit 17.1). A major contributor to these higher prices is ongoing hospital consolidation. Before 2008, the Federal Trade Commission (FTC) was unable to prevent hospital mergers. They were overruled by the courts because the courts believed that if nonprofit hospitals gained market power they would not raise their prices. Subsequent studies by healthcare economists demonstrating that increased consolidation led to higher hospital prices has enabled the FTC to be more successful in blocking anticompetitive hospital mergers.

After reviewing the research literature, Gaynor and Town (2012) concluded that hospital consolidation generally results in higher hospital prices. When hospital mergers occur in markets that are already consolidated, price increases exceed 20 percent. A second important finding is that physician–hospital consolidation was primarily for the purpose of gaining greater bargaining power over insurers and did not lead to more integration. Unless greater integration occurs, physician–hospital consolidation does not lead to improved quality or reduced costs.[6]

The ACA provides for payment of ACOs and illness episodes. Both of these approaches encourage hospital consolidation and vertical integration between hospitals and physicians. Hospitals are employing greater numbers of physicians and purchasing more physician practices. Part of the reason for hospital employment of physicians is that Medicare physician fees are much higher when billed as a hospital outpatient visit than if the same visit were billed at a freestanding physician practice. Similarly, the Medicare fee for an MRI (magnetic resonance imaging) performed by a hospital is several times greater than if the same test were performed at a freestanding physician practice.

Hospitals are moving more of their services to outpatient settings. As new technologies allow patients to be treated less invasively, more inpatient procedures can be performed more effectively in an outpatient setting. About 60 percent to 70 percent of all surgeries are now being done in an outpatient setting, and outpatient services represent about 50 percent of hospital revenue. To remain competitive, hospitals need to be able to offer their services in wider geographic areas and at convenient locations to patients. Patients do not want to travel to a large hospital located in an urban center for all the services they need.

While hospital consolidation and physician integration enables hospitals to raise prices, gain greater leverage with suppliers and pharmaceutical firms, and have better access to capital, hospitals relying on fee-for-service payment will find themselves receiving a smaller part of the pie as government and private payers seek to use less of the most costly component of care.

Expansion of Medicaid and Enrollment on State Health Insurance Exchanges

The ACA sought to expand coverage by broadening Medicaid eligibility and offering income-related subsidies on state health insurance exchanges. Hospitals anticipate receiving additional revenues from 32 million newly covered individuals. However, Medicaid pays hospitals less than private payers do, and insurers offering coverage on state exchanges are using narrow provider networks to limit their costs. High-deductible health plans have been increasing in popularity, given their lower premiums, but they are likely to lead to greater bad debts for hospitals as people may not be able to pay the deductible when they enter the hospital. Further, to reduce their costs, insurers will continue to seek ways to keep their enrollees from entering a hospital, such as by using less expensive settings. The additional enrollment expected from the ACA may not result in as large an increase in hospital revenues as hospitals initially believed.

Changing Payment Systems

Hospital payment has changed over time. When Medicare was enacted in 1965, it paid hospitals according to the hospitals' costs of treating Medicare patients. Starting in 1983, realizing that cost-based payment provides incentives for inefficiency and duplication of facilities and services, Medicare shifted to prospective payment—a fixed price per diagnosis. The ACA changed Medicare hospital payment still further. Greater efficiency incentives could be achieved by including a better continuum of care within that fixed price. Demonstrations using bundled or episode-based payment, payment to ACOs, and not reimbursing hospitals for readmission within 30 days of discharge are forms of prospective payment that give the provider an incentive to keep the patient out of the hospital by anticipating and preventing costly admissions; this is in contrast to fee-for-service, a retrospective fee that pays the provider once the patient is ill. These ACA demonstration projects are a step toward capitation, which is a single payment per enrollee for all their medical services. Medicare already uses capitation for Medicare Advantage plans, which enroll about 28 percent of Medicare enrollees. Kaiser and health maintenance organizations (HMOs) have long relied on capitation in the private sector. Rather than giving Medicare beneficiaries an incentive to use Medicare Advantage plans, the government has reduced payments to these plans and encouraged demonstration projects that offer enrollees or providers few financial incentives to limit high costs. Critics are doubtful these ACO Medicare demonstrations will lead to widespread acceptance by hospitals.

The likely scenario for rising government hospital expenditures is imposing price controls, such as the ACA's assumed hospital productivity increases (hence lower payments) and the IPAB, which limits hospital expenditure increases to GDP plus one percent.

Hospital Strategies

Hospitals face different future scenarios. The underlying assumptions of each scenario is that (1) under the ACA, according to the Medicare actuary, Medicare hospital payments will be reduced to the point that hospitals receive less and less from Medicare; (2) to minimize utilization of inpatient admissions—the most expensive component of care—public and private payers will seek to have more care or services performed in less costly settings, such as outpatient centers or the patients' home; and (3) accelerating the shift from inpatient to outpatient care is the gradual change in payment systems by all types of payers, away from fee-for-service and toward episode-based or capitation reimbursement.

It is generally recognized that fee-for-service does not necessarily promote coordination of care, high-quality outcomes, or efficient use of services. Poor medical performance is not penalized; in fact, providers may receive additional revenues. Organizations that cut unnecessary services and shift patients to lower-cost settings suffer decreased revenues. The financial risk and additional cost of complications and hospital readmissions under fee-for-service is shifted from providers to insurers (and enrollees, in the form of higher insurance premiums). Reforming the delivery system requires reforming the payment system.

Capitation is a single payment per enrollee for all their medical services (but patients may still be required to make copayments for some services). The broader the payment system, the more incentive the organization has to be innovative in reducing medical costs, such as by providing preventive services. Under episode-based payment and capitation, hospitals and physicians have an incentive to form integrated organizations. Further, the measurement of quality and care outcomes becomes easier than under fee-for-service. As Medicare payments for hospitals and physicians are lowered over time, broader payment systems offer providers an opportunity to deliver care in a more efficient and effective manner while enhancing their revenues. Moving the current fee-for-service delivery system to capitation is difficult and will take time.

Status Quo Scenario

Hospitals that continue to primarily rely on inpatient admissions as their major source of revenue under fee-for-service payment will experience declining admissions and falling fee-for-service payments. The annual Medicare DRG payment updates will become insufficient to cover rising hospital costs. Similarly, Medicaid hospital payments will be inadequate to cover the full costs of caring for Medicaid patients. As a consequence, hospital margins will decline and hospitals will be unable to raise the capital to purchase the latest technology. Over time, hospitals will no longer receive enough government funds to pay competitive wages and will have to reduce their staffing ratios. Eventually, publicly funded patients' access to care will be limited and quality of care slowly will deteriorate.

Hospitals that have consolidated and increased their market power will be able to raise their rates to private insurers. Faced with high hospital prices and regulatory and competitive limits on their rate increases, insurers are likely to develop narrow hospital and provider networks (as they did during the 1990s) and try to shift more services to outpatient settings.

Under the status quo scenario, hospitals with market power will perform better than those without such pricing power. However, even for these hospitals, expenditure growth rate will decline.

A New Role For Hospitals

Hospitals need to reinvent themselves with a new business model. Relying solely on a strategy of increasing hospital admissions will not provide hospitals with the necessary revenue and capital to maintain their dominant role in the delivery of medical services. Driven by changes in the payment system (away from fee-for-service and toward capitation), a long-term strategic shift is occurring—from inpatient care to outpatient care. The overriding goal of public and private payers is to reduce the rising cost of medical care while improving patient outcomes.

To become successful under the new payment systems, hospitals must develop a new relationship with their physicians. In the past, hospitals needed physicians to ensure admission referrals and to receive higher payments for outpatient services—such as surgery and imaging tests—when billed by the hospital than by independent physicians. When payment is based on episode of care or capitation, hospitals need physicians to be able to provide coordinated care to reduce medical costs and improve patient outcomes. Physician and hospital incentives must be aligned to achieve these desired outcomes.

Under fee-for-service, insurers and the government bore the risk. As hospitals form ACOs and engage in broader payment systems, risk is transferred from the payer to the ACO. Data are essential for managing risk, understanding costs of caring for different types of patients, and accepting risk-based contracts. "Because insurers pay claims for all doctor visits, lab tests, and other care, they get a full view of their members. Hospital systems say they need direct access to that data, which they can get by offering their own plans, to manage patients better, avoiding duplication and detecting and treating problems early to head off pricey procedures later" (Mathews 2012). Only then will hospitals be able to manage the population health of their enrollees, anticipating and preventing illness particularly among the chronically ill.

Several hospital systems have developed their own health plans, offering HMOs that rely on their own hospitals and physicians while limiting their enrollees' access to out-of-network providers. To survive the trend toward less inpatient care, hospitals must become integrated organizations; develop a capability for data analytics; accept risk contracts; rely on physicians to coordinate care; create integrated delivery systems; expand outpatient capabilities in multiple locations; and provide, in addition to acute care, home health care, telehealth services, and actual as well as virtual services at times convenient to the working population. To control both cost and quality, the hospital needs to have greater control over the entire continuum of care—from wellness and prevention to acute care to post-acute services such as home health care.

Summary

Hospital fortunes have changed over time. Managed care and Medicare DRG payment greatly reduced hospital utilization, created excess capacity, and weakened hospitals' bargaining power with insurers. Over time, hospital capacity was decreased, mergers occurred, and managed care broadened its provider networks; hospitals consolidated and used their increased bargaining power over insurers to raise their prices and profitability.

The future presents threats and opportunities. Technological developments have enabled a greater number of complex procedures to be performed in an outpatient setting. Payment systems have given incentives for performing more services in outpatient settings. Over time, the ACA will lower hospital rates for Medicare patients dramatically. The hospitals' growing reliance on government payment is likely to result in a lower growth rate in hospital expenditures. As the number of publicly insured increases, shrinking the privately insured market, hospital competition for a diminishing pool of privately insured patients will intensify.

Changes in payment systems offer the potential for greater revenues to those hospitals and physicians able to integrate their services over the entire continuum of care. Hospitals unable to do so will rely on fee-for-service and a shrinking revenue base. In preparation for changing payment systems and the necessity of coordinating care, hospitals are employing physicians and purchasing physician practices. Broader payment systems require integrated delivery organizations to manage risk (as they become more like insurers) and collect enrollee data to anticipate and reduce preventable illnesses.

Payment system changes will result in many disruptive innovations in the delivery of medical services. In a $3 trillion industry, huge financial rewards are available to those who are able to cut costs while improving patient outcomes and satisfaction. Providers have traditionally concentrated on their own role in caring for the sick. Will hospitals be able to think in terms of the entire continuum of care? Will hospitals be able to think in terms of managing the health of a population? The future of hospitals will be determined by how well they are able to work with physicians and deliver coordinated care while reducing rising medical costs and improving patient outcomes. Many hospitals will experience difficulty in adjusting to new payment systems.

Discussion Questions

1. What is the outlook for hospital cost increases?
2. How has Medicare hospital payment changed over time?
3. What are the likely economic assumptions hospitals should consider in developing their future strategies?
4. Why do hospital mergers increase hospitals' bargaining power over insurers?
5. What are two different hospital strategies for responding to new payment system changes?

Notes

1. The income of an individual at 133 percent and 400 percent of the federal poverty level in 2014 is $15,521 and $46,680. For a family of four, the income levels are $31,721 and $95,400.

2. Hospitals are expanding their emergency departments (EDs) as a place for lower-acuity patients to have access to care 24 hours a day, 7 days a week. A recent RAND study found that EDs are now responsible for about half of all inpatient admissions and accounted for all the growth in admissions between 2003 and 2009, the period studied (Gonzalez Morganti et al. 2013). The growth in hospital admissions has stagnated. It was previously believed that EDs served mainly the uninsured, but this is no longer the case. Insured patients are also using EDs (which may lead to an admission), and they have become a new source of revenue for the hospital.

3. Under the ACA, hospitals will receive lower payments (3 percent of Medicare revenues) if a Medicare patient is readmitted to the hospital within 30 days for one of five specified diagnoses (heart attack, heart failure, pneumonia, chronic obstructive pulmonary disease, and hip and knee arthroplasty). For example, after being discharged from the hospital for hip replacement surgery, a Medicare patient receives care in a skilled nursing facility and then continues her recovery at home, using physical therapy services and visiting her physician. The hospital's spending per beneficiary would be based on all of these costs. It becomes necessary for the hospital to coordinate all of these elements of care, including if the patient develops an infection and has to be readmitted to the hospital (Pear 2011).

4. Although few payers pay full charges, hospitals will attempt to collect 100 percent of their charges from those who have not previously negotiated a discounted price. Those most likely to be billed full charges are those who are brought to the hospital by an ambulance as a result of an auto accident. At that point, neither the accident victim nor his auto insurance company is in a position to negotiate a discounted rate from the hospital. Billing auto insurance companies full charges is very profitable for hospitals.

5. By merging, hospitals decrease the number of substitutes the insurer can contract with, and their new demand curve will be less price elastic, enabling them to raise price and total revenue. The term *price elasticity of demand* is the percentage change in quantity demanded with a 1 percent change in price. When the percentage change in quantity demanded exceeds the percentage change in price, the good or service is considered to be price elastic. For example, if the price decreases by 5 percent and the quantity demanded increases by 10 percent, the price elasticity equals –2. If the percentage change in price is greater than the percentage change in quantity, the service is *price inelastic* (e.g., price increases by 5 percent and quantity demanded decreases by 2 percent). Price elasticity is important in

determining the effect of a change in price on revenue. When a service is price inelastic, increasing price will raise total revenue; decreasing price will lower total revenue. Conversely, when the demand for a service is price elastic, increasing price decreases total revenue. Price elasticity is mainly determined by the closeness of substitutes. A hospital with good substitutes (i.e., comparable hospitals) will have a price-elastic demand curve; if it raises price, its total revenue will decrease.

6. Hospitals often claim that their merger will achieve greater efficiency and hence lower prices. Economies of scale occur when a firm's output increases by a greater proportion than the increase in its input cost; average total cost per unit, therefore, decreases as output increases. Large firms' unit costs are lower than those of small firms. Economies of scope occur when it is less expensive for a firm to produce certain services (or products) jointly than if separate firms produce each of the same services independently. An example is when the physician who undertakes stem cell research also provides stem cell therapy. In this case, it is less costly to provide the research and therapy together than separately by different firms. When economies of scope exist, multi-product (service) firms are more efficient than single-product (service) firms. Economies of scale are unrelated to economies of scope.

References

American Hospital Association (AHA). n.d. *Hospital Statistics.* Various editions. Chicago: AHA.

———. 2014a. *Hospital Statistics, 2014 ed.* Chicago: AHA.

———. 2014b. "Chapter 4: Trends in Hospital Financing." In *Trendwatch Chartbook: Trends Affecting Hospitals and Health Systems.* Chicago: AHA. www.aha.org/research/reports/tw/chartbook/ch4.shtml.

Centers for Medicare & Medicaid Services (CMS). 2014a. "National Health Expenditure Data." Last modified May. http://cms.gov/Research-Statistics-Data-and-Systems/Statistics-Trends-and-Reports/NationalHealthExpendData/index.html.

———. 2014b. "Tables." Accessed April. http://cms.gov/Research-Statistics-Data-and-Systems/Statistics-Trends-and-Reports/NationalHealthExpendData/Downloads/tables.pdf.

———. 2013. "Tables." In *Medicare & Medicaid Research Review/2013 Statistical Supplement.* Accessed April 2014. www.cms.gov/Research-Statistics-Data-and-Systems/Statistics-Trends-and-Reports/MedicareMedicaidStatSupp/Downloads/2013_Section5.pdf#Table5.1.

Foster, R. 2011. "The Estimated Effect of the Affordable Care Act on Medicare and Medicaid Outlays and Total National Health Care Expenditures." Testimony before the House Committee on the Budget, January 26. http://budget.house.gov/uploadedfiles/fostertestimony1262011.pdf.

Gaynor, M., and R. Town. 2012. "The Impact of Consolidation—Update." *The Synthesis Policy Brief* No. 9, June. www.rwjf.org/content/dam/farm/reports/issue_briefs/2012/rwjf73261.

Gonzalez Morganti, K., S. Bauhoff, J. Blanchard, M. Abir, N. Iyer, A. Smith, J. Vesely, E. Okeke, and A. Kellermann. 2013. *The Evolving Role of Emergency Departments in the United States.* Santa Monica, CA: RAND Corp. www.rand.org/content/dam/rand/pubs/research_reports/RR200/RR280/RAND_RR280.sum.pdf.

Ho, K. 2009. "Insurer–Provider Networks in the Medical Care Market." *American Economic Review* 99 (1): 393–430.

Kaiser Family Foundation. 2013. "Summary of the Affordable Care Act." Last modified April 23. http://kaiserfamilyfoundation.files.wordpress.com/2011/04/8061-021.pdf.

Mathews, A. 2012. "Hospital Systems Branch Out As Insurers." *Wall Street Journal*, December 17, p. B2.

Office of Management and Budget, The White House. 2014. "Fiscal Year 2014 Historical Tables. Budget of the U.S. Government." Accessed April. www.whitehouse.gov/sites/default/files/omb/budget/fy2014/assets/hist.pdf.

Paulus, R., K. Davis, and G. Steele. 2008. "Continuous Innovation in Health Care: Implications of the Geisinger Experience." *Health Affairs* 27 (5): 1235–45.

Pear, R. 2011. "Medicare Plan for Payments Irks Hospitals." *New York Times*, May 30. www.nytimes.com/2011/05/31/health/policy/31hospital.html?pagewanted=all&_r=0.

White, C., A. Bond, and J. Reschovsky. 2013. "High and Varying Prices for Privately Insured Patients Underscore Hospital Market Power." *HSC Research Brief* No. 27, September. www.hschange.org/CONTENT/1375/.

COST SHIFTING

17

T he theory of cost shifting is often used as the basis for public policy proposals, such as an employer mandate and the Affordable Care Act (ACA). Employers and insurers believe one reason for the rise in employees' health insurance premiums is cost shifting. When one purchaser—whether Medicare, Medicaid, or the uninsured patient—does not pay the full charges, many believe hospitals and physicians raise their prices to those who can afford to pay, namely those with private insurance. Cost shifting is considered unfair, and its elimination is an important reason large employers (whose employees have health insurance) favor the mandate that all employers provide their employees with health insurance. One rationale for the ACA used by President Obama to cover the uninsured was that those with insurance pay higher premiums to cover the costs of the uninsured who use the emergency department.

A concern by those favoring the cost-shifting hypothesis is that, to finance expanded Medicaid eligibility and provide subsidies to those buying insurance on state health insurance exchanges, the ACA funds these subsidies—in part by slowing Medicare payment updates to hospitals. These lower hospital payments will, for many hospitals, reduce Medicare prices below the costs of caring for Medicare patients. Will hospitals cost shift to private insurers to make up for these lower payments, resulting in much higher private health insurance premiums?

Evidence of cost shifting is based on the observation that different payers pay different prices for similar services (see Exhibit 17.1). Private payers have always had higher payment-to-cost ratios (higher price markups) than do Medicare and Medicaid, and Medicare has generally paid more than Medicaid has. The payment-to-cost ratios for all three payers have changed over time. Exhibit 17.1 suggests that when Medicare and Medicaid have low payment-to-cost ratios (which result in low profit margins for the providers), private payers have high price-to-cost ratios. Still to be discussed, however, is whether the relationships are causal—that is, whether low public payment–cost relationships lead to high private payment-to-cost ratios.

Although the logic of cost shifting may seem straightforward, it provokes troubling questions. For example, can a hospital or physician merely increase prices to those who can pay to recover losses from those who do not

EXHIBIT 17.1
Aggregate
Hospital
Payment-to-
Cost Ratios for
Private Payers,
Medicare,
and Medicaid,
1980–2012

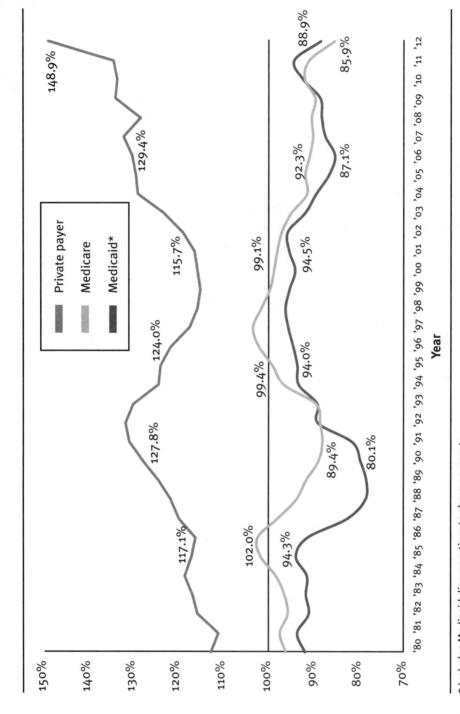

* Includes Medicaid disproportionate share payments
SOURCE: Data from AHA (2014), Table 4.6.

pay? If the provider is able to shift costs, why do hospitals complain about the uncompensated care they are forced to provide? Further, if providers are able to offset their losses by raising prices to those with insurance, why have they not done so previously and thereby earned greater profits?

To better understand cost shifting, we must discuss (1) the provider's objective when it prices its services and (2) how different objectives result in different pricing strategies.

Setting Prices to Maximize Profits

Firms typically price their services to maximize profits—that is, to make as much money as possible. This is the simplest objective to start with in analyzing hospital and physician price setting. Assume that the hospital has two sets of patients: those who can pay and those who cannot pay for services. Exhibit 17.2 illustrates how a profit-maximizing price is set for the insured group of patients. The relationship between price (P) and quantity (Q) is inverse, meaning the lower the price, the more units are likely to be purchased. Total revenue (TR) is price multiplied by quantity. As the price is decreased, more units will be sold and TR will increase; after some point, however, the high number of units sold will not offset the lower price per unit and TR will actually decline. The effect on TR when price is lowered and more units are sold is shown by the TR curve in Exhibit 17.3.

To determine the price and output that result in the largest profit, we must also know the costs for producing that output. Total cost (TC) consists

Price (P)	Quantity (Q)	Total Revenue (TR)	Total Cost (TC)	Profit	TC_2	$Profit_2$
$11	1	$11	$9	$2	$11	$0
10	2	20	13	7	17	3
9	3	27	17	10	23	4
8	4	32	21	11	29	3
7	5	35	25	10	35	0
6	6	36	29	7	41	−5
5	7	35	33	2	47	−12
4	8	32	37	−5	53	−21
3	9	27	41	−14	59	−32

EXHIBIT 17.2
Determining the Profit-Maximizing Price

EXHIBIT 17.3
Profit-
Maximizing
Price With
and Without
a Change in
Variable Cost

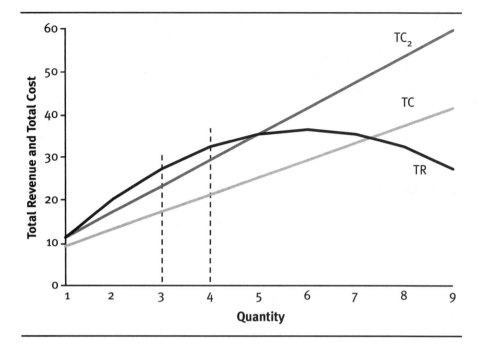

of two parts: (1) fixed costs, which do not vary as output changes (such as rent for an office or depreciation on a building), and (2) variable costs, which do vary. For this example, fixed costs are assumed to be $5 and variable costs are constant at $4 per unit. The difference between TR and TC is profit. According to Exhibit 17.2, the largest amount of profit occurs when the price is $8 and output equals four units. At that price TR is $32, TC is $21 ($5 fixed cost plus $16 variable costs), and profit is $11. According to Exhibit 17.3, the greatest difference between the total cost line (TC) and TR (profit) occurs at four units of output.

Raising or lowering the price will only reduce profits. If the hospital decreases its price from $8 to $7, it will have to cut the price on all units sold. The hospital's volume will increase; TR will rise from $32 to $35 or by only $3. Because the variable cost of the extra unit sold is $4, the hospital will lose money on that last unit. The profit at a price of $7 will be $10. Similarly, if the hospital raises its price from $8 to $9, it will sell one less unit, reducing its variable cost by $4 but forgoing $5 worth of revenue (see Exhibit 17.4).[1] Changing the price once it is at the profit-maximizing price lowers the hospital's profit.

Exhibit 17.2 illustrates several important points. First, establishing a profit-maximizing price means the price is set so that the additional revenue received is equal to the additional cost of serving one more patient. When the change in TR is equal to the change in TC, choosing any other price will result in less profit.

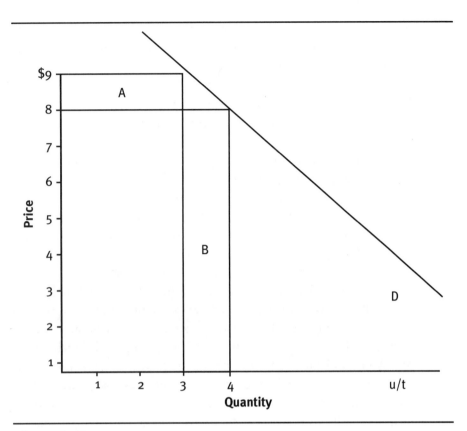

EXHIBIT 17.4
Effect on Total
Revenue of a
Change in Price

u/t: quantity/time

Second, if the hospital's fixed costs go up from $5 to $11, the hospital should not change its price; if it did, it will make even less profit. With an increase in fixed costs, profit will decline by $6 at every quantity sold. At a price of $8, the hospital will make a total profit of $5; TR is $32, while TC is now $27 ($11 plus $16). If the hospital raised its price to $9 to compensate for the higher fixed costs, TR will be $27, TC will be $23 ($11 plus $12), and total profit will fall to $4. Thus, changes in fixed costs should not affect the hospital's profit-maximizing price.

Third, if the hospital's variable costs changed—perhaps because nurses' wages or the cost of supplies increased—the hospital will find it profitable to change its price. For example, if variable costs rise by $2 and the price–quantity relationship is unchanged, the largest profit will occur at a price of $9 (TR − TC_2 = $Profit_2$ in Exhibit 17.2). The higher variable cost is shown in Exhibit 17.3 as TC_2. The distance between TR and TC_2 (which is profit) is greatest at three units of output. If the price per unit remains $8 when variable costs increase to $6 per unit, the addition to TR from producing four rather than three units is only $5. The hospital will lose money on that last unit, the cost of which is $6. Thus, by raising price and producing fewer units, the higher TR slightly exceeds the additional cost of producing that last unit. Hospitals, therefore, will be expected to raise their prices as their variable costs increase. Similarly, if variable costs decrease, the hospital will realize more profit by lowering the price.

Fourth, hospitals will also be expected to change the price they charge if the relationship between price and quantity were to change. The price–quantity relationship is a measure of how price sensitive purchasers are to changes in the hospital's price. When the price is changed and quantity changes by a small percentage, purchasers are not very price sensitive; the demand for the hospital's service is *price inelastic*. Conversely, when quantity changes by a greater percentage than the change in price, purchasers are said to be more price sensitive; the demand is *price elastic*. As the demand for the hospital's services becomes more price sensitive (price elastic), a hospital will be expected to lower its price, even if there is no change in its costs.[2]

For example, if five hospitals exist in a market and each hospital is considered to be a relatively good substitute for the others in terms of location, services, reputation, medical staff, and so on, each hospital's demand is considered to be very price sensitive. In competing to be included in different HMO and insurer provider networks, each hospital will compete on price. If just one hospital lowers price, it will cause large increases in that hospital's patient volume. Similarly, raising its price when the other hospitals do not will cause that hospital to lose a large portion of its market share. Conversely, a hospital that is a sole community provider or that has the only trauma unit, for example, faces a less price-sensitive demand for its services or its trauma unit. That hospital's prices will be higher than if good substitutes were available for its services. If the hospital is already charging a profit-maximizing price to its paying patients and the variable costs of serving paying patients have not changed, the hospital will make even less profit by further increasing prices to paying patients. Referring to Exhibit 17.2, if the hospital raises its price from $8 to $9 simply because other patients did not pay, the hospital will forgo profit. Assuming the hospital wants to make as much money as possible from those who can afford to pay, the hospital will not raise its price to those patients unless there is a change in variable costs or in their price–quantity relationship. Because neither factor changes when another group of patients pays less, it will not make sense for the hospital to charge its paying patients more.

Based on this explanation of how a profit-maximizing price is set, changes in prices can be explained by changes in the variable costs of caring for patients or by a change in the price-sensitivity relationship facing a hospital (or a physician).

Contrary to what many people believe, when the government lowers the price it pays for Medicare or Medicaid patients, physicians will likely reduce the prices they charge to higher-paying patients. For example, assume that a physician serves two types of patients: private patients and Medicaid patients. The government determines the price charged to Medicaid patients, whereas the physician sets the price for private patients. Traditionally, the price received by the physician for treating private patients is higher than that received for treating Medicaid patients. The physician presumably allocates her time so that revenues per unit of time are the same, regardless of the types of patients served. To produce equal returns when the prices for Medicaid and private patients are different, the physician may spend less time on the Medicaid patient.

If the government further decreases the price it pays for Medicaid patients, the physician is likely to decide that she can earn more by shifting some time away from Medicaid patients and toward caring for more private patients. As more physicians limit the time they spend with Medicaid patients and reallocate more time to the private market, the supply of physician time in this market grows. With an increase in supply, physicians will be willing to reduce their prices to receive more private patients. Assuming limited demand creation by physicians, a lower price for Medicaid patients is likely to result in lower physician fees for private patients.

Assuming that the objective of hospitals and physicians is to make as much money as possible, these two examples suggest that prices for private patients will be either unchanged or reduced when another payer—government—pays the provider less.

Origins of Claims of Cost Shifting

Based on the earlier discussion, why do private purchasers claim that they are being charged more to make up for the lower prices paid by the government? The belief that cost shifting is occurring may simply be an artifact of trends over time in rising hospital prices and uncompensated care. Hospitals may appear to be raising prices to compensate for lower prices charged to other patients, but hospital prices to private payers have increased for two reasons: (1) variable costs have increased as expenses for wages and supplies have risen and (2) changes in the hospitals' payer mixes—growth in the proportion of patients who are less price sensitive—may have enabled them to raise their markups on certain types of private patients. This association of rising prices and uncompensated care does not necessarily indicate a causal relationship.

However, a logical explanation, unrelated to cost shifting, does exist for why some purchasers pay more for the same service than do other purchasers: Some purchasers may be more price sensitive than others. Previously, private patients had either indemnity insurance or Blue Cross hospital coverage;

because hospitals had a close relationship with Blue Cross (hospitals started and controlled Blue Cross), Blue Cross was charged a lower price than were indemnity insurers. The price–quantity relationship for those with indemnity insurance represented the average relationship for everyone in the indemnity plan. However, as employers began offering different types of health plans—such as health maintenance organizations (HMOs), preferred provider organizations (PPOs), and managed care—in addition to the traditional indemnity plan and as employees had to pay varying premiums and copayments under these plans, the price–quantity relationships of these plans differed. Those with indemnity insurance could choose whatever hospital and physician they desired. Other plans, however, were more restrictive in deciding which providers their subscribers could use. HMOs and PPOs were likely to bargain with providers for lower prices in return for directing their subscribers to these approved providers.

Faced with different price–quantity relationships with different purchasers, hospitals began charging different prices to each type of payer. These prices take into consideration the price sensitivity of each of these insurance plans. Patients remaining in the traditional indemnity plan are charged the highest prices because they are not restricted in their use of providers. Their insurers cannot promise to direct their subscribers to particular hospitals and are least able to negotiate lower hospital prices. It is the willingness of an insurer to shift its enrollees to another hospital that results in their greater price sensitivity.

Price Discrimination

Charging according to what the market will bear is not really cost shifting but rather simply charging a profit-maximizing price to each group; this is price discrimination. Services for which purchasers are willing to pay more have higher markups. Airlines charge higher prices for first-class seating and lower prices for 21-day advance purchases, for example. Movie theaters charge lower prices for matinees and to senior citizens. Each of these industries is pricing according to different groups' willingness to pay; each group has a different price–quantity relationship. Hospital pricing is no different. Hospitals placing a proportionately higher markup over costs on laboratory tests or drugs used by inpatients than on the room-and-board fee are engaging in price discrimination. Patients who have to pay part of the bill themselves can more easily compare hospital room-and-board rates before they enter the hospital; hospitals, therefore, have to be price competitive on their room rates. Once a patient is hospitalized, however, he has little choice in what he pays for services rendered in the hospital. The price–quantity relationships for inpatient services are quite insensitive to prices charged. Hospitals do not face any competition for laboratory tests or other services provided to their inpatients. Thus, their markup for these services is much higher.

Price discrimination is an important reason some purchasers are able to pay lower hospital prices. A large employer or an HMO willing to direct its employees or enrollees to a particular hospital will receive a lower price for the same service than will a single patient negotiating with the same hospital. The hospital's price–quantity relationship is more price sensitive when the hospital negotiates with a large purchaser than when the hospital deals with a single insured patient. The single insured patient does not pay higher prices because the large purchaser pays a lower price. The hospital is less concerned about losing one patient's business than losing 1,000 patients from a large purchaser.

Even if the government increased its payments to hospitals for treating Medicare patients, the price to the single insured patient is not reduced because the price–quantity relationship for these patients (who are less price sensitive) is unchanged. Only if the patient with indemnity insurance becomes part of a large purchasing group (which is willing to offer a hospital a greater volume of patients in return for lower prices) can that patient receive a lower hospital price. Different prices to different purchasers are related to how price sensitive they are rather than to what other purchasers are paying. As the insurance market has become more segmented with HMOs, PPOs, self-insured employer groups, traditional indemnity-type insurance plans, and so on, hospitals have developed different pricing strategies for each group.

Empirical evidence supports the view that hospital prices are not raised to other purchasers when prices are reduced to large purchasers. Dranove and White (1998) found that hospitals that had a higher proportion of Medicaid patients (20 percent or more of their budgets) did not increase prices to other paying patients when Medicaid decreased its reimbursement; if anything, hospitals lowered their prices to private payers.[3] Research reinforces the finding that hospital cost shifting is minimal, if at all. White (2013) found that when Medicare cut its payment rate by 10 percent, hospital rates charged to private payers were *reduced* by 3 percent to 8 percent. By lowering the prices charged to private payers, hospitals attempt to attract a greater volume of higher-paying patients.

Conditions Under Which Cost Shifting Can Occur

Under certain circumstances, however, cost shifting may occur. Some hospitals may have a different pricing objective—they do not price to maximize their profits. These hospitals may voluntarily forgo some profits to maintain good community relationships. When hospitals do not set profit-maximizing prices, increases in uncompensated care or fixed costs may cause the hospital to raise its prices to those groups who have more ability to pay. For example, *average cost pricing* occurs when a hospital sets its price by relating it to the average cost of caring for all of its patients. If one payer (such as the government) decides to pay the hospital less, the average price goes up for all other payers. For cost shifting to occur, the hospital must have bargaining or market power that it has not used; the purchasers of hospital (or physician) services have to be relatively insensitive to the higher prices. If the purchasers switch to other providers or use fewer services as a result of the provider's cost shifting, the provider's revenues and profits decline.

Is cost shifting an important reason private patients are paying higher medical prices today? Purchasers have become more price sensitive since the mid-1980s. Given the increased competitive market in which providers find themselves, providers are unlikely willing to forgo profits by not setting profit-maximizing prices. Forgoing profits means the hospital has no better use for those funds. Two ways the hospital could use those higher profits are to purchase new equipment or to start new services to increase its revenues. The medical staff, an important constituency within the hospital, also desires new equipment and facilities. Paying higher wages makes attracting needed nursing and technical personnel easier. Hospitals could enhance their community image and market themselves by providing screening and health awareness programs to their communities. Further, additional funds could always be used to provide care to those in the community who cannot afford it and who are not covered by public programs.

The benefits to the hospital of forgoing profit on some payer groups are unlikely to exceed the benefits to the hospital of using that forgone profit in other ways. By not setting profit-maximizing prices, the hospital's decision makers place a greater weight on benefiting some purchaser group than on using those funds for other constituencies.

One type of cost shifting occurs when the government pays hospitals a fixed price for Medicare patients' use of the hospital but reimburses outpatient services on a cost basis. If the hospital has $100 in indirect administrative costs to allocate between inpatient units (paid according to a fixed-price diagnosis-related group) and outpatient units (paid on a cost basis), the hospital will select a cost-allocation method that optimizes its payment from the government—namely the method that allocates a greater portion of the $100 to outpatient units.

Another type of cost shifting occurs when the government shifts its costs to employers, such as when requirements that otherwise cost the government money are imposed on employers. For example, when the government requires all employers to buy health insurance for their employees, the government's Medicaid expenditures for employees and their dependents who are otherwise eligible for Medicaid are reduced.

The Direction of Causality

Payment-to-cost ratios for all three payers—private, Medicare, and Medicaid—have fluctuated over time (see Exhibit 17.1). It appears that the payment-to-cost ratios between public (Medicare and Medicaid) and private payers are inversely related; when public ratios decline (low or negative profit margins), private ratios rise (high profit margins). However, the causality likely goes in the opposite direction—when private payment-to-cost ratios increase, public payment-to-cost ratios decrease.

Stensland, Gaumer, and Miller (2010) found that as hospitals gain market power, they have greater ability to increase their prices to private payers and hence increase their profits. Because nonprofit hospitals cannot distribute their profits to shareholders, the funds are used to expand services, invest in new technology, add staff, purchase physician practices, provide greater patient amenities, and so on. The expenditure of these "profits" increases hospital costs per discharge. The higher costs per discharge affects patients of all payer types—public as well as private. With higher hospital costs per discharge and fixed Medicare and Medicaid prices, the price-to-cost ratio of public payers declines; that is, the higher hospital costs and the same payment result in lower margins from public payers.

Stensland, Gaumer, and Miller found that more profitable hospitals had higher costs per discharge than did less profitable hospitals and that the former also had lower Medicare payment-to-cost ratios. The opposite was also found: Hospitals under financial stress had lower costs per discharge and higher Medicare margins.

Over time, hospitals' market power has changed, leading to different private and public payment-to-cost ratios. During the early 1980s, the payment-to-cost ratios for private payers, Medicare, and Medicaid were relatively close; the economywide recession was ending; and Medicare was beginning to shift from cost-based payment to fixed prices per admission. The late 1980s and early 1990s was a period of economic growth, and hospital private payment-to-cost ratios rose. Managed care had its greatest effect in the mid- to late 1990s, hospitals developed excess capacity, intense price competition occurred among hospitals to be included in managed care's provider networks, hospitals reduced their costs to remain competitive, and managed care plans negotiated large price discounts from hospitals. Private payment-to-cost ratios declined. In the past decade, hospital mergers have increased, hospital capacity has decreased, broadened managed care provider networks have resulted in less insurer bargaining power, and hospitals have developed greater market power. Hospital price markups have increased rapidly, returning to the situation that existed before the managed care period.

Changes in hospital payment-to-cost ratios for each payer regarding trends in hospitals' market power should be examined. Contrary to what many believe—that low Medicare and Medicaid payments lead to increases in hospital prices to private payers—the causality goes in a different direction: Hospitals' market power and their ability to raise prices to private payers result in a higher cost structure, which, with fixed public prices, leads to lower public payment-to-cost ratios.

Summary

The cost-shifting hypothesis has important policy implications regarding how the ACA has relied on reductions in Medicare hospital payment updates to finance its insurance coverage expansions. Will lower Medicare hospital payments cause private insurance premiums to increase faster than would otherwise occur?

Previously, when insurance premiums were paid almost entirely by the employer and managed care was not yet popular, hospitals were probably less interested in making as much money as possible. Many hospitals were reimbursed according to their costs, and they could achieve many of their goals without having to set profit-maximizing prices. However, as occupancy rates dropped and hospitals were left with excess capacity, price competition increased, HMOs and PPOs entered the market, and hospitals could no longer count on having their costs reimbursed—regardless of what those costs were. Hospital profitability declined. Those hospitals that did not price to make as much money as possible began to do so. Some cost shifting occurred during this transition period.

Today, differences in hospital prices for different payer groups are more likely the result of price discrimination rather than cost shifting. The difference between these two explanations is significant. Cost-shifting proponents believe that unless government payments to hospitals and physicians are increased, private payers (such as insurers and employers) will have to pay higher prices for healthcare. Economists, however, predict that with lower government-provider payments, medical prices to private payers will decrease, not increase. As the payment for one type of patient is reduced and becomes less profitable, physicians can earn more money by shifting some time away from less profitable patients. The supply of physician time in the private market will increase, resulting in lower prices to private payers.

Further, as hospitals gain market power through mergers, they will be able to price discriminate and raise their prices to private payers. Because nonprofit hospitals cannot distribute their profits, they use them to increase the hospital's cost structure by adding new facilities and services. These higher costs per discharge affect all payers. Thus, while hospitals are able to raise their payment-to-cost ratios to private payers, higher costs per discharge and fixed government payments result in lower public payment-to-cost ratios.

Discussion Questions

1. Explain why an increase in a hospital's fixed costs or an increase in the number of uninsured cared for by the hospital will not change the hospital's profit-maximizing price.
2. Why would a change in a hospital's variable costs change the hospital's profit-maximizing price?
3. Why are hospitals able to charge different purchasers different prices for the same medical services?
4. Under what circumstances can cost shifting occur?
5. How does cost shifting differ from price discrimination?

Notes

1. Exhibit 17.4 is another way to illustrate how a change in price affects TR. Price is shown along the vertical axis, and quantity (number of units sold each month or year) is shown along the horizontal axis. When the price is $9 per unit, three units are sold. When price is reduced to $8, four units are sold. Cutting the price from $9 to $8 results in a decrease in TR of $1 for each of the three units that would have been sold at $9. This loss of $3 is shown by area A. However, lowering the price to $8 gains $8 for that additional unit sold, shown as area B. The difference between area A (loss of $3) and area B (gain of $8) is $5, which is the increase in TR from selling one additional unit. Increasing the price from $8 to $9 has the opposite effect—a loss of $5 in TR.
2. The effect of price sensitivity (economists use the term *price elasticity*) on hospital prices and markups (percentage increase in price over cost) is based on the following formula:

$$\text{Price} = \frac{MC}{\left[1 - \dfrac{1}{\text{price elasticity}}\right]}$$

MC is the marginal cost of producing an additional unit and is assumed to be equal to the average variable cost. For simplicity, assume MC = $1,000. Thus, if a hospital believes the price sensitivity of a particular employee group is such that a 1 percent increase (decrease) in the hospital's price leads to a 2 percent decrease (increase) in admissions, the hospital's markup—applied to its average variable costs—is 100 percent:

$$\frac{\$1,000}{\left[1 - \dfrac{1}{2}\right]} = \frac{\$1,000}{\dfrac{1}{2}} = \$1,000 \times \frac{2}{1} = \$2,000.$$

If use of services were more price sensitive, such that a 1 percent price increase (decrease) leads to a 3 percent decrease (increase) in admissions, the markup is 50 percent:

$$\frac{\$1,000}{\left[1 - \dfrac{1}{3}\right]} = \frac{\$1,000}{\dfrac{2}{3}} = \$1,000 \times \frac{3}{2} = \$1,000 \times 1.5 = \$1,500.$$

If the hospital's variable costs of serving the patients were the same in both examples, the prices charged to each employee group could vary greatly depending on their price sensitivity. Even those hospitals that have few good substitutes and a less price-elastic demand for their services will always price in the elastic portion of their demand curve. For an explanation see Browning and Zupan (2011, 356).

3. A study by Dranove, Garthwaite, and Ody (2013) analyzed whether nonprofit hospitals increased their prices (cost shifted) as a result of large endowment losses caused by the 2008 recession. The authors reasoned that the losses of endowment revenue would be no different than decreased Medicare or Medicaid revenue. They found that the average hospital did not cost shift; only 10 percent of the hospitals studied that likely had some market power raised their prices compared to what would have occurred in the absence of their financial losses.

Additional Reading

Morrisey, M. 2003. "Cost Shifting: New Myths, Old Confusions, and Enduring Reality." *Health Affairs* (web exclusive): W3-489–W3-491.

References

American Hospital Association (AHA). 2014. "Chapter 4: Trends in Hospital Financing." In *Trendwatch Chartbook: Trends Affecting Hospitals and Health Systems*. Chicago: AHA. www.aha.org/research/reports/tw/chartbook/ch4.shtml.

Browning, E., and M. Zupan. 2011. *Microeconomics: Theory and Applications*, 11th ed. New York: John Wiley & Sons.

Dranove, D., C. Garthwaite, and C. Ody. 2013. "How Do Hospitals Respond to Negative Financial Shocks? The Impact of the 2008 Stock Market Crash." *NBER Working Paper* No. 18853, February. Cambridge, MA: National Bureau of Economic Research. www.nber.org/papers/w18853.pdf?new_window=1.

Dranove, D., and W. White. 1998. "Medicaid-Dependent Hospitals and Their Patients: How Have They Fared?" *Health Services Research* 33 (2, Part I): 163–85.

Stensland, J., Z. Gaumer, and M. Miller, 2010. "Private-Payer Profits Can Induce Negative Medicare Margins." *Health Affairs* web exclusive 29 (5): 1–7.

White, C. 2013. "Contrary to Cost-Shift Theory, Lower Medicare Hospital Payment Rates for Inpatient Care Lead to Lower Private Payment Rates." *Health Affairs* 32 (5): 935–43. http://content.healthaffairs.org/content/32/5/935.full.

CAN PRICE CONTROLS LIMIT MEDICAL EXPENDITURE INCREASES?

I n the continuing debate over how to limit rising medical expenditures, proponents of regulation—such as those who favor a single-payer system—propose placing controls on the prices physicians and hospitals charge. To prevent hospitals and physicians from circumventing such controls by simply performing more services, they would also impose an overall limit (also known as *global budget*) on total medical expenditures.

Price controls and global budgets may seem obvious approaches for limiting rising medical expenditures, but the potential consequences should be examined before placing almost one-fifth (17 percent) of the US economy (more than $2.7 trillion a year, as of 2012) under government control. The healthcare industry in the United States is larger than the economies of most countries. An announcement in any country that price controls would be imposed on the entire economy would seem incredible to all who have observed the past communist economies of Eastern Europe and Russia. Widespread shortages occurred, many of the goods produced were of shoddy quality, and black markets developed. These countries have recognized the inherent failures of a controlled economy, and they have moved toward developing free markets.

Why should we think healthcare is so different that access to care, high quality, and innovation can be better achieved by price controls and regulation than by reliance on competitive markets? What consequences are likely if price controls are imposed on medical services?[1]

Effect of Price Controls in Theory

Imbalances Between Supply and Demand

Imbalances between demands for care and supply of services will occur. The demand for medical services and the cost of providing those services are constantly changing. Prices bring about an equilibrium between the demanders and suppliers in a market. Prices reflect changes in demand or in the costs of producing a service. When demand grows (perhaps because of an aging population or rising income), prices increase. Higher prices cause consumers to curtail some of their demand, but suppliers respond by offering more services. Higher prices serve as a signal (and an incentive) to suppliers that greater investment in personnel and equipment is needed to meet the increased demand (Baumol 1988).

When regulators initially place controls on prices, they are assuming that the conditions that brought about the initial price—namely the demands for service and the costs of producing that service—will not change. However, these conditions do change for many reasons, so the controlled price is no longer an equilibrium price. The problem with price controls is that demand is constantly changing, as is the cost of providing services. Although regulators often allow some increases in prices each year to adjust for inflation, seldom if ever are these price increases sufficient to reflect the changes in demand or costs that are occurring. When prices are not flexible, an imbalance between demand and supply occurs.

Not only do the demand and costs of producing services change, but the product itself—medical care—is also continually changing, which complicates the picture for regulators. For example, the population is aging, and older individuals consume more medical care. Diseases such as AIDS require extensive testing, treatment, and prolonged care. Technology continues to improve. Since the mid-1990s, transplants have become commonplace. Diagnostic equipment has reduced the need for many exploratory surgeries. Very low-birth-weight infants can now survive. Such ongoing advances raise the demand for medical services and require a greater use of skilled labor, expensive monitoring equipment, and new imaging machines. Unless regulators are aware of these changes in the medical product and technology, their controlled prices will be below the costs of providing these services. How will the demand be met? Imbalances will undoubtedly occur because regulators cannot anticipate all the changes in demand, costs, and technology.

Excess Supply

At times, regulators may set prices too high, which occurs when healthcare providers are able to increase their productivity. Surgeons took longer to perform certain procedures, such as heart surgery or transplants, when the procedures were first developed. As surgeons became more experienced in performing these surgeries, their time per procedure decreased and their surgical patients' outcomes improved. Yet for many years, the Medicare price per procedure did not drop as the surgeon's productivity rose. In a competitive market, productivity gains are quickly translated into lower consumer prices.

Medicare, which regulates physician fees, relies on a single committee of the American Medical Association (AMA) to determine the time required for a physician (and different specialties) to perform various procedures, such as colonoscopies. These time requirements become part of the relative values used by Medicare to determine the fee for performing a particular medical service. However, a study has determined that the AMA's estimates of the time involved in many procedures are greatly overstated (Whoriskey and Keating 2013). Some of the physicians in the study performed procedures that, according to the AMA's and Medicare's time estimates, have them working 24, 30, and even 50 hours a day.

Productivity increases lead to decreases in the cost of a service. However, when fees are controlled, it is difficult for the price controller to know when and by how much productivity has increased. As the cost of performing a service declines and the price received for that service remains unchanged (or does not match the decline in costs), the profit per unit of surgeon's time grows; the surgeon responds to that incentive by performing more profitable procedures. The same physician incentive exists for other medical services where the price exceeds costs, such as with diagnostic and imaging services.

The failure of price controllers to accurately change prices in response to changes in physician productivity results in more of these procedures being performed; in some patients receiving too many of such procedures, such as colonoscopies; in higher medical costs; in patients and/or private and public insurers paying too much; and in demand being distorted for different physician specialties because these specialists' income is greater. (Medical students have a financial incentive to enter procedure-oriented specialties that become more profitable as a result of increased productivity and "sticky" prices.)

Service Shortages

Shortages are the inevitable consequence of price controls. Demand for medical services is continually growing, yet price controls limit the expansion of supply. To expand its services, a hospital or a medical group must be able to attract additional employees—by raising wages that will lure skilled and trained employees away from their current employers. As wages increase, trained nurses who are not currently employed as nurses will find returning to their profession financially attractive, and more people will choose a nursing career as its salary becomes comparable to that in other professions. However, if hospitals cannot enlarge wages because they cannot raise prices, they will not be able to hire the nurses needed to expand their services.

In addition, price controls actually cause a reduction in services, which exacerbates the shortage over time. As prices and wages grow throughout the economy, price controls in the health sector make paying competitive wages and high supply costs difficult for hospitals and medical groups. Hospitals must hire nurses and technicians, buy supplies, pay heating and electric bills, and replace or repair equipment. A hospital that cannot pay competitive wages will be unable to attract and retain employees. If the salary of hospital accountants is not similar to that of accountants working in nonhospital settings, fewer accountants will choose to work in hospitals (or those who accept lower wages may not be as qualified as those who do not). As medical costs increase faster than the permitted price growth, hospitals and medical groups will be unable to retain their existing labor forces and to provide their current services. When costs per patient rise faster than government-controlled prices, hospitals, outpatient facilities, and physician practices are faced with two choices: (1) care for fewer but more costly patients or (2) care for the same number of patients but devote fewer resources to each patient.

Eliminating all the waste in the current system would only lead to a one-time savings. If rising expenditures were caused not by waste but by new technologies, aging of the population, and new diseases, medical costs will still rise faster than the rate at which hospitals and other providers would be reimbursed under price controls. Providers will then be faced with the same two choices: (1) care for fewer patients or (2) devote fewer resources to each patient and thus deliver low-quality service.

Price controls on medical services cause the demand for medical services to exceed the supply. The out-of-pocket price the patient pays for a physician visit, an MRI (magnetic resonance imaging), an ultrasound, or laboratory tests will rise more slowly than if the price were not controlled. (The "real," or inflation-adjusted, price to the patient is likely to fall.) Consequently, although patient demand for such services is high, suppliers cannot expand their services if the cost of doing so exceeds the fixed price. In fact, over time, the shortage will become even larger because the fixed price will cover fewer services. We have seen this occur when rent controls are imposed on housing, such as in New York City. The demand for rent-controlled housing continually exceeds its supply, and the supply of existing housing decreases as the costs of upkeep exceed the allowable increases in rent and cause landlords to abandon entire city areas.

Shift of Capital Away from Price-Controlled Services

As profitability is reduced on services subject to price control, capital investment will eventually shift to areas that are not subject to control and in which investors can earn higher returns. Less private capital will be available to develop new delivery systems, invest in computer technology for patient care management, and conduct research and development on breakthrough drugs. Price controls on hospitals cause hospital investment to decline and capital to move into unregulated outpatient services and home health care. Should all health services become subject to controls, capital will move to nonhealth industries and to geographic regions without controls.

Effect of Price Controls in Practice

Medicaid

Price controls have been tried extensively in the United States and other countries. Shortages and decreased access to care, which typify the Medicaid program, are caused by price controls. Once a patient is eligible for Medicaid, the price he has to pay for medical services is greatly reduced, increasing his demand for such services. Government Medicaid payments to physicians are fixed, however, and below what physicians could earn by serving non-Medicaid patients. Low provider payments have decreased the profitability of serving Medicaid patients and resulted in a shortage of Medicaid services. In 2011, 31 percent of physicians were unwilling to accept Medicaid patients (Decker 2012). As the difference in prices for Medicaid and private patients grows, more of the physician's time shifts toward caring for private patients, thereby exacerbating the shortage of medical services faced by Medicaid patients.

Medicare

Hospitals are also subject to price controls on the payments they receive from Medicare. When fixed prices per diagnostic admission were introduced in 1984, hospitals began to "upcode" their Medicare patients' diagnoses to maximize their reimbursements. Medicare hospital payments rose sharply, and 75 percent of the increase was attributed to "code creep" (Sheingold 1989). Eventually, the government reduced Medicare payments so much that more than two-thirds of all hospitals lost money on their Medicare patients. After a few years of losses, payments were raised. The failure of Medicare DRG (diagnosis-related group) payments to accurately measure patient severity of illness has led some hospitals to "dump" on other hospitals those Medicare patients whose costs exceed their payments. Congress has enacted legislation to penalize hospitals that engage in dumping.

In the early 1970s, Medicare limited how rapidly physician fees could rise under Medicare. As the gap between Medicare fees and private fees widened, physicians stopped participating in Medicare and billed their patients directly. To prevent this, Congress changed the rules in the 1990s. Physicians are no longer able to participate for some but not all of their Medicare patients by billing them the balance between what Medicare paid and the physician's normal fee; instead, physicians must participate for all or none of their Medicare patients.

When price controls and fee reductions were imposed on Medicare physician fees in 1992, physicians whose fees were reduced the most showed the largest increases in service volume (Nguyen 1996). For example, radiologists' fees dropped by 12 percent, while their volume rose by 13 percent. Similarly, urologists' fees dropped by 5 percent, while their volume rose by 12 percent. These specialists were apparently able to create demand among their Medicare fee-for-service patients.

Medicare currently uses the sustainable growth rate (SGR) to limit Medicare physician payment increases. The SGR includes, as one of its major components, the growth in gross domestic product (GDP) and is based on the assumption that total Medicare physician expenditures should not rise faster than GDP. The growth in GDP, however, does not accurately reflect changes in the supply of and demand for Medicare physician services. Consequently, Medicare fees for primary care physicians have lagged behind those in the private sector, and each year fewer and fewer primary care physicians are willing to accept new Medicare patients.

When Medicare limited the rise in premiums for Medicare health maintenance organizations (HMOs), a number of HMOs dropped out of the Medicare HMO market. Medicare Advantage plans were subsequently given significant premium incentives in 2003 to reenter the Medicare market (their Medicare payments were about 14 percent higher than the cost of comparable risk-adjusted patients in traditional Medicare). The Affordable Care Act (ACA) removed these higher payments, with the likely consequence that such plans—which enroll about 25 percent of all Medicare beneficiaries—will either again exit the Medicare market or charge their Medicare enrollees' higher premiums and copayments.

The ACA established the Independent Payment Advisory Board (IPAB) to achieve savings in Medicare when Medicare expenditures exceed the rate of growth in per capita GDP plus one percent. The IPAB—by law and for political reasons—is prohibited from submitting proposals that would raise beneficiaries' out-of-pocket costs or premiums, change Medicare benefits, or change Medicare eligibility. Because of the law's constraints on how the IPAB can limit Medicare costs, reducing provider payments is the most likely approach to be used by the government. The IPAB will decrease access to care in two ways. First, by lowering the prices Medicare will pay for certain procedures and drugs, it will become unprofitable for physicians to perform procedures the IPAB believes to be too costly, although such procedures may provide valuable benefits to Medicare beneficiaries. Second, by reducing overall provider payments to achieve their cost-containment goal, Medicare fees will fall greatly below Medicaid fees (which have already caused access problems for Medicaid enrollees) and the fees paid by private health insurers.

The ACA also imposes price reductions on hospitals on the basis of assumed (debatable) productivity increases. Medicare's chief actuary reported that, by 2019, these payment reductions will result in operating losses for 15 percent of hospitals, skilled nursing facilities, and home health agencies. By 2030, 25 percent of those providers will sustain losses, and by 2050, that number will rise to 40 percent (Foster 2011). As these price controls force many hospitals and other providers into bankruptcy, access to care and quality will be greatly diminished.

Rationing

Under price controls, as demand for medical services exceeds supplies, what criteria will be used to ration the supplies that are available? Undoubtedly, emergency cases would take precedence over elective services, but how would elective services be rationed? In some countries where age is a criterion, those above a certain age do not have access to hip replacement, kidney dialysis, heart surgery, and other services. Both quality of life and life expectancy are reduced.

Waiting Lists

Typically, waiting lists are used to ration elective procedures. In countries that rely on this approach, such as Canada and Great Britain, waiting times for surgical procedures—whether for cataracts or open-heart surgery—vary from six months to two years.[2] Delays are costly in terms of reduced quality of life and life expectancy. When resources are limited, acute care has a higher priority than preventive services. Women over age 50 years have a lower use rate of mammograms in Canada, where price controls and global budgets are used, than in the United States (Kadiyala and Strumpf 2011, Figure 1).

Those who can afford to wait—that is, those with lower time costs, such as the retired—are more likely to receive physician services than those with higher time costs. Access to nonemergency physician services will be determined by the value patients place on their time. Waiting is costly in that it uses productive resources (or enjoyable time). A large, but less visible, cost is associated with waiting. Suppose the out-of-pocket price of a physician's office visit is limited to $10, but the patient must take three hours off work to wait and see the physician. If the patient earns $20 an hour, the effective cost of that visit is $70. The "lower" costs of a price-controlled system never explicitly recognize the lost productivity to society or the value of that time to the patient. Patients with high time costs are willing to pay not to wait, but they do not have that option. They cannot buy medical services that are worth more than they are willing to pay.

The effects of price controls are often a great burden on those with low income and those who do not know how to "work the system." Specialists frequently see those with "connections" more quickly, and those with high income can travel elsewhere to receive care.[3] For example, in 2010, the premier of Newfoundland went to the United States for heart surgery at his own expense (Wallace 2010).

Deterioration of Quality

As the costs of providing medical services increase faster than the controlled price, providers may reduce the resources used in treatment, resulting in a deterioration of quality. A physician may prefer a highly sophisticated diagnostic test such as an MRI, but to conserve resources she may order an X-ray instead. The value to the patient of a diagnostic test may exceed its cost, but an overall limit on costs will preclude performing many cost-beneficial tests or procedures. Experience with Medicaid confirms these concerns with quality of care. Large numbers of patients are seen for very short visits in Medicaid "mills." Such short visits are more likely to lead to incorrect diagnosis and treatment. Similarly, in Japan, where physicians' fees are controlled, physicians see many more patients per day than do US physicians and spend 30 percent less time with each patient.[4]

When controlled prices do not reflect quality differences among hospitals or physicians, suppliers have less incentive to provide higher-quality services. If all physicians are paid the same fee, the incentive to invest the time to become board certified is reduced. In a price-controlled environment with excess demand, even low-quality providers can survive and prosper. Similarly, drug and equipment manufacturers have no incentive to invest in higher-quality products if such products could not be priced to reflect their higher value.

Gaming the System

Price controls provide incentives for providers to try to "game" the system to increase their revenues. For example, physicians paid on a fee-for-service basis are likely to decrease the time they devote to each visit, which enables them to see more patients and thus bill for more visits. Less physician time per patient represents a more hurried visit and presumably lower-quality care. Physicians are also likely to "unbundle" their services—tht is, by dividing a treatment or visit into its separate parts, they can charge for each part separately. For example, separate visits may be scheduled for diagnostic tests, for obtaining the results of those tests, and for receiving medications. Price controls also provide physicians and hospitals with an incentive to upcode the type of services they provide—that is, to bill a brief office visit as a comprehensive exam.

Gaming the system results in higher regulatory costs because a larger bureaucracy is needed to administer and monitor compliance with price controls. C. Jackson Grayson (1993), who was in charge of price controls imposed in the United States in 1971, stated, "We started Phase II [from 1971 to 1973] with 3½ pages of regulations and ended with 1,534."

Gaming is also costly to patients. Multiple visits to the physician, which enable the physician to bill for each visit separately, increase patient travel and waiting times, an inefficient use of the patient's resources that may discourage patients from using needed services.

Global Budgets

To ensure that gaming does not increase total expenditures, an expenditure limit (global budget) is often superimposed on price controls. Included in a global budget are all medical expenditures for hospital and physician services, outpatient and inpatient care, health insurance and HMO premiums, and consumer out-of-pocket payments. Unless the global budget is comprehensive, expenditures and investments will shift to unregulated sectors. Additional controls will then be imposed to prevent expenditure growth in these areas, and monitoring compliance with the controls becomes even more costly.

What happens under global budgets when demand for certain providers or managed care organizations increases? The more efficient health plans cannot raise payments to attract a greater number of physicians and facilities to meet increased enrollment demands. Thus, the public is precluded from choosing the more efficient, more responsive health plans that are subject to overall budget limits. Limiting a physician's total revenue discourages the use of physician assistants and nurse practitioners who could boost the physician's productivity because the physician would prefer to receive the limited revenue rather than share it. Once a physician has reached the overall revenue limit, what incentive does he have to continue serving patients? Why not work fewer hours and take longer vacations?

What incentives do hospitals or physicians have to develop innovative, less costly delivery systems—such as managed care, outpatient diagnostics and surgery, or home infusion programs—if the funds must be taken from existing programs and providers? Efficient providers are penalized if they cannot increase expenditures to expand, and patients lose the opportunity to be served by more efficient providers.

To remain within their overall budgets, hospitals will undertake actions that decrease efficiency and access to care. Hospitals adjust to stringent budget limits by keeping patients longer, as this requires fewer resources than does performing procedures on more patients. Strict budget limits will result in greater delays in admitting patients, and patients will have less access to beneficial but costly technology. Hospitals in the Netherlands, under the country's previous global budget payment system (now changed to a more price-competitive system), typically reached the end of their budget in late fall and consequently sharply reduced accepting new admissions, causing long waiting times.

Global budgets are based on the assumption that the government knows exactly the right amount of medical expenditures for the nation.[5] However, a correct percentage of GDP that should be spent on medical care has never been determined, and the fact that other countries spend less than the United States spends does not tell us which country we should emulate or what services we should forgo. Medical expenditures rise for many reasons. No accurate information exists as to how much of that growth is attributable to waste, new diseases, an aging population, and new technology. The quality of healthcare will deteriorate, and long waiting times for treatment will result if price controls and global budgets are set too low. In 1997, Medicare's payment system to physicians was based on the premise that total Medicare physician expenditures should be tied to growth in the economy (adjusted for the number of Medicare beneficiaries)—termed the *sustainable growth rate* (SGR). Even Congress admits that the SGR payment system is badly flawed and has consistently refused to implement the formula's payment reductions.

Whether politicians would permit a strict global budget to continue in the face of shortages and complaints about access to medical services is doubtful. More likely, politicians would respond to their constituents' complaints and relax the budget limit. In fact, this has occurred in other countries, such as Canada, when access to medical services became too limited because of price controls and global budgets. Great Britain, for example, permits "buyouts." A private medical market is allowed to develop, and those with high income who can afford to buy private medical insurance jump the queue to receive medical services from private providers. To the extent that buyouts are permitted, medical expenditures will increase more rapidly and a two-tier system will evolve. If a buyout is envisaged, the rationale for price controls and global budgets is questionable.

Summary

Price controls and global budgets provide the appearance of limiting rising prices and expenditures. In reality, however, they lead to cheating and a reduction in quality, impose large costs on patients and providers, and do little to improve efficiency.

Consumers and producers respond to prices. When government sets prices below costs, hospital and physician economic incentives are to reduce the supply of their services. Regulators should not assume that producers will go against their economic incentives.

If the purpose of regulation is to improve efficiency, eliminate inappropriate services, and decrease the costly duplication of medical technology, government policies should provide incentives to achieve these goals. Such incentives are more likely to occur in a system in which purchasers make cost-conscious choices and providers must compete for those purchasers. Competitive systems provide both purchasers and providers with incentives to weigh the benefits and costs of new medical technology. When patients are willing to pay not to wait and to have access to new technology, medical expenditures will increase faster, but the rate of increase will be more appropriate.

Discussion Questions

1. Why do price controls cause shortages, and why do these shortages increase over time?
2. Why do price controls require hospitals to make a trade-off between quality of medical services and number of patients served?
3. What are the various ways in which a provider can "game" the system under price controls?
4. What costs do price controls impose on patients?
5. What are the advantages and disadvantages of permitting patients to buy out of the price-controlled medical system?
6. How might the IPAB reduce patient access to care?

Notes

1. For a more complete discussion of this subject, see Pope (2013).
2. The Fraser Institute (www.fraserinstitute.ca) collects data annually on waiting times in each of the Canadian provinces by procedure and on waiting time for a referral from a general practitioner to a specialist.
3. The "true" price a patient faces is not just the out-of-pocket price she may have to pay but also the cost of the time she spent waiting (or what she could be doing if she received the care without waiting). For example, a person needing cataract surgery may be unable to drive while waiting six months for such surgery. The cost to the person of being unable to drive may be worth a great deal. Thus, the out-of-

pocket price and the foregone benefits of waiting may be sufficiently high that the person prefers to pay for a substitute service whose out-of-pocket price is high but whose waiting cost is low. A Canadian waiting for cataract or cancer surgery may decide, as many have, that the higher out-of-pocket price of such care in another country (such as the United States) is less expensive.

4. In 1991, Japanese physicians saw an average of 49 patients a day, and 13 percent saw 100 patients a day (Ikegami 1991). The US average was 22 patients per day in 1996. Another study (Ohtaki, Ohtaki, and Fetters 2003) analyzed the amount of time spent by Japanese and US physicians and found that Japanese physicians spent 30 percent less time with each patient.

5. Another expenditure control mechanism is healthcare certificate-of-need (CON) laws, which control capital expenditures on health services and facilities. The rationale for CON laws was that government planning would result in an appropriate and efficient allocation of resources and reduce rising healthcare costs. Economic studies have been unable to find any evidence that CON regulations, which are currently imposed in 36 states, have reduced healthcare expenditures. Instead, such regulations have been found to be used politically by self-interested providers to prevent competitors from entering a market (Yee et al. 2011).

References

Baumol, W. 1988. "Containing Medical Costs: Why Price Controls Won't Work." *Public Interest* 93 (Fall): 37–53.

Decker, S. 2012. "In 2011 Nearly One-Third of Physicians Said They Would Not Accept New Medicaid Patients, But Rising Fees May Help." *Health Affairs* 31 (8): 1673–79.

Foster, R. S. 2011. "The Estimated Effect of the Affordable Care Act on Medicare and Medicaid Outlays and Total National Health Care Expenditures." Testimony before the House Committee on the Budget, January 26. http://budget.house.gov/uploadedfiles/fostertestimony1262011.pdf.

Grayson, C. J. 1993. "Experience Talks: Shun Price Controls." *Wall Street Journal*, March 29, p. A14.

Ikegami, N. 1991. "Japanese Health Care—Low Cost Through Regulated Fees." *Health Affairs* 10 (3): 87–109.

Kadiyala, S., and E. C. Strumpf. 2011. "Are United States and Canadian Cancer Screening Rates Consistent with Guideline Information Regarding the Age of Screening Initiation?" *International Journal for Quality in Health Care* (July 4). http://intqhc.oxfordjournals.org/content/23/6/611/ F1.expansion.html.

Nguyen, X. N. 1996. "Physician Volume Response to Price Controls." *Health Policy* 35 (2): 189–204.

Ohtaki, S., T. Ohtaki, and M. Fetters. 2003. "Doctor–Patient Communication: A Comparison of USA and Japan." *Family Practice* 20 (3): 276–82.

Pope, C. 2013. "Legislating Low Prices: Cutting Costs or Care?" Backgrounder #2834. The Heritage Foundation, August 9. www.heritage.org/research/ reports/2013/08/legislating-low-prices-cutting-costs-or-care.

Sheingold, S. 1989. "The First Three Years of PPS: Impact on Medicare Costs." *Health Affairs* 8 (3): 191–204.

Wallace, K. 2010. "N.L. Premier Williams Set to Have Heart Surgery in U.S." *National Post*, February 2. www.nationalpost.com/news/story .html?id=2510700).

Whoriskey, P., and D. Keating. 2013. "How a Secretive Panel Uses Data That Distort Doctors' Pay." *Washington Post*, July 20. www.washingtonpost.com/ business/economy/how-a-secretive-panel-uses-data-that-distorts-doctors- pay/2013/07/20/ee134e3a-eda8-11e2-9008-61e94a7ea20d_story_4.html.

Yee, T., L. Stark, A. Bond, and E. Carrier. 2011. "Health Care Certificate-of-Need Laws: Policy or Politics." *Research Brief* No. 4. Washington, DC: The National Institute for Health Care Reform.

THE EVOLUTION OF MANAGED CARE

An important policy debate concerns the organization and delivery of medical services—should this country rely on regulation or on market competition to achieve efficiency in the provision of medical services? Market competition can take different forms; one was the emergence and rapid growth of managed care organizations (MCOs) during the 1980s and 1990s. What effect has managed care competition had? Has managed care improved efficiency and reduced the rate of increase in medical expenditures? What happened to patient satisfaction and quality of care? To discuss these issues, we must examine why managed care came about, what managed care means, what types of managed care plans are available, how well managed care has performed and how it has evolved, what recent developments (such as consumer-driven healthcare) it has undergone, and how the Affordable Care Act (ACA) has affected it.

Why Managed Care Came About

Managed care was a market response to the wasteful excesses of the past, which resulted in rapidly rising medical costs in a system widely believed to be inefficient. Traditional indemnity health insurance—with its comprehensive coverage of hospitals and small patient copayments for medical services—lessened patient concerns with hospital and medical expenses. Physicians were paid on a fee-for-service basis and were not fiscally responsible for hospital use, which they prescribed. New medical technology was introduced immediately because the insurer paid for its use and cost; insurers merely passed the higher cost on to employers.

The lack of incentive for insurers, patients, physicians, and hospitals to be concerned about cost led to the sudden rise in cost. Insured patients demanded "too many" services, physicians paid fee-for-service delivered more services, and hospitals competed for physicians by making available the latest technology so that physicians did not have to refer their patients to other hospitals and physicians. Advances in medical technology and the lack of cost incentives led to nonprice competition among hospitals; technology was adopted no matter how small its medical benefits or how infrequently it was used. This led not only to higher costs but also to lower quality, as studies demonstrated that hospitals that performed fewer complex procedures had worse outcomes than hospitals that performed more such procedures (Hughes, Hunt, and Luft 1987).

Large employers sought to slow the increases in health insurance premiums, but physicians, hospitals, and traditional health insurers were not responsive to their cost concerns. Instead, entrepreneurs recognized the potential for reducing medical system inefficiencies and started health maintenance organizations (HMOs), utilization review firms, and preferred provider organizations (PPOs). These innovators, who aggressively marketed their approaches to large employers, were richly rewarded for their efforts.

What Is Managed Care?

Managed care embodies a variety of techniques and types of organizations. Financial incentives, negotiation of large provider discounts, limited provider networks, physician gatekeepers, utilization management, disease management, and drug formularies are some of these techniques.

Managed care health plans were successful in interfering with the traditional physician–patient relationship because employees were willing to switch from traditional insurers in return for lower premiums. Managed care plans contracted with those physicians and hospitals willing to discount their prices, which was a precondition for joining the plan's limited provider network. Because physicians and hospitals had excess capacity in the 1980s and 1990s, they were willing to discount their prices in return for higher patient volume (Wu 2009). The patient's choice of physician was restricted to those in the plan's provider panel, as were the specialists to whom the patient could be referred and the hospitals in which the patient could stay. Decisions about whether to hospitalize a patient, length of stay, specialist referrals, and types of drugs prescribed—formerly made by the physician—were now influenced by the managed care plan.

Managed care techniques have changed over time. First-generation approaches were quite restrictive, relying on selective contracting (which limited the provider panel to those who were willing to discount their prices and who were appropriate users of medical services), a gatekeeper model, and stringent utilization review. In the gatekeeper model, an enrollee in a managed care plan chose a primary care physician from among a panel of physicians to manage that patient's care and control diagnostic and specialist referrals. The primary care physician often did some tasks previously performed by specialists. Utilization review included prior authorization for hospital admission, concurrent review (i.e., length of stay was reviewed to make sure the stay did not exceed what was medically necessary), and retrospective review (i.e., care was reviewed to ensure that appropriate services were provided). The initial sources of managed care savings were less inpatient use (the most expensive component of care) and deep provider price discounts. The HMOs were able to shift large numbers of their enrollees to those physicians who competed to be included in the HMO's provider panel and were able to achieve cost savings relatively easily and without changing the practice of medicine.

To achieve further reductions in medical costs, managed care had to become more innovative and effective in managing patient care. Second-generation managed care approaches rely on changing physicians' practice patterns, such as identifying high-risk enrollees early, decreasing the variation in physicians' utilization patterns, minimizing inappropriate use of services, and substituting less costly in-home services for continued care in the hospital. In addition, second-generation approaches rely on evidence-based medicine to achieve savings. Access to large data sets on physicians' treatment patterns from around the country and information technology to analyze those data allow health plans to determine which treatment decisions have better outcomes. Integrated and coordinated care and disease management can decrease medical costs and improve patient outcomes.

Some managed care plans (particularly in California) have shifted more of the capitation payment—hence risk—to physicians and hospitals; providers are, thereby, given an incentive to innovate in delivering medical services. Furthermore, with risk shifting from employers to HMOs, large employers place greater emphasis on report cards. Because, under capitation, managed care plans and their providers have a financial incentive to perform fewer services, both the plans and their providers have to be continually monitored for patient satisfaction and medical outcomes. Health plans and their providers are being held accountable for the health status of their enrolled populations.

What Are the Types of Managed Care Plans?

Managed care health plans vary in the degree to which they use a select network of providers and limit access to specialists. Typically, the more restrictive the managed care plan, the lower its premium. The most restrictive type of managed care plan is an HMO, which offers the most comprehensive health benefits. An HMO relies on a restricted provider network, and the patient is responsible for the full costs of going to non-network providers. Cost control by an HMO is achieved through stringent utilization management, financial incentives to physicians, and limited access to providers.

Managed fee-for-service indemnity insurance plans include a PPO, which is a closed provider panel. Providers are paid fee-for-service, and enrollees have a financial incentive (low copayment) to use the PPO providers versus going out of network. Costs are controlled through utilization management, patient copayments, and discounted fees from PPO providers.

Specialist referrals also vary. In an HMO, the primary care physician must recommend specialist referrals. In a PPO, the patient may self-refer to a specialist, but the copayment is lower if the specialist is in the PPO.

Traditional HMOs began to offer a point-of-service option in the early 1990s to counter the growing popularity of PPOs. A point-of-service plan is an HMO that permits its enrollees to use nonparticipating providers if the enrollees are willing to pay a high copayment (e.g., 40 percent) each time they use such providers.

Exhibit 19.1 shows, for the working population, the market share of each type of managed care plan and how that share has changed over time. In the early 1980s, managed care was just beginning to grow. Traditional indemnity insurance (or conventional health insurance), with free access to all providers (called *unmanaged care*), was the dominant form (95 percent) of health insurance. Since that time, the distribution of different types of health plans has changed rapidly. By 2013, traditional insurance had virtually disappeared, and various types of managed care had become the predominant form of insurance.

The premium in a typical managed care plan is allocated as shown in Exhibit 19.2. In this example, the ABC Managed Care Health Plan retains 15 percent of the premium to cover expenses associated with marketing, administration, and profit. About 35 percent of the premium is allocated for hospital and other medical facility expenses, 40 percent is set aside for physician services, and 10 percent is allocated for pharmacy and ancillary services. Use of services by enrollees outside the plan's area and certain catastrophic expenses may also be included in the health plan's retained 15 percent.

Providers within each of these budgetary allocations may be paid in several ways. Some managed care plans (e.g., Kaiser Health Plan) place their physicians on a salary, others pay discounted fee-for-service, and still others capitate their physicians. (Capitation means to pay an annual amount to the physician group for each enrollee for whom they are responsible. Capitated medical groups are primarily found in California.) Within each of these payment arrangements, the organization at financial risk withholds a certain percentage of the budget allocated to the providers to ensure that sufficient funds are available to provide all the necessary services. Funds remaining at the end of the year are divided among the members of that provider group. When medical groups and hospitals are capitated, a shared risk pool exists between them. Part of the hospital's capitated payment is set aside to be shared between the hospital and medical group to give the latter an incentive to minimize use of the hospital.

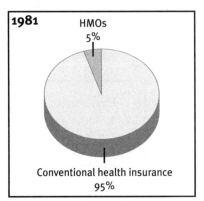

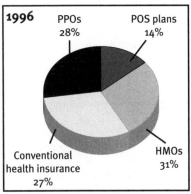

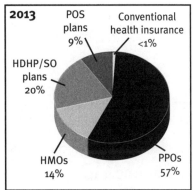

EXHIBIT 19.1
The Trend
Toward
Managed Care

NOTES:
HMO: health maintenance organization, an organization that provides comprehensive healthcare services to a voluntarily enrolled membership for a prepaid fee. HMOs control costs through stringent utilization management, payment incentives to its physicians, and restricted access to its providers.
PPO: preferred provider organization in which a third-party payer contracts with a group of medical providers that agrees to furnish services at negotiated fees in return for prompt payment and increased patient volume. PPOs control costs by keeping fees down and curbing excessive service through utilization management.
POS: point of service, an HMO that permits its enrollees access to nonparticipating providers if the enrollees are willing to pay a high copayment each time they use such providers.
Conventional health insurance: a plan that permits patients to go to any provider, and the provider is paid fee-for-service. The patient normally pays a small annual deductible plus 20 percent of the provider's charge, up to an annual out-of-pocket limit of $3,000.
HDHP/SO: high-deductible health plan with savings option, a consumer-driven health plan that works like a PPO plan with an in-network and out-of-network benefits for covered services. Patients can see a specialist without a referral. Selection of a primary care physician is not required. HDHP plan has higher annual deductibles and out-of-pocket maximums but lower premiums. Patients with HDHP plans are able to set up a tax-deductible health savings account.
SOURCES: Data from Kaiser/HRET (2013); KPMG Peat Marwick (1982, 1991).

How Has Managed Care Performed?

Managed care did not spread equally to all parts of the country or to all population groups. It moved faster into those areas that had high healthcare

EXHIBIT 19.2
How an HMO
Allocates the
Premium Dollar

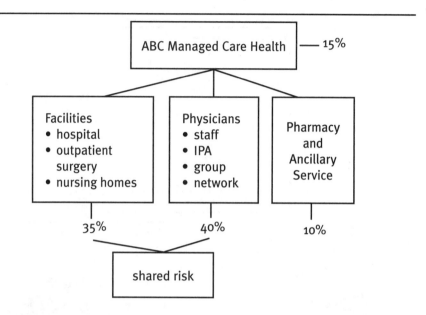

Staff model: An HMO that delivers health services through a physician group that is controlled by the HMO unit.

IPA: An HMO that contracts directly with physicians in independent practices.

Group: An HMO that contracts with one independent group practice to provide health services.

Network: An HMO that contracts with two or more independent group practices.

costs, where the potential for cost reductions was greatest. Managed care plans were more likely to enter urban than rural areas. The West—particularly California—introduced managed care earlier and had a greater percentage of its population enrolled in managed care than did the East or Southeast. Those employed in large firms moved more rapidly into managed care than did those on Medicare and Medicaid, who had limited price incentives to enroll in managed care plans.

While almost all the privately insured are in some form of managed care, only 29 percent of the 52 million aged are in Medicare managed care plans (referred to as Medicare Advantage plans) as of 2013. However, 75 percent of the 57 million who are on Medicaid were in managed care (CMS 2013).

To determine the performance of managed care competition, population groups subject to managed care should be compared to comparable populations not in managed care. Thus, earlier studies compared enrollees in managed care plans with those in traditional fee-for-service plans in the private sector. Such comparisons of the privately insured are more difficult to conduct today. Instead current studies evaluate the performance of managed care plans by comparing enrollees in Medicare Advantage plans to those enrolled in traditional Medicare.

The Issue of Biased Selection

A concern with all studies on managed care is the issue of biased selection. Managed care plans initially attracted younger enrollees, persons new to an area, and fewer persons who were chronically ill—people who did not have long-standing physician relationships. If HMOs and managed care plans enrolled a healthier population group, a comparison of their performance relative to traditional health insurers would be biased. Better health outcomes and lower healthcare costs in an HMO are more related to the population enrolled than to the HMO's performance. Thus, crucial to any study determining whether managed care plans are better at controlling growth in costs and improving treatment outcomes is the ability to control for low-risk groups enrolled in managed care.

A large number and wide variety of studies have been conducted on the performance of HMOs, managed care plans, and traditional insurers serving the privately insured (Glied 2000). Following is a brief summary of the results of these earlier studies and also of those serving Medicare enrollees (which have controlled for biased selection).

Rise in Health Insurance Premiums

Managed care competition worked in the following manner. As managed care plans entered a market and enrolled a significant number of members, hospitals and physicians competed on price to be included in the plan's provider network. Given their excess capacity and need for more patients, providers were also willing to accept utilization review, which decreases hospital use. These cost savings—discounted prices and lower hospital use rates—enabled the managed care plan to cut its premium relative to those of non–managed care health plans. When employees are required to pay the additional cost of more expensive health plans, studies show that premium differences as small as $5 to $10 a month will cause 25 percent of a health plan's employees to switch (Buchmueller and Feldstein 1996). Employees are very price sensitive. Health plans, therefore, have to be very price competitive.

To prevent further losses in their market share, indemnity, non–managed care insurers adopted managed care techniques—such as utilization review and PPOs—to limit the rise in their premiums. Managed care plans not only reduced their own medical costs but, by their competitive effect, forced other insurers to adopt managed care techniques to reduce their costs and remain price competitive.

Managed care competition dramatically slowed the rise in health insurance premiums, particularly during the mid-1990s. Exhibit 19.3 shows the national trend in employer-paid health insurance premiums and the annual percentage change in the Consumer Price Index. Also included are premium data from California, where managed care competition started earlier and was more extensive than in the rest of the country. Clearly, as managed care market share increased (see Exhibit 19.1), insurance premiums rose more slowly. (In California, the managed care effect was even more pronounced; it occurred earlier and included a greater percentage of the population. During the mid-1990s, health insurance premiums in California actually declined.)

A major source of the early savings from managed care was decreased hospital use, which is shown in Exhibit 19.4. Hospital patient days per 1,000 population declined from 1,302 in 1977 to 591 by 2012. Also shown is the earlier and larger decline in hospital use rates in California, where rates declined from 996 to 445 per 1,000 population over that same period. New York, whose hospital use rate was higher than the national average, also saw a decline—although at 858 in 2012 it was still much higher than the national average and almost twice as high as the rate in California. Hospital admissions per 1,000 population have also fallen, although not as dramatically as patient days. Admission rates in 1978 were 162 nationally, 147 in New York, and 141 in California. By 2012, these rates had declined to 110, 125, and 87, respectively. As a consequence of managed care, hospitals' share of total medical expenditures fell. The decline in hospital use rates that occurred in California indicates the reductions in hospital use that are still possible in other parts of the country.

Onetime Versus Continual Cost Savings

Managed care achieved the easiest cost reductions, such as decreased hospital days, substitution of less costly settings for expensive inpatient stays, and lower provider prices. These reductions, however, are onetime cost savings, although they occur over a period of years and are instituted at different times in different parts of the country. An important policy question is whether managed care competition is only able to produce these onetime savings or whether it can achieve continual cost reductions.

The two most important factors that determine the rate at which medical expenditures will increase are (1) demographics—an older population has more costly care needs—and (2) the development and adoption of new medical technology. Whether managed care is able to achieve continual cost decreases will depend on whether it is able to innovate in managing the care of the aged and the chronically ill and whether it can lower the rate of new technology diffusion while encouraging the development of cost-reducing technology.

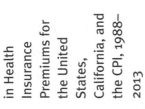

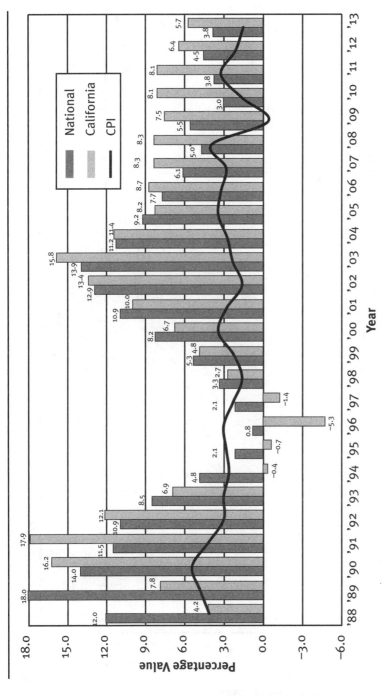

EXHIBIT 19.3
Annual
Percentage
Increase
in Health
Insurance
Premiums for
the United
States,
California, and
the CPI, 1988–
2013

* 2011 national percentage increase is estimated.

NOTE: In 2008, Kaiser/HRET changed its method for reporting the US annual percentage premium increase. Before 2008, percentage increase was calculated as the average of percentage changes in premium for a family of four in the largest plan of each plan type. Since 2008, percentage increase reflects the overall percentage increase in premium for family coverage using the average of the premium dollar amounts for a family of four in the largest plan of each plan type and weighted by covered workers.

SOURCES:

1. National data: 1988–2007 data from Kaiser/HRET (2007); 2008–2013 data from Kaiser/HRET (2013).
2. California data: 1988–2012, CALPERS and CHCF (2013); Gable (2014).
3. CPI data: BLS (2014).

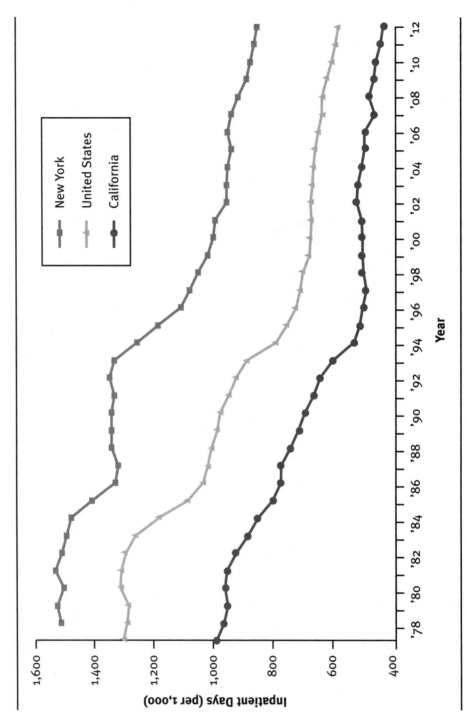

EXHIBIT 19.4
Trends in
Hospital
Utilization per
Thousands:
United States,
California,
and New York,
1977–2012

SOURCE: Utilization data from AHA (n.d.).

Under unmanaged fee-for-service indemnity insurance, new technology was adopted as long as it provided some additional benefit—no matter how small—regardless of its cost. Developing cost-reducing technology offered little financial incentive. For managed care to produce continual savings, new technology must be justified on its costs as well as its benefits. To the extent that investment in technology can be directed to reducing the use of more costly procedures, using less invasive procedures, enabling care to be provided in the home or an outpatient setting, and preventing the need for costly acute care, continual reductions in medical costs are possible.[1] Based on a limited number of studies, managed care slowed the rate at which new technology was adopted (Baker and Wheeler 1998). Furthermore, as managed care penetration increased in an area, capacity use of the equipment rose; consequently, fewer facilities were needed than under the unmanaged fee-for-service system. Managed care appears to have been able to achieve continual reductions in the cost of medical care.

Managed care achieved one of the main goals it was meant to accomplish: It restrained the rise in healthcare expenditures. Without managed care, insurance premiums would have increased more rapidly. Higher insurance premiums make health insurance less affordable; consequently, the number of uninsured would have been greater because the demand for insurance is inversely related to its price. Further, the lower rate of increase in insurance premiums resulted in a redistribution of income from hospitals and physicians (an important reason for their opposition to managed care) to employees. Lower health insurance premiums meant that employees had greater take-home pay. Reduced premiums also meant, however, that less revenue was available for physicians, hospitals employed fewer people, and provider wages grew more slowly.

Patient Satisfaction and Quality of Care

An evaluation of managed care performance should be broader than just examining whether it results in lower insurance premiums. Managed care competition (and any system for organizing the delivery of medical services) should also be evaluated on whether it promotes efficiency (the rate at which premiums increase), desired treatment outcomes, and patient satisfaction.

Many studies have examined member satisfaction in managed care plans, such as HMOs and non-HMOs (Glied 2000). (These studies typically compare the most restrictive form of managed care—an HMO—to less restrictive forms or to non–managed care insurance plans.) Measures of member satisfaction typically include waiting times for an appointment, referrals to a specialist, and travel times to a panel provider. These results typically show a high degree of member satisfaction in HMOs. Such studies, however, have limited usefulness because most people do not have health problems and therefore do not make costly demands on the HMO.

More recent surveys attempt to measure patient satisfaction by those who are chronically ill and have serious health problems. Such studies have examined access to care by those with low income, those who are HIV positive, and those who are chronically ill. The results of these studies are mixed: either no significant differences exist between the health plans or patient satisfaction is better in some HMOs than in others. On one hand, in traditional unmanaged health plans, the patient has easier access to specialists and fewer restrictions on hospital use. In managed care plans, however, coordination of care is better for those with chronic illness; otherwise, a chronically ill patient can be hospitalized multiple times, increasing the managed care plan's costs. Early managed care plans were not experienced in caring for those with chronic illness, and as a result of anecdotal stories of access problems, regulatory restrictions were placed on managed care plans; this has since changed in most managed care plans.

With regard to quality of care in managed care versus traditional insurance, the empirical literature suggests little difference between the two. Some studies indicate that traditional insurance may perform better for those who have serious health conditions, particularly those with low income. Given the large number and the different types of managed care plans, generalizations are difficult to make about which type of health plan results in greater or worse patient satisfaction and treatment outcomes. The provider payment system (fee-for-service, salary, or capitation), the party responsible for financial risk, the decision-making structure, and the managed care culture of the medical group are likely to be more important determinants of patient satisfaction and outcomes than the type of health plan.

To the extent that risk-adjusted premiums are used to pay for high-risk patients and those who have serious illnesses, a higher capitation rate paid by the employer to the health plan for such groups provides managed care plans with an incentive to compete for such patients, improve their access to care, and innovate in devising new treatment methods. An example of these types of managed care plans are Medicare demonstration projects that pay such firms risk-adjusted premiums to care for special needs populations, such as frail elderly. The HMO has an incentive to provide the necessary services, including preventive care, to keep their enrollees in the community rather than admitted to nursing homes.

Medicare Advantage HMOs Versus Traditional Medicare

Landon and colleagues (2012) compared enrollees' utilization patterns in Medicare Advantage HMOs with those of enrollees in traditional fee-for-service Medicare during 2003 to 2009 to determine whether the difference in utilization patterns reflected more integrated care received by the HMO enrollees. Utilization rates in several major categories, including emergency departments and ambulatory surgery, were 20 percent to 30 percent lower in Medicare Advantage HMOs during each of the years studied. Further, Medicare Advantage HMO enrollees underwent more coronary bypass surgery than did patients in traditional Medicare. The authors concluded that their "findings suggest that overall, Medicare Advantage HMO enrollees might use fewer services and be experiencing more appropriate use of services than enrollees in traditional Medicare."

Managed Care's Spillover Effect

Medicare Advantage plans have different financial incentives than do providers in traditional Medicare. These plans receive from Medicare a risk-adjusted payment per enrollee for providing at least the same coverage as does traditional Medicare. More efficient plans—that is, the same coverage for less than the Medicare payment—can offer their enrollees greater coverage and thereby increase their market share over traditional Medicare. However, they have a "spillover" effect. When they improve the efficiency of delivering medical care to their enrollees, their providers apply the same efficiencies when caring for non–Medicare Advantage plan patients. Baicker, Chernew, and Robbins (2013) found that as the market share of Medicare Advantage plans in an area increases, their providers begin to adopt the same approaches when caring for traditional Medicare patients and for younger, privately insured patients. The growth of Medicare Advantage plans has led to a decrease in intensity of care (hence lower hospitalization costs) and a decrease in length of stay for non-Medicare patients.

How Has Managed Care Evolved?

Managed care underwent a change starting in the late 1990s. Several events occurred that resulted in a loosening of managed care's tight cost-containment measures.

Economic Prosperity of the 1990s

In the late 1990s, the US economy was expanding, the stock market was reaching new highs, dot-com companies were launching, and firms were having difficulty attracting and retaining skilled employees. In that prosperous period, employees wanted health plans that were less restrictive on specialist referrals and that offered broader provider networks. Given the tight labor market, employers were more concerned with keeping their employees than with the costs of healthcare; employers were willing to pay higher insurance premiums for more generous health plans. Enrollment growth in HMOs began to decline, and PPO plans became more popular.

As health plans restructured themselves to accommodate employees' demands, they encountered more difficulty controlling medical costs. Changing from limited to broader networks meant that health plans had less leverage over the provider to negotiate large price discounts. The removal of physician gatekeepers meant higher numbers of self-referrals to specialists and more procedures. Less utilization review by health plans led to greater use of medical services. Greater use of specialists, more procedures, and reliance on fee-for-service payment over a broader network not only made coordinating and monitoring patient care difficult but also raised the cost of care and consequently premiums.

Further, to the extent that managed care plans have broader networks and providers participate in multiple health plans, holding the health plan accountable for the performance of its providers is difficult. Similarly, a single health plan has difficulty collecting data from providers, monitoring their performance, and changing their practice patterns. The broader the network and the fewer the restrictions on specialist referrals, the less control health plans have over providers.

Higher Prices for Hospitals, Physicians, and Prescription Drugs

The industry structure was also changing during the late 1990s. To improve their bargaining power with fewer but larger health plans, hospitals and physicians began merging and consolidating into fewer, larger organizations. Hospital mergers within a market meant fewer competitors among which the health plan could negotiate discounts. In addition, excess capacity among hospitals was reduced as a result of hospital closures and mergers. Hospitals, therefore, were able to charge the health plans' higher prices. Drug costs began to rise sharply as new, more effective drugs became available and pharmaceutical companies were successful in stimulating demand with direct-to-consumer advertising. Health plans had to raise their premiums to pay for these higher costs.

Regulation of Managed Care

By the end of the 1990s, a backlash by providers and patients forced many managed care plans to abandon the strict cost-containment methods, such as gatekeepers and specialist referral requirements, and adopt less-restrictive options. More government regulation of managed care occurred for several reasons:

- Widespread media attention was given to certain cases of denial of care by HMOs.
- The public wanted more access to specialists (without paying more).

- The American Medical Association wanted to redress the balance of power between managed care plans and physicians; physicians' bargaining power would be increased if limited provider networks could be opened to all physicians, thereby allowing patients greater choice of physician (*any willing provider* laws).
- Some were opposed to managed care because they wanted a single-payer system, and regulation would eliminate managed care's success in reducing medical costs.

Legislators saw an opportunity to gain visibility by holding hearings on HMO practices and receive the public's support by enacting laws making certain managed care practices (e.g., outpatient mastectomies and "drive-through deliveries") illegal. Lawmakers did not discuss the trade-offs between legislating freer access to care and the more expensive premiums that would result. The public was led to believe greater access would come at no additional cost, and Congress and the states increased regulation. To the extent that government intervenes in the practice of medicine (establishing minimum lengths of stay and determining which procedures can be performed in an outpatient setting) and regulates how managed care plans structure their delivery systems, treatment innovation is inhibited and health insurance premiums will rise by more than they would otherwise.

In October 1999, a class-action lawsuit requesting billions of dollars in damages was filed against a managed care firm (Humana), alleging that by using cost-containment methods the firm reneged on its promise to pay for all medically necessary care. Although the lawsuit was dismissed three years later, along with similar suits against other managed care plans, managed care plans relaxed their cost-containment methods.

What Recent Developments Managed Care Has Undergone

As managed care's stringent cost-containment methods and limited provider networks were loosened, premiums began increasing rapidly in the late 1990s. Employers and their employees once again became concerned with rising premiums. Employers started shifting a greater portion of the insurance premium to their employees and pressured managed care firms to better control high healthcare costs.

Changing Cost-Containment Approaches

Managed care's cost-control approaches have evolved from restricting access to developing innovative approaches for managing care and reducing medical costs. Approaches being used today include the early management of diseases such as diabetes, hypertension, and congestive heart failure, as these diseases can lead to catastrophic medical expenses (Berenson et al. 2008). Managing chronic illness includes developing clinical guidelines or protocols, clinical integration and coordination of care, and early identification and treatment of high-risk patients. With the aging of the population, managed care firms are learning how to manage chronic care needs for which they are at financial risk.

Assisting in the development of innovative approaches are computer information systems and large databases, which can revolutionize treatment patterns (known as *evidence-based medicine*). Large data sets that track specific diseases over long periods will enable providers to determine which variations in treatment methods have the most desired patient outcomes; this information could be used to promote changes in physicians' practice patterns. Information technology and large amounts of data will also enable managers to enhance efficiency by better understanding their enrollees' medical costs and to improve clinical outcomes and quality of care. Provider performance will be evaluated in terms of patient outcomes, satisfaction, and cost of care.

Report Cards

Previously, consumers had little or no information by which to judge the quality of different providers or the quality of care they received. The development of managed care made it possible to evaluate patient satisfaction and treatment outcomes of enrolled population groups. By having limited provider panels of physicians and hospitals, together with a defined group of enrollees, a managed care plan is able to develop information on the practice patterns of and patient satisfaction with its providers and the care received by its enrollees.

Under pressure from employer coalitions for more information by which their employees can judge different managed care plans and their participating providers, managed care plans have supplied data to independent organizations for developing report cards. These report cards include information on patient satisfaction, quality process measures, and outcomes data on health plans and their participating providers. When these report cards are made available to employees during open-enrollment periods, the additional information influences their choice of health plan (Kolstad and Chernew 2009). Public information increases the pressure on health plans and their providers to compete on satisfaction and outcome measures as well as on premiums. Employees can then make a more informed trade-off between lower premiums and desirable plan characteristics.

Pay for Performance

Incentive-based provider payments, referred to as *pay for performance,* began around 2000. Insurers typically pay physicians and hospitals for providing services and little if any attempt has been made to reward providers who perform higher-quality services or reduce treatment costs. This is beginning to change. Although quality of medical care is difficult to measure, medical experts agree that certain standards should be met for preventive care and specified diagnoses (Rosenthal et al. 2005). Although the measures used for incentive payments are not standardized across different health plans, three types of measures are being used: (1) clinical quality, including childhood immunization rates, breast cancer and cervical cancer screening rates, and measures related to the management of chronic diseases such as diabetes and asthma; (2) patient satisfaction measures; and (3) measures related to investment in information technology that enables clinical data integration.

The pay-for-performance experiments have been started by those managed care plans having a large market share (and therefore greater bargaining power over their providers). Incentive payments paid to providers represent 1 percent to 5 percent of a provider's total revenue. Pay for performance is still in its early stages. Medical societies have generally been opposed on grounds that the quality measures are not fully developed and that the implication is that providers are not delivering high-quality care. Although these incentive payments have been widely adopted by health plans, studies examining their impact have found mixed results depending on the size of the incentive bonus, the competitiveness of the market, and the financial situation of participating providers (James 2012).

Pay-for-performance programs will continue to evolve; the amount of the incentive payment will likely grow, standards for judging providers will become uniform across health plans, and medical groups will have to invest more in information technology to be able to supply the data by which they will be measured.

Consumer-Driven Healthcare

A popular approach to curbing rising insurance premiums is consumer-driven healthcare (CDHC). More of the financial risk and responsibility for controlling cost—such as seeking lower provider prices and using fewer services—are placed on the consumer. A CDHC plan relies on a large-deductible insurance policy, making the enrollee responsible for large out-of-pocket payments. The Medicare Modernization Act of 2003 provided tax advantages to employees who establish health savings accounts (HSAs). An HSA has two parts: (1) a high-deductible health insurance policy and (2) a tax-free savings account for the employee. Each year, funds in the savings account that are not spent on medical services can be accumulated. When the employee retires, the accumulated funds and the earnings on those funds belong to the employee. A number of websites provide information on hospital and physician quality rankings and prices for different treatments to help employees with high-deductible plans choose their providers.

As of 2013, 9.7 percent of the US population (11.8 million adults aged 21 to 64 years with private insurance) have CDHC plans, which are achieving greater acceptance among employees. Enrollment in managed care plans appears to have stabilized, and more managed care plans have begun marketing CDHC plans. Evidence on these plans indicate that they are associated with lower costs and lower cost increases; however, some studies suggest that CDHC plans may also attract healthier enrollees (Fronstin 2013).

How the Affordable Care Act Affects Managed Care

The ACA established insurance exchanges whereby individuals and employees could purchase health insurance. Those whose income is between 133 percent and 400 percent of the federal poverty level are eligible for subsidies. The initial (2014) groups purchasing insurance on the exchange were those who were previously uninsured and those who had purchased coverage in the individual insurance market. In subsequent years, larger numbers of employees become eligible to purchase insurance on the exchanges. Health plans competing on the exchanges are required to offer a very comprehensive set of benefits.

To limit the size of their enrollees' premiums, insurers have several choices. They may offer fewer benefits, increase patient deductibles and cost sharing, and/or limit their provider networks. Required by the ACA to offer comprehensive and costly benefits, insurers offered plans on the exchanges that contained high deductibles and very limited provider networks. The narrow networks excluded prominent and costly hospitals and many physicians, thereby disrupting the care patterns of many patients.

Managed care firms previously used limited provider networks to reduce their enrollees' medical costs. Participating hospitals and doctors agreed to price discounts in return for a greater number of patients. In the earlier managed care period, many excluded hospitals and physicians were successful in having their state enact any willing provider laws permitting them to participate in the insurer's network. These anticompetitive laws made it less likely for providers to discount their prices if they could not be assured of receiving more patients.

The trend toward narrow provider networks being offered on the exchanges may be a sign of the future also for those who are privately insured and not buying insurance on the exchange. Unable to reduce the ACA's costly mandated benefits, insurers have little choice in how they can control their costs. Rather than base their networks on providers who provide the largest discounts, managed care's approach over time will be to use their narrow networks to direct patients to high-quality facilities and physicians who are able to cut their costs by providing integrated and coordinated care.

Accountable Care Organizations

The ACA included funds for experimenting with new provider payment systems. One such approach is to encourage providers to organize as accountable care organizations (ACOs), which provide primary care, specialty services, and inpatient care for a defined population of Medicare beneficiaries. An ACO and its physicians are responsible for the overall care of their Medicare beneficiaries, adequate participation of primary care physicians, coordinated care, evidence-based medicine, and quality and costs of care. ACOs that meet their quality and cost thresholds share in the cost savings they achieve for the Medicare program. The hope is that ACOs will transform not only the Medicare system but also the delivery of medical services in the private sector, improving the quality of care and reducing rising medical costs.

To become an ACO, hospitals have been consolidating and employing physicians so as to provide integrated and coordinated care to their Medicare enrollees. However, unlike Medicare Advantage plans, Medicare enrollees do not choose to join an ACO nor are they provided with a financial incentive to do so. In fact, *enrollees are unaware that they are being assigned to an ACO.* As such, the Medicare patient incurs no financial penalty if they use providers unaffiliated with the ACO. As of 2013, 360 ACOs are operating within the Medicare program, serving about 5.3 million beneficiaries (about 12 percent to 13 percent of all people with Medicare). Results of early studies on the effectiveness of ACOs are not promising; the number of participating ACOs is few, and little evidence exists that ACOs are able to improve quality or cut costs (Epstein et al. 2014; McWilliams, Landon, and Chernew 2013).

Instead, opponents of the ACO concept have two concerns. First, permitting combinations of hospital and physician groups to form large ACOs may lessen competition, thereby raising prices to the private sector. Second, it will be easier for the government to impose price controls on large organizations than on large numbers of independently practicing providers.

Summary

Health insurance premiums once again began to rise sharply as a consequence of the economic prosperity that led to employee demands for less restrictive health plans in the 1990s, hospital mergers and physician consolidations that resulted in higher provider prices and drug prices, regulations imposed on managed care plans, and advances in medical technology. Managed care plans have demonstrated less ability to control costs today than they had previously.

Employers and employees are searching for new approaches to limit their premium increases. Employers are shifting more of the insurance premium to their employees, and health plans are developing new cost-containment strategies, such as disease management and evidence-based medicine. Under pressure from employers, health plans are using report cards to enable employees to make more informed choices of health plans and participating providers. Health plans are also beginning to use incentive-based payment to encourage their participating providers to improve quality of care, patient satisfaction, and the use of information technology to integrate clinical data.

A recent trend affecting the growth of managed care plans is CDHC. These high-deductible plans, sold at low premiums, shift more financial risk to consumers and require them to become more informed about their purchases of healthcare services and their choice of providers.

The market is responding to rising premiums by offering a variety of health plans, as consumers have different preferences and abilities to pay. Greater emphasis is being placed on consumer cost sharing to hold down costs and use of services.

The ACA established health insurance exchanges with subsidies for those with low income. Insurers competing on these exchanges are required to offer a very comprehensive set of benefits and have formed very narrow provider networks to limit the size of their enrollees' premiums. These narrow networks, which may be a sign of future managed care plans, have disrupted the care patterns of many patients. In addition, the ACA has given demonstration funds for providers to form ACOs that deliver coordinated care to Medicare patients while decreasing Medicare costs. These ACOs have led to greater provider consolidation and hospital employment of physicians. It is too early to judge whether ACOs will be able to achieve their objectives, given the lack of financial incentives for Medicare enrollees to choose lower-cost ACOs.

Discussion Questions

1. What is managed care, and what are managed care techniques?
2. When managed care enrollment increases in a market, how does it affect other insurers and providers?
3. Why did managed care emerge?
4. What are the different types of managed care plans?

5. What are report cards, and what effects are they expected to have on managed care competition?
6. How has the growth of managed care affected the performance of the medical sector?
7. Why have hospitals and physicians agreed to participate in insurers' narrow provider networks?

Note

1. On balance, new technology has led to increased, not decreased, medical expenditures. However, increased medical expenditures resulting from new technology are not the same as inflation in medical costs. The medical treatment the patient receives is different and improved. Further, as long as the public is willing to pay for those increased benefits, it is appropriate for medical costs to rise.

Additional Reading

Dranove, D. 2000. *The Economic Evolution of American Health Care: From Marcus Welby to Managed Care*. Princeton, NJ: Princeton University Press.

References

American Hospital Association (AHA). n.d. *Hospital Statistics*. Various editions. Chicago: AHA.

Baicker, K., M. Chernew, and J. Robbins. 2013. "The Spillover Effects of Medicare Managed Care: Medicare Advantage and Hospital Utilization." *NBER Working Paper* No. 19070, May. Cambridge, MA: National Bureau of Economic Research. www.nber.org/papers/w19070?utm_campaign=ntw&utm_medium=email&utm_source=ntw.

Baker, L., and S. Wheeler. 1998. "Managed Care and Technology Diffusion: The Case of MRI." *Health Affairs* 17 (5): 195–207.

Berenson, R., M. Hash, T. Ault, B. Fuchs, S. Maxwell, L. Potetz, and S. Zuckerman. 2008. *Cost Containment in Medicare: A Review What Works and What Doesn't*. Washington, DC: AARP Public Policy Institute. http://assets.aarp.org/rgcenter/health/2008_18_medicare.pdf.

Buchmueller, T., and P. Feldstein. 1996. "Consumers' Sensitivity to Health Plan Premiums: Evidence from a Natural Experiment in California." *Health Affairs* 15 (1): 143–51.

Bureau of Labor Statistics (BLS). 2014. "Consumer Price Index. CPI Databases." Accessed March. www.bls.gov.

California Public Employees Retirement System (CALPERS) and California HealthCare Foundation (CHCF). 2013. *California Employer Health Benefits Survey.* Accessed 2014. www.chcf.org/publications/2013/04/employer-health-benefits.

Centers for Medicare & Medicaid Services (CMS). 2013. *Brief Summaries of Medicare and Medicaid.* Published November 1. http://cms.hhs.gov/Research-Statistics-Data-and-Systems/Statistics-Trends-and-Reports/MedicareProgramRatesStats/Downloads/MedicareMedicaidSummaries2013.pdf.

Epstein, A., A. Jha, E. Orav, D. Liebman, A. Audet, M. Zezza, and S. Guterman. 2014. "Analysis of Early Accountable Care Organizations Defines Patient, Structural, Cost, and Quality-of-Care Characteristics." *Health Affairs* 33 (1): 95–102.

Fronstin, P. 2013. "Findings from the 2013 EBRI/Greenwald & Associates Consumer Engagement in Health Care Survey." *EBRI Issue Brief* No. 393, December. www.ebri.org/pdf/briefspdf/EBRI_IB_012-13.No393.CEHCS.pdf.

Gable, J. 2014. Personal correspondence with the author, February.

Glied, S. 2000. "Managed Care." In *The Handbook of Health Economics*, edited by J. P. Newhouse and A. J. Culyer, 707–53. New York: North-Holland Press.

Hughes, R., S. Hunt, and H. Luft. 1987. "Effects of Surgeon Volume and Hospital Volume on Quality of Care in Hospitals." *Medical Care* 25 (6): 489–503.

James, J. 2012. "Pay-for-Performance. New Payment Systems Reward Doctors and Hospitals for Improving the Quality of Care, But Studies To Date Show Mixed Results." *Health Affairs Health Policy Brief,* October 11. http://healthaffairs.org/healthpolicybriefs/brief_pdfs/healthpolicybrief_78.pdf.

Kaiser Family Foundation and Health Research & Educational Trust (HRET). 2013. *Employer Health Benefits. 2013 Annual Survey.* Accessed 2014. http://kaiserfamilyfoundation.files.wordpress.com/2013/08/8465-employer-health-benefits-20131.pdf.

———. 2007. *2007 Kaiser/HRET Employer Health Benefits Survey.* Accessed 2014. www.kff.org/insurance/7672/upload/7693.pdf.

Kolstad, J. T., and M. E. Chernew. 2009. "Quality and Consumer Decision Making in the Market for Health Insurance and Health Care Services." *Medical Care Research and Review* 66 (1 Suppl): 28S–52S.

KPMG Peat Marwick. 1982; 1991. *Survey of Employer-Sponsored Health Benefits.* Amstelveen, Netherlands: KPMG Peat Marwick.

Landon, B., A. Zaslavsky, R. Saunders, L. Pawlson, J. Newhouse, and J. Ayanian. 2012. "Analysis of Medicare Advantage HMOs Compared with Traditional Medicare Shows Lower Use of Many Services During 2003–09." *Health Affairs* 31 (12): 2609–17.

McWilliams, J. M., B. E. Landon, and M. E. Chernew. 2013. "Changes in Health Care Spending and Quality for Medicare Beneficiaries Associated with a Commercial ACO Contract." *JAMA* 310 (8): 829–36. http://jama.jamanetwork.com/article.aspx?articleid=1733718.

Rosenthal, M., R. Frank, Z. Li, and A. Epstein. 2005. "Early Experience with Pay-for-Performance." *JAMA* 294 (14): 1788–93.

Wu, V. 2009. "Managed Care's Price Bargaining with Hospitals." *Journal of Health Economics* 28 (2): 350–60.

HAS COMPETITION BEEN TRIED—AND HAS IT FAILED—TO IMPROVE THE US HEALTHCARE SYSTEM?

C ritics claim that market competition has been tried but has failed to improve the US healthcare system. Healthcare costs are rising rapidly and per capita healthcare spending is the highest in the world—yet many Americans are without health insurance. More of the middle class are finding that health insurance has become too expensive, life expectancy is lower than in other countries, and the infant mortality rate is higher than in some countries with lower per capita healthcare expenditures. In other words, is it time to try something different? Specifically, is it time for more government regulation and control of the healthcare system? "Some say that competition has failed, I say that competition has not yet been tried." Alain Enthoven (1993, 28) wrote that statement in 1993, and it continues to be correct today.

This chapter discusses how medical markets differ from competitive markets, why making medical markets more competitive is desirable, what changes are needed to bring about greater competition, whether competitive markets are responsible for the growing numbers of uninsured, and what role the government plays in a competitive medical care environment.

Criteria for Judging Performance of a Country's Medical Sector

The health of a population, as measured by life expectancy or infant mortality rates, is not solely the consequence of the country's medical system. How people live and eat are more important determinants of life expectancy than whether they have good access to medical services when they become ill. Life expectancy is related to a number of factors, such as smoking, diet, marital status, exercise, drug use, and cultural values. Although universal access to health insurance is desirable, studies have shown that medical care has a smaller effect on health levels than personal health habits and lifestyle (see Chapter 3). Therefore, assessing the medical care system on measures that are more affected by lifestyle factors is inappropriate. After all, the financing and delivery of medical services has been based on treating people when they are ill and not on keeping them well.

Several healthcare organizations in the United States have gone beyond treating people when they become ill and have tried to lower costs by preventing illnesses that are expensive to treat. Reducing hip fractures among the elderly and instituting monitoring mechanisms for diabetes patients, for example, have been shown to prevent more costly treatments later. The financial incentives of these organizations differ from the typical fee-for-service payment methods predominantly used in the United States and other countries.

Assuming the purpose of a medical care system is more narrowly defined—that is, treating those who become ill—what criteria should be used to evaluate how well that system performs? The criteria should be the same as those used to evaluate the performance of other markets, such as housing, food, automobiles, and electronics—markets that produce necessities and luxuries. The following are the performance criteria of a medical care system:

1. Information. Do consumers have sufficient information to choose the quantity and type of services based on price, quality, and other characteristics of the services being supplied?
2. Consumer incentives. Do consumers have incentives to ensure that the value of the services used is not less than the cost of producing those services?
3. Consumer choices. Does the market respond to what consumers are willing to pay? If consumers demand more of some services, will the market provide more of those services? If consumers differ in how much they are willing to spend or want different types of services, will the market respond to those varied consumer demands?
4. Supplier incentives. Do suppliers of goods and services have an incentive to produce those goods and services (for a given level of quality) at the lowest cost?
5. Price markups. Do the prices suppliers charge for their services reflect their costs of production? (This occurs when suppliers compete on price to supply their services.)
6. Redistribution. Do those who cannot afford to pay for their medical services receive medically necessary services?

To the extent that the medical sector approximates the first five criteria, the system will produce its output efficiently, and medical costs will rise at a rate that reflects the cost of producing those services.[1] The type of services available, as well as the new medical technology adopted, will be based on what consumers are willing to pay.

Competitive markets—compared with monopoly markets or markets with government controls on prices and investment—come closest to achieving the first five criteria. Competitive markets are the yardstick by which all markets are evaluated, and they underlie the antitrust laws. Proponents of competition believe the same benefits can be achieved by applying competitive principles to medical care. Competitive markets, however, do not help those unable to afford the goods and services produced. It is government's role, not the market's, to subsidize those with low income so that they can receive the necessary amounts of food, housing, and medical services. When subsidies in the form of vouchers for health insurance are provided, through a competitive market, to those with low income, the value of the subsidies is greater; providers have incentives to produce those services efficiently, and patients have a greater choice when using them.

Market forces are powerful in motivating purchasers and suppliers. The search for profits is an incentive for suppliers to invest a great deal of money to satisfy purchaser demands. Suppliers innovate to become more efficient, develop new services, and differentiate themselves from competitors, thereby increasing their market share and becoming more profitable. Incentives exist in both competitive and regulated markets. The incentives appropriate to a competitive market are those where both the purchaser and the supplier bear the cost and receive the benefits of their actions. When a purchaser's and a supplier's costs and benefits are not equal, the market becomes less competitive and its performance suffers.

How Medical Markets Differ from Competitive Markets

The Period Before Managed Care

Before managed care began to grow in the 1980s, health insurance coverage was predominantly traditional indemnity insurance. Patients had little or no out-of-pocket cost when they used medical services, and hospitals and physicians were paid on a fee-for-service basis. Information on providers was nonexistent, as it was prohibited by medical and hospital associations, and accrediting agencies (such as The Joint Commission) did not make their findings public. Insurance companies merely passed higher provider costs on to employers, who paid their employees' insurance premiums. Medicare and Medicaid greatly reduced their beneficiaries' concern with medical prices. Medicare paid hospitals according to their costs, and physicians were paid on a fee-for-service basis. Medicaid paid hospitals and physicians fee-for-service.

Regulatory policies at the state and federal levels, enacted at the behest of provider groups, led to greater market inefficiency. Restrictions were imposed on any form of advertising; on the tasks different health professionals were permitted to perform; on entry by new hospitals and freestanding outpatient surgery centers into hospital markets; on requiring health maintenance organizations (HMOs) to be not-for-profit; and on which healthcare providers were eligible for payment under Medicare, Medicaid, and even Blue Cross and Blue Shield. Neither patients nor physicians had any incentive to be concerned with the use or cost of services. Comprehensive health insurance results in a "moral hazard" problem; patients use more services because their insurance has greatly reduced the price they have to pay. The additional benefit of using more services is much less than if the patient had to pay more of the cost. Exhibit 20.1 illustrates how payment for medical services has changed since 1960.

Currently (2013), private insurance and government pay for most medical services; out-of-pocket payments by patients have declined from almost 50 percent of total medical expenditures to just 11.7 percent. Furthermore, physicians, because they are paid on a fee-for-service basis, have a financial incentive to provide more services. Given the lack of patient and provider incentives to be concerned about the cost and use of services, "too many" services are delivered. Wide variations in care occur because factors other than clinical value are used to decide whether the services should be provided, and rapid increases have occurred in the growth of medical spending.

To control rapidly rising medical costs from the late 1960s to the early 1980s, federal and state governments used regulatory approaches. The medical sector was placed under wage and price controls from 1971 to 1974,

EXHIBIT 20.1
Trends in Payment for Medical Services, 1960–2012

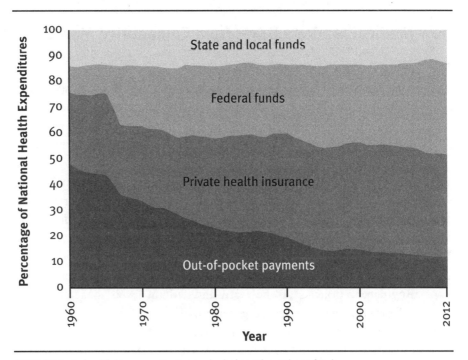

NOTE: "Private health insurance" category includes other private funds.
SOURCE: Data from CMS (2014).

health-planning legislation placed controls on hospital investment, many states used hospital rate regulation, and Medicare instituted hospital utilization review and limited physicians' fee increases. Medicaid simply reduced payments to hospitals and physicians. These regulatory approaches failed to limit rising medical costs.

Managed Care

Managed care was the reaction of large employers against a medical care system that was out of control and had brought about rapidly rising health insurance premiums. Under pressure from large employers and unions, health insurers and providers became adversaries. Health plans negotiated price discounts with providers and instituted cost-containment measures that reduced use of services (gatekeepers, prior authorization for specialist and hospital services, and covering care in settings less expensive than the hospital). These cost-reduction measures achieved large savings in insurance premiums, as shown in Exhibit 19.3. When employees were offered a choice of health plans and given an opportunity to save on their monthly premiums, they switched plans. Price competition penalized high-cost plans.

A backlash against managed care and its cost-containment methods occurred by the end of the 1990s. As more low-risk users switched to HMOs for less expensive premiums, those remaining in traditional indemnity plans (patients with chronic illnesses and patients with established physician and specialist relationships) faced high premiums. (Adverse selection caused premiums to rise more in traditional indemnity plans.) They joined HMOs to reduce their premiums but were dissatisfied with the restrictions on access to providers. The backlash against managed care was likely driven by those forced to join HMOs.

Managed care was, at most, an example of partial market competition. Although managed care competition achieved large private-sector cost savings for a limited time, much of the previous regulatory and economic framework under which competition occurred was unchanged. Any framework includes a set of consumer and supplier incentives, and market performance responds to these incentives. When these incentives influence consumers and suppliers to consider the full costs and benefits of their decisions, market outcomes are efficient. At times, however, the legal and economic framework within which consumers and producers make their choices distorts the costs and benefits of these incentives, in which case markets perform inefficiently.

The following sections provide examples of how the medical care market's legal and economic framework has distorted consumer and producer incentives—and hence their choices—and has led to inefficient market outcomes.

Demand-Side Market Failures

These market failures on the demand side have limited the expansion of more competitive managed care firms.

Tax-Exempt Employer-Paid Health Insurance

When an employer purchases health insurance on behalf of employees, these contributions are not considered taxable income to the employee. Compared with other employee purchases paid for with after-tax income, the purchase of insurance is subsidized; employees do not pay the full price of their insurance as they would if they had to buy the same amount with after-tax income. When the price of a good or service is reduced, consumers will purchase a greater quantity of that service (known as the *law of demand*).[2] The price of insurance, when purchased by the employer, is not the same for all employees. Those in the highest income-tax brackets receive the largest tax subsidies. On average, changes in the out-of-pocket price of health insurance result in an approximate proportional change in the quantity of insurance demanded.[3] (A 5 percent decrease in price leads to about a 5 percent increase in the quantity demanded.) The tax subsidy for health insurance results in employees purchasing more comprehensive coverage with fewer deductibles and lower cost sharing (and additional benefits, such as vision and dental care) than they would if they had to pay the entire premium themselves.

Consumer incentives have been distorted because consumers do not pay the full cost of health insurance or their use of medical services. When consumers pay only a small fraction of the provider's price out of pocket, they are less aware of and concerned with the prices charged by medical providers.

Health Plan Choices

Health plan competition could have been stronger for several reasons. First, many employers limited their employees' choice to only one health plan.[4] For competition to occur among plans, employees must be offered a choice. Yet during the 1990s almost 80 percent of insured employees were offered only one health plan (Marquis and Long 1999). By 2010, about 60 percent of employed insured workers were still offered only one health plan (Janicki 2013). When employees are unable to choose among substitutes, the single plan being offered has less incentive to respond to employees' preferences or to lower prices.

Second, many employers that offer their employees a choice of health plans either contribute more to the higher-cost health plan or contribute a fixed percentage of the premium to the plan the employee chooses. A fixed-percentage contribution provides a greater dollar subsidy to the more expensive plan, thereby reducing the employee's incentive to select the less costly plan.

(If the employer pays 80 percent, the employee opting for the more expensive plan pays only 20 percent of the price difference, not 100 percent.) The more efficient health plan is at a competitive disadvantage because the more expensive competitor is more heavily subsidized. When employees have a choice of plans, and the employer pays a fixed-dollar contribution to the chosen plan, most employees will select a more restrictive plan—such as an HMO. "For example, 70–80 percent of active employees and dependents covered by the University of California, CalPERS, and Wells Fargo in California [each company makes a fixed-dollar contribution] choose HMOs" (Enthoven and Tollen 2005, w5-429).

Third, when competing managed care plans offer broad networks with overlapping providers, the plans are not sufficiently differentiated and do not offer employees real choices. Overlapping provider networks make it difficult for the plan to control costs (because it cannot exclude providers) and for employees to observe quality differences. The plans are not competing on their provider's ability to manage care, on the quality of their providers, or on patient satisfaction and have little incentive to invest resources to do so—because all plans with the same providers will benefit. Consumers should be able to select among health plans that vary in premiums, quality of care, access to providers, provider network, and so on.

Fourth, few employers pay insurers risk-adjusted premiums for their employees. Paying the same premium for an employee who is older and has more risk factors as for a younger employee who is less likely to incur a large medical expense gives insurers an incentive to engage in risk selection by seeking out younger employees. Paying risk-adjusted premiums gives insurers an incentive to compete on price for higher-risk employees. Insurers also have to compete on how well they can manage the care of high-risk enrollees rather than on how well they can entice low-risk employees to join their plans.

Lack of Information

Historically, healthcare providers have been opposed to being compared with one another. The Federal Trade Commission's (FTC) antitrust suit against the American Medical Association—affirmed by the US Supreme Court in 1982—concerned the association's prohibitions on advertising. A consumer seeking information on a provider's prices and quality was unable to find it. (Consumers with limited cost sharing also had little incentive to search for a lower price.) Lack of information on how good a substitute one competitor is for another enables each competitor to charge higher prices or produce lower quality of care than they could if consumers were informed on the prices and quality of both providers.

Wide price variations—unrelated to quality or other attributes of the service—are unlikely to persist in a price-competitive market. Knowledgeable purchasers will shun overpriced suppliers of a service. Currently, price information for medical services is difficult to determine, and the services included in the stated price are not transparent. For example, a study by Rosenthal, Lu, and Cram (2013) tried to determine elective pricing data (bundled payment that includes hospital and physician fees) for total hip arthroplasty, a common elective surgical procedure. The authors found obtaining price information difficult and observed a wide variation in the prices quoted.

One of the tenets of a competitive market is that consumers not only bear the cost of their choices but also are informed purchasers. If consumers do not have access to information on provider quality, providers have little incentive to invest in higher-quality care because they receive the same fee as those who do not. In recent years, quality and patient satisfaction measures on providers have been collected in report cards and disseminated to employees when they choose their health plans.[5] One study found that two years after the publication of a report card, "more than 20 percent of bottom-quartile surgeons stopped practicing CABG surgery in New York ... whereas only about 5 percent of surgeons in the top three quartiles did so" (Jha and Epstein 2006).

Tax subsidies for purchasing health insurance have led to a demand for more comprehensive insurance—with lower out-of-pocket payments and larger employer subsidies for more expensive health plans—and have lessened consumer incentives to choose more efficient health plans. Subsidies, combined with a lack of information on health plans and providers, have resulted in a medical care market where purchasers have insufficient incentives and limited opportunity to make informed choices.

Medicare and Medicaid

About half of all medical expenditures are made by federal and state governments. Incentives for those beneficiaries and Medicare and Medicaid's provider payment policies have an important effect on the market's performance, similar to the impact of tax subsidies. Most Medicare beneficiaries have supplementary health insurance to cover their Medicare cost-sharing requirements. Because low-income persons are covered by Medicaid, there is no cost sharing. Thus, neither Medicare nor Medicaid beneficiaries have any incentive to be concerned about provider prices or their use of medical services.

Although Medicare allows beneficiaries a choice of health plans, the aged have not had a strong financial incentive to choose lower-cost, restrictive Medicare Advantage plans. Only if Medicare were to provide a fixed dollar contribution, with the aged paying the additional cost of a more expensive health plan, would beneficiaries have an incentive to switch from the more costly, traditional fee-for-service plan. Medicaid enrollees, on the other hand, are not given a choice of health plans. Instead, Medicaid may enroll some of its (young, low-cost) enrollees in a health plan, but most Medicaid expenditures on behalf of the aged and disabled are paid on a fee-for-service basis to hospitals, physicians, and nursing homes.

Supply-Side Market Failures

Provider Consolidation
The greater the number of healthcare providers in a market, the greater the competition among them to respond to purchaser demands. Conversely, when only one provider is available in a market, the patient has no choice but to go to that provider. Providers respond when the purchaser has a substitute provider to choose from. A monopolist provider has no incentive to innovate, improve quality, respond to patients' needs, or offer lower prices.

A great deal of provider consolidation has been occurring. Insurers have fewer hospitals to negotiate with when hospitals in a market merge. The antitrust laws are meant to prevent suppliers—such as hospitals and physicians—from gaining market power. Unfortunately, the FTC had been unsuccessful in preventing hospital mergers that decrease competition. Federal judges, ruling in the merged hospitals' favor, believed merged nonprofit hospitals would not exercise their market power as for-profit hospitals would. Consolidated hospitals and single-specialty groups dominate certain markets (Berenson, Ginsburg, and Kemper 2010). Only recently has the FTC been successful in winning an antitrust suit against a nonprofit hospital merger that occurred years earlier. As the number of competitors has declined, health plans have been forced to pay higher prices, which are passed on to consumers in the form of higher insurance premiums (White, Bond, and Reschovsky 2013).

State Regulations
The states have enacted a number of anticompetitive regulations that limit price competition and result in higher health insurance premiums. These regulations address such areas as the training of health professionals and the tasks they are permitted to perform, entry into medical markets, pricing of health insurance policies, health insurance benefit coverage, and rules covering provider networks.

More than 2,200 state mandates (as of 2012) have been enacted that specify the benefits, population groups, and healthcare providers that must be included in health insurance policies. Large business firms are legally exempt from these state mandates when they self-insure their employees, which most large organizations do. The higher cost burden of these state mandates falls predominantly on individuals and small businesses, raising the cost of insurance and thereby making health insurance unaffordable to those who prefer less expensive health plans. Although some of these state mandates may be beneficial, many individuals and small businesses prefer to have insurance they can afford than no insurance at all. Many states regulate health insurance premiums charged to individuals and small businesses.

Community rating includes all types of individuals or small businesses in a common risk pool, and all are charged the same premium. Firms whose employees are engaged in high-risk jobs are charged the same as organizations with employees who have low-risk jobs. Firms that provide incentives to employees to engage in healthy lifestyles are charged the same premium as those that do not. Community rating eliminates price competition among insurers. Instead, insurers have an incentive to engage in favorable risk selection. Community rating increases the price of insurance to low-risk individuals, thereby leading many to drop their insurance.

Certificate-of-need (CON) laws prohibit competitors from entering a market. A CON protects existing providers from competition, thereby giving monopoly power to the existing hospital, home health agency, hospice, and nursing home.

Training of health professionals emphasizes process measures of quality as a prerequisite for licensure. Re-examination for relicensure is not used, and physicians are rarely evaluated on outcomes-based measures of quality. Innovative methods of training health professionals are inhibited when rigid professional rules specify training requirements. The tasks health professionals are permitted to perform are specified in state practice acts, based on political competition by different health associations over which a profession is permitted to perform certain tasks. A greater supply of health manpower can be obtained and care can be produced less expensively when performance is monitored and flexibility is allowed in the tasks health professionals are qualified to perform.

Any willing provider (AWP) laws limit price competition among physicians (and dentists). Health plans were able to negotiate large price discounts from physicians by offering them exclusivity over their enrollees. The AWP laws enable any physician to have access to a health plan's enrollees at the negotiated price. As a result of AWP laws, physicians have no incentive to compete on price for a health plan's enrollees because they cannot be assured of a higher volume of patients in return for a lower price.

Lack of Physician Information

Competitive markets assume that demand-side and supply-side participants are well informed. Physicians—who act as the patient's agent and as a supplier of a service—are considered to be knowledgeable about their patients' diagnosis and treatment. Further, physicians are assumed to act in their patients' best interest. If these assumptions are incorrect, medical services are not being provided efficiently, quality of care is lower, and the cost of medical services is higher than it would otherwise be.

Wide variations exist in the medical services provided by physicians in the same specialty, to patients with the same diagnosis, and across different geographic regions (IOM 2013). These variations in medical services are likely attributable to two factors. First, physicians are not equally proficient in their diagnostic ability or in their knowledge of the latest treatment methods. These wide variations have given rise to evidence-based medicine, whereby large insurers analyze large data sets to determine best practices and disseminate clinical guidelines to their network physicians.

Second, physicians have a financial interest in the quantity and type of care they provide. Most physicians are paid fee-for-service; thus, the more they do, the more they earn. *Supplier-induced demand* is the term economists use to explain physicians' financial incentive to increase their services. When combined with the lack of consumer incentives regarding prices and use of medical services and consumers' lack of knowledge regarding physicians' practice methods, both the use and the cost of medical services are greatly increased. Medicare—under which most aged have supplementary insurance to cover their cost sharing—is a prime example of how lack of patient price sensitivity and medical information, together with some physicians' lack of knowledge and the incentives inherent in fee-for-service, have resulted in large variations in the cost and number of services provided.

Based on the preceding discussion, market forces have been greatly weakened. Given the lack of effective market competition in medical markets, one cannot claim that competition has been tried and has failed.

How Can Medical Markets Be More Competitive?

Markets always exist, but, depending on government rules, they can be efficient or inefficient. To improve market efficiency in medical care, several changes are needed in government regulations and in the private sector.

Government tax policy that excludes employer-paid health insurance from an employee's taxable income should be changed. Employer contributions should be treated as regular income; however, it is more politically feasible to limit the amount that is tax free.[6] This change will affect how much insurance consumers buy, what health plans they choose, and how much medical care they use. Additional needed government reforms include removing restrictions on market entry and on laws promoting anticompetitive behavior, such as CON and AWP laws; overriding state mandates that raise health insurance costs; eliminating state insurance regulations requiring community rating; enforcing antitrust laws; and reforming Medicare and Medicaid so that beneficiaries pay the additional cost of more expensive health plans, thereby giving these beneficiaries incentives to choose health plans on the basis of costs and benefits.[7] These policies should stimulate greater competition in the private and public medical sectors.

In the private sector, employers who subsidize their employees' health insurance should be encouraged to offer a choice of health plans, to give fixed-dollar contributions, and to use risk-adjusted premiums in making such payments. With more plan choices and employee incentives to be concerned about the costs and benefits of a health plan, information is more accessible to help employees make a selection. When consumers can choose, information has a value and private sources will develop to provide that information—as has occurred in other markets.

In competitive markets, not all purchasers have to be informed or switch in response to changes in prices and quality for suppliers to respond and for markets to perform efficiently.[8] In competitive medical markets, as in other markets, more responsive purchasers and suppliers drive the market toward greater efficiency.

Are the Poor Disadvantaged in a Competitive Market?

Opponents of competitive medical care markets claim that the poor will be unable to afford medical services. Competitive markets produce the most goods and services (with a given amount of resources) and sell them at the lowest possible price to consumers willing to buy. By doing so, competitive markets make goods and services more affordable to those with low income. However, competitive markets should not be evaluated on whether the poor receive all the medical services needed.

Achieving market efficiency has little to do with ensuring that everyone's needs are met or that everyone receives the same quantity of services. It is the role of government, based on voters' preferences, to subsidize the healthcare of the poor—just as is done with the need for food and housing. Providing the poor with subsidies (such as vouchers for a health plan) to be exercised in a competitive market is more likely than any other approach to ensure that they receive the greatest value for those subsidies.

Competitive medical markets may be considered unfair because those with high income are able to buy more than those with low income. The wealthy always have been, and always will be, able to buy more than the poor can. Even in the Canadian single-payer health system, patients with more money are able to skip the waiting lines and travel to the United States for their diagnostics and surgery.

Patient Incentives Drive Price Competition in Government and Private Markets

The following examples illustrate how a change in patient incentives resulted in a price competitive healthcare market.

Medicare Part D Prescription Drug Benefit

In 2004, the Congressional Budget Office (CBO) projected that the federal budgetary cost of the Medicare prescription drug benefit—Part D—for 2012 would be $122 billion. In 2012, the actual federal cost was $55 billion and was relatively constant for each year since 2004 (Cook 2013). It is rare that a federal entitlement program would come in below its projected cost and not increase over time.

The design of the Part D benefit is different from the design of Medicare Parts A and B in that Part D makes the beneficiary responsible for the additional cost of choosing a more expensive drug plan. Under Part D, drug plans submit bids to the federal government for providing the basic prescription drug benefit to a beneficiary. The federal government calculates a national average bid and pays 75 percent of the national average bid to the drug plan chosen by the beneficiary, who is then responsible for the remaining 25 percent of the monthly premium. If a beneficiary enrolls in a plan that submitted a bid higher than the national average, the beneficiary pays the difference in addition to the base premium.

Plans understand that any difference between a plan's bid and the national average bid translates directly into a price difference that will be paid by beneficiaries.[9] Beneficiaries have access to a wide choice of drug plans and have to choose among lower premium plans or more costly plans that may offer greater benefits, such as a more preferable drug formulary. Because competing plans vary in the brand name drugs offered in their formulary, a person can choose the plan in which their preferred drug is covered. Beneficiaries have an incentive to make a trade-off between additional plan benefits versus the additional costs of a higher-priced plan.

Drug plans compete for enrollees by offering lower premiums. By relying on a drug formulary, rather than including all brand name drugs within a disease category, the plan is able to negotiate discounted prices with a pharmaceutical firm to include only their drug in their formulary. Drug plans also encourage their enrollees to use less costly generics when appropriate by using lower cost sharing for generics compared to brand name drugs.

These cost-saving strategies by the drug plans are passed on to beneficiaries in the form of lower premiums and cost sharing.

Drug plan negotiation with drug manufacturers and encouraging generic substitution when appropriate is the direct result of plans competing for price-sensitive enrollees who have to pay out of pocket the additional cost of higher-price drug plans.

Value-Based Purchasing and Reference Pricing

In recent years, employers and insurance have begun to provide patients with financial incentives to choose higher-quality, lower-priced hospitals for their surgery. Several employers (such as Walmart, Safeway, and Lowe's) and insurers (such as WellPoint) have used value-based purchasing or reference pricing to give their employees a financial incentive to choose among competing providers (Robinson and MacPherson 2012). Under these approaches, the employer or insurer contracts for a fixed price with several centers of excellence (such as the Cleveland Clinic) for elective surgical procedures (such as orthopedic joint replacement, interventional cardiology, and cardiac surgery). These are expensive procedures, whose prices vary widely, and differences in their outcomes when performed by different providers are relatively small. Patients are then given a fixed amount (such as $30,000) to cover the cost of their surgery. A patient can go to providers other than those on his employer's preferred list, but if the price is greater than $30,000, then the patient pays the additional cost himself.

Robinson and Brown (2013) found that when patients are provided with a financial incentive, reference pricing results in significant savings. The most dramatic price reductions occurred in higher-priced hospitals. Also interesting is that when patients went to providers other than those on their employers' or insurers' preferred list and when they had only $30,000 to spend, the patients were able to negotiate large price reductions. The insurer did not negotiate with these providers, the patients did. The authors concluded that it is important to change financial incentives of patients and not just rely on direct price negotiations between insurers and providers. When patients are responsible for the additional cost of their care, healthcare markets become price competitive.[10]

What Might Competitive Medical Markets Look Like?

If medical care markets were to become more like a competitive market, what might one observe? As consumers (and Medicare and Medicaid enrollees) have to pay the additional cost of more expensive health plans and become more cost conscious, the variety and number of plan choices will increase;

plans will attempt to match purchasers' preferences and willingness to pay. Some people would prefer to choose among health plans, which is less expensive than choosing and evaluating different providers.

Competitive markets may evolve in several ways. Integrated delivery systems, as articulated by Enthoven (2004), are organizations with their own provider networks that offer coordinated care to their enrollees. These integrated delivery systems may be built around large multispecialty medical groups with relationships to hospitals and other care settings and may be paid a risk-adjusted annual capitation amount per enrollee. Health plans would compete for consumers on the basis of risk-adjusted premiums. These systems would select healthcare providers, be responsible for monitoring quality, examine large data sets to develop evidence-based medicine guidelines, reduce widespread variations in physicians' practice patterns, provide coordinated care across different care settings (the physician's office, hospital, ambulatory care facility, and the patient's home), have incentives to innovate ways to care for patients with chronic conditions, and minimize total treatment costs (not just the costs of providing care in one setting while shifting costs to other settings). In addition, health plans would be responsible for evaluating new technologies and, in turn, would be evaluated by how well they perform in improving the health of their enrolled populations, their premiums, and patient satisfaction.

At the other end of the spectrum of financing and delivering medical services is consumer-directed healthcare (CDHC). Under the CDHC, consumers purchase a high-deductible (catastrophic) plan, which provides them with the incentive to be concerned about the use of medical services and the prices of different healthcare providers. The health savings account (HSA) approach combines a high-deductible plan with a savings account; money saved in the HSA belongs to the individual and can accumulate year after year.

Health plans preferred by consumers will expand their market share, while others will decline. Health plans and large multispecialty medical groups will have an incentive to innovate ways to reduce costs, improve quality and treatment outcomes, and achieve better patient satisfaction; by doing so, they will differentiate themselves from competitors and gain a competitive advantage. Other health plans will copy the methods applied by successful competitors, and the process of innovation and differentiation will start over again. (Economist Joseph Schumpeter referred to this as the process of *creative destruction*.)

Summary

Markets are evaluated by how closely they approximate a competitive market. The closer the approximation, the more likely the market will produce products efficiently and be responsive to consumer demands. Medical markets are not inherently different from other markets in their ability to efficiently allocate resources. It is the regulatory framework of medical markets that leads to inefficient outcomes.

Medical markets differ from competitive markets in significant ways. The tax treatment of health insurance lessens consumer incentives to be concerned about the price and use of medical services. Consumers lack the necessary information to make economic and medical choices; often, they are not offered choices. Competition among suppliers is limited by laws barring market entry, restricting the tasks health professionals are permitted to perform, preventing price competition, and regulating market prices.

These market failures have resulted in inefficiency, inappropriate care, less-than-optimal medical outcomes, and rapidly rising medical costs. Increased government regulation has been shown to worsen rather than improve market performance. Several of the major inefficiencies in medical care markets are the result of government intervention. Regulation to limit rising medical prices was tried in the 1970s and failed. Medicare, which controls hospital and physician fees, fails to limit overuse of services and gaming of the system; upcoding and unbundling of services are common.[11] Under a system of government regulation of prices, budgets, and entry restrictions, interest groups—such as hospitals, physicians, unions, and large employers—are more effective in representing their economic interests than (and at the expense of) consumers. Organized interest groups are more effective than consumers in the political marketplace. Consumer interests are best served in competitive economic markets.

Government has an important role to play. Government sets the rules for competitive markets, such as eliminating practices that result in anticompetitive behavior, monitoring inaccurate information, and enforcing antitrust laws. It is also government's responsibility to raise the funds to subsidize those unable to afford medical care; those subsidies can be provided at lower cost and higher quality in a competitive market.

Market competition has not failed in medical care. It just has not had a full opportunity to work. Consumer incentives must be changed so that consumers consider the costs and the benefits of their choices. When Medicare beneficiaries had to pay the additional cost of more expensive drug plans, drug plan competition responded by greatly lowering the projected cost of the Medicare drug benefit. Similarly, when employees were provided with a fixed amount for their surgeries (reference pricing) and had to pay the additional cost themselves, they were able to negotiate reduced prices. Medicare enrollees should be offered a choice of health plans and given the option to pay the additional cost of a more expensive plan, and restrictions on providers' ability to compete on price should be removed. Without competition, providers have no incentive to be efficient, innovate, invest in new facilities and services, improve quality, develop best practices and clinical guidelines, or lower prices.

Discussion Questions

1. Why is it said that competition in medical care has failed?
2. What are the criteria for a competitive market?
3. How well does medical care meet the criteria of a competitive market?
4. Is it the responsibility of a competitive market to subsidize care for those with low income?
5. Explain why the cost of the Medicare Part D drug benefit has been lower than its projections.
6. What changes are required for medical care to more closely approximate a competitive market?

Notes

1. Growth of demand may result in temporary increases in prices (high price markups over cost), which equilibrate demand and supply so that shortages do not occur while signaling suppliers to raise their production to meet the greater demand. Over time, as supply grows, prices will again reflect the cost of providing those services.
2. Not every consumer necessarily purchases more when the price is reduced, but, on average, the quantity demanded will rise.
3. The tax exclusion for employer-purchased health insurance is unfair because employees in a higher tax bracket receive a greater subsidy (see Exhibit 6.2). It is also unfair to individuals who are not part of an employer group, as they do not qualify for the same tax exclusion. Individual coverage is more expensive, not only because of higher marketing costs and insurers' concern about adverse selection but also because it is paid for with after-tax dollars.
4. Many small and medium-sized businesses were unable to offer their employees a choice of health plans; the indemnity plan was concerned that it would receive a higher-risk group. Thus, small businesses were typically offered only one plan for all of their employees.

5. Data on hospital quality—and to a lesser degree physician quality—have become available from more public sector and private sector sources. Such sources include Medicare's Hospital Compare (www.medicare.gov/hospitalcompare), the New York State Hospital Report Card (www.myhealthfinder.com), and Health Grades (www.healthgrades.com).

6. The ACA imposes a 40 percent tax on insurers of employer-sponsored health plans on the amount of employer-paid health insurance that exceeds $10,200 for individuals and $27,500 for family coverage starting in 2018.

7. Recent unsuccessful legislative proposals seeking to lower insurance premiums in the individual and small-group markets included permitting association health plans—organizations, such as non-employer groups, ethnic organizations, and small business associations—to form and negotiate with insurers on behalf of their members. These associations will have stable insurance pools and greater bargaining power with insurers. Further, legislation permitting insurers to sell their products across state lines will enable them to bypass costly state mandates.

8. In some markets, such as rural areas, competition among health plans is unlikely to be strong enough to achieve the same efficiency as in large urban areas. Rural populations do not have the same choices with regard to other services, either.

9. When a Medicare Advantage plan's bid is below the benchmark premium, the plan must provide additional benefits rather than pass the price difference on to the enrollee in the form of lower premiums. This difference results in drug plan enrollees paying lower premiums while Medicare Advantage plan enrollees must receive more benefits rather than have a choice of benefits versus lower premiums.

10. Goodman (2011) discusses how price competition also leads to quality competition.

11. Unbundling occurs when a provider charges separately for each of the services previously provided together as part of a treatment. Upcoding occurs when the provider bills for a higher-priced diagnosis or service than was provided.

References

Berenson, R., P. Ginsburg, and N. Kemper. 2010. "Unchecked Provider Clout in California Foreshadows Challenges to Health Reform." *Health Affairs* 29 (4): 699–705.

Centers for Medicare & Medicaid Services (CMS). 2014. "Tables." Accessed March. http://cms.gov/Research-Statistics-Data-and-Systems/Statistics-Trends-and-Reports/NationalHealthExpendData/Downloads/tables.pdf.

Cook, A. 2013. *Costs Under Medicare's Prescription Drug Benefit and a Comparison with the Cost of Drugs Under Medicaid Fee-for-Service.* Washington, DC: Congressional Budget Office. Published June 23. www.cbo.gov/sites/default/files/cbofiles/attachments/44366_AcademyHealthPresentation_Cook.pdf.

Enthoven, A. 2004. "Market Forces and Efficient Health Care Systems." *Health Affairs* 23 (2): 25–27.

———. 1993. "Why Managed Care Has Failed to Contain Health Costs." *Health Affairs* 12 (3): 27–43.

Enthoven, A., and L. Tollen. 2005. "Competition in Health Care: It Takes Systems to Pursue Quality and Efficiency." *Health Affairs* (web exclusive): W5-420–W5-433. http://content.healthaffairs.org/cgi/reprint/hlthaff.w5.420v1.

Goodman, J. 2011. "Will Price Competition Lead to Quality Competition?" *Health Affairs* blog, April 21. http://healthaffairs.org/blog/2011/04/21/will-price-competition-lead-to-quality-competition/.

Institute of Medicine (IOM). 2013. *Variation in Health Care Spending: Target Decision Making, Not Geography.* Washington, DC: National Academies Press. www.iom.edu/Reports/2013/Variation-in-Health-Care-Spending-Target-Decision-Making-Not-Geography.aspx.

Janicki, H. 2013. "Employment-Based Health Insurance: 2010." *Household Economic Studies.* Issued February. www.census.gov/prod/2013pubs/p70-134.pdf.

Jha, A., and A. Epstein. 2006. "The Predictive Accuracy of the New York State Coronary Artery Bypass Surgery Report-Card System." *Health Affairs* 25 (3): 844–55.

Marquis, S., and S. Long. 1999. "Trends in Managed Care and Managed Competition, 1993–1997." *Health Affairs* 18 (6): 75–88.

Robinson, J., and T. Brown. 2013. "Increases in Consumer Cost Sharing Redirect Patient Volumes and Reduce Hospital Prices for Orthopedic Surgery." *Health Affairs* 32 (8): 1392–97.

Robinson, J., and K. MacPherson. 2012. "Payers Test Reference Pricing and Centers of Excellence to Steer Patients to Low-Price and High-Quality Providers." *Health Affairs* 31 (9): 2028–36. http://content.healthaffairs .org/content/31/9/2028.full.

Rosenthal, J., X. Lu, and P. Cram. 2013. "Availability of Consumer Prices from US Hospitals for a Common Surgical Procedure." *JAMA Internal Medicine* 173 (6): 427–32. http://archinte.jamanetwork.com/article .aspx?articleID=1569848.

White, C., A. M. Bond, and J. D. Reschovsky. 2013. "High and Varying Prices for Privately Insured Patients Underscore Hospital Market Power." *HSC Research Brief* No. 27, September. Washington, DC: Center for Studying Health System Change. www.hschange.org/CONTENT/1375/.

COMPARATIVE EFFECTIVENESS RESEARCH

A s part of the $787 billion stimulus bill passed in 2010, $1.1 billion was allocated for comparative effectiveness research (CER). Included in the Affordable Care Act (ACA) of 2010 was an additional $3 billion for studies to compare the effectiveness of different treatments for the same illness. The different treatments to be analyzed include drugs, medical devices, surgery, and other ways of treating a specific medical condition.

CER and the Role of Government

What Is CER?

The scope of CER includes conducting, supporting, and synthesizing research that compares the clinical outcomes, effectiveness, and appropriateness of services and procedures used to prevent, diagnose, and treat diseases and other health conditions. CER involves three major areas: (1) comparing new treatments for an illness to the best available alternatives for treating that illness, (2) using the information from CER to improve joint physician and patient decision making, and (3) basing the data on which these comparative studies are to be conducted on a sufficiently large population.

Physicians lack information on the effectiveness of alternative treatments for many different diseases. For some illnesses, the relative effectiveness of alternative treatments has not been studied; for others, the results of effectiveness studies have not been disseminated to all physicians. The CER's federal coordinating council has developed a priority list of diseases and is awarding grants to study the comparative effectiveness of alternative treatments for diseases highest on the priority list. CER is a continuing process as it is conducted on more conditions and as new treatments become available for illnesses whose alternative treatments have since been studied (Conway and Clancy 2009).

Why Is the Government Supporting CER?

Public insurance programs, such as Medicare, and private health insurance pay for any medical treatment no matter how small the benefit or how large the cost. Under fee-for-service payment, neither insured patients nor their physicians have any incentive not to seek the most advanced medical treatments in search of a cure. Further, many policy experts acknowledge that insufficient information exists on which treatments work best for different diseases. New drugs are typically compared to a placebo rather than to an existing drug currently on the market.

Given the soaring cost of healthcare and the belief that each year hundreds of billions of dollars are spent on care that is of no value, more accurate information on which treatments perform better will improve quality of care and reduce the wide variations that occur in treatment methods, thereby reducing rising medical expenditures. Few people are opposed to providing consumers, physicians, and insurers with additional information on which treatments are more effective.

As shown in Exhibit 21.1, several well-known academic medical centers were compared according to their total reimbursements per decedent, hospital days per decedent, and reimbursement per day for treating a patient during the last two years of his or her life. Wide variations exist among these medical centers in each of these measures. The study authors further show that wide variations also exist among the underlying resources, such as nurse staffing and physician hours, used in treating these patients in the different

EXHIBIT 21.1
Medicare
Spending
per Decedent
During the Last
Two Years of
Life (Deaths
Occurring in
2010), Selected
Academic
Medical Centers

Academic Medical Center	Inpatient Reimbursements per Decedent	Hospital Days per Decedent	Reimbursements per Day
Johns Hopkins Hospital	$88,750	26.8	$3,311
Ronald Reagan UCLA Medical Center	$78,196	28.5	$2,740
University of Maryland Medical Center	$78,156	24.9	$3,135
Hahnemann University Hospital	$69,304	36.3	$1,909
Massachusetts General Hospital	$51,385	26.7	$1,925
Cleveland Clinic Foundation	$46,100	25.5	$1,807
Mayo Clinic–St. Mary's Hospital	$36,411	17.5	$2,082
Scott & White Memorial Hospital	$32,354	15.2	$2,127

SOURCE: Data from The Dartmouth Institute for Health Policy & Clinical Practice (2013).

institutions. The federal government can play a crucial role in aggregating information about the effectiveness of various medicines and treatments and disseminating that information to physicians and their patients.

Advocates of public funding for CER claim that such information has the characteristics of a public good—that is, everyone benefits from the information generated and that information cannot be denied to anyone once it becomes available. Because the information cannot be restricted to just those who pay for it, the private sector (health plans) will invest too little to develop such information. Many, therefore, want government to fund CER and assist in the dissemination of such information.

Concerns Over How CER Will Be Used

Using CER for Reimbursement

Funding for CER generated a great deal of controversy when it was enacted. Critics were concerned that once the effectiveness of two treatments or drugs were determined, the relative costs of the two treatments would also be used to determine which drugs should be used. Fearful of being accused of promoting "death panels," Congress prohibited the use of information based on CER for mandating coverage, reimbursement, or treatment decisions for public and private payers. However, many remain concerned that under the fiscal pressures of rising medical costs, use of results of the CER effort will eventually move closer to how European countries use their findings on comparative effectiveness (Nix 2012).

Some of the opponents of government-funded CER believe that the government would ultimately use the findings from such research to establish medical practice guidelines, limit access to treatments, and refuse to pay for expensive new drugs. Reinforcing this concern was the book by Tom Daschle, who was nominated by President Obama to become secretary of the Department of Health and Human Services (HHS). (He subsequently withdrew his name amid a growing controversy over his failure to accurately report and pay income taxes.) Daschle had proposed a federal health board that would promote high-value medical care by recommending coverage of drugs and procedures based on the board's research (Daschle, Greenberger, and Lambrew 2008).

Differences in Patient Responses to the Same Treatment

CER is a one-size-fits-all approach to medicine; however, widespread variation occurs in patient responses to different drugs. Patients who do not respond well to the recommended treatment are disadvantaged. For example, for most patients a generic drug is cheaper and works as well as a brand-name drug. However, for some patients the generic version may cause serious side effects or have little effect. Thus, although a branded and a generic drug may be equally effective on average, not paying for the newer, more expensive drug leads to increased hospitalization costs and worse health outcomes for those patients who do not respond well to the cheaper drug.

The problem of a one-size-fits-all approach is illustrated by a CER analysis of antipsychotic drugs, which found little difference existed between the effectiveness of older, less costly antipsychotic drugs and newer, more costly drugs. Using the older drugs could have saved Medicaid $1.2 billion (out of the $5.5 billion spent on these drugs in 2005). Basu, Jena, and Philipson (2011) concluded, however, that the mental health of thousands of patients would have been worse and that societal costs would have been greater than any savings in Medicaid costs from using the less costly drugs.

Variations in Medical Practice

While most agree that wide variation occurs in medical practice, huge amounts of money are wasted on ineffective treatments and testing, and more information is obviously beneficial, there is opposition to moving from information generation and dissemination to basing payment on CER.

A recent study attempted to explain why wide variations in medical spending occur. Using data on Medicare beneficiaries, Zuckerman and colleagues (2010) found that unadjusted Medicare spending per beneficiary was 52 percent greater in the highest-spending than in the lowest-spending geographic region. The authors then adjusted the regions based on demographics, baseline health characteristics, and changes in health status. After these adjustments, the difference between the highest and lowest regions decreased to 33 percent. Health status was found to explain an important part of this variation. Although inefficiency in spending per Medicare beneficiary exists, wide cost differences across geographic areas in Medicare spending are not the result of inefficiency alone.

Policies to decrease spending differences per beneficiary between high- and low-cost areas by reimbursing physicians only for treatments that follow certain protocols or guidelines should not ignore the legitimate reasons for some of these variations.

Accuracy and Timeliness of Comparative Effectiveness Studies

One study generally does not provide a definitive answer; several studies will likely have to be undertaken. For example, bone marrow transplantation for breast cancer was widely accepted as beneficial, and patients won lawsuits because some health plans refused to cover it. Subsequently, it was found that this treatment was ineffective.

Comparative effectiveness studies may not adequately evaluate alternative treatments for patients with multiple chronic diseases or rare illnesses. Similarly, CER often does not include sufficient numbers of women, African Americans, and Hispanics. Some drugs appear to be more effective in women than in men, while other medicines are more likely to cause serious complications in women. CER has to include larger numbers of patients in clinical trials so that gender and minority differences can be considered. As CER studies are expanded to account for such differences, the time and money needed to complete these clinical trials will increase (Chandra, Jena, and Skinner 2011).

Because it takes time to complete CER and for guidelines to be approved by the government, physicians and their patients may be willing to try untested therapies, as occurred for AIDS patients. Will they be permitted to do so? Will these therapies be reimbursed?

CER and Innovation

An additional concern is that CER might lead to slower adoption of new, more effective technologies. As new treatments and prescription drugs are developed, will reimbursement for them be delayed until their comparative effectiveness has been determined? Physicians might be willing to try new surgical techniques that offer improved patient outcomes; will they and the hospital have to forgo payment because these possibly innovative techniques have not undergone CER? Will the healthcare system become more rigid and less innovative because physicians fear repercussions if their treatments differ from the official guidelines? And will health plans refuse to reimburse for procedures and treatments that are not within the federal recommendations?

Medical device and pharmaceutical companies are also likely to face another layer of government approval that would increase their cost to bring a product to market, thereby decreasing their incentive for innovation.

Dissemination of CER Findings

CER results have to be disseminated. Will dissemination of information, which is often slow and may go against the financial interest of different physicians, be sufficient to have the CER adopted? Or will financial incentives and reporting requirements be necessary? A concern with providing information to physicians is that their adoption rate of new practices is very slow. If information is to change medical practice, lower costs, and improve quality, physician practice behavior will have to change more rapidly. However, without appropriate incentives, new information often takes years to change physician behavior.

Exhibit 21.2 provides several examples of the time it takes for treatment information to be disseminated to physicians. In 1988, the Food

EXHIBIT 21.2
Use of Acute
Interventions
(Pharmaceuticals)
for Myocardial
Infarction

Pharmaceuticals	Year of Innovation	Pharmaceutical Use[a]				
		1973–1977	1978–1982	1983–1987	1988–1992	1993–1996
Beta-blockers	1962	20.6	41.5	47.5	47.3	49.8
Calcium-channel blockers[b]	1971	0	0	63.9	59.0	31.0
ACE inhibitors	1979	0	—	—	—	56.0
Aspirin	1988[c]	15.0	14.1	20.1	62.0	75.0

[a] In hospital or 30-day use
[b] Calcium-channel blocker use increased rapidly in the early 1980s and then fell, following the publication of studies documenting potentially harmful effects of their use in acute management.
[c] In 1988, the Food and Drug Administration (FDA) proposed the use of aspirin for reducing the risk of recurrent myocardial infarction (MI) or heart attack and preventing first MI in patients with unstable angina. The FDA also approved the use of aspirin for the prevention of recurrent transient-ischemic attacks or "mini-strokes" in men and made aspirin standard therapy for previous strokes in men.
SOURCE: Data from Cutler, McClellan, and Newhouse (1999), tables 3 and 5.

and Drug Administration approved the use of aspirin for the treatment of heart attacks. Use of aspirin by physicians for the treatment of heart attacks increased from 20 percent to 62 percent. However, by the mid-1990s it had only increased to 75 percent. After studies were published indicating the potential harmful effects of calcium-channel blockers, their use declined but still remained above 30 percent ten years later.

Possible Stages in the Use of CER

Again, the legislation providing government funding for CER states that CER will not be used for reimbursement or coverage decisions. However, some people believe that government funding of CER is just the first stage of its evolution. These opponents foresee the following stages. First, CER provides information on the clinical effectiveness of different treatments and drugs for a particular disease. Second, their cost-effectiveness is compared. Third, given the rising costs of medical care and its increasing burden on the federal deficit, the federal government only pays for those drugs and treatments that are cost-effective, even though the effects may differ among people or population groups. Fourth, instead of deciding which drug to pay for on the basis of cost-effectiveness, the government decides which drugs and treatments to pay for by comparing the cost of the drug with the value of an additional year of life (as occurs in Great Britain).

The following sections discuss cost-effectiveness, how it might be used for reimbursement, and how it is used in Great Britain.

Cost-Effectiveness Analysis

Cost-effectiveness analysis compares the additional costs of alternative approaches to achieve a specific outcome designed to improve health. For example, an organization interested in decreasing hip fractures would want to know the different programs that can reduce hip fractures, the cost of expanding each program, and the extent of reduction in hip fractures each would achieve. Results from a cost-effectiveness analysis are typically presented in the form of a cost-effectiveness ratio, where the numerator of the ratio is the additional cost of the intervention and the denominator is some measure of the outcome of interest.

Alternative approaches for decreasing hip fractures are likely to differ in costs and effectiveness. Thus, they can be compared according to their cost-effectiveness ratio, which is the additional cost per averted hip fracture. (For an example of cost-effectiveness analysis, see Exhibit 3.3.)

Calculating the cost-effectiveness ratio for each alternative method of achieving a given health outcome allows the trade-offs of choosing one alternative over another to be compared. Decision makers—whether they are administrators in government agencies such as Medicaid or HMO managers—can make better-informed choices about the relative costs and effectiveness of alternative interventions by using cost-effectiveness analysis. When selecting among alternative expenditures to improve health, alternative interventions can be ranked according to their cost-effectiveness ratios (such as cost per death averted), giving the intervention with the lowest ratio the highest priority. Choosing according to those with the lowest cost-effectiveness ratio maximizes the outcome for a given budget.

Many cost-effectiveness studies have been conducted on the relative effectiveness of a new drug compared to existing drugs for treating the same disease. The originators of such studies include health plans seeking to determine which drugs to include in their formularies and pharmaceutical firms hoping to use their results to demonstrate to large purchasers the greater effectiveness of their new drugs when compared to the drugs of competitors.

A concern with cost-effectiveness analysis if it were used for reimbursement by the government is that, as discussed earlier, patients may differ in their response to different drugs or treatments. Medical costs could be higher if patients respond poorly to certain drugs and have to be hospitalized. Further, the cost-effectiveness ratio to the government may be different than the patient's cost or evaluation of the treatment's effectiveness.

Quality-Adjusted Life Years

A specific type of cost-effectiveness analysis uses quality-adjusted life years (QALYs) as an outcome measure. QALYs are an outcome measure indicating the increased utility achieved as the result of an intervention, such as comparing a new drug to an existing one. The cost-effectiveness ratios are in terms of the cost per QALYs gained. The advantage of using QALYs rather than, for example, life expectancy is that QALY incorporates multiple outcomes—increase in length of life and quality of life. Using QALYs as an outcome measure also enables comparisons to be made across different disease conditions.

QALY is calculated as follows: Each additional year of perfect health for an individual is assigned a value of 1.0, which is the highest value of a complete QALY. The assigned value decreases as health decreases, with death equal to 0.0. If the patient has various limitations—such as a disability, physical pain, or being on kidney dialysis—the extra life years are assigned a value between 1.0 and 0.0. Thus, if new intervention A enables a person to live an additional five years, but with a quality of life weight of 0.7, then the QALY score for that intervention is 5 × 0.7 = 3.5 QALYs. If intervention B extends life for four years with a quality of life weight of 0.6, the additional QALYs provided are 4 × 0.6 = 2.4. The net benefit of intervention A over intervention B is 3.5 QALYs – 2.4 QALYs = 1.1 QALYs.

When comparing alternative interventions according to their additional cost per QALY, those with a lower cost per QALY are preferred to those with a higher cost per QALY.

A common approach for developing QALYs involves the use of an Activities of Daily Living (ADL) scale. Patients are asked to rate their ability to function independently, such as dressing, bathing, and walking. Patient responses range from unable to perform the function to able to perform the function without difficulty. These scores are summed up over all the ADL categories to arrive at a patient's overall functional status.

The calculation of QALYs is the same regardless of a person's income, wealth, or age, and QALYs that occur in later years may be valued less than QALYs that occur earlier in life.[1]

QALYs have several drawbacks. For example, QALY does not include the effects of a patient's disability on the quality of life of others, such as family members. Assigning a quantitative value to a disability may not be accurate because people differ in their perception of the severity of various limitations to their normal activity. Further, applying these utility measures across a large, diverse population having differing utility preferences is unlikely to reflect many individuals' utility preferences. And yet developing QALY to be used for a large population is necessary if alternative medical treatments are to be compared.

Applications of QALYs

QALYs have been used in two types of policy analysis. First, QALYs are used as an outcome measure in cost-effectiveness analysis to compare alternative interventions in determining which intervention offers the lowest cost per QALY. Second, and more controversial, cost per QALY has been used to determine benefit coverage—for example, to decide whether a costly treatment, such as an expensive new drug, should be provided to a breast cancer patient.

Exhibit 21.3 shows the results of several cost-effectiveness studies examining different drug therapies potentially applicable for the Medicare

Intervention vs. Base Case in Target Population	Dollars per QALY Gained
Captopril therapy vs. No captopril in 80-year-old patients surviving myocardial infarction	4,000
Treatment with mesalazine vs. No treatment to maintain remission in Crohn's disease	6,000
One-year course of isoniazid (INH) chemoprophylaxis vs. No INH chemoprophylaxis in 55-year-old white male tuberculin reactors with no other risk factors	18,000
Treatment to reduce the incidence of osteoporotic hip fracture vs. No treatment in 62-year-old woman with established osteoporosis	34,000
Ticlopidine vs. Aspirin in 65-year-old with high risk of stroke	48,000
Chemotherapy vs. No chemotherapy in 75-year-old with breast cancer	58,000
Captopril vs. Propranolol in persons in the US population aged 35–64 without the diagnosis of coronary heart disease but with essential hypertension	150,000
Antiemetic therapy with ondansetron vs. Antiemetic therapy with metoclopramide in 70-kg. patient receiving cisplatin chemotherapy who had not been previously exposed to antineoplastic agents	$460,000

EXHIBIT 21.3
Selected Cost-Effectiveness Ratios for Pharmaceuticals, with a Focus on the Medicare Population

SOURCE: Adapted from Neumann and colleagues (2000), Exhibit 3.

population. Each of the studies describes an intervention compared to the alternative of no treatment. The results—in the form of cost per QALY gained—are ranked from lowest to highest cost per QALY. Therapies whose cost per QALY is relatively low (such as $4,000) are very favorable. Therapies with a relatively high cost per QALY (such as $460,000) are considered unfavorable and less likely to be adopted.

The National Institute for Health and Clinical Excellence

Great Britain established the National Health Service (NHS) in 1948 as a single-payer system, administered by the government, funded through taxation, and provided by public institutions. The British government has a long history of underfunding the NHS, resulting in long waiting lines and failure to provide certain types of treatments. To limit expenditures on expensive innovative medical technology and drugs and to attempt to rationalize its limited budget, in 1999 the government formed the National Institute for Health and Clinical Excellence (NICE)—a private, independent organization in the Department of Health—to provide guidance on health technology, clinical medicine, and new prescription drugs, basing its decisions on clinical efficacy and cost-effectiveness (NICE 2013; Rawlins 2013).

NICE uses QALYs to determine which treatments to cover in the NHS. Given that budget constraints exist on the amount the government can spend for medical services, NICE undertakes cost-effectiveness analysis for new drugs and treatments in an attempt to provide patients, health professionals, and the public with scientifically based guidance on current best practices. A NICE committee consisting of medical and other professionals—such as health economists, statisticians, managers, patient advocates, and manufacturer representatives—assists in its decision making.

Before NICE was established, availability of costly treatments varied greatly throughout the country, as did the level of medical services. NICE has made the availability of drugs and treatments more uniform throughout the NHS. Decisions by NICE are transparent to all, and the information used by NICE for its decisions is also publicly available. Further, when NICE believes that a particular treatment or drug is cost-beneficial, it will attempt to ensure that the treatment or drug becomes widely available.

The main criticism of NICE is that it bases its recommendations more on cost-effectiveness than on clinical effectiveness (Hope 2011; Steinbrook 2008). The criticism of NICE for being "coldhearted" stems from the fact that it uses cost per QALY to determine cost-effectiveness. One of NICE's most contentious criteria is how much should be paid per additional year of life that a drug is expected to provide. NICE's general threshold is about

$48,000 per QALY. If a treatment has a cost per QALY above that, NICE will generally deny the treatment.

The following example illustrates how NICE uses its cost per QALY to determine approval for costly treatments. A *New York Times* article tells the story of patient Bruce Hardy, who was fighting kidney cancer that was spreading throughout his body (Harris 2008). His physician wanted to prescribe a new drug from Pfizer called Sutent, which delays cancer progression for six months at a cost of $54,000. NICE, however, decided that the drug was too costly to be offered free to all those who needed it. According to NICE, the cost of saving six months of life should be no more than $22,750; therefore, Hardy could not receive the drug. When NICE rejected Sutent, some patients mortgaged their homes to pay for the drug on their own. (After much protest, NICE reversed its decision and approved the drug.) NICE has also limited the use of certain breast cancer drugs, such as Herceptin, and drugs for osteoporosis and multiple sclerosis.

Great Britain has been explicit in recognizing that resources are scarce and that choices must be made on how to allocate those scarce resources. At some point, with rising medical costs and a huge government deficit, will the United States become as explicit or, more likely, make such decisions implicitly by limiting healthcare provider reimbursement and thereby limiting the resources available for new technology and expensive drugs?

Summary

CER should provide additional information to physicians and their patients regarding the effectiveness of alternative treatments. To the extent that wide variations in medical practice are the result of lack of information, CER should improve patient outcomes and reduce medical costs. However, if the findings from CER are used for reimbursement or coverage decisions, some patients may suffer adverse health consequences and the medical system could become less innovative.

Some policy experts are concerned that federal funding for CER is but the first step toward limiting government payment for treatments considered less effective than others or for treatments that are too expensive for their return in extending life expectancy. If CER studies demonstrate that a new drug for $1,000 a year provides greater benefits than a $50,000 surgical procedure, but the financial incentive for many surgeons is to continue performing the more expensive treatment, will insurers and the government continue to pay for both treatments? Great Britain's NICE is often cited as an example of a government agency that determines which medical treatments will be covered based on cost-effectiveness. Using cost-effectiveness, NICE covers only those treatments that do not exceed a certain threshold, such as the cost per QALY not exceeding the value of a life. Although the ACA states that CER shall not be used as a basis for payment, some are concerned that the United States may eventually use cost-effectiveness in reimbursement of medical services.

Society cannot spend an infinite amount of money to extend each person's life; society must make choices. Economics requires trade-offs because resources are scarce and can be spent on enhancing life in other ways. The opportunity cost of spending $100,000 on a new drug that would extend the life of a terminally ill patient by three months is that those same funds could have been spent on prenatal care or to increase the life expectancy of very low–birth-weight infants. Spending resources on additional medical services to extend one person's life involves having fewer resources to spend on extending the lives of others. States and the federal government, faced with higher limits on their expenditures and increasing demands for costly medical services, will have to make difficult choices in coming years.

The proposal to have a separate federal health board to make difficult political decisions regarding which medical services and prescription drugs to fund insulates legislators from making these difficult choices, such as denying expensive but potentially life-extending services to a patient whose need for the treatment is discussed in the media.

Discussion Questions

1. What are the advantages of CER?
2. What are disadvantages of using CER for federal payment?
3. What are QALYs?
4. How are QALYs used in cost-effectiveness analysis?
5. How does NICE use QALYs in determining whether to approve a new drug?

Note

1. When interventions produce QALYs over different time periods, discounting may be used to convert them into equivalently valued units at the present period, similar to discounting future income streams (as is done in a cost–benefit analysis). To determine the present value of future QALYs, the number of QALYs in each future year should be multiplied by $(1/1 + rt)$, where r is the discount rate—such as 0.05—and t represents the number of years from the future to the present.

Additional Reading

Health Affairs volume 31, issue number 10 (October 2012) as well as volume 29, issue number 10 (October 2010) contain many excellent articles on CER. See http://content.healthaffairs.org/content/31/10/.toc http://content .healthaffairs.org/content/vol29/issue10/index.dtl?etoc.

References

Basu, A., A. Jena, and T. Philipson. 2011. "Impact of Comparative Effectiveness Research on Health and Healthcare Spending." *Journal of Health Economics* 30 (4): 695–706.

Chandra, A., A. Jena, and J. Skinner. 2011. "The Pragmatist's Guide to Comparative Effectiveness Research." *Journal of Economic Perspectives* 25 (2): 27–46.

Conway, P., and C. Clancy. 2009. "Comparative-Effectiveness Research— Implications of the Federal Coordinating Council's Report." *New England Journal of Medicine* 361: 328–30. www.nejm.org/doi/full/10.1056/ NEJMp0905631.

Cutler, D., M. McClellan, and J. Newhouse. 1999. "The Costs and Benefits of Intensive Treatment for Cardiovascular Disease." In *Measuring the Prices of Medical Treatments*, edited by J. Triplett, pp. 34–71. Washington, DC: The Brookings Institution.

The Dartmouth Institute for Health Policy & Clinical Practice, Center for Health Policy Research. 2013. "Care of Chronically Ill Patients During the Last Two Years of Life." *The Dartmouth Atlas of Health Care*. www .dartmouthatlas.org/tools/downloads.aspx#l2ychron.

Daschle, T., S. Greenberger, and J. Lambrew. 2008. *Critical: What We Can Do About the Health-Care Crisis*. New York: Thomas Dunne Books.

Harris, G. 2008. "British Balance Benefit vs. Cost of Latest Drugs." *New York Times*, December 2. www.nytimes.com/2008/12/03/health/03nice. html?pagewanted=all&_r=0.

Hope, J. 2011. "Breakthrough MS Pill Rejected as too Expensive by NHS Watchdog (But You Can Get It in U.S. and Germany." *Mail Online*, August 5. www.dailymail.co.uk/health/article-2022767/Miracle-MS-pill- rejected-expensive-NHS-watchdog-available-U-S-Germany.html.

National Institute for Health and Care Excellence (NICE). 2013. "About." Copyright 2014. www.nice.org.uk/aboutnice/.

Neumann, P. J., E. A. Sandberg, C. M. Bell, P. W. Stone, and R. H. Chapman. 2000. "Are Pharmaceuticals Cost-Effective? A Review of the Evidence." *Health Affairs* (19) 2: 98.

Nix, K. 2012. "Comparative Effectiveness Research Under Obamacare: A Slippery Slope to Health Care Rationing." *Backgrounder* No. 2679. Washington, DC: The Heritage Foundation. www.heritage.org/research/reports/2012/04/comparative-effectiveness-research-under-obamacare-a-slippery-slope-to-health-care-rationing.

Rawlins, M. 2013. "NICE-Moving Onward." *New England Journal of Medicine* 369: 3–5. www.nejm.org/doi/full/10.1056/NEJMp1303907?query=health-policy-and-reform.

Steinbrook, R. 2008. "Saying No Isn't NICE—The Travails of Britain's National Institute of Health and Clinical Effectiveness." *New England Journal of Medicine* 359 (19): 1977–81. www.uiowa.edu/~ibl/documents/Steinbrook.pdf.

Zuckerman, S., T. Waldman, R. Berenson, and J. Hadley. 2010. "Clarifying Sources of Geographic Differences in Medicare Spending." *New England Journal of Medicine* 363: 54–62.

US COMPETITIVENESS AND RISING HEALTHCARE COSTS

One of the oft-cited reasons for controlling the rise in healthcare costs has been that it makes American business less competitive internationally. Automobile manufacturing executives, for example, have complained that their competitors in other countries have lower healthcare costs per employee, enabling them to sell their products at a lower price than US manufacturers do.[1] After labor costs, healthcare is often the largest cost for many firms. GM estimated that its employees' healthcare expenses were increasing faster than any other single cost incurred in producing a vehicle (Storm n.d.). Unless healthcare costs can be controlled, the executives claim, US business will be priced out of international markets and foreign producers will increase their market share in the United States.

Do rising healthcare costs really make US industries less competitive than their foreign counterparts? To understand this controversy, we must consider who actually bears the burden of higher employee medical costs—the employee, the firm, or the consumer?

Who Pays for Higher Employee Medical Costs?

The market for labor is competitive. Firms compete for different types of labor, and employees compete for jobs. This competition results in similar prices for specific types of labor. For example, if a hospital pays its nurses less than do other hospitals in the area, the nurses will move to the hospital that pays the highest wages. Not all nurses have to change jobs to bring about similar pay among hospitals. Some nurses will move, and the hospital will find it difficult to replace them. The hospital will soon realize that its pay levels are below what nurses are receiving elsewhere. In reality, not all firms have the same working conditions, nor are they located next to one another. Employees are willing to accept lower pay for more pleasant conditions and require higher pay to travel longer distances. The greater the similarity in how firms treat their employees and the more closely they are located, the more quickly wage differences disappear.

When an employer hires an additional employee, the cost of that addition cannot exceed the value of the employee to the firm; otherwise, the firm will not profit from the hiring. The total cost to the firm of an employee consists of two parts: cash wages and noncash fringe benefits. The cost of hiring an additional worker is the total compensation—cash and noncash benefits—that the employer has to pay to that employee. The employer does not care whether employees want 90 percent of their total compensation in cash and 10 percent in noncash fringe benefits or a cash–noncash ratio of 60 to 40. The employer is only interested in an employee's total cost.

Employees working in high-wage industries typically prefer a higher ratio of fringe benefits to cash wages because of the tax advantages of having benefits purchased with pretax income. Low-wage industries typically provide their employees with few benefits; most of their compensation is in cash income. The combination of cash and noncash income reflects the preferences of employees, not employers. If an employer compensates its low-wage employees with a high proportion of fringe benefits, the employees will seek the same total compensation at another firm that pays them a higher ratio of cash wages.

What happens when the fringe benefits portion of total compensation rises sharply, as occurs when health insurance premiums increase? For example, assume that employees in a particular industry are expected to receive a 5 percent increase in compensation next year, but health insurance premiums—which are paid by the employer and represent 10 percent of the employees' total compensation—are expected to rise by 20 percent. The employer is always concerned with the total cost of its employees; thus, cash wages in that industry would rise by only 3.3 percent. There is a trade-off between fringe benefits and cash wages.[2]

If one firm in the industry paid its employees 5 percent higher wages plus the 20 percent increase in insurance premiums, that firm would have higher labor costs than all the other firms in the industry. What are the consequences to the firm? To incur above-market labor costs, the firm would either have to make less profit or raise the prices of the products it sells. If the firm were to make less profit, it would earn a lower return on invested capital. A lower return on invested capital will lead investors to move their capital to other firms in the industry, to other industries, or to other countries where they can earn a higher return. Capital knows no loyalties or geographic boundaries; it will move to receive the highest return (consistent with a given level of risk). Thus, higher labor costs cannot impose a permanently lower return to a firm; otherwise, the firm will shrink as it loses capital. The same would be true if labor costs among all firms in the industry increased and profits declined.

What if the firm or industry passes the higher labor costs on to consumers by raising its prices? As long as the firm's products have competitors—either from other firms in the industry or from manufacturers in other countries—and as long as consumers are price sensitive to the firm's product, the firm will lose sales.[3] Good substitutes to any firm's (or industry's) product are generally available, either from other products or other manufacturers. Thus, large price differences for the same or similar products cannot be maintained. The failure to keep prices in line with a competitor's prices will reduce sales, with a consequent flight of capital from that firm or industry.

As long as competition from other firms or from foreign competitors (or both) is possible and capital can move to other industries and countries, rising medical costs will not result in lower profits or higher prices but will be borne by employees in the form of lower cash wages.

Short-Term Effects

Although rising medical costs are typically carried by the employee in the form of lower cash wages, an employer could experience a short-term effect on its profits. Shifting the cost of health insurance back to employees is difficult in the short run. For example, if an employer did not anticipate how rapidly medical costs would increase and (perhaps because of a long-term labor agreement) the firm is unable to lower its employees' wages to compensate for the higher-than-expected medical costs, profitability could decline.

Few firms, however, have been unaware of how rapidly medical costs have been rising; thus, these growing costs are built into labor agreements. However, medical costs could also rise less rapidly than anticipated, boosting profitability. In any case, unanticipated cost increases will be reflected in future wage agreements and will not affect profitability over time.

An Example

The following example illustrates why labor bears the burden of higher insurance premiums. Automobiles can be produced in Michigan or in the southern part of the United States. Unless the prices of cars produced in Michigan and in the South are the same, consumers will purchase the least expensive cars, assuming their quality is similar. Unless labor costs and productivity were similar in both places, the automobile manufacturers would move their production facilities to the less costly location to produce the car. Yet we observe that, in the automobile industry, employees' medical costs and insurance premiums are higher in Detroit than in the South. How can cars produced in the North compete with cars produced in the South?

Medical costs per employee could be higher in the North as long as northern employees' cash wages are lower. Unless total compensation per employee is the same in both places, the cars produced in different locations could not be sold at the same price and manufacturers would shift their production to the lower-cost site.

Effect of Unions

What if an industry was strongly unionized and the firms in that industry were not permitted to hire nonunion labor? Could the union then shift its higher medical costs to the firm or consumers? The extent to which a union can increase labor costs is always limited by the potential loss of its members' jobs. If US manufacturers raise their prices relative to their competitors, foreign competition and price-sensitive consumers will cause them to suffer declines in sales and profits. Even when foreign competitors are prevented from competing with US manufacturers, consumers will demand fewer automobiles as prices rise, although the declines would be less than if greater competition were permitted. Firms facing decreased demands for their products would hire fewer employees. A powerful union that is willing to accept a certain loss of its members' jobs by forcing firms to raise its members' compensation would do so regardless of whether the increase was for medical benefits or wages. Thus, greater medical benefits to the union members still come at the expense of higher wages.

Exhibit 22.1 illustrates the effect of rising medical costs on employees' wages. After 1973, total employee compensation rose less rapidly than previously because of a slowdown in employee productivity. The difference between total compensation and wages grew as a greater portion of employees' total compensation went to pay for fringe benefits. Between 1973 and 1990, employers' contributions to their employees' health insurance premiums "absorbed more than half of workers' real (adjusted for inflation) gains in compensation, even though health insurance represented 5 percent or less of total compensation" (CBO 1992, 5).

Total employee compensation increased in the 1990s, reflecting growth in productivity. However, wages and salaries remained relatively constant from the late 1980s until the mid-1990s, reflecting the greater importance of health insurance and retirement plans in employee compensation. Until the mid-1990s, employees' wages rose very slowly because most of the increase in compensation went to pay for higher health and retirement benefits.

From the late 1990s to 2000, total employee compensation and wages soared, again reflecting greater productivity. However, in contrast to the earlier period of the late 1980s to the mid-1990s, wages increased at a slightly faster rate than total compensation; cost-containment activities by managed care plans resulted in a slower growth in premiums and greater wage increases for employees (see Exhibit 19.3). The late 1990s, however, saw a backlash against restrictive managed care plans, with the consequence that between 2001 and 2012, total compensation once again rose faster than wages.

Rising medical costs have had a large effect on employees' take-home pay; employees have had less to spend on other goods and services. For this

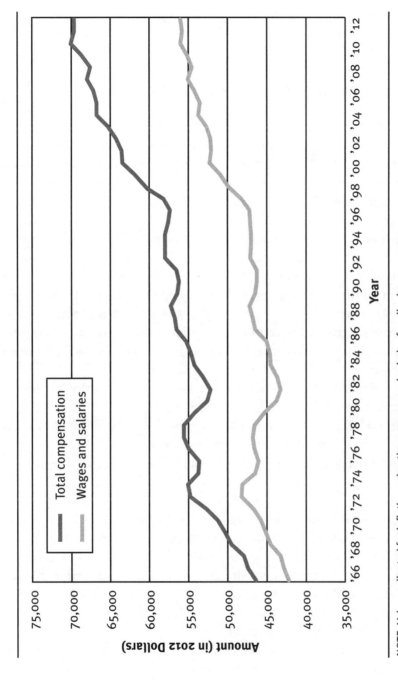

EXHIBIT 22.1
Inflation-Adjusted Compensation and Wages per Full-Time Employee, 1965–2012

NOTE: Values adjusted for inflation using the consumer price index for all urban consumers.
SOURCE: Data from Bureau of Economic Analysis (2013).

reason, unions have been strong advocates of using government controls to limit rising healthcare costs.

Who Pays for Retiree Medical Costs?

During labor negotiations in past years, many employers agreed to provide their employees with medical benefits when they retire, in return for wage concessions.[4] In 2013, 28 percent of large firms—those with 200 or more workers—that offered health benefits to their employees provided retiree coverage (down from 66 percent in 1988 and 34 percent in 2000). Only about 5 percent of small firms—those with 3 to 199 workers—offer retiree health benefits (Kaiser Family Foundation and HRET 2013, exhibits 11.1 and 11.2). At the time, employers agreed to provide their employees with medical benefits, retiree medical costs were much lower than they are today, and employers undoubtedly underestimated how costly they could become. Instead of setting aside funds to pay these retiree obligations, as one would do with a pension obligation, firms paid their retirees' medical costs on a "pay-as-you-go" basis; that is, they paid their retirees' medical costs when they were incurred, out of current operating expenses.

Funding retiree medical costs changed as a result of a ruling by the Financial Accounting Standards Board that, starting in 1993, firms had to set aside funds for such benefits as they are earned. That is, retiree medical benefits must be treated similarly to pension benefits; as employees earn credit toward their retirement, the firm must set aside funds to pay for those employees' medical costs when they retire. Further, the unfunded liability for current and future retirees must be accounted for on the firm's balance sheet. Firms were shocked by the size of their unfunded obligations. GM, for example, in 2005 had an unfunded liability for its current and future retirees' medical costs of $77 billion (Seider and Williamson 2005). This liability had to be listed on its balance sheet, and an equivalent amount had to be deducted from the firm's net worth. GM's stockholders' equity was thereby decreased by $77 billion. In addition, GM had to expense part of that liability each year. For 2005, GM's earnings had to be reduced by $5.6 billion.

How did firms such as GM pay off these huge unfunded liabilities? Did they raise the prices of their products, harming US competitiveness? If they raised their prices, they would lose sales to competitors, both in the United States and overseas, that did not make such commitments to their employees. That evidently did not happen. Thus, US competitiveness is not harmed by firms having to list unfunded retiree medical benefits on their balance sheets. (In view of the automobile industry's deteriorating financial condition, in 2008 GM—together with Ford and Chrysler—reached an agreement with the UAW to form a union-run retiree healthcare fund called Voluntary Employee Beneficiary Association. GM was released from UAW retiree healthcare claims incurred after 2009. The total value of the healthcare trust was about $60 billion, with GM providing around $33 billion, Ford roughly $15 billion, and Chrysler about $9 billion [Smerd 2008].)

Employers also cannot reduce the wages of current employees to pay for unfunded obligations to current retirees. If they were to do so, the firm would lose its employees. The labor market is competitive. If a firm decides to reduce its employees' wages, those employees will move to firms whose retirees have not been promised medical benefits. Instead, firms are likely to use current and future profits to pay off this liability, in which case the stockholders will be the losers.

Some firms have reneged on their promises to their retirees by either reducing benefits or requiring them to pay part of the cost; they have tried to shift these obligations from their stockholders back to their retirees. Retirees responded by bringing lawsuits against their former employers. Court rulings, however, have generally allowed employers to reduce or eliminate the benefits for salaried, nonunion retirees, even years after they have retired. When a firm declares bankruptcy and is reorganized, it is able to reduce its obligations to its unionized employees and retirees. If firms with large retiree liabilities declare bankruptcy, the stockholders, bondholders, employees, and retirees will all have to make some sacrifice for the firm to be viable again. Another option for lowering retiree medical costs is for the firm and its union to agree to such a reduction to prevent the firm from having to declare bankruptcy, in which case the retirees, the current employees, and the firm's stockholders would likely suffer greater losses. GM's renegotiation of retiree health benefits with its union to form a union-run fund is an example of this approach.

Rising medical costs will not directly affect US competitiveness by forcing firms to increase their prices. Instead, these higher costs will be borne by the employees themselves, who will receive lower cash wages. Similarly, the huge unfunded retiree medical liabilities will also not affect US competitiveness because these liabilities will not be paid off by raising prices but will be shifted to the firm's stockholders in the form of less equity. Do rising medical costs have any adverse effects on the economy and US competitiveness?

Possible Adverse Effects of Rising Medical Costs on the US Economy

Rising medical costs could adversely affect the US balance of trade if they were the major cause of the increased federal deficit or decreased private savings.

Increase in the Federal Deficit

The argument on the deficit is as follows. Government expenditures for Medicare and Medicaid are the fastest-increasing portion of the federal deficit. In 1970, federal spending on these two programs represented 1 percent of gross domestic product (GDP). The Congressional Budget Office (CBO) estimated that spending on these programs would represent 5.3 percent of GDP in 2013 (up from 5.2 percent in 2012). This figure is expected to reach 6.4 percent by 2023 (CBO 2013, tables 1.1 and 1.3). If left unchanged, these two programs will represent an increasing percentage of the federal government's nonhealth spending. To fund these additional expenditures, the government will have to increase its borrowing.

A higher level of government borrowing to finance a larger federal deficit will increase the value of the dollar relative to other currencies because interest rates in the United States will rise with the greater government demand for savings. In the process of moving their funds to the United States to take advantage of the higher interest rates, foreign investors will demand more dollars, which will increase their value. With a higher exchange value of the dollar, the prices of US-produced goods rise and foreign goods become less expensive. As the relative prices of US and foreign goods change, domestic manufacturers will sell less overseas, and imports into this country will go up as the price of foreign goods falls. American competitiveness and the trade balance will worsen.

However, the blame for the rising budget deficit need not be placed only on rising medical costs. Many government programs contribute to the deficit, and many are of less value than Medicare and Medicaid. The deficit could be lowered by reducing expenditures on these other programs, such as farm subsidies, tax exempt employer paid health insurance, and those military projects whose sole purpose is to maintain jobs in a community. Emphasizing medical spending as the cause of the growing federal deficit shifts attention from these other programs and decreases the government's incentives for eliminating wasteful programs that provide less benefit than medical expenditures. Reducing expenditures on Medicare and Medicaid could also merely result in shifting these savings into expanding other or creating new government programs. (To the extent medical services are inefficiently provided, patient and provider incentives should be changed so that patients and third-party payers receive more value for their money.)

Decrease in Private Savings

The second way increased medical spending could adversely affect the American economy is if private savings were reduced. To finance the federal deficit, the government has had to borrow, which has left less savings available for the private sector to invest in plant, equipment, and new ventures.

Lower private investment eventually means lower productivity and lower real income. The CBO (1992) estimated that if federal spending on Medicare and Medicaid had been limited to its 1991 share of GDP, real income would have been 2.4 percent higher by the year 2002.

Similar to the effects of government spending, rising medical costs cause the public to spend more on medical services, decreasing the amount it has available to save. Consequently, savings in the private sector decline, as do private investments. The argument blaming the lower rate of savings on rising medical expenditures is similar to blaming the growing federal deficit just on Medicare and Medicaid. The government could cut the deficit by eliminating and reducing other government programs. Medicare and Medicaid, while being significant contributors, are not the sole cause of large federal deficits.

It is not clear that rising medical costs decrease or increase the private savings rate. Having health insurance may lessen the need for a person to save for his medical expenses. However, medical expenses increase with age, more out-of-pocket payments may be required; as people live longer, they will have to save for their long-term care needs if they do not want to rely on Medicaid (and have to spend down their assets to qualify). The expectation of higher medical costs and new technology may cause people to raise their savings. The effect of rising medical expenses on savings is uncertain.

The notion that the growth in medical expenditures should be limited because it raises consumption and reduces savings for investment is also a fallacy. Some medical expenditures are, in fact, investments that increase productivity, such as preventive measures and certain surgical procedures that enable a person to resume normal activity. More important, if increasing the savings rate by decreasing consumption is desired, many other consumer activities—some of which are harmful, such as alcohol and cigarette consumption—should probably be reduced before limits are placed on medical spending. Many people would place a higher value on medical services than on other goods and services.

Summary

It is not clear that increased spending on healthcare, efficiently provided, has harmful effects on the economy, the budget deficit, or American competitiveness, as some have suggested. The fact that employees rather than employers bear the cost of rising healthcare benefits should not mean, however, that employers are absolved of the responsibility of ensuring that those funds are well spent. As Uwe Reinhardt (1989, 20) stated,

> Even if every increase in the cost of employer-paid healthcare benefits could immediately be financed by the firm with commensurate reductions

in the cash compensation of its employees—so that "competitiveness" in the firm's product market is not impaired—it would leave employees worse off unless the added health spending is valued at least as highly as the cash wages they would forego [sic] to finance these benefits. Because it is the perceived value of a firm's compensation package that lures workers to the firm and away from competing opportunities, the typical business firm has every economic incentive to maximize this perceived value per dollar of healthcare expenditure debited to the firm's payroll expense account. Therein, and not in "competitiveness" on the product side, lies the most powerful rationale for vigorous healthcare cost containment on the part of the American business community.

Discussion Questions

1. What determines the ratio of cash to noncash (fringe benefits) compensation that an employer will pay to its employees?
2. What are the consequences of an employer raising its prices to pay for its employees' higher medical costs?
3. How can employees of automobile companies in Michigan receive more costly health benefits than their counterparts in the South while automobiles produced in both locations sell for the same price?
4. Even if employees bear the entire cost (in terms of lower cash wages) of rising medical costs, why should employers still be concerned with cost containment?
5. Evaluate the following statement: Rising healthcare costs are harmful to the economy because greater consumption expenditures on medical services result in lower savings, hence reduced private investment.
6. Evaluate the following statement: Rising Medicare and Medicaid expenditures contribute to the growing federal deficit. To finance this larger deficit, the government must borrow more, which in turn increases interest rates, raises the value of the dollar, and consequently makes US goods more expensive than foreign-produced goods.

Notes

1. At a meeting of the National Governors Association, former Ford Motor Company vice chairman Allan Gilmour stated that high healthcare costs could force Detroit automakers to invest overseas rather than in the United States to remain profitable. Ford spent $3.2 billion on healthcare in 2003 for 560,000 employees, retirees,

and dependents. These costs added $1,000 to the price of every Ford vehicle built in the United States, up from $700 three years previously. Gilmour stated that their foreign competitors do not share these problems, and if healthcare costs are not controlled, investment will be driven overseas. He called on state governors to pass legislation to control healthcare costs (Mayne 2004).

2. Tax-exempt employer-paid health insurance disguises the cost of health insurance to the employee. Because the federal government taxes wages and not health benefits, many employees are unaware of how much they have forgone in wages as a result of rising health benefit costs. If employees were more aware of the trade-off between wages and health benefits, they would become more cost conscious in their choice of health plans.

3. The following is an example of how global competitiveness affects a firm's sales and labor costs. Delphi, a US firm that sells automotive components, was forced into bankruptcy because of its high labor costs. To emerge from bankruptcy, it had to reduce its US labor costs. The firm paid its US unionized employees $27 an hour, but when health and retirement benefits were included, its labor costs rose to $65 an hour. Delphi's Asian operations were highly profitable. In China, it paid its workers about $3 an hour, about a third of which was for medical and pension benefits (Sapsford and Areddy 2005).

4. Early retirees who are not eligible for Medicare are more costly than those who are eligible. Early-retiree health benefits cost, on average, $14,988 in 2010, whereas Medicare-eligible retirees cost firms $7,848 on average. For retirees on Medicare, the firm usually pays for the portion of the retiree's medical expenses not covered by Medicare, such as deductibles and copayments (Towers Perrin 2009, Exhibit 1).

References

Bureau of Economic Analysis. 2013. "National Data: GDP and Personal Income." www.bea.gov/iTable/index_nipa.cfm.

Congressional Budget Office (CBO). 2013. *The Budget and Economic Outlook: Fiscal Years 2013 to 2023*. Washington, DC: CBO. www.cbo.gov/sites/default/files/cbofiles/attachments/43907-BudgetOutlook.pdf.

———. 1992. *Economic Implications of Rising Health Care Costs*. Washington, DC: CBO.

Kaiser Family Foundation and Health Research & Educational Trust (HRET). 2013. *2013 Employer Health Benefits Survey*. Posted August 20. http://kff.org/private-insurance/report/2013-employer-health-benefits/.

Mayne, E. 2004. "Ford: Health Costs Could Drive Investment Overseas." *The Detroit News*, July 20. www.pnhp.org/news/ 2004/july/ford_health_costs_c.php.

Reinhardt, U. E. 1989. "Health Care Spending and American Competitiveness." *Health Affairs* 8 (4): 5–21.

Sapsford, J., and J. Areddy. 2005. "Why Dephi's Asia Operations Are Booming." *Wall Street Journal*, October 17, p. B1.

Seider, M. A., and B. L. Williamson. 2005. "Pension and OPEB Obligations in U.S. Bankruptcies: Answers to the Most Frequently Asked Questions." Accessed May 2014. http://lw.com/upload/pubContent/_pdf/pub1410_1.pdf.

Smerd, J. 2008. "UAW's VEBA Board: Autoworkers' Health Care Benefits in Peril." Posted November 10. www.workforce.com/articles/12504.

Storm, P. n.d. "VEBA Accounts and Health Insurance." Online Powerpoint presentation. Accessed November 2013. www.pptfilesearch.com/single/17946/veba-accounts-and-health-insurance.

Towers Perrin. 2009. *2010 Retiree Health Care Cost Survey Shows Continuing Affordability and Access Concerns*. Posted November 18. www.towersperrin.com/tp/showdctmdoc.jsp?url=Master_Brand_2/USA/Press_Releases/2009/20091118/2009_11_18.htm&country=global.

WHY IS GETTING INTO MEDICAL SCHOOL SO DIFFICULT?

23

In 2013, only 21,070 of the 48,010 students who applied to 126 medical schools in the United States were accepted, for an applicant-to-acceptance ratio of 2.3:1. (The number of matriculants was 1,015 fewer because some applicants are accepted at more than one school.) The ratio—having reached a high of 2.8:1 in 1973—steadily declined to 1.58:1 in 1988; rose again in the mid-1990s; and, after falling again and reaching a low of 1.9:1 in 2002, has increased to 2.3:1. As shown in Exhibit 23.1, first-year medical school enrollments grew sharply in the early 1970s, mostly because federal legislation (the Health Manpower Training Act of 1964) gave medical schools strong financial incentives to increase their enrollments. When these federal subsidies phased out, enrollments leveled out. They have remained relatively steady since the early 1980s and have only recently started to rise. Since 2009, four new medical schools have started and several schools have expanded their class size, which will lead to further growth in student enrollment. However, even with greater school capacity, a large excess demand for a medical education will continue.

Many qualified students are rejected each year because of the limited number of medical school spaces. Some rejected students choose to enroll in medical schools in other countries, such as Mexico. Medical schools overseas often charge higher tuition and require longer training periods than do US medical schools, which require four years of college before the four years of medical school. Residency training requires an additional three to seven years of graduate medical education. Unfortunately, academic excellence is not a sufficient qualification for admission to medical school. Other types of graduate-level professional education programs have experienced sharp increases in demand, but not the continual excess demands medical schools experience. Although every well-qualified student who wants to become a physicist, a mathematician, an economist, or a lawyer cannot realistically expect to be admitted to her first choice in graduate schools, if she has good academic qualifications (as do most medical students) she will likely be admitted to a US graduate school.[1]

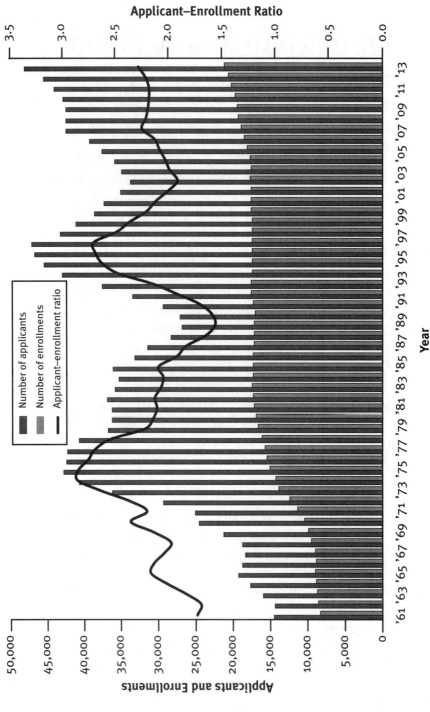

EXHIBIT 23.1
Medical School
Applicants and
Enrollments,
1960–2013

Applicant–Enrollment Ratio

Year

Applicants and Enrollments

- Number of applicants
- Number of enrollments
- Applicant–enrollment ratio

SOURCE: Data from AAMC (n.d.).

The Market for Medical Education in Theory

When medicine is perceived as relatively more attractive than other careers, demand for medical schools exceeds the available number of spaces. If the market for medical education were like other markets, this shortage will be only temporary while more medical schools are built and existing schools recruit additional faculty and add physical facilities to meet the greater demand. Over time, the temporary shortage will be resolved as the supply of spaces increases. Crucial in eliminating a temporary shortage is a rise in price (tuition). Higher tuition will serve to ration student demand for the existing number of spaces and provide medical schools with a financial incentive (and the funds) to invest in facilities and faculty so that they could accommodate larger enrollments. Subsidies and loan programs could be made available directly to low-income students faced with high tuition rates.

The Market for Medical Education in Practice

The market for medical education, however, differs from other markets. The medical education industry produces its output inefficiently (at high cost and using too many years of a student's time), and the method used to finance medical education is inequitable (large subsidies go to students from high-income families, who then go on to earn high salaries). If medical education were similar to other industries, more efficient competitors would have driven out less efficient competitors and transformed the industry. How has this industry, with its record of such poor performance, been able to survive?

The producers of medical education have been insulated from the marketplace. Tuition, established at an arbitrarily low level, represents less than one-third of the costs of education and approximately 3.7 percent (as of 2012) of medical school revenues (AAMC 2013).

Medical schools can maintain low tuition because large state subsidies and research grants offset educational costs. Tuition, being such a small fraction of educational costs and not rising with higher demand, neither serves to ration excess demand among students nor provides an incentive to medical schools to expand their capacity. Medical schools—particularly public ones—do not depend on tuition revenue to even cover their operating expenses. Lacking a financial incentive to expand, medical schools do nothing to alleviate the temporary shortage. Instead, the shortage becomes permanent, which is a far more serious situation.

For-profit businesses respond to greater consumer demands by raising prices and increasing supplies because they want to make more profit. New firms enter industries in which they perceive they can earn more on their investments than they can earn elsewhere. When prices are prevented from rising or barriers exist to new firms entering an expanding market, temporary shortages can become permanent. Typically, barriers to entry are legal rather than economic and protect existing firms from competition. Protected firms are better able to maintain higher prices and receive above-normal profit than if new firms were permitted to enter the market.

Medical schools, being not-for-profit, are motivated by more "noble" goals, such as the prestige associated with training tomorrow's medical educators. Most medical schools share the goal of having renowned, research-oriented faculty members who teach a few small classes of academically gifted students, who in turn will be their successors as super-specialist researchers. Few, if any, medical schools seek acclaim for graduating large numbers of primary care physicians who practice in underserved areas.

Only by maintaining an excess demand for admissions can medical schools choose the type of student who will become the type of physician they prefer (i.e., someone who will meet their prestige goals). Both the type of student selected and the design of the educational curriculum are determined by the desires of the medical school faculty, not by what is needed to train quality physicians efficiently (in terms of student time and cost per student). As long as a permanent shortage of medical school spaces exists, medical schools will continue to "profit" by selecting the type of student the faculty desires, establishing educational requirements the faculty deems most appropriate, and producing graduates who mirror the faculty's preferences. The current system of medical education contains inadequate incentives for medical schools to respond cost-effectively to changes in the demand for medical education.

How likely is it that an organization, perhaps a health plan, could start its own self-supporting medical school—one that admits students after only two years of undergraduate training (as is done in Great Britain), with a revised curriculum and residency requirement that combines the last two years of medical school with the first two years of graduate medical education (reducing the graduate medical education requirement by one year, as proposed by the former dean of the Harvard Medical School), and financed either by tuition or by graduates repaying their tuition by practicing for a number of years in the organization (Ebert and Ginzberg 1988)? Emanuel and Fuchs (2012) claim that the average length of training could be reduced by 30 percent without any loss of physician competence or quality of care. Further, they argue that "there is no evidence that graduates of 6-year programs perform more poorly on standardized board examinations or as practicing physicians." Schools with shorter training times could satisfy the excess demands for a medical education, reduce the educational process by three to four years, and at the same time teach students to be practitioners in a managed care environment.[2]

Accreditation for Medical Schools

Not surprisingly, starting new and innovative medical schools is very difficult. The Liaison Committee on Medical Education (LCME) accredits programs leading to the MD (doctor of medicine) degree and establishes the criteria to which a school must adhere to receive accreditation (LCME 2013). For example, a minimum number of weeks of instruction and calendar years (four) for the instruction to occur are specified, and an undergraduate education (usually four years) is required for admission to a medical school. Innovations in curriculum and changes in the length of time for becoming a physician (and to prepare for admission to medical school) must be approved by the LCME. The LCME further states that the cost of a medical education should be supported from diverse sources: tuition, endowment, faculty earnings, government grants and appropriations, parent universities, and gifts. Through its belief that too great a reliance should not be placed on tuition, the LCME encourages schools to pursue revenue sources and goals unrelated to educational concerns.

To be accredited, medical schools must also be not-for-profit. The LCME's accreditation criteria in effect eliminate all incentives for health plans and similar organizations to invest in medical schools in hopes of earning a profit or having a steady supply of practitioners. Private organizations have no incentive to invest capital to start a new medical school.

The status quo of the current high-cost medical education system would be threatened if graduates of these new medical schools proved as qualified as those trained in more traditional schools (as evidenced by their licensure examination scores and performance in residencies offered to them) and could enter practice three years earlier.

Instead, to bring about medical education reforms, nine commissions have been set up since the 1960s to recommend changes. In a 1989 survey, medical school deans, department chairs, and faculty members overwhelmingly endorsed the need for "fundamental changes" or "thorough reform" in medical student education. One examination of the lack of medical education reform indicated that faculties lack sufficient incentives to participate in reforming medical education programs because promotion and tenure are based primarily on research productivity and clinical practice expertise: "[There is] the relegation of students' education to a secondary position within the medical school.... Faculty have tended to think of the goals of their own academic specialty and department rather than the educational goals of the school as a whole" (Enarson and Burg 1992, 1142).

Recommended Changes

Not surprisingly, without financial incentives the not-for-profit sector will fail to respond to increased student demands for a medical education and will not be concerned with the efficiency by which medical education is provided. Instead of relying on innumerable commissions whose proposed reforms go largely unimplemented, three changes in the current system of medical education and quality assurance should be considered: (1) ease the entry requirements for starting new medical schools, (2) reduce medical school subsidies, and (3) place more emphasis on monitoring physician practice patterns.

Ease the Entry Requirements for Starting New Medical Schools

The accreditation criteria of the LCME should be changed to permit other organizations, such as managed care organizations (MCOs) (including those that are for-profit) to start medical schools. A larger number of schools competing for students would pressure medical schools to be more innovative and efficient. With easier entry into the medical education market, the emphasis on quality would be to shift from the process of becoming a physician toward quality outcomes—namely toward examining physicians and monitoring their practice behavior. Directly monitoring physicians' practice behavior is the most effective way to protect the public against unethical and incompetent physicians.

As more physicians participate in MCOs and physicians and as hospitals become more integrated, physician peer review will be enhanced. Peer review organizations have a financial incentive to evaluate the quality and appropriateness of care given by physicians under their auspices, as these organizations compete with similar groups according to their premiums, quality of care provided, and access to services. Report cards documenting physician quality of care and patient satisfaction are increasingly required by large employers and consumer groups. Quality assurance of physician services will increase as a result of competition among medical groups, integrated organizations, and health plans.

Reduce Medical School Subsidies

Reducing government subsidies would cause medical schools to become more efficient by shortening the time required for a medical degree and lowering the costs of providing it. Medical students should not be subsidized to a greater extent than students in other graduate or professional schools. A decrease in state subsidies to medical schools would force medical schools to reexamine and cut the costs of their education. Medical schools that merely raise their tuition to make up the lost revenues would find it difficult to attract a sufficient number of highly qualified applicants once more schools are competing for students. As tuition more accurately reflects the cost of education, applicants would comparison shop and evaluate schools with a range of tuition levels. To be competitive, schools with lesser reputations would have to have correspondingly lower tuition levels. The need to reduce students' educational costs most likely would result in innovative curricula, new teaching methods, and better use of the medical student's time.

To ensure that every qualified student would have an equal opportunity to become a physician once subsidies are decreased, student loan and subsidy programs must be made available. Current low-tuition rates, in effect, subsidize the medical education of all medical students, even those who come from high-income families; once these students graduate, they enter one of the highest-income professions. Providing subsidies directly to qualified students according to their family income levels would be more equitable.

Furthermore, instead of providing subsidies directly to medical schools, the subsidies should be given directly to students in the form of a voucher (to be used only in a medical school). Giving the state subsidies to students would be an incentive for them to select a medical school according to its reputation, total costs of education, and number of years of education required to graduate (college and medical school). Medical schools would then be forced to compete for students on the basis of these criteria.

Place More Emphasis on Monitoring Physician Practice Patterns

Currently, the process for ensuring physician quality relies wholly on graduating from an approved medical school and passing a licensing examination. Once a physician is licensed, no reexamination is required to maintain that license, although specialty boards may impose their own requirements for admission and maintenance of membership. State licensing boards are responsible for monitoring physicians' behavior and penalizing physicians whose performance is inadequate or whose conduct is unethical. Unfortunately, this approach for ensuring physician quality and competence is completely unreliable.

State licensing boards discipline very few physicians. In 1972, the disciplinary rate was only 0.74 per 1,000 physicians; a number of states did not undertake any disciplinary actions against their physicians. Between 1980 and 1982, the disciplinary rate rose to 1.3 per 1,000 physicians, or about one-tenth of 1 percent of all physicians. Although some improvements in certain states have been observed in recent years, the number of disciplinary actions against physicians varies greatly among states. As of 2011, the number of disciplinary actions per 1,000 practicing physicians was 5.2 in New York, 5.1 in California, 7.9 in Ohio, 12.7 in Texas, and 8.9 in Colorado. Many states had much lower disciplinary rates. Two of the states with the lowest serious disciplinary action rates for 2011—Minnesota (2.4 actions per 1,000 physicians) and Massachusetts (2.4 actions per 1,000 physicians)—have been consistently among the bottom ten states for each of the past five years. (The lowest serious disciplinary actions rate in 2011 was in Washington state (2.2 actions per 1,000 physicians) (Federation of State Medical Boards of the United States 2012).

It is unlikely that Texas, which had 12.7 prejudicial acts per 1,000 physicians, has a greater percentage of more unethical or incompetent physicians or more physicians requiring disciplinary actions than many other states. Instead, the considerable variability among states represents the uneven efforts by the states' medical licensing boards (which are mainly composed of physicians) to monitor and discipline physicians in their states. In fact, even when physicians lose their licenses in one state, they can move to another state and practice; some state medical boards encourage physicians to move to another state in exchange for dropping charges. Only five states permit their licensing boards to act based solely on another state's findings. The public is not as protected from incompetent and unethical medical practitioners as the medical profession has led it to believe.[3]

Monitoring the care provided by physicians through the use of claims and medical records data would more directly determine the quality and competence of a physician. And state licensing boards need to devote more resources to monitoring physician behavior. Requiring periodic reexamination and relicensure of all physicians would make physicians update their skills and knowledge. Rather than require physicians to take a minimum number of hours of continuing education, states should require reexamination, which would determine the appropriate amount of continuing education on an individual basis. (Continuing education by itself is a process measure for ensuring quality and does not ensure that physicians actually maintain and update their skills and knowledge bases.) Reexamination is a more useful and direct measure for assessing whether a physician has achieved the objectives of continuing education.

Periodic reexamination and relicensure would determine what tasks an individual physician is proficient in performing. Currently, all licensed physicians are permitted to perform a wide range of tasks, although they may have insufficient training in some of these tasks. Physicians may designate themselves as specialists whether or not they are certified by a specialty board. At present, any physician can legally perform surgery, provide anesthesia services, and diagnose patients. Reexamination could result in a physician's practice being limited to those tasks for which she continues to demonstrate proficiency. Instead of all-or-nothing licenses, physicians would be granted specific-purpose licenses. Such a licensing process would acknowledge that licensing physicians to perform a wide range of medical tasks does not serve the best interests of the public because not all physicians are qualified to perform all tasks adequately.

Specific-purpose licensure would mean that not all physicians would need to take the same educational training; training in some specialties would take much less time, whereas training to become a super-specialist would take longer. Shorter educational requirements for family practitioners would lower the cost of their medical education and enable them to graduate earlier and earn an income sooner. Even with higher tuition, family practitioners would incur a smaller debt and could begin paying it off at least three years earlier.[4] The number of family practitioners would increase because they would incur a much smaller investment (fewer years of schooling and lost income) in their medical education, and that would more than compensate for not receiving as high an income as a specialist. When a physician wants an additional specific-purpose license, he can receive additional training and take the qualifying examination for that license. Training requirements for entering the medical profession would be determined not by the medical profession but by the demand for different types of physicians and the lowest-cost manner of producing them.

Summary

The competition among medical schools that would result from reducing their subsidies (or providing the subsidies directly to students) and permitting the opening of new schools would improve the performance of the market for medical education. Easing entry restrictions would make opening nontraditional schools (and innovating in existing schools) easier, allowing more qualified students to be admitted to a medical school. Qualified students would no longer have to incur the higher expense and longer training times of attending a foreign medical school.

Emphasizing outcome measures and appropriateness of care would better protect the public from incompetent and unethical physicians. Reducing government subsidies to medical schools would force medical schools to be more efficient and innovative in structuring and producing a medical education. Further, distributing subsidies to students according to family income rather than to the medical school (which results in a subsidy to all students) would enhance equity among students receiving a medical education and force medical schools to compete for those students.

Discussion Questions

1. Evaluate the performance of the current market for medical education in terms of the number of qualified students admitted and the cost (both medical education and student forgone income) of becoming a physician.
2. The current approach to subsidizing medical schools results in all medical students being subsidized. Contrast this approach with one that awards the same amount of subsidy directly to students (according to their family income) for use in any medical school.
3. Medical schools are typically interested in prestige. How would medical school behavior change if schools had to survive in a competitive market (with free entry of new competitors) and without subsidies?
4. An important reason that so few family practitioners exist is their much lower economic returns than specialists. How would a competitive market in medical education increase the relative profitability of becoming a family practitioner?
5. Currently, the public is protected from incompetent and unethical physicians by the requirement that physicians graduate from an approved medical school, pass a one-time licensing examination, and receive continuing education. What are alternative, lower-cost approaches to protecting the public's interest?

Notes

1. Medical education also differs from other graduate programs in that, once accepted to medical school, a student is virtually assured of graduating. The attrition rate is approximately 2 percent, compared with attrition rates of 50 percent in other graduate programs.
2. About 30 medical schools admit a small number of students who completed only two to three years of college.
3. Improvements have been occurring slowly over time. All states now share formal action information with other states and report disciplinary actions to the National Practitioner Data Bank.
4. Youngclaus and Fresne (2013) estimate that the median graduating-student debt levels for public and private medical schools in 2012 was $160,000 and $190,000, respectively.

References

Association of American Medical Colleges (AAMC). n.d. *Medical School Admission Requirements, United States and Canada*. Various editions. Washington, DC: AAMC.

———. 2013. *LCME Part I-A Annual Medical School Financial Questionnaire (AFQ), FY2012*. Prepared June. www.aamc.org/download/344948/data/fy2012_medical_school_financial_tables.pdf.

Ebert, R. H., and E. Ginzberg. 1988. "The Reform of Medical Education." *Health Affairs* 7 (2 Suppl.): 5–38.

Emanuel, E., and V. Fuchs. 2012. "Shortening Medical Training by 30%." *JAMA* 307 (11): 1143–44.

Enarson, C., and F. Burg. 1992. "An Overview of Reform Initiatives in Medical Education: 1906 Through 1992." *JAMA* 268 (9): 1141–43.

Federation of State Medical Boards of the United States, Inc. 2012. *Summary of 2011 Board Actions*. Accessed January 2014. www.fsmb.org/pdf/2011-summary-of-board-actions.pdf.

Liaison Committee on Medical Education (LCME). 2013. *Rules of Procedure*. Prepared June. www.lcme.org/publications/rules-of-procedure.pdf.

Youngclaus, J., and J. A. Fresne. 2013. *Physician Education Debt and the Cost to Attend Medical School, 2012 Update*. Published February. www.aamc.org/download/328322/data/statedebtreport.pdf.

WILL A SHORTAGE OF REGISTERED NURSES REOCCUR?

24

Since World War II, concerns over a national shortage of registered nurses (RNs) have been recurrent. At times, the shortage seems particularly acute; at other times, it appears to be resolved, only to reassert itself several years later. Government and private commissions have attempted to quantify the magnitude of the shortage and have proposed remedies. Since 1964, the federal government has spent billions of dollars to alleviate the nursing shortage. The Great Recession this country experienced between 2007 and 2009 (and the subsequent slow recovery) eliminated the RN shortage and resulted in an RN surplus (NBER 2010). Once the economy fully recovers, will a shortage of RNs occur once again? Given the concern over a possible future shortage and the large federal subsidies that have supported nursing education, it is useful to examine why shortages of nurses recur, whether they are likely to occur again, and what, if anything, should be done about it.

Measuring Nursing Shortages

The measure commonly used to indicate a shortage of nurses is the nurse vacancy rate in hospitals—the percentage of unfilled nursing positions for which hospitals are recruiting. The vacancy rate attained a high of 23 percent in 1962, steadily declined throughout the 1960s, and reached single digits by the early 1970s. It rose in the late 1970s, reaching 14 percent in 1979, but by 1983 it had fallen to approximately 4.4 percent. By the mid-1980s, the vacancy rate was climbing again. It shot up to 12.7 percent by 1989, after which it sunk to 4 percent in 1998 and then rose sharply to 13 percent in 2001. Once again it declined to 4 percent in 2009. See Exhibit 24.1.

Each of these periods of high or rising RN vacancy rates brought forth commissions to study the problem and make recommendations. The high vacancy rates in the early 1960s led to the start of federal support for nursing education called the Nurse Training Act of 1964, which has been renewed many times.

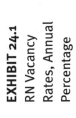

EXHIBIT 24.1
RN Vacancy
Rates, Annual
Percentage
Changes
in Real RN
Earnings, and
the National
Unemployment
Rate, 1979–
2012

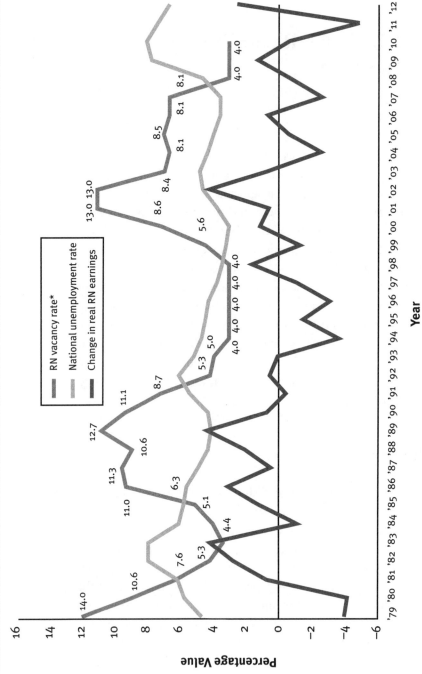

* Estimated data for 1997–1998, 2006, and 2008–2009.
SOURCES: 1979–2008 data on RN vacancy rates and the national unemployment rates compiled in 2009 by Peter I. Buerhaus, Vanderbilt University School of Nursing, and Douglas O. Staiger, Dartmouth College and Research Associate, National Bureau of Economic Research; 2009 data on RN vacancy rate from AHA (2010); data on real RN earnings and national unemployment rates from BLS (2014b).

Nursing Shortages in Theory

What are the reasons for a shortage of RNs? The definition of a nurse short-age is hospitals' inability to hire all the nurses they want at the current wage. In other words, the demand for nurses exceeds the number of nurses willing to work at the existing market wage. However, economic theory claims that if the demand for nurses exceeds the supply of nurses, hospitals will compete for nurses and then nurses' wages will increase. As nurses' wages rise, nurses who are not working will seek employment, and part-time nurses will be will-ing to increase the hours they work. Those hospitals willing to pay the new, higher wage will be able to hire all the nurses they want and will no longer have vacancies for nurses.[1]

Thus, economic theory predicts that once shortages begin, we observe rising wages for nurses followed by declining vacancy rates. Nurse employ-ment will expand (more nurses will enter the labor force and others will work longer hours), and as nurses' wages increase, hospitals will not hire as many nurses at the higher wage as they initially wanted. Shortages could recur if the demand for nurses once again grows (more rapidly than supply). With higher demand, the process starts over: Hospitals find they cannot hire all the nurses they want at the current wage, and so on. Clearly, wages are not the only reason nurses work or increase their hours of work. The nurse's age, whether she has young children, and overall family income are also important considerations. A change in the nurse's wage, however, will affect the benefits of working versus not working and thereby affect the number of hours the nurse chooses to work.

Nursing Shortages in Practice

How well does economic theory that relies on increased demand for nurses explain the recurrent shortages of nurses? Nurse shortages must be separated into two periods: (1) before the 1965 passage of Medicare and Medicaid and (2) after that.

Before the Passage of Medicare and Medicaid

Before Medicare, the vacancy rate kept rising, exceeding 20 percent by the early 1960s. Hospital demand for nurses continued to exceed the supply of nurses at a given wage. Surprisingly, however, nurses' wages did not rise as rapidly as wages in comparable occupations, which were not even subject to the same shortage pressures. Worsening shortages of nurses and limited growth of nurse wages over a period of years could only have resulted from interference with the process by which wages were determined.

Working on the hypothesis that nurse wages were being artificially held down, economist Donald Yett (1975) found that hospitals were colluding to prevent nurses' wages from rising. The hospitals believed competing for nurses would merely result in large nurse wage hikes—hence, a large increase in hospital costs without a large increase in the number of employed nurses. This collusive behavior by hospitals on the setting of nurses' wages prevented the shortage from being resolved. (For additional references on the nursing shortage and a more complete discussion of the shortage over time, see Buerhaus, Staiger, and Auerbach [2009] and Feldstein [2011].)

After the Passage of Medicare and Medicaid

Once Medicare and Medicaid were enacted, hospitals began to be reimbursed according to their costs for treating Medicare and Medicaid patients. Consequently, hospitals were more willing to raise nurses' wages, which they did rapidly in the mid- to late 1960s. The vacancy rate declined from 23 percent in 1962 to approximately 9 percent by 1971. The nurses' wage hike brought about a large increase in the number of employed nurses, contrary to hospitals' earlier expectations. Trained nurses who were not working decided to reenter nursing. The percentage of all trained nurses who were working rose from 55 percent in 1960 to 65 percent in 1966 and 70 percent in 1972. Higher wages had an important effect on expanding nurse participation rates.

The artificial shortages created by hospitals before the mid-1960s are no longer possible. The antitrust laws make collusion by hospitals to hold down nurses' wages illegal. Therefore, the recurrent shortage of nurses since that time has been of a different type.

The lack of information in the market for nurses lengthens the time necessary to resolve shortages. For example, if a hospital experiences growth in its admissions or a higher acuity level in its patients, it will try to hire more nurses. The hospital may, however, find that its personnel department cannot hire more nurses at the current wage. The hospital's vacancy rate goes up. Other hospitals in the community may have the same experience. The hospital then has to decide whether and by how much to raise the wage to attract additional nurses. If the hospital decides to raise nurses' wages, it will have to pay the higher wage to its existing nurses as well. The hospital must then decide how many additional nurses it can afford to hire at the higher wage. The cost of a new nurse is not only the higher wage a hospital must pay that new nurse but also the cost of increasing wages to all of the other nurses.

The hospital may decide that other approaches for recruiting new nurses, such as providing child care and a more supportive environment, may be less costly than raising wages. Thus, a lag exists between the decision to hire more nurses, the wage hike, and the point at which the hospital is satisfied with the number of nurses it has.

A lag also exists before the supply of nurses responds to changed market conditions. Once nurses' wages are increased, it takes time for this information to become widely disseminated. Nurses who are not working may decide to return to nursing at the higher wage; this would be indicated by a greater nurse participation rate. Other nurses who are working part time may decide to increase the number of hours they work, and higher wages may make more high school graduates decide to undertake the educational requirements to become a nurse. The most rapid response to higher wages will come from those who work part time, followed by those who are already trained but not working as nurses. The long-run supply of nurses is determined by those who decide to enter nursing schools (and by the immigration of foreign-trained nurses). Short- and long-run supply responses to an increase in nurses' wages thus occur.

Let us now return to an examination of how well economic theory explains the recurrent shortage of nurses. Throughout the late 1960s and early 1970s, nurses' wages rose more rapidly than wages in comparable professions, such as teaching. This resulted in lower vacancy rates and higher nurse participation rate. Within several years, enrollments in nursing schools (offering either a bachelor's, associate, or diploma degree) climbed (a lag of several years always exists before the information on nurses' wages is transmitted to high school graduates and nursing school enrollments change). See Exhibit 24.2.

By the late 1970s, concerns surfaced about a new shortage of nurses. The basis of this shortage began in 1971, when President Nixon imposed wage and price controls on the economy. Although these controls were removed from all other industries in 1972, they remained in effect for medical care until 1974. The wage controls, together with the increased supply of nurse graduates, began to have an effect by the late 1970s—well after the controls were lifted because of the lag in transmission time mentioned earlier. Demand for nurses continued to grow throughout the 1970s, while the wage controls led to lower relative wages for nurses and, by the late 1970s, declining nursing school enrollments. By 1979, the vacancy rate reached 14 percent.

Trends in the 1980s

The shortage in 1979 and 1980, however, was short lived. As shown in Exhibit 24.1, nurses' wages rose sharply at the same time the economy entered a severe recession in the early 1980s. The rising unemployment rate caused more nurses to seek employment and increase their hours of work. Because 70 percent of RNs are married, the loss of a spouse's job or even the fear of it is likely to cause nurses to participate in the labor force to maintain their family income (Buerhaus, Staiger, and Auerbach 2009, 201).

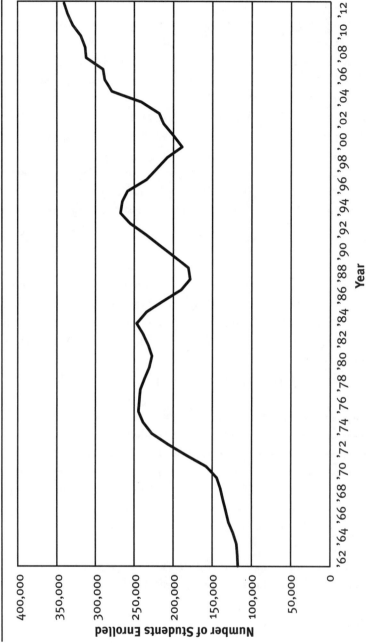

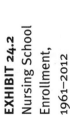

EXHIBIT 24.2
Nursing School
Enrollment,
1961–2012

Number of Students Enrolled

400,000
350,000
300,000
250,000
200,000
150,000
100,000
50,000
0

'62 '64 '66 '68 '70 '72 '74 '76 '78 '80 '82 '84 '86 '88 '90 '92 '94 '96 '98 '00 '02 '04 '06 '08 '10 '12

Year

NOTE: Data for 1997 and 2009–2012 are unavailable and are based on author's extrapolations.
SOURCES: Data from ANA (n.d.); National League for Nursing (2009); Census Bureau (n.d.); NCHS (n.d.).

Higher wages and unemployment rate increased nurse participation rates from 76 percent in 1980 to 79 percent by 1984. As a consequence, vacancy rates dropped to 4.4 percent by 1983. The nursing shortage had once again been resolved through a combination of wage hike, greater nurse participation rate, and high national unemployment rate. RN wages remained stable (and actually decreased in real dollars) between 1983 and 1985 and the vacancy rate fell, and nursing school enrollments began a sharp decline through the late 1980s.

In the 1980s, the market for hospital services underwent drastic changes, which affected the market for nurses. Medicare changed hospital payment from cost-based to a fixed price per admission, and private insurers started utilization management. The trend by government and private insurers to reduce use of the hospital resulted in shorter hospital lengths of stay. Patients required more intensive treatment for the shorter time they were in the hospital. Hospitalized patients were more severely ill, a greater number of transplants were being performed, and the number of low-birth-weight babies went up. The recovery period, which requires less-intensive care, was occurring outside the hospital. As a result, hospitals began to use more RNs per patient. The higher demand by hospitals for RNs during this period is indicated by the fact that in 1975 there were 0.65 RNs per patient; this figure climbed to 0.88 by 1980, to 1.31 by 1990, and to 1.6 by 2000. The percentage increase in RNs per patient exceeded the decline in patient days.

The demand for nurses also rose in outpatient and nonhospital settings. As the use of the hospital decreased, use of outpatient care, nursing homes, home care, and hospices for terminally ill Medicare patients increased. From 1980 to 2010, annual outpatient visits (ambulatory care visits to physicians' offices, hospital outpatient departments, and emergency departments) skyrocketed from 262 million to 1.24 billion (CDC 2010a; 2010b; 2010c). Use of skilled nursing homes by Medicare patients grew substantially from 8.6 million days in 1980 to 71.6 million days in 2010 (CMS 2014, Table v.15). In addition to providing care in these alternative settings, cost-containment companies raised their demand for RNs to conduct utilization review and case management.

As the demand for nurses in these different settings increased faster than supply in the mid- to late 1980s, nurses' wages were slow to respond. Nursing school enrollments had been falling, and the national unemployment rate dropped as the economy began to improve. Consequently, vacancy rates began to rise once more—from 5.1 percent in 1984 to 12.7 percent in 1989. By the late 1980s, concern emerged over a shortage of nurses.

Hospitals again lobbied Congress for subsidies to increase nurse education programs and to ease immigration rules on foreign-trained nurses. The nursing shortage of the late 1980s resulted in Congress enacting the

Nursing Shortage Reduction and Education Extension Act of 1988 and the Immigration Nursing Relief Act of 1989, which made it easier for foreign nurses to receive working visas.

Trends in the 1990s

Neither of these legislative acts was needed, however, as economic incentives again eliminated the shortage. As the economy weakened in the early 1990s and the unemployment rate began to rise, nurse participation rates increased to 82 percent by 1992. Nursing school enrollment had continued to grow in the early 1990s as a result of prior nurse wage hikes. With the growth in supply of new nurses and the higher participation rate, vacancy rates dropped to 4 percent by 1994. The nursing shortage ended.

One could have forecasted that another shortage would occur by the end of the decade. As shown in Exhibit 24.1, nurses' real wages (adjusted for inflation) declined starting in 1994 and did not rise again until 1998. During this time, hospitals were trying to be more price competitive by reducing their costs so as to be included in managed care's provider networks. Only by 1998 did nurse wage increases finally begin to grow faster than inflation. The national unemployment rate also fell throughout the late 1990s, as the US economy was doing very well.

Nursing school enrollments typically drop several years after a decline in wages and vacancy rates. As shown in Exhibit 24.2, nursing school enrollments peaked at 270,000 in 1994 and then slumped for the remainder of the 1990s. The reduction in nurse wages during the mid- to late 1990s led to a large decrease in nursing school enrollments and, consequently, in the number of nurse graduates.

Current Supply and Demand for RNs

After years of declining (adjusted for inflation) nurse wages during the latter part of the 1990s, shrinking nursing school enrollments, and the aging of the nurse population, one would have expected to read newspaper articles about the new shortage of nurses and hospitals once again paying bonuses to attract nurses. After years of low vacancy rates, the vacancy rate started increasing in 1999 (from 4 percent in 1998 to 5.6 percent) and quickly rose to 13 percent by 2001.

As hospitals recognized the difficulty of attracting nurses in the beginning of the decade, nurses' real wages went up. With the wage hike, RN supply started to expand faster. Nursing school enrollments grew, part-time RNs increased their hours of work, trained RNs rejoined the workforce, and immigration of RNs from other countries escalated. Further stimulating the greater supply of nurses in the beginning of the decade was the slowdown of the economy in 2001, leading to growth in unemployment. Those states experiencing the greatest spikes in unemployment saw the largest number of married RNs reentering the workforce (Buerhaus, Auerbach, and Staiger 2009). Almost all of the increase in RNs in 2002 (94 percent) occurred among married nurses. The nurse vacancy rate then declined, but it was still relatively high (at 8.1 percent) by the middle of the decade.

In 2006, the Health Resources and Services Administration of the US Department of Health and Human Services projected that by 2020 there would be a shortage of one million nurses—mainly as a result of the medical needs of retiring baby boomers. Shortage warnings of such a large magnitude led to the establishment of more nurse education programs and a concern of a shortage of nursing instructors. Not long after these shortage warnings, the United States slipped into a severe recession in 2007. A sharp rise in the unemployment rate occurred; the number of uninsured patients multiplied, as did hospital bad debts; and hospitals saw a decrease in the number of elective procedures. The Great Recession led to a large growth in the supply of nurses. As occurred in previous periods of high unemployment, nurses' need to maintain their family income resulted in more of them entering or reentering the nursing workforce. Part-time RNs increased the number of hours they worked, and more trained RNs returned to the workforce (to protect their families against their spouses' job insecurity). Large numbers of nursing graduates, as a result of the previous increases in nursing school enrollments, started their nursing careers. The nurse vacancy rate fell to 4 percent in 2010 (the most current data available). The shortage of RNs was once again resolved. But not only did the shortage end, a nursing *surplus* occurred; many new nurse graduates could not find a job.

The Outlook for Registered Nurses

Disagreement exists over the outlook for nurses. The conventional view is that, as soon as the current slow economic recovery (for the Great Recession that officially ended in 2010) expands more rapidly, older nurses would retire as they had originally planned and nurses who had returned to nursing to shore up their family's income would again leave nursing. A shortage of nurses would again occur, so support for expanded numbers of nursing programs should not be diminished.

The contrary view claims that the effects of the Great Recession would continue longer than the effects of previous recessions, the jobs recovery would be slow, and financial uncertainties would make older nurses and those who reentered nursing reluctant to leave nursing. Further, the sharp increase in nursing graduates from baccalaureate programs would—particularly if this trend continues—mitigate the loss of retiring nurses.

A new nursing shortage is unlikely for some time. Some analysts even claim that new nursing shortages may be a thing of the past as the development of new technology might result in a lower demand for nurses; monitoring equipment and even robots would substitute for some of the tasks performed by nurses.

Several uncertainties affect the outlook for nurses; these involve changes in the demand for nurses and supply of nurses.

Factors Affecting the Demand for Nurses

The demand for RNs is expected to continue to increase. The population is growing—and a greater percentage of the population is getting older; the oldest of the baby boomers began to retire in 2011. Medical advances will continue to stimulate the demand for expensive medical services provided by hospitals, increasing the demand for hospital nurses. As more medical services are provided in outpatient settings and in patients' homes, the demand for RNs in these settings will continue to rise. New payment systems, such as episode-based payment and capitation, and cost-containment efforts are expanding the use of less expensive in-home and outpatient settings. Further, the shortage of primary care physicians will raise the use of nurse practitioners.

In discussing the future role of RNs, Auerbach and colleagues (2013) stated, "The importance of RNs is expected to increase in the coming decades, as new models of care delivery, global payment, and a greater emphasis on prevention are embraced. These and other changes associated with health care reform will require the provision of holistic care, greater care coordination, greater adherence to protocols, and improved management of chronic disease—roles that are inherently aligned with the nursing model of care."

Legislation and regulatory policies are also likely to affect the demand for RNs—in both a positive and a negative way. The Affordable Care Act (ACA) may have an adverse effect on the demand for RNs. Included in the legislation are significant reductions in hospital payment, which will limit hospitals' ability to raise nurse wages. Whether these payment decreases will actually occur is uncertain, given that scheduled Medicare physician payment reductions (according to the sustainable growth rate formula) have been continually postponed for fear of limiting seniors' access to physicians. Should these reductions in hospital payments occur, however, hospitals will be unable to attract additional RNs by increasing wage rates. RN wages that fall behind wages in other careers available to potential nurses will result in a *permanent* shortage of hospital nurses; the demand for nurses will exceed supply at the wage hospitals can afford to pay given their lower budget.

Finally, in coming years, greater state regulation may cause hospital demand for RNs to increase.

In 2004, the California Nurses Association (CNA) was successful in having the state enact a law mandating minimum RN-to-patient ratios in California hospitals. These mandated nurse–patient ratios varied according to whether the patient was in a medical or surgical unit. Nurse ratio laws boost the demand for nurses. The CNA claimed that the higher ratios would reduce patient deaths and improve patient safety. Hospitals in the state objected to the minimum staff ratios, claiming their nurse–patient ratios were adequate; they were concerned that the mandated higher ratios would raise their costs. The CNA and other state nurse associations are lobbying other states to enact similar nurse–patient ratios.

Do the patient benefits of higher RN staffing ratios exceed their additional cost? Because California was the only state (as of 2013) to have enacted minimum nurse staffing ratios, several studies compared patient quality in California hospitals before and after the law. Before the law was passed, some California hospitals had already achieved the minimum staffing ratios, while others did not meet the mandated standards. Cook and colleagues (2012) found that, in hospitals that had to increase their staffing ratios, patient outcomes did not disproportionately improve; the authors concluded that they found no evidence that the law had a causal impact on patient safety, such as failure-to-rescue rates.[2] (It is possible that the finding of no change in patient outcomes resulted from those hospitals that raised their staffing ratio to meet the minimum ratio by reducing the use of non-RNs and relying instead on newly hired RNs to perform tasks previously undertaken by non-RNs. The effect of this substitution would be higher hospital costs with limited if any change in patient outcomes.) Researchers acknowledge that more research using specific staffing and outcomes data by nursing unit is needed to determine the effects of minimum ratios on patient outcomes.[3]

Factors Affecting the Supply of Nurses

Important to determining whether shortages will reoccur is the question of whether supply of RNs will grow faster than demand for RNs. Several trends are emerging. The RN workforce is aging, and as these nurses retire and the economy recovers, the supply of RNs will be reduced.

An important source of RNs has been and will continue to be immigration of foreign-born RNs. Foreign-trained RNs have strong financial incentives to immigrate. In the United States, foreign-trained RNs have more opportunities to earn much higher pay (allowing them to send money home to assist their families), to have better working conditions, and to learn and practice. In 2012, the median annual wage for RNs in the United States was $65,470, which is 20 to 30 times greater than what RNs earn in the Philippines (BLS 2014a; Healthcare Salaries n.d.). (These higher wages in the United States have even led physicians in the Philippines to train as RNs to be able to immigrate to the United States.) In several countries, including the Philippines, RNs are trained for the purpose of being able to immigrate to the United States, as they provide a major source of remittances of hard currency to their countries of origin (Aiken et al. 2004, 72). To facilitate the immigration of foreign-trained nurses to the United States, for-profit firms have emerged to serve as brokers between US hospitals and foreign-trained RNs.[4] An increase in supply of foreign-trained RNs will depress RN wages (wages will not increase as high as they would with a smaller supply). Lower wages will eventually affect the demand for a nursing education and hence reduce future supply of US nursing graduates.

Men also could eventually be a major source of RN supply. Male RNs represent about 9 percent of the RN workforce. The stereotype of nursing as a female-dominated profession is an important reason men have not chosen to become nurses. Also underrepresented in the nursing profession are Hispanics, who account for 5 percent of RNs. Increases in the proportion of both these groups would lead to large increases in the supply of RNs (Buerhaus, Auerbach, and Staiger 2009, w666).

Federal Subsidies to Nursing Schools and Students

The supply of RNs is importantly affected by the number of new nursing graduates. Each time a new nursing shortage occurs, various bills are introduced in Congress to address different aspects of the shortage, such as more funding for nurse scholarships, financial support for nurses seeking advanced degrees, and funding for increasing faculty in nursing schools. Proposals for federal funding to expand the supply of nurses have been made since the enactment of the Nurse Training Act of 1964. These recommendations ignore the important role played by higher wages in multiplying the short- and long-run supply of nurses.

Federal subsidies to nursing schools and students cannot be directed only to those students who would otherwise have chosen a different career. Nurse education subsidies take years to affect the supply of nurses. More important, to the extent that federal programs are successful in increasing the number of nursing school graduates, nurses' wages rise more slowly. A larger supply of new graduates causes a lower rate of growth in nurses' wages, which in turn results in a smaller increase in the nurse participation rate. Nurses would be more reluctant to return to nursing or work more hours if their wages did not go up.

The supply of US-trained RNs has been limited by the inadequate response by nursing schools to the high demand for nursing education. In 2011, only 39.5 percent of student applicants were admitted to nursing programs; this represents a decrease from 45 percent in recent years (AACN 2012). Nursing programs complain that they cannot admit more students because they do not have enough faculty members. Colleges and universities attempting to expand their nursing faculties operate in a highly competitive market for RNs with graduate degrees who can receive much higher salaries from hospitals and health systems. A significant factor in the shortage of nurse faculty is the salary, which is lower than the market wage. It is surprising that nursing schools are unable to resolve a problem of attracting new faculty, a problem that other academic programs must contend with and appear to have resolved. The not-for-profit market for nursing education does not appear to be performing efficiently.

Greater reliance on market mechanisms would negate the need for federal nurse-education subsidies to increase the supply of nurses. For example, higher wages will bring about an increase in the number of hours part-time nurses work; about 25 percent of all employed nurses work part time. Higher wages also attract qualified RNs from other countries, such as the Philippines. Higher wages for nurses will cause hospitals and other demanders of nurses to rethink how they use their nurses. As nurses become more expensive to employ, hospitals will use nurses in higher-skilled tasks and delegate certain housekeeping and other tasks currently performed by RNs to less-trained nursing personnel, such as licensed practical nurses. Higher wages and new roles for nurses would make nursing a more attractive profession, thereby boosting the demand for a nursing career. Finally, nursing is predominantly a female profession. Higher wages and new nursing roles will increase the attractiveness of nursing to a larger segment of the population.

Since the mid-1960s, the recurrent shortages of nurses have been caused by greater demands for nurses and the failure of hospitals to immediately recognize that, at the higher demand, nurses' wages must be increased. Once hospitals realize market conditions for nurses have changed, the process once again brings equilibrium to the market. The supply of nurses is responsive to changes in nurse wages and economic conditions.

In coming years, uncertainty exists regarding how the factors affecting the demand and supply of nurses are likely to change. Will the large increase in nurse graduates continue? Will older RNs decide to retire? Will the slow economic recovery improve more rapidly? Will more states adopt higher minimum nurse-staffing ratios? Will more care be shifted outside the hospital, the predominant setting for nurse employment? Will government hospital payments be so reduced that it limits hospitals' ability to pay nurses market wages? Finally, will nurses adapt to the new payment and delivery systems by undertaking new roles with greater responsibilities in care of the patient? The remainder of the decade should clarify the direction of each of these forces.

Summary

The nursing profession faces challenges and opportunities in coming years. The major reason for recurrent RN shortages has been the cyclical pattern of nurse wages. As nurse wages stagnated, the rate of return on a nursing career fell and enrollments in nursing schools declined, as did the number of graduates. With a smaller supply of nurses and greater acuity level of patients, hospitals eventually found that they could not attract as many nurses as they wanted at the current nurse wage rate and RN vacancy rates increased. Each of these shortages was resolved when nurse wages rose; nursing school enrollments grew, older RNs reentered the workforce, and more foreign-trained RNs immigrated to the United States; all of these expanded the supply of nurses.

To forestall future shortages and make the nurse market function more smoothly, better information must be provided to the demanders and suppliers of nursing services. Information will facilitate the market's adjustment process by eliminating the time lags in wage increases and enrollments that have caused these cyclical shortages. Hospitals and other demanders of nursing services must be made more aware of approaches that increase nurses' productivity and improve the wages and other working conditions necessary to attract more nurses. To realize the full potential of nursing as a profession and enlarge the supply of nurses, potential nursing students need to be provided with timely information that allows them to make informed career choices. Nurses—particularly those who are not employed or are working part time—have to be aware of opportunities in nursing as well as wages and working conditions being offered. Efforts to disseminate more information are more likely to eliminate shortages and lead to a greater supply of nurses than are policies that merely rely on large federal subsidies to nursing education.

Both public policy and private initiatives are directed at reducing the rising costs of medical care. If the outcome of public policy is to place arbitrary budget limits on hospitals and total medical expenditures, nurses' wages will not rise as rapidly as wages for comparably trained professions in the nonregulated health sector, and a permanent nurse shortage will occur. Innovation in the use of RNs and provision of new medical services will be stifled for lack of funds.

If, however, public policy reinforces what is occurring in the private sector—namely competition among managed care organizations on the basis of their premiums and quality of care—the demand for RNs will be determined by their productivity, the tasks they are permitted to perform, the improved patient outcomes they provide, and their wages relative to the wages of other types of nursing personnel. To the extent that RNs are able to perform more highly valued tasks—such as assuming responsibility for more primary care services, utilization management, and management of home health care—as is currently the case in many competitive organizations, they become more valuable to such organizations. In competitive markets, these organizations will be willing to increase their use of RNs and their wages to reflect the higher value of services rendered. The future roles, responsibilities, and income of RNs will be affected by the incentives created by a competitive healthcare system.

Discussion Questions

1. Why was the demand for RNs rising faster than supply during the 1980s?
2. How have the last several shortages of nurses been resolved?
3. How does an increase in nurses' wages affect hospitals' demand for nurses and the supply of nurses?
4. Why was the shortage of nurses that occurred before Medicare different from subsequent shortages?
5. Contrast the following two approaches for eliminating the shortage of nurses:
   a. Providing federal subsidies to nursing schools
   b. Providing more information on nurse demand and supply to prospective nursing students and demanders of nursing services, such as hospitals

Notes

1. Even when hospitals are able to hire all the nurses they want at the prevailing wage, a nurse vacancy rate will still exist because of normal turnover.
2. Cook and colleagues (2012) state that, although a statistically significant positive cross-sectional relationship exists between nurse staffing ratios and failure to rescue in California hospitals and hospitals in other states, we cannot assume there is a causal relationship. Higher staffing ratios and better patient outcomes may be correlated with other hospital inputs and policies.
3. Spetz and colleagues (2013) found that the mandated minimum nurse staffing ratios had a limited impact on patient safety in California hospitals, while McHugh, Berez, and Small (2013) found that hospitals with higher RN staffing ratios had a lower hospital readmission rate.

4. Foreign-trained RNs are limited in their entry to the United States by US immigration and licensure policies. According to Aiken and colleagues (2004, 72), "All U.S. nurses must pass the National Council Licensure Examination (NCLEX-RN) to practice as RNs. To take the exam, foreign applicants must demonstrate that their education meets U.S. standards—most notably, that their education was at the postsecondary level. Also, nurses trained in countries in which English is not the primary language must also pass an English proficiency test (the Test of English as a Foreign Language, or TOEFL). The Commission on Graduates of Foreign Nursing Schools (CGFNS) offers an exam in many countries that is an excellent predictor of passing the NCLEX-RN. The CGFNS exam reduces the number of foreign-trained nurses who travel to the United States expecting to work as RNs who cannot pass the licensing exam."

References

Aiken, L., J. Buchan, J. Sochalski, B. Nichols, and M. Powell. 2004. "Trends in International Nurse Migration." *Health Affairs* 23 (3): 69–77.

American Association of Colleges of Nursing (AACN). 2012. "New AACN Data Show an Enrollment Surge in Baccalaureate and Graduate Programs Amid Calls for More Highly Educated Nurses." Press release. www.aacn.nche.edu/news/articles/2012/enrollment-data.

American Hospital Association (AHA). 2010. *The State of America's Hospitals—Taking the Pulse*. www.aha.org/aha/content/2010/pdf/100524-thschartpk.pdf.

American Nurses Association. n.d. *Facts About Nursing*. Various editions. Silver Springs, MD: ANA.

Auerbach, D., D. Staiger, U. Muench, and P. Buerhaus. 2013. "The Nursing Workforce in an Era of Health Care Reform." *New England Journal of Medicine* 368: 1470–72. www.nejm.org/doi/full/10.1056/NEJMp1301694.

Buerhaus, P., D. Auerbach, and D. Staiger. 2009. "The Recent Surge in Nurse Employment: Causes and Implications." *Health Affairs* (web exclusive) 28 (4): w657–w668.

Buerhaus, P., D. Staiger, and D. Auerbach. 2009. *The Future of the Nursing Workforce in the United States: Data, Trends, and Implications*. Boston: Jones and Bartlett.

Bureau of Labor Statistics (BLS). 2014a. "Registered Nurses: Summary." In *Occupational Outlook Handbook*. Published January 8. www.bls.gov/ooh/healthcare/registered-nurses.htm.

———. 2014b. "Labor Force Statistics from the Current Population Survey." Last modified February 26. www.bls.gov/cps/tables.htm.

Centers for Disease Control and Prevention (CDC). 2010a. *National Ambulatory Medical Care Survey: 2010 Summary Tables*. Accessed March 2014. www .cdc.gov/nchs/data/ahcd/namcs_summary/2010_namcs_web_tables.pdf.

———. 2010b. *National Hospital Ambulatory Medical Care Survey: 2010 Emergency Department Summary Tables*. Accessed March 2014. www.cdc .gov/nchs/data/ahcd/nhamcs_emergency/2010_ed_web_tables.pdf.

———. 2010c. *National Hospital Ambulatory Medical Care Survey: 2010 Outpatient Department Summary Tables*. Accessed March 2014. www.cdc .gov/nchs/data/ahcd/nhamcs_outpatient/2010_opd_web_tables.pdf.

Centers for Medicare & Medicaid Services (CMS). 2014. *Data Compendium, 2011 edition*. Accessed March. www.cms.gov/Research-Statistics-Data-and-Systems/Statistics-Trends-and-Reports/DataCompendium/2011_Data_Compendium.html.

Cook, A., M. Gaynor, M. Stephens, and L. Taylor. 2012. "The Effect of a Hospital Nurse Staffing Mandate on Patient Health Outcomes: Evidence from California's Minimum Staffing Regulation." *Journal of Health Economics* 31 (2): 340–48.

Feldstein, P. 2011. "The Market for Registered Nurses." In *Health Care Economics*, 7th ed., Albany, NY: Delmar.

Healthcare Salaries. n.d. "Average Nurse Salary." Accessed March 2014. www.healthcare-salaries.com/nursing/average-nurse-salary.

McHugh, M., J. Berez, and D. Small. 2013. "Hospitals with Higher Nurse Staffing Had Lower Odds of Readmissions Penalties Than Hospitals with Lower Staffing." *Health Affairs* 32 (10): 1740–47. http://content.healthaffairs .org/content/32/10/1740.full.

National Bureau of Economic Research (NBER). 2010. "Business Cycle Dating Committee." Published September 20. www.nber.org/cycles/sept2010.html.

National Center for Health Statistics (NCHS). n.d. *Health United States*. Various editions. Hyattsville, MD: NCHS.

National League for Nursing. 2009. "Nursing Education Statistics." Accessed March 2014. www.nln.org/researchgrants/slides/index.htm.

Spetz, J., D. Harless, C. Herrera, and B. Mark. 2013. "Using Minimum Nurse Staffing Regulations to Measure the Relationship Between Nursing and Hospital Quality of Care." *Medical Care Research and Review* 70 (4): 380–99.

US Census Bureau. n.d. *Statistical Abstract of the United States*. Various editions. Washington, DC: Census Bureau.

Yett, D. 1975. *An Economic Analysis of the Nurse Shortage*. Lexington, MA: D.C. Heath.

THE HIGH PRICE OF PRESCRIPTION DRUGS **25**

Spending on prescription drugs has greatly increased since 1990, when drug expenditures were $40 billion. As of 2012, drug expenditures reached $260 billion (CMS 2014a). In the late 1990s and the early part of the past decade, drug expenditures rose more rapidly than did other medical expenditures. After reaching a peak rate of 18 percent in 1999, the annual rate of increase in drug expenditures has been declining and climbed by only 0.4 percent in 2012, compared with the 4.9 percent and 4.6 percent growth in hospital and physician expenditures, respectively. The annual percentage increases in prescription drug expenditures and drug prices since 1980 are shown in Exhibit 25.1. Prescription drug expenditures represent a smaller percentage of total health expenditures (9.4 percent) than do hospital or physician services (31.6 percent and 20.2 percent, respectively).

Despite this and the fact that the annual rate of increase has slowed, drug expenditures are a cause for concern in the public and private sectors. Higher drug expenditures are a growing burden to state Medicaid programs, the federal deficit, and private insurance premiums. Further, patients pay a higher percentage of drug expenditures out of pocket than they do for other major health expenditures. Not surprisingly, patients are more likely to complain about paying $50 for a prescription drug than about $20,000 to stay in the hospital, which is covered by insurance.

Reasons for the Increase in Pharmaceutical Expenditures

The major factors causing the high drug expenditures are the surge in drug prescription utilization, the rise in drug prices, and the changes in the types of drugs prescribed.

Surge in Drug Prescription Use

As shown in Exhibit 25.2, the total number of prescriptions filled (including refills) nearly doubled in just ten years—from 1.9 billion in 1992 to 4.1 billion in 2012. On a per capita basis, the average number of retail prescriptions went up from 7.3 in 1992 to 10.4 in 2000 and to 13.0 in 2012. The

EXHIBIT 25.1
Annual
Percentage
Changes in the
Prescription
Drug Price
Index and
Prescription
Drug
Expenditures,
1980–2012

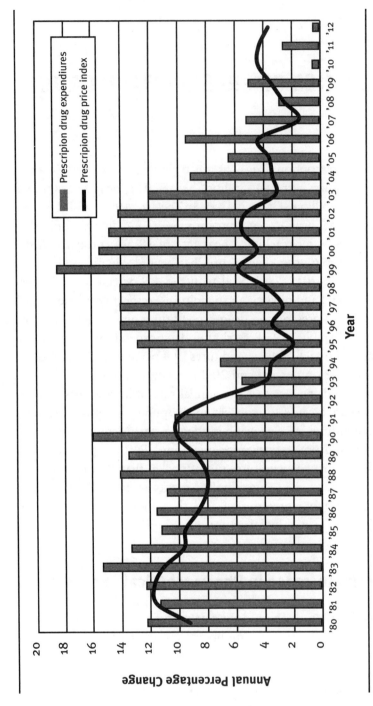

SOURCES: Data from BLS (2014); CMS (2014b).

EXHIBIT 25.2

Total
Prescriptions
Dispensed and
Prescriptions
per Capita,
1992–2012

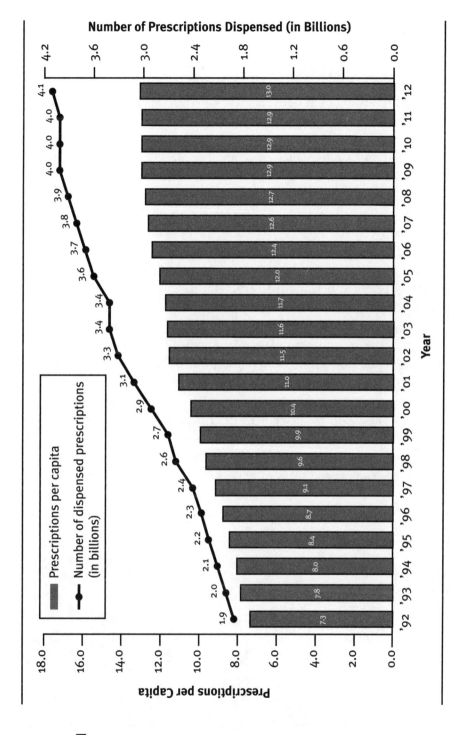

SOURCES: 1992–2001 data from the National Institute for Health Care Management (2002); 2002–2012 from IMS Health (2013) and Census Bureau (2013).

two important reasons for this escalation over time are (1) the growth in the number of aged and (2) the proliferation of insurance coverage for prescription drugs.

Although population growth is about 1 percent per year, the number of aged has been rising even faster, and the elderly's use of prescription medication is the highest among the US populace. With regard to prescriptions, including refills, purchased in an outpatient setting only, those between the ages of 18 and 44 each uses an average number of 5.3 prescriptions per year, while those between the ages of 45 and 64 each uses an average of about 16.4 prescriptions per year. In contrast, for those between the ages of 65 and 74, the average number of prescriptions increases to more than 24.9 per person, and those between the ages of 75 and 84 each receives 29.7 prescriptions (see Exhibit 25.3). As the population continues to age, the volume of prescriptions is expected to stay large. Given the greater number of seniors and prescriptions per aged person, drug expenditures in general (and among the aged in particular) will continue to expand.

The growth in private and public insurance coverage for prescription drugs is the second reason that drug expenditures have grown. The percentage of the population with some form of third-party payment for prescription drugs has been growing for some time. Conversely, out-of-pocket expenditures on these medicines have been falling. As shown in Exhibit 25.4, in 1990, 57 percent of drug expenditures were paid out of pocket, 27 percent were covered by private insurance, and the remaining 16 percent were covered by public funds (primarily Medicaid). As of 2012, only 18 percent of drug expenditures were paid out of pocket by consumers, and

EXHIBIT 25.3
Average
Number of
Prescription
Drug Purchases,
by Age, 2011

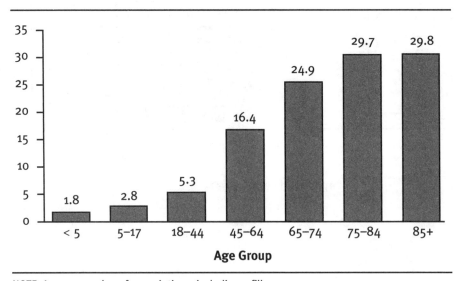

NOTE: Average number of prescriptions, including refills
SOURCE: Data from AHRQ (2013).

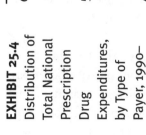

EXHIBIT 25.4
Distribution of
Total National
Prescription
Drug
Expenditures,
by Type of
Payer, 1990–
2012

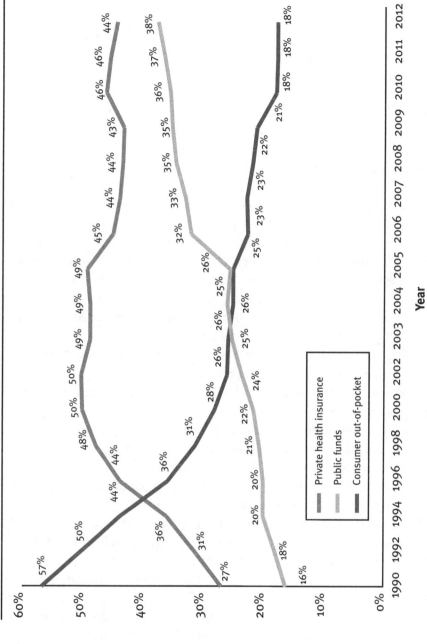

SOURCE: Data from CMS (2014b).

the remaining 44 percent was paid by private insurance and 38 percent was paid by public funds (primarily Medicaid and Medicare). A drug benefit in which the patient's copayment is only $5 per prescription represents a deep price decrease, and drug plans offered by health plans led to large increases in the use of prescription drugs.

The Medicare prescription drug benefit (Part D), which became effective in 2006, stimulated greater use of prescription drugs among the elderly. (As shown in Exhibit 25.1, drug expenditures jumped in 2006.) With Part D, Medicare became the primary payer for many of the aged who were on Medicaid. Medicare drug expenditures rose slower than expected because of the way the benefit is provided.

Drug plans submit bids to the federal government for providing the basic prescription drug benefit to a beneficiary. The federal government calculates a national average bid and pays 75 percent of the national average bid to the drug plan chosen by the beneficiary. The beneficiary is then responsible for the remaining 25 percent of the monthly premium. If a beneficiary enrolls in a plan that submitted a bid higher than the national average, he or she pays the difference—in addition to the base premium. Any difference between a plan's bid and the national average bid translates directly into a price difference that becomes the responsibility of beneficiaries. Beneficiaries choose between plans with a low premium and plans that are more expensive but offer more benefits (such as whether the beneficiary's drugs are included in the insurer's formulary).

Drug plans compete for enrollees by offering low premiums, and the premiums are held down through several cost-containment approaches. One example is the use of formularies (which exclude certain drugs from coverage) requiring prior authorization for approval of certain drugs and tiered cost sharing, such as 25 percent (or $10) copayment for generics, 30 percent (or $25) for branded drugs in the formulary, and 40 to 50 percent (or $50) for branded drugs not in the formulary. Prices and expenditures would have increased more rapidly without the financial incentive that beneficiaries have to choose among competing drug plans, the competition among firms providing the benefit, and the ability of these firms to negotiate price discounts from pharmaceutical companies to include their branded drugs in the plans' formularies. The estimated federal cost of the drug benefit has been much less than anticipated.

As part of the 2010 Affordable Care Act (ACA), the Part D "donut hole" is reduced and Medicare beneficiaries have smaller out-of-pocket payments for their prescription drugs. This change, which is phased in over time, is likely to increase prescription drug utilization and Medicare drug expenditures.

Exhibit 25.5 illustrates both the changing share of spending on prescription drugs and the growth in drug expenditures over time. Previously, the largest share of spending on drugs came from private health insurance and health plans. After Part D became available, the share of total drug expenditures by private health plans shrank and the number of firms serving Medicare beneficiaries grew.

Rise in Drug Prices

Drug prices (which are less of a contributing factor to expenditure increases than drug utilization) rose at double-digit rates annually during the 1980s but moderated to 4 percent to 5 percent annually during the 1990s. Recent annual drug price increases have been less than the price hikes for hospital and physician services, and they (as measured by the Bureau of Labor Statistics) appear to be less of a contributing factor to the higher drug expenditures today than before the mid-1990s.

An important reason for the slowdown in drug price increases is that patents for many top-selling drugs have expired and these drugs have been subject to competition from cheaper generics, resulting in lower prices (and profits). Further, fewer high-priced new drugs have entered the market, resulting in an overall slowdown. Health plans have tried to control expenditure growth by creating stronger incentives for their enrollees to choose generic or cheaper brand-name drugs.

Several studies have examined the relationship between the out-of-pocket drug price (copayments) and drug expenditures. These studies (such as Goodell and Swartz 2010) have found that more cost sharing leads to more adverse health events, such as emergency department visits and inpatient admissions. Conversely, the use of newer drugs results in less inpatient care. Understanding the effect of price on drug utilization has important consequences on both drug and total medical expenditures. A substitution effect occurs between drug use and use of other medical services. Raising the copayments for certain drugs not only reduces the demand for those drugs but also likely encourages the use of expensive medical services, thereby increasing medical expenditures.[1] Health plans, aware of the high price sensitivity between copayments and drug usage, have lowered the copayments for patients taking prescription drugs for chronic illnesses (and have also applied various methods to remind those patients to take their medications) to reduce costly hospitalizations.

Changes in Types of Drugs Prescribed

Over time, the composition of the types of prescription drugs used changes, which in turn affects how fast drug expenditures grow. When a new, innovative drug enters the market, its price is higher than the drug it replaces. When a

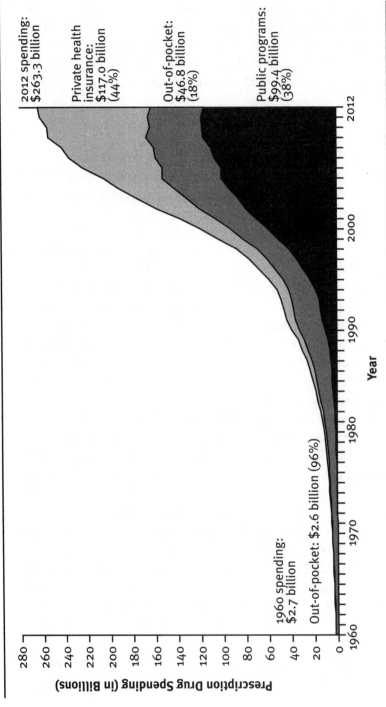

EXHIBIT 25.5
Share of Prescription Drug Spending, by Source of Funds, Selected Years, 1960–2012

Prescription Drug Spending (in Billions)

Year

2012 spending: $263.3 billion

Private health insurance: $117.0 billion (44%)

Out-of-pocket: $46.8 billion (18%)

Public programs: $99.4 billion (38%)

1960 spending: $2.7 billion

Out-of-pocket: $2.6 billion (96%)

NOTE: "Public programs" cover federal, state, and local spending for prescription drugs, including Medicare, workers' compensation, temporary disability, public assistance (Medicaid and CHIP), Department of Defense, maternal/child health, Veterans' Administration, and Indian Health Services.
SOURCE: Data from CMS (2014b).

"me-too" drug enters the market, it becomes a good substitute for an innovative drug, which in turn lowers the price of both drugs. Similarly, when the patent on a drug expires and a generic version of the drug enters the market, many switch from the expensive brand-name drug to the cheaper generic. (About 50 percent of drugs approved by the Food and Drug Administration (FDA) have generic versions.) Drug expenditures may increase more or less rapidly depending on the number of innovative, high-priced drugs brought to market, the entry of me-too drugs, whether (and how many) branded drugs lose their patent protection, and how rapidly generic substitutes become available.

The 1990s saw a large addition to the market of innovative but costly new drugs that have preventive and curative effects, which resulted in greater use. These drugs can treat previously untreatable illnesses and have substituted for expensive invasive medical procedures, which lowered overall treatment costs. New drugs reduce nonpharmaceutical medical costs, such as new antidepressants that have minimized costly psychotherapy as well as beta-blockers and blood pressure drugs that have lessened expensive cardiovascular-related hospital admissions and surgeries. Lichtenberg (2007, 2012) concluded that replacing older drugs with newer drugs has resulted in greater life expectancy at birth and lower mortality, morbidity (as indicated by fewer days lost from work), and total treatment costs (particularly for inpatient care). The use of new drugs has brought about large hospital savings because it shortened lengths of stay and cut down on the number of admissions. The total reduction in nondrug medical expenses is about seven times the increase in drug costs.

Some new drugs also have fewer adverse side effects. Many lifestyle drugs—such as Viagra (treatment of male impotence), Claritin (relief from allergies), Prilosec (relief from stomach upsets), and pain relievers—improve quality of life. However, they may be much more expensive than older drugs. For example, new pain relievers treat severe arthritis, but they cost $150 a month, nearly 20 times more than older pain relievers. Enbrel, a biotech drug that treats rheumatoid arthritis, can cost $1,500 a month. Whereas drugs such as penicillin would be prescribed for a brief period to cure an infection, some modern drugs (including lifestyle drugs) can be taken for decades. The prospect of better health and better quality of life has led to a proliferation of prescriptions and boosted the price of new drugs.

Over the past several years, many well-known brand-name prescription drugs, such as Lipitor (an anticholesterol drug), lost their patent protection. As generic substitutes entered the market, prices for these drugs declined along with the growth rate of drug expenditures. In coming years, additional innovative specialty drugs will become available. These specialty drugs—referred to as *biologics*—are "complex proteins that are made in living cells that treat a range of diseases, from various types of cancer to rare hereditary diseases. Increasingly, they come with jaw-dropping price tags: four drugs approved in 2012 carry a yearly cost of more than $200,000 per patient" (Thomas 2013). In 2012, expenditures on specialty drugs for privately insured patients rose by 18.4 percent, while spending on traditional prescription drugs has barely changed.

Although many patients relying on traditional prescription drugs will have smaller out-of-pocket costs, the expense of specialty drugs will be a financial hardship for patients who have to incur large copayments to use these drugs. Insurers will also face a major financial expense as the use of specialty drugs becomes common.

Rising drug expenditures should be viewed favorably when innovative drugs become available to extend life, substitute for more costly treatments, and improve the quality of life. Further, a greater number of prescriptions per person (particularly for the aged) may indicate that chronic diseases can be better managed, the elderly can live longer, and their quality of life can be enhanced.

Pricing Practices of US Pharmaceutical Companies

Drug manufacturers sell their drugs to different purchasers (intermediaries), who in turn sell them to patients. Retail (independent and chain) pharmacies sell about 45 percent of all prescription drugs; healthcare organizations such as health maintenance organizations (HMOs), hospitals, long-term care facilities, home health care agencies, federal facilities, and clinics sell 28 percent; mail-order pharmacies sell 20 percent; and food stores sell 7 percent (see Exhibit 25.6). (HMO and insurance company patients rely on mail-order and retail pharmacies that are in their insurers' networks for their drugs.)

Pharmaceutical companies sell the same prescription drug to different purchasers at different prices. An HMO pays less for its drugs than does an independent retail pharmacy, although the latter sells a much greater volume of drugs. Similarly, patients without any prescription drug coverage (often the poor and sick) pay more for the same drug at a retail pharmacy than patients who are part of a managed care plan.

Two aspects of the pricing practices of pharmaceutical companies have been criticized as unfair and have led to proposals for government intervention. First, different purchasers are charged different prices for the same drug. Second, prescription drugs have a high price markup.

Pricing According to Cost

A new prescription drug is priced many times higher than its actual costs of production. This high markup over cost has generated a great deal of criticism. If

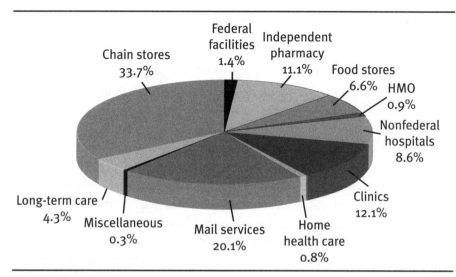

SOURCE: Data from IMS Health (2013).

EXHIBIT 25.6
Prescription
Sales by Outlet,
US Market,
2012

the drug were priced closer to its production cost, it would be less of a financial burden on those with low income, those without prescription drug coverage, and state Medicaid budgets.

Drug manufacturers often claim that their prices are determined by the high costs of developing the drugs. High research and development (or R&D) costs, however, are not the reason for high or rising drug prices. Large fixed (or sunk) costs are those that have already been incurred; hence, they are not relevant for setting a drug's price. Fixed costs must eventually be recovered, or the drug company will lose money; however, a new drug that is no different than drugs already on the market could not sell for more than these competing drugs—regardless of how much that drug cost to develop.

Pricing According to Demand

When price differences for the same drug cannot be entirely explained by cost variations, according to economic theory the reason must be related to the differences in the purchaser's price sensitivity or willingness to pay. Purchasers who are not price sensitive will be charged higher prices than those who are. A purchaser who is willing to buy less or switch to another drug when the price increases is more price sensitive than one who is not.

The higher price charged to one purchaser is not meant to make up for the lower price charged to another purchaser. Instead, the reason for different prices is that the seller can simply make more money by charging according to each purchaser's willingness to pay (Frank 2001).

The ability to shift market share rather than just the volume purchased drives discounts. Not all large-volume purchasers receive price discounts. Retail pharmacies in total sell a large volume of drugs, but they do not receive the same price discounts as managed care plans do. When an HMO negotiates with a drug company on one of several competing brand-name drugs within a therapeutic class, the HMO's willingness to place the drug on its formulary while excluding a competitor's drugs can result in substantial discounts for the HMO.[2] Medicare prescription drug plans use the same strategy as HMOs use. Similarly, pharmacy benefit managers (PBMs), who manage health plans' drug benefits for drugs sold through retail pharmacies, can promote brand-name substitution and thereby receive large discounts.[3]

Retail pharmacies pay the highest prices for their prescription drugs because they must carry all branded drugs. Furthermore, the pharmacy cannot promote substitution between branded drugs because the physician may be prescribing according to a health plan's formulary. Because pharmacies cannot shift volume, drug manufacturers see no need to give them a price discount.[4] (To receive price discounts, government entities have resorted to price regulation; see Chapter 28.) For a pharmacy to be included in a health plan or a PBM network it must charge lower dispensing fees, which also results in lower prices to the PBM and to health plan enrollees.

Price discrimination—whereby a seller charges different prices to different purchasers—occurs in many other areas of the economy. For example, seniors and students pay lower prices at the movies and other events. Prices may differ by time of day, such as early-bird dinner specials and drinks, and airlines charge business travelers more than they do vacationers because the former group books flights on short notice. Those who are less likely to switch are less price sensitive and are charged more for the same service.

Price discrimination actually promotes price competition between drug manufacturers for more price-sensitive purchasers, which results in lower prices for purchasers and consumers. To price discriminate, a seller must prevent low-price buyers from reselling the product to those who are charged more. A 1987 federal law prevented resale of prescription drugs on the basis of preserving the safety and integrity of those drugs.

Pricing Innovative Drugs

Pharmaceutical manufacturers are strategic in how they mark up the price of their drugs (price-to-cost ratio) and negotiate price discounts. A drug's price markup is determined by demand. New drugs are priced according to their therapeutic value and the availability of good substitutes. When a new drug for which there is no close substitute comes on the market and is clearly therapeutically superior to existing drugs, it will have a higher price markup. Sometimes a drug is priced according to some concept of value, such as comparing it to the surgical procedure it replaces. Approving an existing drug for a new use also raises its value, as its therapeutic effects for that new use are greater than the effects of existing drugs; thus, the drug company is able to increase its price.

The greater the price markup over costs, the more innovative the drug and the fewer the close substitutes to it. Innovative drugs command higher price markups than do imitative drugs. Ultimately, the price of a new drug is determined by a purchaser's willingness to pay for its greater therapeutic benefits. A new breakthrough drug is priced much higher than any other drug in its therapeutic class (typically, more than three times the price) because no good substitutes are available. New drugs with modest therapeutic gains are priced about two times the average for available drug substitutes. New drugs with little or no gain over existing drugs are priced at about the same level as existing substitutes. Once the patent has expired on a branded drug, generic drugs are introduced and are typically priced at about 30 percent to 70 percent of the branded drug's price before the patent expired. As more generic versions become available, the prices of generic drugs drop.

New, higher-priced drugs will fail commercially if their therapeutic benefits are similar to those of existing drugs. As health plans evaluate drugs (on the basis of therapeutic benefits and price) for inclusion in their formularies, differences in drug prices will reflect differences in therapeutic benefits. Knowledgeable purchasers evaluating a more expensive new drug will pay a higher price only if its therapeutic benefits are greater than those of the older drug.

A new drug that is similar to an existing drug (a me-too drug) cannot be priced much higher than the existing drug because purchasers will switch to a good substitute (the existing drug) at a lower price. Although drug companies have been criticized for producing me-too drugs, their availability contributes to price competition. (Me-too drugs also provide value in that they may have fewer side effects than the existing drugs have.)

Once competitors enter the market originally served by an innovative drug, prices decline. Interestingly, when generic versions enter the market after the patent on a branded drug has expired, the branded drug loses market share to the generic drug, but the price of the branded product actually increases; the price-sensitive customers switch to the generic drug, and those who do not switch are not price sensitive. Therefore, the seller of the branded drug is able to raise its price. Some physicians (and consumers) have strong preferences for the branded drug and do not want it substituted with the generic version; they are willing to pay more for the perceived security of the brand-name drug.[5] Drug manufacturers have determined that serving a smaller market at a higher price is more profitable than reducing the price of the branded drug to compete with generic versions.[6]

Thus, the pricing strategy of pharmaceutical companies is based on two principles. First, the greater the price sensitivity of the purchaser—such as an HMO willing to shift its drug purchases to a competitor's drug—the lower the price. Second, the more innovative the drug, the higher the price markup will be. These pricing strategies are designed to maximize profits for the drug manufacturer.

Drug Companies' Marketing Response to Managed Care Plans

Purchaser decision making regarding pharmaceuticals has changed. Previously, physicians chose a patient's prescription drug. As a result, drug manufacturers spent a great deal of money marketing directly to physicians. With the growth of managed care and its use of closed formularies, drug companies began to develop new marketing strategies. As the purchasing decision over prescription drugs shifted from the individual physician to the committee overseeing the organization's formulary, sending sales representatives to individual physicians caring for an HMO's patients was less useful than marketing to the HMO itself. Drug companies have had to demonstrate that their drugs are not only therapeutically superior to competing drugs but also cost-effective—namely that the additional benefits of their drug are worth its higher price. Physicians continue to be important in prescribing drugs to their patients, but PBMs and health plans determine which brand-name drugs the physician is able to prescribe and the prices paid for those drugs.

To counteract the closed formularies, drug manufacturers started direct-to-consumer television and newspaper advertising to generate consumer demand for certain drugs from their physicians. Direct-to-consumer advertising—the cost of which increased from about $600 million in 1997 (the first year it was permitted by the FDA) to $2.5 billion in 2000 and to $3.2 billion in 2012—initially proved effective in boosting sales of advertised prescription drugs. Physicians almost never wrote prescriptions for drugs requested by patients because most patients did not know enough to demand drugs by name or therapeutic class. As more medical information has become available to patients, they have begun demanding more input into the therapeutic decisions that affect their lives. Drug companies claim that ads are meant to inform the patient and stimulate a discussion between the patient and her physician. Critics claim that the ads do not inform patients about who is most likely to benefit from that drug, its possible side effects, or other treatment options.[7]

Prescription drug plan formularies include a tiered set of copayments for a drug—a small copayment for a less costly generic version of the drug and a higher copayment for the branded version. Brand-name drug firms have made coupons available to patients at the physician's office, and on their websites they give patients an opportunity to pay the difference in copayment between the generic and branded version. These coupons make the out-of-pocket costs to the patients the same, regardless of whether they choose the generic or branded version of the drug. The coupons are subsidized by the firm when the patient redeems the coupon at the pharmacy (Ross and Kesselheim 2013).

Brand-name drug firms benefit from the use of coupons through increased sales of branded drugs, given that the out-of-pocket price to the patient of a branded drug is reduced and is the same as the generic version. Further, coupons are generally available for branded drugs that are used for long periods, such as for chronic diseases. The availability of coupons, however, is limited, typically for several months and less than a year at which time the out-of-pocket copayment to the patient for the branded drug rises. Presumably, after the patient has become used to the branded drug, he may be less likely to switch to the generic version.

By using coupons, drug firms have been able to undercut insurers' tiered formularies of shifting patients to cheaper generics through the use of different copayments. Although the cost of the branded drug to the patient has been reduced, insurers must pay the higher cost of the branded drug. The cost, and subsequently the premium, for the drug plan is raised to all of the plan's enrollees.

Although drug costs have become a large expense for health plans, and health plans have introduced tiered copayments to provide their enrollees with an incentive to use less costly drugs, health plans have also reduced or eliminated copays for the use of certain drugs. Given the inverse relationship between price and use of drugs, health plans are lowering drug copayments to encourage the use of drugs that reduce expensive medical episodes. If decreasing copayments—or even providing the drug for free—makes a patient more likely to follow the recommended drug therapy and thereby prevent recurrence of a heart attack or a stroke, the health plan is able to reduce its cost and benefit the patient.

Summary

Prescription drug expenditures will continue to grow partly because of greater drug utilization, which results from the introduction of costly drugs. New drugs have a high markup in relation to their cost of production. To those without drug coverage and to large purchasers of drugs—such as health plans, Medicare drug plans, and state Medicaid agencies—these facts are a cause for concern. However, the public should view rising drug expenditures and even high price markups favorably. Rising drug prices are often an indication that new drugs are more effective than existing drugs or alternative treatments. (When new drugs are of higher quality—that is, when they provide greater benefits than the drugs they replace—their "quality-adjusted" price may well be lower than the price of older drugs. Thus, considering the higher prices of new drugs as mere price increases is misleading.) Further, when new drugs replace old drugs, purchasers value the therapeutic benefits of the new drugs more and are willing to pay the cost for that value. Clearly, the consumers are better off.

Replacing old drugs with new drugs is just one important factor in the growth of drug expenditures. Also contributing factors are the increase in third-party payment for prescription drugs, population growth, and the aging of the population. All of these will likely cause drug expenditures to continue to stay enormous in the future.

Drug manufacturers charge different prices to different buyers for the same drug (price discrimination) so as to give price discounts to purchasers who are willing to switch their drug purchases and charge higher prices to those who are less price sensitive (unwilling to switch). The cost-containment strategies of health plans and PBMs have caused pharmaceutical firms to compete on price to have their drugs included in the formularies of large purchasers and to emphasize the cost-effectiveness of their drugs. These firms have rolled out direct-to-consumer advertising that puts pressure on consumers to demand the firms' drugs from their physicians.[8] To limit the effect of such tactics, health plans have instituted tiered copayment systems that give consumers incentives to use drugs on the health plan's formulary.

Discussion Questions

1. Which factors have contributed most to the increase in drug expenditures?
2. Are rising drug expenditures necessarily bad?
3. Is the high price of drugs determined by the high cost of developing a new drug?
4. Why do drug manufacturers charge different purchasers different prices for the same prescription drug?
5. What methods have managed care plans used to limit their enrollees' drug costs?
6. What are the likely consequences of the ACA closing the "donut hole"?

Notes

1. The relationship between the out-of-pocket price of drugs and drug expenditures has been estimated to be −1.13; that is, a 1 percent *increase* in price will result in a 1.13 percent *decrease* in drug expenditures over time (Gaynor, Li, and Vogt 2006).

2. As HMOs and health plans seek volume discounts from drug companies, they are willing to limit their subscribers' choice of drugs in return for lower drug prices. Drug formulary committees focus on drugs for which therapeutic substitutes exist and evaluate different drugs according to their therapeutic value and price; higher-priced drugs are used only when justified by greater therapeutic benefits. Restrictions are then placed on their physicians' prescribing behavior. These organizations are also using computer technology to conduct drug utilization review; each physician's prescription is instantly checked against the formulary, and data are gathered on the performance of each physician and the health plan's use of specific drugs.

3. PBMs are firms that provide administrative services and process outpatient prescription drug claims for health insurers' prescription drug plans. To control growth in prescription drug expenditures, PBMs also contract with a network of pharmacies, negotiate pharmacy payments, negotiate with drug manufacturers for drug discounts and rebates, develop a drug formulary listing preferred drugs for treating an illness, encourage use of generic drugs instead of high-priced brand-name drugs, operate a mail-order pharmacy, and analyze and monitor patient compliance programs. Some PBMs have been very aggressive in switching physicians' prescriptions; they may call a physician and tell her that a less expensive drug is available for the same medical condition and suggest that the physician switch drugs to one on which the PBM receives a large price discount or rebate.

4. In 1993, an antitrust suit was filed by 31,000 retail pharmacies against 24 pharmaceutical manufacturers, claiming that the drug companies conspired to charge HMOs, PBMs, and hospitals lower prices while denying price discounts to retail pharmacies. Most of the drug companies settled by paying a relatively small average amount per retail pharmacy and said they would give the same discounts to retail pharmacies if they could demonstrate that the pharmacies were able to shift the market share of their drugs. Five drug companies refused to settle. The retail pharmacies had to prove that price discrimination harmed competition and that the discounts were not a competitive

response to another drug firm's lower prices. At the trial in 1998, the judge dismissed the lawsuit; the decision was upheld on appeal (Culyer and Newhouse 2000).

5. The drug companies claimed they did not offer a price discount to retail pharmacies because the discounts would not increase the drug companies' market share. Retail pharmacies had to carry a wide selection of drugs because they merely filled orders of prescribing physicians. The greater the ability of the buyer to switch market share away from one drug manufacturer to a competitor's drug, the greater the discount. The drug companies claimed that retail pharmacies were unable to switch volume from one drug company to another; therefore, there was no reason to give them a discount.

6. The Bureau of Labor Statistics drug price index overstates drug price increases when a generic equivalent of a branded drug enters the market. The lower-priced generic drug rapidly expands the market share at the expense of the branded drug for which the generic drug is a substitute. As the branded drug loses market share to the generic drug, its price is raised to the remaining patients who are less price sensitive and more reluctant to use the generic version of the drug. The drug price index picks up the price increase of the branded drug but does not measure the price decline experienced by the large proportion of consumers who switch to the generic version. Thus, the drug price index fails to reflect the sharp price decline with the introduction of the generic drug.

7. When the patent on a branded drug expires, the first generic version of that drug has a six-month period of exclusivity over other generics; the first generic can capture up to 90 percent of the market from the branded drug. Typically, the branded drug manufacturer does not produce the generic version when its patent expires.

8. Direct-to-consumer advertising has recently declined. Advertisers believe that such advertising is effective only for new brand-name drugs and for new drug categories (Pharma Marketing Network 2013).

References

Agency for Healthcare Research and Quality (AHRQ). 2013. "Medical Expenditure Panel Survey (MEPS) Household Component, 2011." MEPSnet/HC Trend Query. Last updated November 1. http://meps.ahrq.gov/mepsweb/data_stats/MEPSnetHC.jsp.

Bureau of Labor Statistics (BLS). 2014. "Consumer Price Index." Accessed
    January. www.bls.gov/cpi/home.htm.

Centers for Medicare & Medicaid Services (CMS). 2014a. "National
    Health Expenditure Data." Last modified May 5. www.cms.gov/
    NationalHealthExpendData/.

———. 2014b. "Tables." Accessed January. www.cms.gov/NationalHealthExpend
    Data/downloads/tables.pdf.

Culyer, A., and J. Newhouse. 2000. *Handbook of Health Economics*, vol. 1B. New
    York: North-Holland.

Frank, R. G. 2001. "Prescription Drug Prices: Why Do Some Pay More Than
    Others Do?" *Health Affairs* 20 (2): 115–28.

Gaynor, M., J. Li, and W. Vogt. 2006. "Is Drug Coverage a Free Lunch? Cross-
    Price Elasticities and the Design of Prescription Drug Benefits." *NBER
    Working Paper* No. 12758, December. Cambridge, MA: National Bureau of
    Economic Research.

Goodell, S., and K. Swartz. 2010. "Cost Sharing: Effects on Spending and
    Outcomes." *Policy Brief* No. 20. Robert Wood Johnson Foundation.
    Accessed December 2013. www.rwjf.org/content/dam/farm/reports/
    issue_briefs/2010/rwjf402103.

IMS Health. 2013. *Top-Line Industry Data*. www.imshealth.com.

Lichtenberg, F. 2012. "Pharmaceutical Innovation and Longevity Growth in 30
    Developing and High-Income Countries, 2000–2009." *NBER Working
    Paper* No. 18235, July. Cambridge, MA: National Bureau of Economic
    Research.

———. 2007. "The Benefits and Costs of Newer Drugs: An Update." *Managerial
    and Decision Economics* 28 (4–5): 485–90.

National Institute for Health Care Management. 2002. "Prescription Drug
    Expenditures in 2001: Another Year of Escalating Costs." Revised May 6.
    www.nihcm.org/pdf/spending2001.pdf.

Pharma Marketing Network. 2013. "Spending on Direct-to-Consumer Advertising
    Takes a Nosedive." *Pharma Marketing News* 12 (3). www.pharma-mkting
    .com/news/pmn1203-article03.pdf.

Ross, J., and A. Kesselheim. 2013. "Prescription-Drug Coupons—No Such Thing
    as a Free Lunch." *New England Journal of Medicine* 369: 1188–89. www
    .nejm.org/doi/full/10.1056/NEJMp1301993?query=health-policy-and-
    reform.

Thomas, K. 2013. "U.S. Drug Costs Dropped in 2012, but Rises Loom." *New
    York Times*, March 18. www.nytimes.com/2013/03/19/business/use-of-
    generics-produces-an-unusual-drop-in-drug-spending.html.

US Census Bureau. 2013. "Population Estimates." Accessed January 2014.
    www.census.gov.

ENSURING SAFETY AND EFFICACY OF NEW DRUGS: TOO MUCH OF A GOOD THING?

26

Innovative new drugs have decreased mortality, increased life expectancy, and improved the quality of life for many millions of people. New drugs have also reduced the cost of medical care, substituting for more costly surgeries and long hospital stays. At the time of discovery, however, the effects of new drugs are not fully known. Powerful drugs that have the potential for curing cancer may also have harmful side effects. Some drugs may cause illness or even death for some people but may provide beneficial effects to others. New drugs offer a trade-off: improvements in the quality and length of life versus possible serious adverse consequences.

Approval by the Food and Drug Administration (FDA) is required before any new drug may be marketed in the United States. The FDA's objective should be to achieve a balance between the concerns of drug safety and the prospective benefits of pharmaceutical innovation. Ensuring that a new drug does not harm anyone delays the introduction of a beneficial drug that may save many lives. This delay may result in the deaths of thousands of people whose lives could have been saved had the new drug been approved earlier. On the other hand, introducing potential breakthrough drugs immediately may cause the deaths of many, as the full effects of the new drug are not completely understood.

How should this trade-off in lives be evaluated? Is each type of life—those potentially saved by early introduction of a new drug versus those who might die from early approval—valued equally? Regulatory delay increases the time and cost of bringing a new drug to market. Thus, excessive caution and excessive expediency both incur risks. Either may cause a loss of lives. This chapter discusses the FDA and its history and performance regarding the drug-approval process.

History of Regulation of Prescription Drugs

The Pure Food and Drug Act of 1906 was the federal government's first major effort at regulating the pharmaceutical industry. The supporters of this act, however, were primarily concerned with the quality of food, not drugs. Pure food acts had been submitted to Congress for at least ten years before one was finally passed. Media publicity on the ingredients of food and drugs generated popular support for legislative action. A great deal of publicity was generated by newspapers; magazine articles; and Upton Sinclair's 1906 book *The Jungle*, with its graphic descriptions of what was being included in the foods the public was eating. The result was public outrage, to which Congress responded by passing the Pure Food and Drug Act.

The act required drug companies to provide accurate labeling information, including whether the drug was addictive. (A number of medicines contained alcohol, opium, heroin, and cocaine, which were legal at that time.) The government could verify the accuracy of the drug's contents. Subsequent court cases resolved that therapeutic claims made by the sellers of a drug would not be considered fraudulent if the sellers believed their therapeutic claims. Thus, the drug-related portion of the act was quite limited and was modeled by the public's concern with the contents of food.

In the 1930s, the modern drug era began with the development of sulfa drugs. As these drugs were introduced, a tragedy provided the impetus for new legislation. A company seeking to make a liquid form of sulfanilamide for children dissolved it with diethylene glycol (a component of antifreeze), unaware of the toxic effects. As a result, more than 100 children died before the drug was recalled. Responding to the public outcry, Congress passed the Food, Drug, and Cosmetic Act in 1938. This law, which created the FDA, was intended to protect the public from unsafe, potentially harmful drugs. A company had to seek approval from the FDA before it could market a new drug. Drug companies determined the necessary amount and type of pre-marketing test to prove to the government that the drug was safe for its intended use.

A 1950 amendment to the 1938 act authorized the FDA to distinguish prescription from nonprescription drugs by stating that some types of drugs could only be sold by prescription, as they could be harmful to the individual if bought on their own.

The 1962 Amendments to the Food, Drug, and Cosmetic Act

In 1959, Senator Estes Kefauver (who was running for the Democratic nomination for president at that time) held hearings on the drug industry. Critics of the industry were concerned that drug prices were too high, that drug companies undertook unnecessary and wasteful advertising expenditures, and that the drug industry earned excessive profits.

In the late 1950s, a new drug was introduced in Europe to treat morning sickness for pregnant women. After the introduction of thalidomide in Europe, an FDA staff member expressed doubts about the safety of the drug because of reported side effects and delayed its approval. An American drug company, however, was able to introduce it into the United States on an experimental basis. (The 1938 FDA amendments permitted such limited distribution to qualified experts so long as the drug was labeled as being under investigation.) As soon as reports began to appear in Europe that deformed babies were born to mothers who had taken the drug during pregnancy, the American company withdrew the drug.

The resulting media attention given to thalidomide and its effects in Europe shifted Congress's concern about high drug prices, wasteful expenditures, and excessive profits to concern with public safety. Congress responded to the public's fears about drug safety and passed the 1962 amendments to the Food, Drug, and Cosmetic Act. (Richard Harris [1964] provides a history of the 1962 amendments.)

The 1962 amendments resulted in a major change in the regulation of pharmaceuticals. Drug companies were now required to prove the safety of their new drugs and their efficacy (beyond a placebo effect) for the indications claimed for them in treating a particular disease or condition. (Effectiveness must be determined by a controlled study in which some patients are given the new drug and others are given a placebo, an inactive substance such as a salt or sugar pill.) Once the FDA approves a new drug for marketing, the drug is approved only for specific claims. If the drug company wants to broaden those claims, it must file a new application with the FDA and provide evidence to support the new uses of that drug. (Physicians may, however, prescribe a drug for a use for which the FDA has not approved it.)

The steps that a drug company must take to meet the FDA's safety and efficacy standards are costly and time consuming. The FDA specifies the type of pre-marketing tests that are required. Before undertaking clinical trials using humans, animal trials are used to determine whether the drug is sufficiently safe and promising to justify human trials. Based on this evidence, the FDA will approve clinical trials using humans. Each of the three different stages of clinical trials uses a greater number of subjects so that more dangerous drugs are identified before they can affect more patients. Stage 1 introduces the drug to a small number (20 to 80) of healthy individuals to evaluate its safety and to identify side effects. Stage 2 uses a large number (100 to 300) of persons with the disease to determine appropriate medication dosage and preliminary effectiveness. Stage 3 uses a great number (1,000 to 3,000) of patients, half of whom take a placebo, and is designed to confirm the drug's effectiveness, demonstrate efficacy, and provide additional evidence of safety. Clinical trials take, on average, six years to complete once animal and laboratory studies have been undertaken. Once completed, the drug firm must receive FDA approval, which can take an additional several years.[1] Once approved by the FDA, the new drug must be manufactured according to specified standards.

Easier Entry for Generic Drugs

After the 1962 amendments were enacted, generic and patented drugs were treated in the same manner. Both had to meet the same stringent FDA requirements as a new drug seeking a patent. Manufacturers of generic drugs had to independently prove the safety and efficacy of their products to receive FDA approval. Because the research of generic drugs had to be undertaken in the same process as the patented drug, the cost and time for developing generic drugs increased. Once a new drug received its patent and was approved by the FDA, the drug had no competition for a longer period and the price could be kept high for a longer time. Consumers continued to face high prices for prescription drugs for which the patents had expired because of FDA requirements that delayed the entry of generic substitutes.

The Drug Price Competition and Patent Term Restoration (Hatch-Waxman) Act of 1984 simplified and streamlined the process for FDA approval of generic drugs in exchange for granting patent extensions to innovative drugs. Generic drugs no longer had to replicate many of the clinical trials performed by the original manufacturer to prove safety and efficacy. Instead, the generic drug manufacturer was only required to demonstrate that the generic drug was "bioequivalent" to the already approved patented drug, which was much less costly than proving safety and efficacy. (Bioequivalence means the active ingredient is absorbed at the same rate and to the same extent for the generic drug as for the patented drug.) The effect of the Hatch-Waxman act was to reduce the delay between patent expiration and generic entry from more than three years to less than three months. Generic substitutes for branded drugs with expired patents are now quickly available at much-reduced prices. Previously, only 35 percent of top-selling drugs whose patents expired had generic copies; currently, almost all do.[2]

Although the Hatch-Waxman act made generic-drug entry easier and less costly once a patent expired, it also extended the patent life of branded drugs to compensate for patent life lost during the long FDA approval process. (Effective patent life is measured from the time the FDA approves a new drug to the end of the patent.) The act permitted drugs that contain a new chemical entity to qualify for a patent life extension. These patent extensions postpone generic entry by an average of about 2.8 years. The act was a compromise between the generic-drug manufacturers (which wanted easier entry) and the brand-name drug manufacturers (which wanted a longer patent life).[3]

State legislation in the 1970s and 1980s also enabled generic drugs to rapidly increase their market share. Through the early 1970s, pharmacists in many states could not legally dispense a generic drug when a prescription specified a brand-name drug. By 1984, all states had enacted drug substitution legislation that permitted a pharmacist to substitute a generic drug even when a brand-name drug was specified, as long as the physician had not indicated otherwise on the prescription.

Accelerated Approval for Lifesaving Drugs

During the 1980s and 1990s, AIDS activists were critical of the FDA's approval process. AIDS patients were dying from the disease and wanted promising new drugs to be immediately available. Approval would be too late for many if these drugs were delayed for years because of research protocols required by the FDA. Giving half of terminally ill AIDS patients a placebo was believed to be immoral, as they would be denied a possible lifesaving drug. Many terminally ill AIDS patients were willing to bear the risk of taking drugs that might prove to be unsafe or to have adverse side effects.

AIDS activists pressured Congress and the FDA for an accelerated approval process. As a result, new laws and regulations were enacted between 1987 and 1992 that enabled seriously ill patients to have access to experimental drugs. These types of drugs were provided with a "fast-track" approval process. For other serious or life-threatening diseases, drugs in the clinical trial stages that were shown to have meaningful therapeutic benefit compared with existing treatments were also given an expedited review. In return for early approval of these new drugs, the drug firm had to periodically notify the FDA about any adverse reactions to the drug that were not detected during the clinical trial periods.

In 1992, Congress enacted the Prescription Drug User Fee Act (renewable every five years), which authorized the FDA to collect fees from drug manufacturers seeking a drug approval. The revenues from these fees were to be used to increase the number of FDA staff reviewing drug approvals. As a result, the approval process took less time and the number of new drugs approved rose, compared to figures in previous years.[4]

Both the fast-tracking approval process and the funds from user fees reduced the time for FDA approvals of new drugs. As shown in Exhibit 26.1, in the late 1980s, the FDA took about 32 months to approve a new drug. By 1998, the average approval time was less than 12 months. Unfortunately, over the past decade, the average FDA approval time has increased to almost a year and a half; in 2011, it was 15.8 months.

FDA's Stringent Guidelines for Safety and Efficacy

It is difficult to oppose greater drug safety. As a consequence of FDA regulatory requirements, physicians and the public are better informed about

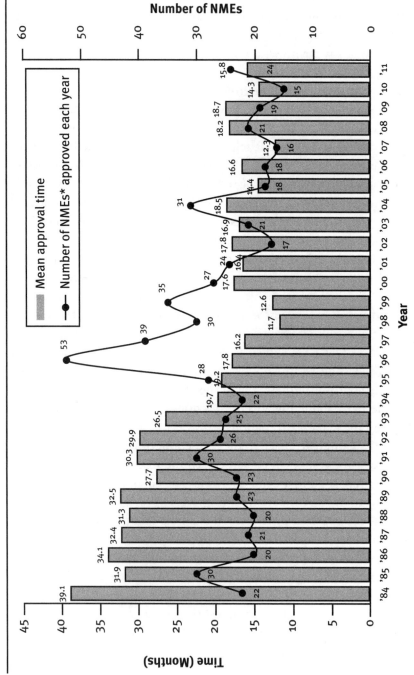

Number of NMEs

EXHIBIT 26.1
Number of and
Mean Approval
Times for New
Molecular
Entities in the
United States,
1984–2011

* NMEs: new molecular entities
NOTE: NMEs are new medicines that have never been marketed before. They include diagnostic and nondiagnostic drugs.
SOURCE: Data from PAREXEL International (2013), p. 293.

approved drug uses and possible side effects. However, FDA regulation has had some adverse consequences.

The US Drug Lag

One measure of the FDA's performance is how long it takes to approve a drug in the United States versus in other countries. After the 1962 amendments were enacted, a long lag developed between the time drugs were available for use in other countries and the time they could be used in the United States. For example, drugs proven effective for treating heart disease and hypertension were used in Great Britain as early as 1965, but they were not fully approved for use in the United States until 1976. Approximately 7,500 to 15,000 people died in 1988 alone from gastric ulcers while waiting for the FDA to approve misoprostol, which was already available in 43 countries. Furthermore, about 20,000 people are estimated to have died between 1985 and 1987 while waiting for approval of streptokinase, the first drug that could be intravenously administered to reopen the blocked coronary arteries of heart attack victims (Gottlieb 2004).

The drug lag—the time it takes for a new drug to be approved in the United States after it has been approved in another country—has two effects. First, the longer the approval time, the greater the cost of producing a new drug and the fewer years that remain on the patent life of that drug; both of these factors reduce research and development (R&D) profitability and the number of new drugs likely to be developed. Second, and perhaps most important, the longer it takes to approve a new drug, the greater the harm to patients who would have benefited by having access to that drug sooner.[5]

Studies looking at data through the 1970s concluded that a drug lag existed. Researchers compared drugs approved in the United Kingdom and the United States and concluded that drugs approved in the United States lagged behind those approved in the United Kingdom by about two years. However, in more recent years, the US drug lag has decreased. As shown in Exhibit 26.1, the approval rate of new drugs by the FDA was 50 percent faster in the mid-1990s than in the previous decade. Since then, approval times have increased: Between 2000 and 2011, the average approval time has varied from 12.2 to 19.6 months. Understanding changes in the FDA's drug approval rate requires an understanding of the FDA's decision-making process.

FDA's Incentives

The two main criticisms of FDA regulation are the long delays before new drugs are approved (currently about 15.8 months) and the increasing R&D cost imposed on drug companies for bringing a new drug to market. The FDA makes a choice when it decides how much emphasis to place on drug safety and efficacy versus approval delays and increased R&D cost. It is important to understand the political incentives that the FDA faces in making this trade-off.

Politically, a large difference exists between statistical (or invisible) persons who could have been saved and identifiable persons who died as a result of a new drug. When the FDA approves a drug that subsequently results in the deaths of a number of individuals, these deaths will be publicized in the media. Congress is likely to become involved as the publicity increases. The congressional committee that has oversight of the FDA will have hearings at which the relatives of the deceased patients testify. The FDA staff will have to explain why they approved an unsafe drug. As then–FDA commissioner Schmidt stated in 1974 (Grabowski 1976):

> In all of the FDA's history, I am unable to find a single instance where a Congressional Committee investigated the failure of the FDA to approve a new drug. But, the times when hearings have been held to criticize our approval of new drugs have been so frequent that we aren't able to count them…. The message to FDA staff could not be clearer. Whenever a controversy over a new drug is resolved by its approval, the Agency and the individual involved likely will be investigated. Whenever such a drug is disapproved, no inquiry will be made.

Deaths caused by a drug are "visible" or "identifiable" deaths because the individuals affected can be readily identified. Minimizing identifiable deaths, however, delays the FDA approval process. Each day a lifesaving drug is unavailable is a day someone may die because of the lack of that drug. Deaths of persons who may die because a lifesaving drug is unavailable are referred to as *statistical deaths*.[6]

People who die because a lifesaving drug has not yet received FDA approval, although it may be available in Europe, are difficult to identify and are not as visible. The media do not publicize all the nameless people who may have died because a new drug was too costly to be developed or was slow in receiving FDA approval. No media attention is given to the thousands of individuals in need of the drug and their families. Deaths that can be attributed to drug lag, particularly with the early beta-blockers that prevent heart attacks, number in the tens of thousands. The large number of these statistical deaths has greatly outweighed the number of victims of all drug tragedies before the 1962 amendments, including those deaths caused by elixir sulfanilamide in the 1930s.

Statistical lives and identifiable lives are not politically equal. The media and members of Congress place a great deal more pressure on the FDA when a loss of identifiable lives results from a prematurely approved drug than if a much greater loss of statistical lives occurs as a result of the

FDA delaying approval of a new drug. The FDA's incentives are clearly to minimize the loss of identifiable lives at the expense of a greater loss of statistical lives. The FDA can make one of two types of errors, as shown in Exhibit 26.2. Type I error occurs when the FDA approves a drug that is found to have harmful effects; type II error occurs when the FDA either delays or does not approve a beneficial drug. These types of errors are not weighted equally by the FDA. The FDA places greater emphasis on preventing type I errors.

Although a human life is a human life, the decision maker's calculation of the costs and benefits of early versus delayed approval is on the side of delayed approval. The political pressure on FDA staff to justify their decisions will cause them to be overly cautious in approving new drugs until they can be sure no loss of life will occur.

However, the cost–benefit decision to the FDA of when to approve a drug has undergone a change in the past decade. Previously, the FDA bore little cost of delaying approval of a drug (from those who would have benefited from the drug), while it benefited by gathering more and more information on the drug's safety; the FDA minimized the chances that Congress would criticize it for endangering the public's safety. Under these cost–benefit calculations, it was in the FDA's interest to delay approval until it was much more certain about the drug's safety. In recent years, the cost to the FDA of delaying approval has increased. Patient advocacy groups, at times allied with the drug company whose drug is being reviewed, have pressured the FDA for accelerated approval of drugs. Advocacy groups for AIDS patients were among the first to publicize the cost of delays in drug approval. (Pharmaceutical firms supported these patient advocacy groups because they wanted to start earning revenues sooner.)

The effect of patient advocacy groups and media publicity on drug approval times is illustrated by data on approval times for different types of cancer drugs (Carpenter 2004). Although lung cancer has a higher mortality

	Drug Is Beneficial	Drug Is Harmful
FDA Approves Drug	Correct decision	Type I error Allowing a harmful drug; victims are identifiable, and FDA staff must explain to Congress
FDA Does Not Approve Drug	Type II error Disallowing a beneficial drug; victims are not identifiable	Correct decision

EXHIBIT 26.2
The FDA and Type I and Type II Errors

rate and is more costly to treat (requiring more hospitalizations and longer hospital stays) than breast cancer, breast cancer has more advocacy groups who were able to generate greater media attention; consequently, breast cancer drugs were more quickly approved than lung cancer drugs. The same relationship between media publicity and drug approval times exists for other drugs as well.

Patient advocacy groups that are able to generate a great deal of media attention have increased the visibility of the consequences of delay. In doing so, they have raised the political cost to the FDA of drug approval delays (type II errors). However, whenever an approved drug is shown to be less safe than originally believed—as occurred with the arthritis drug Vioxx, which was traced to a small but higher risk of heart attacks among patients who used it (type I error)—the FDA staff will come under much criticism and will revert toward excessive caution in approving new drugs.

Increased Cost of Drug Development

Stringent FDA guidelines and long approval times have greatly raised the cost of developing new drugs. After the 1962 amendments required more rigorous clinical testing, proof of efficacy, and safety criteria for FDA approval, the cost and time for bringing a new drug to market increased sharply. Before the 1962 amendments, the cost of a new drug (including the cost of failed drugs) was $7.9 million in 2013 dollars. The median time between starting clinical testing and receiving FDA approval has gone up over time, from 4.7 years on average during the 1960s (after the 1962 amendments) to 6.7 years in the 1970s, to 8.5 years in the 1980s, and to 9 years in 2010. In the past decade, the time from research idea to marketing a drug took between 10 and 15 years on average (PhRMA 2013).

The cost of developing a new drug has increased dramatically. In 1987, drug companies spent about $231 million to develop a new drug; if the costs had increased at the same rate as inflation, this would have been $467 million in 2012. A study conducted by DiMasi and Grabowski (2007) estimated that the cost has soared to $1.2 billion. More recent estimates range from $1.5 billion to more than $1.8 billion (Mestre-Ferrandiz, Sussex, and Towse 2012). An important reason for the rapidly rising cost of drug development is the cost of human trials. The typical clinical trial currently involves 4,000 people, compared with 1,300 in the 1980s. Managed care companies are demanding that drug companies prove the value of their drugs in larger and longer clinical trials.

Included in the costs of drug development are actual expenditures as well as the opportunity cost of the interest forgone on these investment costs. For example, only about half of the cost of drug development represents actual out-of-pocket costs. The rest is the estimated cost of capital, or the amount that would have been earned over time if the same amount of money were invested and earned interest. This opportunity cost of capital is significant, as long time lags exist between investment expenditures and revenues generated by new drugs.

These investment costs include expenditures on many drugs that will never make it to market (failures). Of every 5,000 potential new drugs tested in animals, only five are likely to reach human clinical trials; of those five, only one will eventually be marketed.

Also important to a drug firm's profitability is the fact that the longer it takes to achieve the FDA's stringent research guidelines and receive FDA approval, the shorter the remaining patent life on the drug and the period in which to make profits. Profit is the principal motivating factor behind drug companies' willingness to assume risk and invest large amounts in R&D. The pharmaceutical manufacturers' profitability over time is determined by their investment in R&D. As shown in Exhibit 26.3, R&D expenditures as a percentage of US sales are about 23 percent of revenue (as of 2013). This rate of investment is one of the highest of any industry.

Profitability over time (as a percentage of revenue) for pharmaceutical firms has also been higher than for companies in any other industry. Although profits are high, so are the risks. The high rates of profit earned by drug manufacturers to finance R&D result from the few breakthrough drugs discovered. Even those that are marketed may not be financially successful; about three out of ten drugs marketed make a profit, and about 10 percent of all drugs marketed provide 52 percent of the industry's profits.

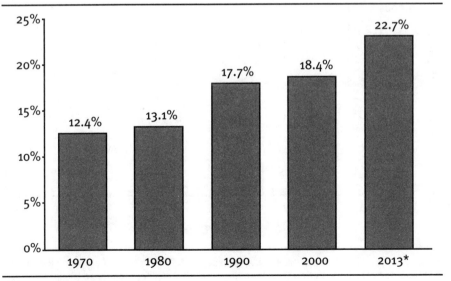

EXHIBIT 26.3
Domestic R&D Expenditures as a Percentage of US Domestic Sales, Pharmaceutical Companies, 1970–2013

* Estimated data for 2013
SOURCE: Data from PhRMA (2014).

Exhibit 26.4 describes the percentage of drugs the profits of which exceed average R&D costs. As can be seen, the distribution of profits is skewed. Very few drugs offer a profitable return, but for the 10 percent of drugs considered "blockbuster" drugs the profits are substantial. Thus, a drug company needs a few "winners"—especially blockbusters—to repay the costs on the majority of drugs that do not even repay their R&D investments.

Patent protection is essential for protecting a drug manufacturer's investments in R&D. Once a new drug is discovered, it can be reproduced relatively easily. Without the period of market exclusivity that patents provide, drug manufacturers could not recover their R&D investments. Patents provide a drug manufacturer with market power, the ability to price above costs of production. Breakthrough drugs have a great deal more market power than a "me-too" drug. Although a new breakthrough drug (the first drug to treat an illness) may initially have a great deal of market power, other companies can eventually patent drugs that use the same mechanism to treat the illness. Once patent protection expires, generic versions priced much below the branded drug quickly take a large part of the market. For example, in 1997, the patent on Zantac expired, and the generic version captured 90 percent of the market served by Zantac within two years (Berndt 2001). Currently, about 84 percent of all prescription drugs dispensed are off-patent generic drugs (IMS Health 2013).

EXHIBIT 26.4
Decile Distribution of Present Values of Postlaunch Returns for the Sample of 1990–1994 New Chemical Entities

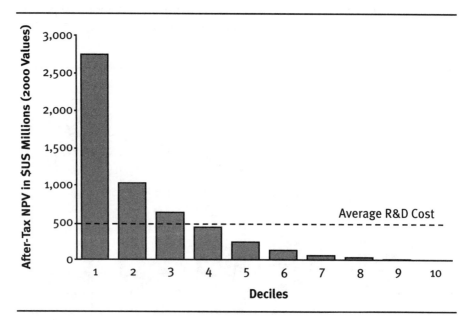

SOURCE: Grabowski, H., J. Vernon, and J. A. DiMasi. 2002. "Figure 7." In "Returns on Research and Development for 1990s New Drug Introductions." *Pharmacoeconomics* 20 (Suppl. 3): 11–29. With kind permission from Springer Science and Business Media.

Public policy with respect to the drug industry must deal with the following trade-off. To increase R&D investments, drug manufacturers must earn high profits on innovative drugs that provide significant increases in therapeutic value. However, the cost of producing these drugs is but a small fraction of their selling price. If prices on these breakthrough drugs were made more affordable (closer to their production costs) to alleviate the large burden on those with low income, the high profits that provide the incentive to invest in R&D would disappear. Lower drug prices that benefit today's patients mean fewer innovative drugs in the future.

Orphan Drugs

As R&D costs and the time for drug approval have increased, long and costly clinical trials to develop *orphan drugs*—those that benefit only small population groups—became unprofitable. The potential revenue for a new orphan drug may be small because these drugs are designed to treat diseases that only affect a small number of people (or treat the small percentage of people who do not respond to standard treatments for common illnesses). Congress enacted the Orphan Drug Act in 1984 to provide drug companies with a financial incentive (tax incentives or exclusive marketing rights) to develop drugs that provide therapeutic benefits for fewer than 200,000 patients.

Similar to the orphan drug issue is the concern that drug development is targeted toward people living in wealthy countries. Only 5 percent of global R&D is directed at health problems unique to developing nations, although 90 percent of the global disease burden is in the developing world (Hotez et al. 2013). Private-sector R&D is determined by prospective demand conditions. For example, malaria is a parasitic disease that has a global incidence of 200 to 300 million cases annually. About 1 million deaths are caused by malaria each year, and the majority of these deaths involve children under age 5 years living in sub-Saharan Africa (Bloom et al. 2006). Drug development aimed at health problems of people in poor countries will need to be subsidized from government sources.

Summary

The rationale for FDA regulation of drugs is presumably to provide a remedy for the lack of information that exists among physicians and consumers when buying drugs. Lack of information on a drug's safety could cause serious harm to patients. Given this serious information problem, what should the FDA's role be? Should the FDA continue to be the sole decision maker on the availability of new drugs? Or should the FDA play a more passive role by merely providing information on the safety and efficacy of new drugs and leave the decision about whether to use a new drug to the physician and the patient?

What is the optimum trade-off between statistical and identifiable deaths? Who should make that decision? Decreased identifiable deaths means more testing, high R&D costs, delays in FDA approval, and a consequent increase in statistical deaths. Clearly, for saving lives and treating serious illnesses the choice should be less concern with drug safety and efficacy and quicker approval to minimize the number of statistical deaths. The costs of delay vary depending on the seriousness of the illness. Even two patients with the same disease will differ on the types of risks they are willing to accept. Under the current system the FDA is determining the level of risk acceptable to society, while some patients would be willing to go above that level.

Proponents of strengthening the FDA's current role (rather than changing it to be merely a provider of information) are concerned that physicians and patients would still have incomplete information to make appropriate decisions on new drugs. Physicians may be too busy or unwilling to invest the time to fully understand the safety and efficacy information on new drugs and may even be influenced by drug company advertising. Changing the FDA's role from that of a decision maker to simply a provider of information does not appear to have much public support. Instead, public policy is more concerned with speeding up the FDA's approval process. Various proposals have been made to speed up the FDA's review process for drug approval, such as having the FDA also rely on evidence gathered from other countries that have high approval standards, dropping the proof-of-efficacy requirement, and requiring less evidence of a drug's safety for lifesaving drugs that have no alternative therapy.

Speeding up the FDA's approval process will require greater post-marketing surveillance of drug interactions and safety. Evidence of the effects of a new drug may not be known for several years. The long preapproval process continues to miss dangerous drugs. For example, Trovan, an antibiotic drug, had to be withdrawn because of unforeseen liver injuries. Only after a drug has been on the market and used by a large number of people can its safety and efficacy be truly evaluated.

In addition to speeding up the FDA's approval process and expanding post-marketing surveillance of new drugs, concerns exist about the time and cost required to bring a new drug to market. High R&D costs (such as longer times for approval that shorten patent life) decrease the profitability of an investment in new drugs. Low profitability leads to a lower investment and results in fewer new drugs being discovered. As the costs of drug discovery are increased, drug companies are less likely to develop drugs that have small market potential. An additional consequence of the high cost and long time requirements to introduce a new drug is that, with fewer new drugs being introduced, drug prices are higher because less competition exists than would if the process were easier.

High R&D costs also have a great effect on small drug firms. Large drug firms have many new drugs in the discovery pipeline and on the market. Small firms invest their capital in the particular drug that is going through the R&D and approval process. The longer the delay in being able to market their drug, the greater their capital requirement is. To minimize its chance of running out of money, a small firm with a promising new drug will merge or partner with a large firm that has greater capital resources and experience with the drug approval process.

Economics is concerned with trade-offs. Choosing one policy (namely increased drug safety and efficacy) has a "cost" (namely fewer new drugs being developed). More statistical deaths will occur, the drug industry will become more consolidated, and drug prices will be higher because fewer new drugs will compete with existing drugs. Thus, merely favoring increased drug safety and efficacy is not a simple choice without consequences. The issue is how to strike an appropriate balance between these choices.

Discussion Questions

1. How have the 1962 amendments to the Food, Drug, and Cosmetic Act affected the profitability of new drugs?
2. What is the consequence of the FDA providing the public with greater assurance that a new drug is safe?
3. What is the difference between identifiable death and statistical death?
4. What are orphan drugs, and why are drug firms less likely to develop such drugs today?
5. Why has the FDA's drug approval process sped up in recent years?
6. What are the advantages and disadvantages of greater reliance on pre-marketing test versus post-marketing surveillance?

Notes

1. Once the FDA approves a new drug as being safe and efficacious for its intended use, the new drug must also pass the health plan's review process to show that it is also cost-effective. Unless the new drug can pass this review, it may not be added to the health plan's drug formulary.

2. The Federal Trade Commission has been investigating anticompetitive behavior in the drug industry. Drug companies that hold patents on brand-name drugs have been accused of making special deals with generic-drug manufacturers to keep the generic drugs off the market (thereby not competing with the branded drug) for longer than the Hatch-Waxman Act intended. Specifically, drug manufacturers have been accused of paying generic-drug firms to delay introducing their products. Congress and the FDA are also examining whether changes to the Hatch-Waxman Act are required to close loopholes in the law. Industry critics claim that another tactic drug firms use to delay the entry of generic drugs is to sue the generic manufacturers, allowing the branded drugs several more months of lucrative, exclusive sales.

3. Olson (1994) described why, after several years of failure, the Hatch-Waxman legislation was ultimately enacted. Her analysis included the proposals of different interest groups, turnover in key Senate committees, and a change in the majority party.

4. In 1994, federal legislation (called the Uruguay Round Agreements Act) changed the patent life of prescription drugs and all types of inventions from 17 years from the date a patent is granted to 20 years from the date the application is filed. Between two and three years elapse from the time an application is filed until a patent is granted. The average period for which a new drug can be marketed under patent protection has risen from about 9 years to 12.4 years (Grabowski et al. 2011).

5. One analyst who examined the 1962 amendments concluded that they made the public worse off. Sam Peltzman (1974) attempted to quantify the benefits of the 1962 amendments by comparing the estimated effect of the new regulations on keeping ineffective and dangerous drugs (of which there were very few before 1962) off the market with the lost benefits of having fewer new drugs, higher prices for existing drugs (because of less competition from new drugs), and reduced availability of drugs because of the time lag. The decline in the development of new drugs was the greatest disadvantage of the amendments; this factor alone, according to Peltzman, made the costs of the new amendments greatly exceed the potential benefits.

6. Statistical deaths are calculated as follows. Assume that a new drug is introduced in Europe and two years elapse before that same drug receives FDA approval to be marketed in the United States. Further assume that the new drug is more effective than the drug currently on the market to treat that same disease, such that the new drug is able to decrease mortality from 5 percent to 1 percent. Suppose 100,000 persons each year are affected by that illness. The number of lives that

would have been saved by earlier FDA approval is 8,000. The percentage difference in mortality rate (0.05 − 0.01 = 0.04), multiplied by the two-year lag when the drug could have been on the market (0.04 × 2 = 0.08), multiplied by the number of people at risk each year (0.08 × 100,000) equals 8,000 statistical deaths because of the two-year delay.

References

Berndt, E. 2001. "The U.S. Pharmaceutical Industry: Why Major Growth in Times of Cost Containment?" Accessed November 2013. http://contenthealthaffairs.org/content/20/2/100.full.

Bloom, B., C. Michaud, J. Montagne, and L. Simonsen. 2006. "Priorities for Global Research and Development of Interventions." Accessed November 2013. www.ncbi.nlm.nih.gov/books/NBK11751/.

Carpenter, D. 2004. "The Political Economy of FDA Drug Review: Processing, Politics, and Lessons for Policy." *Health Affairs* 23 (1): 52–63.

DiMasi, J. A., and H. G. Grabowski. 2007. "The Cost of Biopharmaceutical R&D: Is Biotech Different?" *Managerial and Decision Economics* 28 (4–5): 469–79.

Gottlieb, S. 2004. "The Price of Too Much Caution." *New York Sun,* December 22. www.aei.org/news/newsID.21746, filter./news_detail.asp.

Grabowski, H. 1976. *Drug Regulation and Innovation.* Washington, DC: AEI Press.

Grabowski, H., M. Kyle, R. Mortimer, G. Long, and N. Kirson. 2011. "Evolving Brand-Name and Generic Drug Competition May Warrant a Revision of the Hatch-Waxman Act." *Health Affairs* 30 (11): 2157–66.

Grabowski, H., J. Vernon, and J. A. DiMasi. 2002. "Returns on Research and Development for 1990s New Drug Introductions." *Pharmacoeconomics* 20 (Suppl. 3): 11–29.

Harris, R. 1964. *The Real Voice.* New York: MacMillan.

Hotez, P., R. Cohen, C. Mimura, T. Yamada, and S. Hoffman. 2013. "Strengthening Mechanisms to Prioritize, Coordinate, Finance, and Execute R&D to Meet Health Needs in Developing Countries." Discussion paper. Washington, DC: Institute of Medicine. www.iom.edu/StrengtheningMechanismsRD.

IMS Health. 2013. "IMS Health Study Points to a Declining Cost Curve for U.S. Medicines in 2012." Press release. Danbury, CT: IMS Health. www.imshealth.com/portal/site/imshealth/menuitem.c76283e8bf81e98f53c753c71ad8c22a/?vgnextoid=8659cf4add48e310VgnVCM10000076192ca2RCRD&vgnextchannel=2e11e590cb4dc310VgnVCM100000a48d2ca2RCRD&vgnextfmt=default.

Mestre-Ferrandiz, J., J. Sussex, and A. Towse. 2012. *The R&D Cost of a New Medicine*. London: Office of Health Economics. http://ohematerials.org/NMECost/index.html#/0.

Pharmaceutical Research and Manufacturers of America (PhRMA). 2014. *2014 Biopharmaceutical Research Industry Profile*. Published April. www.phrma.org/sites/default/files/pdf/2014_PhRMA_PROFILE.pdf.

———. 2013. *2013 Biopharmaceutical Research Industry Profile*. Published July. www.phrma.org/sites/default/files/pdf/PhRMA%20Profile%202013.pdf.

Olson, M. K. 1994. "Political Influence and Regulatory Policy: The 1984 Drug Legislation." *Economic Inquiry* 32 (3): 363–82.

PAREXEL International. 2013. *PAREXEL Biopharmaceutical R&D Statistical Sourcebook, 2012–13 Edition*. Deerfield, IL: PAREXEL International.

Peltzman, S. 1974. *Regulation of Pharmaceutical Innovation*. Washington, DC: American Enterprise Institute.

WHY ARE PRESCRIPTION DRUGS LESS EXPENSIVE OVERSEAS?

27

necdotes abound about people traveling to Canada or Mexico to buy a prescription drug at a much lower price than that offered by retail pharmacies in the United States. In addition, studies by the US Government Accountability Office (GAO 1992, 1994) have shown that branded prescription drugs are more expensive in the United States than in other countries. The studies concluded that US prices were 32 percent higher than prices in Canada and 60 percent higher than prices in the United Kingdom. A 2012 report found that the average price of Celebrex, a drug commonly prescribed for pain, was $258 in United States but only $53 in Canada or $116 in United Kingdom (see Exhibit 27.1) (International Federation of Health Plans 2012).

Cross-national comparison studies of branded (prescription) drug prices generally conclude that lower prices in other countries are a result of regulatory price controls, which implies that the United States can similarly lower drug prices by using price controls. The following sections discuss the

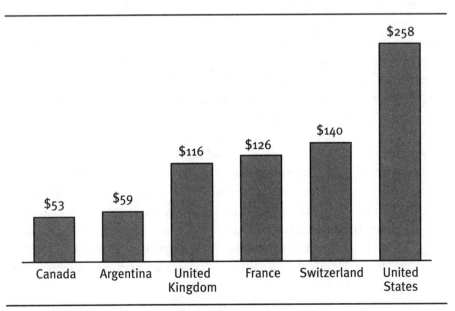

EXHIBIT 27.1
Prices for Celebrex, Selected Countries, 2012

NOTE: Celebrex is commonly prescribed for pain.
SOURCE: Data from International Federation of Health Plans (2012).

accuracy of cross-national drug price studies, the reason higher prices for prescription drugs in the United States are not surprising, and the implications of requiring US drug manufacturers to charge a single uniform price overseas and in this country.

Accuracy of Studies on International Variations in Drug Prices

The methodology used in the 1994 GAO studies and in similar studies concluding that prescription drug prices are higher in the United States than in other countries has been widely criticized. What these studies purport to analyze and the methods used should be subject to greater examination before their implications for the United States are accepted.

Retail Price Comparisons

Typically, cross-national studies compare the retail prices of selected prescription drugs that are bought by cash-paying patients in the United States to the retail prices of those same drugs in another country. (The GAO studies used listed wholesale prices in the United States, which were intended to approximate prices charged to retail pharmacies.) These comparisons greatly overstate US drug prices because they assume that all purchasers of the same prescription drug in the United States pay the same price. Using retail (or even wholesale) prices as the prescription drug price in the United States does not account for the large discounts and rebates received by large US purchasers such as managed care organizations (MCOs), pharmacy benefit managers, mail-order drug firms, private drug plans, and federal government programs such as Medicaid. Patients in these organizations merely pay a copayment that is a small fraction of the price the organizations pay for the drug. Not only do these large purchasers make up the majority of the US prescription drug market, large purchasers also represent a larger percentage of the purchasers in the United States than in comparison countries.

These large purchasers pay substantially less for prescription drugs than cash-paying US patients who do not have prescription drug insurance and buy directly from a retail pharmacy. Cash-paying patients represent a small segment of the prescription drug buyers in the United States, so comparisons using these patients greatly overstate prices. Rather than assuming a single US retail price, comparing prices paid on average by all those purchasing drugs in the United States to the prices paid by overseas patients would be more appropriate.[1]

Cost of Drug Therapy

Given the public policy implications of cross-national studies, the purpose of these comparisons must be clarified so that an appropriate study design can be determined. One objective of such studies might be to estimate the cost of drug therapy (by disease) in different countries, not just the differences in prices for specific prescription products. To accurately examine differences in drug therapy costs across countries, such studies should adjust for the use of generic substitutes and weighting of the different drugs used in a country's drug price index.

Cross-national studies have excluded generic drugs, which are priced between 40 and 80 percent lower than branded drugs. Furthermore, US purchasers rely much more on generic drugs than do patients in other countries. (Generics accounted for 84 percent of prescriptions in the United States in 2012 [IMS Health 2013a], whereas use of generics in countries with strict drug price regulation, such as France and Italy, is very low.) If generic drugs are more frequently substituted for expensive branded drugs in the United States than in other countries, a comparison based solely on branded drugs overstates the cost of a prescription for US patients.

Another important issue in cross-national comparisons is the mix or consumption pattern of drugs used in different countries. Comparisons of drug prices between countries rely on a simple average of the prices paid for several leading brand-name drugs. For example, the 1992 GAO study merely compared US prices to Canadian prices for a number of branded drugs. (The Canadian prices were added up and compared to the sum of the US retail prices for those same drugs. Dividing the sum of the prices of one country by the sum of prices in the other country resulted in a ratio of prices between the two countries.) In doing so, the study gave an equal weight to each branded drug being compared. Whether some branded drugs were widely or infrequently used did not matter; each received an equal weight.

Because the United States and other countries have different drug consumption patterns, any price index should reflect these differences by weighting the volume of use of different branded drugs. Some branded drugs represent a greater percentage of purchased branded drugs than others; these percentages differ by country.

Cross-national comparisons should use a weighted average of the prices of branded drugs. The index should also include the use of generic drugs and the average prices paid for all drugs, including the discounted prices paid by MCOs and other large purchasers in the United States and the volume they purchase. This would result in a much lower weighted average price than simply observing the price of the branded drug (and its volume) sold to retail customers. Further, for some branded drugs a great deal of substitution of the generic version, which is sold at a lower price, occurs. A weighted average price of that drug would include the branded and generic versions, which would result in a much lower price than simply using the branded version. Each drug should also be given a weight in the index according to its use in that country.

Drug Price Index

Research conducted by Danzon and Chao (2000) determined that when a drug price index is constructed for each country using average prices paid by different purchasers and weighting drug prices by the drugs' (including generic drugs) frequency of use, the index may be no higher in the United States than in other countries. Although individual prescription drugs may be more expensive in the United States, the costs of drug therapy across countries (based on an accurately constructed drug price index) are not much different. (For a detailed discussion of cross-national comparisons, including additional limitations such as the unit of measurement and the availability of branded drugs, as well as appropriate methodologies and results, see Danzon and Furukawa [2003].)

Why Prescription Drugs Are Expected to Be Priced Lower Overseas

Numerous examples can be found of prescription drugs that are less expensive in other countries than in the United States. Why would a manufacturer of a patented prescription drug be willing to sell the same drug at greatly reduced prices overseas? This pricing behavior is based on two characteristics of the drug industry, its cost structure and differences in each country's bargaining power.

The costs of developing and bringing to market a new innovative drug are high; ten years ago the estimate was $800 million (DiMasi, Hansen, and Grabowski 2003). A 2012 estimate indicates the research and development (R&D) costs for a new prescription drug can go as high as $1.5 million to $1.8 billion (Mestre-Ferrandiz, Sussex, and Towse 2012). Experimental trials must be conducted, and the Food and Drug Administration's (FDA's) approval is required. It may take seven to ten years to develop a new drug and receive FDA approval. The R&D costs—including the interest that could have been earned on those funds and the costs involved in receiving FDA approval—are known as *fixed costs*. These development costs are the same regardless of how much of the patented new drug is produced and sold. The actual costs of producing the new drug, once its chemical entities have been determined through the R&D process and once it has received FDA approval, are relatively small. Thus, patented drugs are characterized by large fixed costs and relatively small variable costs (the actual costs of producing the drug).

The drug manufacturer would like to receive the highest possible price for that new drug. For some purchasers, however, the manufacturer would be willing to accept any price that exceeds its variable costs. A price in excess of variable costs contributes to covering those large fixed costs and to profit. The manufacturer is better off receiving $5 even if it costs $4 to produce that drug; the $1 revenue from some purchasers is better than nothing.

The drug industry is sophisticated in its pricing of the same medicine across different countries. A drug manufacturer would like to add new users (sell the drug in different countries) because the variable costs of producing the drug are so low, but it is not willing to add new users if it has to reduce the price and revenues it earns in higher-priced markets. The single largest market for new innovative drugs is the United States, which accounts for 33.9 percent of the world pharmaceutical market (North America, or the United States and Canada, represents 36.3 percent [Exhibit 27.2]). People in the United States are, on average, wealthier than those in other countries and want access to innovative drugs as soon as possible, so they are less price sensitive to high drug prices; about 85 percent of the US population in 2012 had insurance to pay for prescription drugs (Rowan 2012). Not surprisingly, drug manufacturers charge higher prices when consumers are less price sensitive.

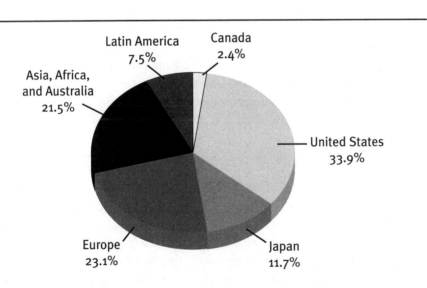

EXHIBIT 27.2
World Pharmaceutical Market, 2012

Latin America
7.5%

Canada
2.4%

Asia, Africa, and Australia
21.5%

United States
33.9%

Europe
23.1%

Japan
11.7%

Total World Pharmaceutical Market = $962 Billion

SOURCE: Data from IMS Health (2013b).

In countries that regulate the price of drugs, the same manufacturer is willing to sell the same drug at a lower price as long as the regulated price exceeds the manufacturer's variable cost of producing that drug. The drug manufacturer would be concerned if purchasers in the lower-priced countries were to resell the drug in the higher-priced markets. If resale from the lower-priced countries to the higher-priced countries were possible, a differential pricing system could not persist.

As long as the manufacturer is able to prevent resale of the same drug from low- to high-priced markets, this system of differential pricing allows markets that would otherwise be neglected to be served. Differential pricing—whereby a drug manufacturer charges different prices to different countries for the same medicine—results in the greatest number of people gaining access to a drug. The manufacturer is willing to reduce its price to countries that regulate drugs and to poor countries that cannot afford to pay much for drugs; the manufacturer does this not because it has a social conscience but because any sales at a price that exceeds the drug's variable cost contribute to profits. By trying to increase profits, however, the drug manufacturer also provides the greatest number of people with access to its drug.

Canadian and European governments, which pay for most of their populations' health expenditures, keep drug prices down because they have limited budgets for healthcare. These tight budgets for drug expenditures have had unintended side effects. The introduction of new innovative and cost-effective drugs has been delayed and restrictions have been placed on patient's eligibility for new prescription drugs because the budget for drugs would be exceeded (Kanavos et al. 2013). Consequently, surgical and hospital expenditures have been greater than if costly new innovative drugs had been used, and delays have occurred in approving lifesaving drugs for citizens of these countries. For example, "Herceptin, which was considered to be a breakthrough drug for about a third of all breast cancer patients...was approved two years [earlier] by regulators in the US, where it benefited from an accelerated review offered to novel cancer therapies" (Moore 2000). Further,

> Many European countries also attempt to restrict demand after new medicines reach pharmacy shelves. European...countries with tight pharmaceutical budgets have made it difficult for cancer patients to have access to older cancer drugs (Taxol) that were top selling anti-cancer drugs. One study (industry funded) examining prescribing patterns between 1996 and 1998 finds the following: while 99.9% of patients with advanced breast cancer in the US received treatment with taxane, the comparable [rate] was 48% for the Netherlands and only 25% for Britain.

Another consequence of regulated lower drug prices overseas is that total drug expenditures represent a higher portion of total medical expenditures in those countries than in the United States (see Exhibit 27.3) because the prices for drugs in those countries are quite low (generally for older molecules), and neither patients nor their physicians have any incentive to use fewer drugs. For example, to reduce drug expenditures, the German government imposed financial penalties on physicians to limit their prescriptions. The United States spends a smaller portion on drugs (11.7 percent of total health expenditures) than France (15.6 percent), Japan (20.3 percent), Canada (16.6 percent), or Germany (14.1 percent).

Public Policy Issues

Cross-national studies that have found that the United States has higher prescription drug prices imply that the United States should institute a price-control system similar to those of countries that have lower drug prices. By publicizing these study findings, along with examples of persons who cannot afford to pay high retail drug prices, advocates of price controls hope to build political support for imposing controls on US prescription drugs.

Two methods for equalizing US and overseas prices on prescription drugs are favored by proponents of a regulatory approach. The first is having the US government require that the retail price of prescription drugs

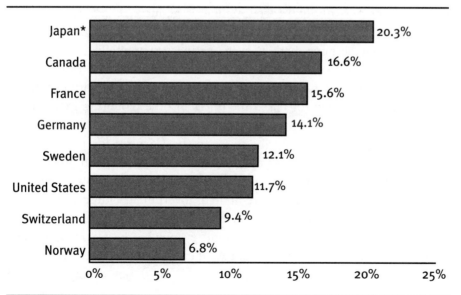

EXHIBIT 27.3
Pharmaceutical Expenditures as a Percentage of Total Health Expenditures, Selected Countries, 2011

* 2010 data
NOTE: Pharmaceuticals include prescription and nonprescription drugs.
SOURCE: Data from OECD (2013).

sold in the United States be no different from the price at which those same drugs are sold in other countries, such as Canada and Mexico. The second approach is to allow pharmacists to import FDA-approved US prescription drugs to the United States from other countries where they sell for substantially less. Each of these proposals has short-term effects as well as indirect, or unintended, long-term consequences.

A Single Price for Prescription Drugs Across Countries

What would happen to prescription drug prices in the United States and overseas if US drug manufacturers were required to price US-branded drugs at the same price at which they are sold to other countries? Proponents of a single price for the same medicine assume that the uniform price will be the lowest of the different prices charged for that same drug. Assume that a prescription drug, called ABC, sells for $10 in the United States and $5 in Canada. Further assume that the United States enacts a law stating that the manufacturer of ABC must charge the same price regardless of the country in which ABC is sold. Would the price of ABC be reduced to $5 and US consumers receive a $5 benefit?

The answer is no.

The manufacturer of ABC would have to determine which single price would result in the greatest amount of profit. Because the United States is the largest single market for innovative branded drugs and its consumers are less price sensitive, greatly reducing ABC's price in the US market would not result in a large increase in the number of ABC users. Consequently, a large decrease in price (without a corresponding large increase in volume) would cause a large drop in revenue.[2] Given the substantial profits earned in the United States (the price markup over variable cost multiplied by the large number of users), the uniform price of ABC would likely be closer to the US price than to the lower prices paid in other countries. The drug company would lose less money if it raised the prices in other countries by a greater amount than if it lowered the US price.

Keeping the uniform price closer to the US price for a drug would mean the new uniform price of the drug would be increased in other countries. Raising the price in these countries would likely cause a decrease in use. These countries typically have limited government budgets for healthcare, and a large increase in the price of drugs would cause the government to restrict their use. Whether total revenue to the US manufacturer from sales of the drug in other countries increases or decreases depends on whether the percentage increase in price exceeds the percentage decrease in use in those countries.

In either case, requiring a uniform price for ABC in the United States and other countries means overseas patients who need the drug will be worse off. Whereas formerly they (or the government on their behalf) paid $5, they will now have to pay a higher price. Some patients will no longer have access to ABC. If close substitute drugs were available, patients will buy these other drugs (assuming the price of these other drugs had not similarly increased). If close substitutes were not available for innovative drugs, patients/government will have to spend more of their income on ABC. If patients could not afford to buy ABC or their government restricted its use because of its higher price, adverse health consequences will occur.

Thus, requiring a uniform pricing policy in the United States and other countries would likely lead to a small reduction in the US price of a drug and an increase in the drug's overseas price so that it would be equal to the new US price. This policy would inflict a loss on many patients in other countries, who would have to go without innovative drugs.

Reimportation

The second regulatory approach to reducing US retail prices for prescription drugs is to allow US pharmacists and drug wholesalers to buy lower-priced supplies of FDA-approved medicines in Canada and other nations for resale in the United States. Drugs reimported into the United States from Canada would likely be less expensive than the same drugs sold in the United States because of Canadian price controls on those drugs. The presumed effect of this policy would be to reduce the US retail price of drugs to prices comparable to those in the countries from which they are reimported.

A federal law permitting reimportation was enacted in October 2000. This law overturned a 1988 law that permitted only pharmaceutical manufacturers to reimport prescription drugs based on the concern that drugs were being improperly stored and repackaged overseas. Although reimportation was vigorously opposed by the pharmaceutical industry, senators and congressional candidates from both political parties running for reelection in 2000 voted for the bill, which was then signed into law by President Clinton. As both political parties could not agree on a Medicare prescription drug benefit, legislators running for reelection believed voting for reimportation would be viewed by the public as being in favor of helping the aged with their prescription drug costs.

In December 2000, Donna Shalala, then-secretary of the Department of Health and Human Services (HHS), refused to implement the new law, claiming that it was unworkable and would not lower drug costs (Kaufman 2000). (Since then, no secretary of the HHS under Republican or Democratic administrations has agreed to implement the law.) At the time of the debate, the FDA said it could oversee the drug reimportation system—but only at considerable cost. Unless funding was provided ($93 million a year), the safety of the reimported drugs could not be monitored; full funding was not included in the legislation. Further, the Clinton Administration believed the bill had several fatal flaws that would deter reimportation—namely that the drug companies would retaliate against reimporters and would not provide the reimporters with the necessary package labeling inserts.

A US manufacturer of a branded prescription drug would be unlikely to increase its sales to a country that resells that drug in the United States. Drug manufacturers could easily monitor drug sales to each country to determine whether sales of a particular drug had suddenly increased. (If the drug importer in a country resold the country's limited supply of that drug back to the United States, patients in that country would be harmed by not having access to that drug.)

Thus, to be able to reimport drugs into the United States, US pharmacists and wholesalers would have to buy those chemical entities from a foreign producer of those drugs. When a drug is manufactured in the United States, the manufacturer must adhere to strict FDA guidelines to ensure that the drug is produced with certain quality standards. If a drug is manufactured in another country without extensive monitoring of the reimported drug by the FDA, no guarantee can be given that the drug will meet the same quality standards. The concern over drug safety resulted in 11 former FDA commissioners opposing the reimportation bill (Dalzell 2000).

Thousands of illegal shipments of prescription drugs enter the United States each month through the postal service. This growth in overseas sales to US patients has dramatically increased because of the Internet. The sheer volume of these shipments has overwhelmed the ability of the FDA and customs officials to verify the safety of the imported drugs. Finally, on June 7, 2001, the FDA proposed stopping overseas drug products from being mailed to individuals unless the products met certain strict conditions. The FDA claimed that these products could be counterfeit or even dangerous and that the volume is so large that it no longer has the ability to inspect them.

Reimportation is unlikely to be effective in reducing US prescription drug prices for several reasons. First, US drug manufacturers would be unwilling to sell large quantities of their drugs at greatly reduced prices to other countries so that these countries could sell the same drugs back to US pharmacists at lower prices.[3] Second, if foreign drug manufacturers are permitted to produce a drug patented by a US manufacturer and sell that drug to customers in the United States, those foreign producers would be violating US patent laws and the imports would be prohibited. Third, if other countries were unable to receive sufficient supplies of US-produced drugs to sell back to the United States, counterfeit drugs would likely be produced and sold to US patients, resulting in significant safety issues, which would eventually halt mail-order drug sales from overseas.

The pressure to enact a stronger drug importation law that would permit reimportation without the consent of the secretary of the HHS (as some in Congress have proposed) decreased once Medicare beneficiaries were provided with a prescription drug benefit as part of the Medicare Modernization Act, which lowered beneficiaries' out-of-pocket costs for prescription drugs.

Summary

Cross-national comparison studies that claim drug prices are lower in other countries have been seriously misleading. Although the retail prices of certain prescription drugs may be lower overseas than in the United States, the more relevant comparison is the cost of drug therapy in different countries. Only a small percentage of the US population pays retail prices for drugs. The majority of the US population has some form of third-party payment for drugs, and these large purchasers buy their drugs at discounted prices. Generic drugs are also much more widely used in the United States than in other countries. Absent from these cross-national comparisons is any discussion of the availability of innovative drugs overseas.

Public policy affecting prescription drugs should be evaluated on its effect on R&D expenditures. The incentive for drug manufacturers to invest large sums in R&D and develop breakthrough drugs is based on the prospect of earning large profits. Once a drug has been discovered and approved by the FDA for marketing, the actual cost of producing that drug is low. Not surprisingly, therefore, countries can regulate the price of drugs and still have access to US drugs. (Evidence exists that other countries' regulation of drug prices resulted in a decline in R&D by drug firms in those countries.) These countries can receive a "free ride" on the large R&D expenditures by US drug firms. However, if the United States were to regulate its drug prices as do other countries or permit reimportation by foreign drug producers, R&D investment would decline, as would the supply of innovative drugs. Without government enforcement of patent rights and pricing freedom, the drug industry would decrease its investment in R&D—as drugs are easy to copy but expensive to develop. Consumers in the United States and other countries benefit from differential pricing policies. In other countries more consumers benefit by having access to lower-priced drugs, whereas in the United States the higher prices generate greater profits for the drug companies and provide them with an incentive to invest more in R&D.

If the objective of cross-national studies is to pressure legislators to lower the retail prices of drugs so that cash-paying seniors can buy them at lower prices, a better alternative than mandating uniform prices across all countries or permitting reimportation has become available. Seniors were provided with a prescription drug benefit as part of the 2003 Medicare Modernization Act; they have a financial incentive to choose among competing drug plans based on the premiums charged and the plan's drug formulary. The competing plans negotiate lower drug prices from the drug manufacturer, substitute generic drugs when appropriate, and manage the drug benefit to reduce the total cost of drug therapy. The cost to the government of this Medicare drug benefit was much lower than projected. Seniors now have better access to needed drugs, and competition has reduced their prescription drug prices as well as their monthly premium (CBO 2011; Hoadley 2012).

Discussion Questions

1. What are some criticisms of cross-national studies of drug prices?
2. Although some prescription drugs are priced lower in other countries, is the cost of a drug treatment also lower in those countries?
3. Why would a drug manufacturer be willing to sell a drug that is priced high (in relation to its variable costs) in the United States at a low price overseas?
4. What would be the consequences—in terms of drug prices and drug users—if prices of prescription drugs sold in the United States had to equal the price at which those same drugs are sold in other countries?
5. Why would a policy of reimportation of prescription drugs be ineffective?

Notes

1. A number of other issues are involved in examining retail drug prices, such as dosage form; strength; and pack size—for example, price per gram of active ingredient or price per dose (standard unit), which may be one tablet, one capsule, or 10 mL of a liquid. Differences in prescription drug prices also occur because of differences in dosage form, strength, and pack size used in the comparison countries.
2. When consumers are less price sensitive, changes in price cause smaller proportionate changes in volume. By increasing price, total revenue increases because the percentage change in price is greater than the percentage change in volume. Similarly, lowering price when consumers are not price sensitive will result in a decrease in total revenue. Conversely, when consumers are price sensitive, the percentage

change in price is less than the percentage change in volume. With price-sensitive consumers, total revenue increases when prices are reduced, up to a certain point.

3. In an effort to eliminate drug shipments to Canadian Internet pharmacies that sell lower-cost US-produced drugs to US consumers, Pfizer notified all Canadian drug retailers of its policy to halt all sales of Pfizer drugs to them if they sell Pfizer drugs to US consumers. Pfizer receives information on all drug orders from individual drug stores from its distributors (Carlisle 2004).

Additional Readings

Congressional Budget Office (CBO). 2004. "Would Prescription Drug Importation Reduce US Drug Spending?" *Economic and Budget Issue Brief*, April 29. www.cbo.gov/showdoc.cfm?index=5406&sequence=0#F4.

Danzon, P., and M. Furukawa. 2008. "International Prices and Availability of Pharmaceuticals in 2005." *Health Affairs* 27 (1): 221–33.

Perron, M. 2012. "Drug Approval Faster in U.S. than Canada, Europe: Study." Posted May 16. www.huffingtonpost.com/2012/05/17/drug-approval-faster-united-states-canada-europe_n_1524527.html.

US Government Accountability Office (GAO). 2012. "Drug Pricing: Research on Savings from Generic Drug Use." GAO-12-371R. www.gao.gov/assets/590/588064.pdf.

References

Carlisle, T. 2004. "Pfizer Pressures Canadian Sellers of Drugs to U.S." *Wall Street Journal*, January 14, p. A6.

Congressional Budget Office (CBO). 2011. "Spending Patterns for Prescription Drugs Under Medicare Part D." *Economic and Budget Issue Brief*, December. www.cbo.gov/sites/default/files/cbofiles/attachments/12-01-MedicarePartD.pdf.

Dalzell, M. 2000. "Prescription Drug Reimportation: Panacea or Problem?" Accessed November 2013. www.managedcaremag.com/archives/0012/0012.reimport.html.

Danzon, P. M., and L. W. Chao. 2000. "Cross-National Price Differences for Pharmaceuticals: How Large, and Why?" *Journal of Health Economics* 19 (2): 159–95.

Danzon, P., and M. Furukawa. 2003. "Prices and Availability of Pharmaceuticals: Evidence from Nine Countries." *Health Affairs* (web exclusive): W3-521–W3-536. http://content.healthaffairs.org/cgi/ reprint/hlthaff.w3.521v1.

DiMasi, J., R. Hansen, and H. Grabowski. 2003. "The Price of Innovation: New Estimates of Drug Development Cost." *Journal of Health Economics* 22 (2): 151–85.

Hoadley, J. 2012. "Medicare Part D Spending Trends: Understanding Key Drivers and the Role of Competition." *Issue Brief*, May. http:// kaiserfamilyfoundation.files.wordpress.com/2013/01/8308.pdf.

IMS Health. 2013a. "IMS Health Study Points to a Declining Cost Curve for U.S. Medicines in 2012." Press release. www.imshealth.com/portal/site/ imshealth/menuitem.c76283e8bf81e98f53c753c71ad8c22a/?vgnextoid=86 59cf4add48e310VgnVCM10000076192ca2RCRD&vgnextchannel=2e11e5 90cb4dc310VgnVCM100000a48d2ca2RCRD&vgnextfmt=default.

———. 2013b. *Total Unaudited and Audited Global Pharmaceutical Market by Region, 2012–2017.* Accessed April 2014. www.imshealth.com/ deployedfiles/imshealth/Global/Content/Corporate/Press%20Room/ Total_World_Pharma_Market_Topline_metrics_2012-17_regions.pdf.

International Federation of Health Plans. 2012. *2012 Comparative Price Report: Variation in Hospital and Medical Prices by Country.* https:// static.squarespace.com/static/518a3cfee4b0a77d03a62c98/ t/51dfd9f9e4b0d1d8067dcde2/1373624825901/2012%20iFHP%20 Price%20Report%20FINAL%20April%203.pdf.

Kanavos, P., A. Ferrario, S. Vandoros, and G. F. Anderson. 2013. "Higher US Branded Drug Prices and Spending Compared to Other Countries May Stem Partly from Quick Uptake of New Drugs." *Health Affairs* 32 (4): 753–61.

Kaufman, M. 2000. "Shalala Halts Bid to Lower Drug Costs." *Washington Post*, December 27, p. 1.

Mestre-Ferrandiz, J., J. Sussex, and A. Towse. 2012. *The R&D Cost of a New Medicine.* London: Office of Health Economics. www.ohe.org/ publications/article/the-rd-cost-of-a-new-medicine-124.cfm.

Moore, S. D. 2000. "In Drug-Cost Debate Europe Offers U.S. a Telling Side Effect." *Wall Street Journal,* July 21, p. 1.

Organisation for Economic Co-operation and Development (OECD). 2013. *OECD Health Data 2013.* Paris: OECD.

Rowan, K. 2012. "Why Americans' Prescriptions Are Going Unfilled." *Livescience.* Posted September 13. www.livescience.com/23179-why-americans-prescriptions-are-going-unfilled.html.

US Government Accountability Office (GAO). 1994. *Prescription Drugs: Companies Typically Charge More in the United States than in the United Kingdom*. GAO/HEHS 94–29. Washington, DC: US Government Printing Office.

———. 1992. *Prescription Drugs: Companies Typically Charge More in the United States than in Canada*. GAO/HRD 92–110. Washington, DC: US Government Printing Office.

THE PHARMACEUTICAL INDUSTRY: A PUBLIC POLICY DILEMMA

The pharmaceutical industry is subject to a great deal of criticism regarding the high prices charged for its drugs, its large (some would say "wasteful") marketing expenditures, and its emphasis on "lifestyle" and "me-too" drugs over drugs to cure infectious diseases and chronic conditions. Yet the industry has developed important drugs that have saved lives, reduced pain, and improved the lives of many. Public policy that attempts to respond to industry critics may at the same time change the industry's incentives for research and development (R&D) and thereby reduce the number of potential blockbuster drugs. To evaluate the criticisms of this profitable industry and the consequences of public policy directed toward it, an understanding of the structure of this industry is needed.

The pharmaceutical industry is made up of two distinct types of drug manufacturers: (1) pharmaceutical manufacturers, who engage in R&D and market brand-name drugs, and (2) generic manufacturers. Pharmaceutical manufacturers invest large sums in R&D, whereas generic manufacturers do not. Consequently, the former group develops innovative branded drugs for new therapeutic uses, while generic firms sell copies of branded drugs (when their patents expire) at greatly reduced prices. These two industries differ in their economic performance and in the public policies directed toward them. Most public policy is directed at pharmaceutical manufacturers.

Understanding the distribution channel for prescription drugs is also essential in understanding the structure of the industry. Manufacturers produce the drugs and, for the most part, sell them to wholesalers, who then sell them to pharmacies, where the drugs are purchased by patients. Pharmacies can take many forms and can be found in various places, including chain drug stores such as Walgreens, mass merchandisers such as Walmart and Target, grocery store pharmacies such as Albertsons, mail-order or retail pharmacies, or pharmacy websites. Over time, the number of independent retail pharmacies has declined. Wholesalers and retail pharmacies are each competitive industries.

Public Policy Dilemma

An important characteristic of the drug industry is the low cost of actually producing a drug once it has been discovered. Very large costs are incurred by the pharmaceutical manufacturer in the R&D phase and in marketing the new drug once it has been approved by the Food and Drug Administration (FDA). A new drug's price is not determined by its R&D costs, however, because these costs have already been incurred. Instead, the price is based on the demand for that drug, which is determined by its therapeutic value and whether it has close substitutes. Because the production costs of a drug (marginal costs) are low, a drug with great therapeutic value and few, if any, substitutes will command a high price. The resulting markup of price over production costs will therefore be high, leading to criticism of the drug company that the drug is priced too high for those who need it.

The public policy dilemma is that if the high price markups over cost are decreased so that more people can buy the drug, profits for R&D will also be lowered, thereby reducing future R&D investment and the discovery of new drugs with great therapeutic value.

Structure of the Pharmaceutical Industry

The structure of the pharmaceutical industry, together with regulatory restraints and government payment policies, affects drug prices and the rate of investment in new innovative drugs. Industry performance is generally measured by the number of blockbuster drugs produced. High price markups for innovative, high-value drugs with no existing substitutes appear justified; high price markups on older drugs are simply an indication of lack of price competition, because the industry is unable (or lacks the incentive) to produce new innovative drugs to take their place. Industry performance is also affected by regulations that raise the cost of developing new drugs, the time it takes for a new drug to receive FDA approval, and whether the government establishes the prices it will pay for new drugs; each of these government policies affects the profitability of new drugs and hence incentives for R&D investment.

The growth in regulatory requirements over the past several decades has adversely affected the discovery of new drugs by increasing the cost of developing them. The costs of enrolling patients in phase three of clinical trials (representing about 90 percent of the total cost of clinical trials), as well as the length of time spent in clinical trials, have been increasing; bringing a new drug to market can take about 12 years and cost a billion dollars. Given the time to bring the drug to market and the size of the investment required, little time is available to recoup the investment because the patent expires in 20 years.

Drug firms are also experiencing a more difficult reimbursement climate. The patent periods on several blockbuster drugs (such as Lipitor) have expired, and the drugs have been replaced by competition from generic substitutes. Medicare Part D drug plans use formularies, forcing drug firms to compete on price to have their drug included in the formulary. Managed care plans use similar approaches to reducing their enrollees' pharmacy costs.

Mergers and Acquisitions

Since the mid-1990s, many mergers have occurred among pharmaceutical companies. These mergers have been of two types.

The first type is a vertical merger, whereby a firm diversifies into another product line. The growth of managed care and the greater importance of pharmacy benefit managers (PBMs) led several large drug manufacturers to spend many billions of dollars to buy PBMs in the early 1990s. (Merck, for example, paid $6.6 billion for the PBM Medco in 1993.) These drug firms believed that, by buying PBMs, they could gain more control over the market for their drugs; the PBMs would presumably substitute their drugs for those of their competitors, increasing their market share and drug sales. PBMs, however, were unable to merely include their owners' drugs to the exclusion of others because their credibility in serving health plans would have been adversely affected. The drug firms' PBM strategy does not appear to have been worthwhile. Pharmaceutical companies that did not buy PBMs were also able to increase their drug sales, and some companies that bought PBMs sold them. The growth of managed care turned out to be a benefit rather than a threat to drug manufacturers. As more people enrolled in managed care, they received prescription drug coverage, use of prescription drugs grew, and sales at all drug firms sharply rose.

The second type is horizontal merger, where one drug manufacturer purchases another. There are several reasons for horizontal mergers. First, by becoming larger, firms expect that economies of scale will increase efficiency and decrease costs. Merging two companies can lower administrative costs and raise the efficiency of the two companies' sales forces, which is critical to the success of any drug firm. Drug firms with distinctive products are able to use a single distribution system and sales force when they merge, which results in significant cost savings. Consolidating research units can eliminate competing efforts, and mergers can reduce duplicative manufacturing costs.

Second, for some large firms, mergers are a response to patent expirations and gaps in a firm's product pipeline (Danzon, Epstein, and Nicholson

2007). A wider array of prescription drugs diversifies the financial risk of a firm that has just a few best-selling drugs. Third, for small pharmaceutical firms, mergers are primarily an exit strategy, an indication of financial trouble. Fourth, horizontal mergers can improve the combined drug firms' market power. However, few mergers have occurred between firms with drugs in the same therapeutic category. Instead, the types of drugs offered by the combined drug firms are in different therapeutic categories, offering a broader range of prescription drugs across many therapeutic categories to large purchasers.

Pharmaceutical Firms' New Research Strategy

The pharmaceutical industry has undergone major changes in the past several decades. Previously, most pharmaceutical firms were large; able to take advantage of economies of scale; and vertically integrated—that is, most activities were performed in-house, from drug discovery to clinical trials to regulatory approval processes to marketing. The firm's investments in R&D were financed by internally generated funds. Large drug firms' drug development emphasized having very large research staffs to screen millions of compounds to discover the next blockbuster drug that would be used by large population groups. This strategy, however, resulted in finding very few new blockbuster drugs.

Revolutionary discoveries in biologic sciences in the 1970s changed the structure of the industry. Thousands of new biotechnology firms were started. Venture capital funded many of these startups, which were not expected to be profitable for a number of years. Although the risk was high, the profit potential from new drug discoveries was believed to be so large that investors were willing to risk substantial sums on these new firms. The biotechnology industry became a major source of drug innovation (Cockburn, Stern, and Zausner 2011).

Scientific advances in genetics and biology enabled drug discovery to become more focused, targeting the particular pathway that causes a disease for relatively small population groups. Biotechnology firms attempt to discover genetically targeted drugs that treat relatively small populations, but because of the effectiveness of these new drugs, the drug's price can be as high as $100,000 a year. Insurers are more willing to pay higher prices because there are no close substitutes, compared to what they would pay for drugs for common diseases, such as high cholesterol, which have many generic substitutes. These specialty drugs are generally able to receive regulatory approval in a shorter period; the time required to bring a new drug to market is reduced to about 6 years from the previous 12 years.

Large drug firms were concerned that they had fallen behind small biotechnology firms in their ability to develop innovative drugs. Small companies were more likely to take greater scientific risks and have a greater number of researchers devoted to a particular research idea, while large companies became more bureaucratic in their scientific decision making. Large drug firms began to depend on small biotechnology firms to fill their drug pipelines.

The new approach to drug discovery also changed the size of a drug manufacturer's research efforts. Large research staffs have been downsized and reorganized. The size of a research team has been greatly reduced to about 20 to 40 focused teams. Drug companies believe that smaller research units may be willing to take greater risks and be more innovative than might large bureaucracies.

Another major change in drug firms' research strategy has been to become venture capitalists. Rather than investing a billion dollars to find the next blockbuster drug, large drug firms are minimizing their financial risks by developing contractual relationships with and investing in a number of small biotechnology companies to find promising new drugs (Walker and Loftus 2013).

Most of the small, new biotechnology firms did not have the capabilities of large drug firms to bring a new product to market. At the same time, large drug firms recognized the profit potential of the drug research being undertaken by these small firms. Both types of firms realized that developing relationships would capitalize on each of their strengths. These small firms face large risks and huge investment costs before their products can be marketed. The process of discovery, clinical trials, and drug approval is lengthy and costs hundreds of millions of dollars. Larger firms are able to bear these costs and have the expertise to navigate the drug-approval process. Greater risk pooling also occurs when many different drugs are in the discovery and development phase, as only a few of the many drugs developed will be successful. Only a large firm can afford to undertake these large research efforts. Small firms may not have the financial resources to complete the long drug-approval process or the expertise to perform all of the steps required (Golec and Vernon 2009; Lazonick and Tulum 2011).

Although the research innovation is being generated by small firms, large firms have an advantage when it comes to marketing and selling their drugs. They are able to offer health plans and PBMs (which contract with large employers and medical plans) as well as prescription drugs for almost all therapeutic categories at a package discount. Providing a full line of drugs for different therapeutic areas at a discount lowers the cost to the PBM, by removing the need to negotiate with multiple firms while enabling the large pharmaceutical firm to include drugs in its package that the PBM might not otherwise select. The Medicare Part D drug benefit reinforces these marketing advantages for the large firm; they are better able to provide the range of drugs used in the restricted formularies by the drug plans offering the Part D benefit to Medicare beneficiaries.

Scientific advances have changed the structure of the pharmaceutical industry by stimulating the growth of many small biotechnology firms, shifting the direction of drug research, downsizing the size of research teams, and creating a new role for large drug firms as venture capitalists.

Industry Competitiveness

The pharmaceutical industry appears to be relatively competitive, as measured by the degree of market concentration. Concentration—which is measured by the combined market share of the top four firms—was only about 23 percent in 2012, based on data from IMS Health (2014). However, when therapeutic categories are used, the degree of market concentration is much higher (in some cases 100 percent) as a therapeutic category may include only one drug. Thus, the competitiveness of the pharmaceutical industry depends on the definition of the market.

Markets that are less concentrated (i.e., have more competitors) are typically more price competitive. The higher the degree of market concentration and the fewer the substitutes available for a particular drug, the greater the firm's market power—that is, the ability to raise price without losing sales. Thus, the manufacturer of the first breakthrough drug in a therapeutic category has a great deal of market power. As additional branded drugs are developed in that therapeutic category, substitutes become available and price competition increases. When the patents on those drugs expire and generic versions are introduced, a great deal of price competition occurs. At each of these stages purchasers are able to buy the prescription drug at a lower price.

Development of New Drugs by the US Pharmaceutical Industry

Several measures are used to indicate the productivity of the US pharmaceutical industry. One measure is designation as a *global new chemical entity* (NCE), a drug that is marketed to a majority of the world's leading purchasers of drugs; this designation is preferred over total NCEs as an indicator of a drug's commercial and therapeutic importance. *First in* (a therapeutic) *class* is another designation that reveals how innovative a drug is. In addition, the introduction of biotechnology and orphan drugs is examined, as both are major sources of industry growth and innovation.

Grabowski and Wang (2006) analyzed all NCEs introduced worldwide between 1982 and 2003. During that period, 919 NCEs were introduced:

42 percent were global NCEs, 13 percent were first in class, 10 percent were biotechnology drugs, and 8 percent were orphan drugs. Over this period, the total number of NCEs introduced each year showed a downward trend. However, the measures of the drugs' importance (global NCEs, first in class, biotechnology drugs, and orphan drugs) increased over the same time period. Grabowski and Wang concluded that although the trend in total NCEs declined, the relative quality of new drugs had been increasing, and most of the biotechnology and orphan drugs were introduced from 1993 to 2003. The number of NCEs considered global or first in class varied by therapeutic category, the highest number being oncology drugs, which is an emphasis of the biotechnology industry. (The United States is the dominant source of biotechnology drugs.)

When the introduction of drugs was analyzed by country, the United States was found to be a leader in the development of innovative drugs, particularly from 1993 to 2003. As shown in Exhibit 28.1, 30 out of 62 first-in-class drugs, 37 out of 71 biotechnology products, and 27 out of 49 orphan drugs are manufactured in the United States. These ratios translate to 48 percent of first-in-class drugs, 52 percent of biotechnology products, and 55 percent of orphan drugs. Further, when the countries in which important new drugs were first introduced (as opposed to developed) were examined, the United States was again a strong leader compared with the rest

Country	All NCEs		Global NCEs		First-in-Class NCEs		Biotech NCEs		Orphan NCEs	
	82–92	93–03	82–92	93–03	82–92	93–03	82–92	93–03	82–92	93–03
EU* Total	230	183	99	112	23	27	6	23	9	20
France	35	18	9	11	2	3	0	3	0	4
Germany	53	42	21	27	5	5	2	6	2	5
Italy	29	14	4	1	1	0	0	0	0	0
Switzerland	42	41	26	30	8	11	3	8	1	8
United Kingdom	34	36	23	27	6	7	0	3	5	2
Others	38	33	17	16	2	2	1	3	1	2
Japan	125	88	12	12	5	3	5	9	1	0
United States	120	152	66	81	24	30	9	37	10	27
ROW**	7	13	3	1	0	2	0	2	0	2
Total	482	437	179	206	53	62	19	71	20	49

EXHIBIT 28.1
Country-Level Output of New Chemical Entities (NCEs) by Category and Time Period, 1982–1992 and 1993–2003

* EU: European Union; ** ROW: rest of the world
SOURCE: Reprinted with permission as it appeared in Henry G. Grabowski and Y. Richard Wang, "The Quantity and Quality of Worldwide New Drug Introductions, 1982–2003," *Health Affairs*, 25(2), March/April 2006: 425–460, Exhibit 4. © 2006 Project HOPE—The People-to-People Health Foundation, Inc.

of the world in the most recent period that data were available (i.e., 1993 to 2003). Both foreign and domestic drug firms preferred to introduce their important new drugs first in the US market. US patients benefit from having earlier access to important new drugs (although there is an associated risk with being the first users of such drugs). Unfortunately, no updates to these figures are available; different results/interpretation of these findings can be found in Light (2009).

The decrease in the total number of NCEs appears to indicate that the productivity of the US drug industry has declined. However, when measures of important new drugs are used, productivity in the US drug industry has increased. Biotechnology drugs, in which the United States is a leader, have been a source of important new drugs and industry productivity growth.

The US market provides greater incentives to drug firms than do other countries for developing important new drugs and for first introducing innovative drugs. Whether the US's predominance in drug innovation and first choice of introduction will continue depends on government payment policies to reduce the costs of new drugs.

The Political Attractiveness of Price Controls on Prescription Drugs

For many years the high price of prescription drugs was a major concern of the elderly. When Medicare was enacted in 1965 prescription drugs were not included as a benefit. Many of the elderly, who are the highest users of prescription drugs, could not afford to buy needed prescription drugs; having a prescription drug benefit became their highest political priority. In 2003, the Medicare Modernization Act was enacted. It included a new Medicare Part D prescription drug benefit, which became effective in 2006 (see Chapter 8). Part D increased the demand for prescription drugs by the aged, and pharmaceutical manufacturers benefited from higher revenues. However, increased revenues to the pharmaceutical companies meant higher federal expenditures for the aged's prescription drugs, 75 percent of which were being subsidized by the government. Part D, similar to Medicare Part B, became another unfunded federal entitlement; no matter how much was spent on drugs by the elderly, Medicare was committed to paying 75 percent of those expenditures. (As part of the 2010 Affordable Care Act [ACA] the aged's cost sharing for prescription drugs is reduced over time, leading to greater use of prescription drugs and higher drug expenditures.)

The Medicare Modernization Act and the ACA prohibited the federal government from negotiating drug prices with pharmaceutical firms. The elderly enroll in a private drug plan, which then negotiates drug prices with the drug manufacturer. As the cost of Part D to the federal government continues to rise, the pharmaceutical companies are concerned that Congress will change the law and have the government regulate drug prices. (A number of legislators have proposed changing the law to allow the government to negotiate directly with pharmaceutical companies.) Part D creates a huge unfunded federal liability at a time when the federal government's budget deficit is already very large. As long as the government is ultimately responsible for paying for the elderly's drug expenses, regardless of who administers the benefit, there is concern that drug expenditures will eventually be regulated, as the government currently regulates payment for each type of provider participating in Medicare.

Proponents of government regulation of drug prices claim that in addition to reducing federal expenditures, the aged would also benefit by lowering their out-of-pocket drug expenses and their premium for the Medicare drug benefit, which equals 25 percent of total Medicare drug expenditures. As evidence of the benefits of price controls, proponents claim that prices on branded drugs are as much as 30 percent higher in the United States than in Canada, which uses price controls.

Price controls on new breakthrough drugs are politically attractive. Politicians try to provide their constituents with short-term visible benefits, seemingly at no cost. In the short run, drug prices would be reduced and there would be no decrease in access to drugs currently on the market. Because the costs of R&D have already been incurred, the only cost of producing an existing drug is its relatively small variable costs. As long as the regulated drug price is greater than the drug's variable costs, the firm will continue selling the drug. Profits from that drug will be lower, but the drug firm will make more money by continuing to sell the drug, even at the regulated price, than by not selling it.

Consequences of Price Controls on Prescription Drugs

Price controls would not decrease access to innovative drugs currently on the market or even to those currently in the drug-approval process. Those who would benefit include patients who cannot afford expensive drugs, states with rapidly increasing Medicaid expenditures, and the federal government, which is responsible for bearing 75 percent of the cost of the prescription drug benefit. The aged (who have the highest voting-participation rate), state Medicaid programs, and legislators interested in decreasing federal drug expenditures are likely to favor legislation to reduce drug prices. The only apparent loser would be drug companies.

The real concern with price controls is their effects not on current drugs but on R&D for future drugs. Price controls reduce the profitability of new drugs. With lower expected profits, drug companies would be less willing to risk hundreds of millions of dollars on R&D. Most new drugs (about 70 percent to 80 percent) are not therapeutic breakthroughs and, although their price may exceed their variable costs, do not generate sufficient profit to cover their R&D investments. Thus, the drug company loses money on these drugs. (See Exhibit 26.3.) The small percentage that are considered to be blockbuster drugs have high price markups over their variable costs. The large profits generated by these blockbuster drugs generate the funding used for the drugs that lose money. Although there is a short-term visible benefit to price controls, they impose a long-term cost on patients. This long-term cost is not obvious because it occurs in the future, and the public would be unaware of breakthrough drugs that were never developed.

Blockbuster drugs, with their high price markups, would be targeted by price controls. With price controls, profit would be insufficient to provide R&D funding for new drugs. Fewer breakthrough drugs would mean treating a disease would be more costly; these drugs might make surgical intervention unnecessary or might even prevent the disease from occurring. Through R&D and the development of new drugs, the total cost of medical treatment is lowered. With price controls, R&D investments would decline. Drug companies would also reallocate their R&D efforts away from diseases affecting the elderly (where price controls limit profits) toward diseases affecting other population groups (where profits are not limited).

Exhibits 28.2 and 28.3 illustrate the effects of imposing price controls on the product life cycle of a blockbuster drug (Helms 2004). During the beginning phases of R&D, including clinical trials, the company incurs a negative cash flow. Once the FDA approves the drug and the drug company markets the drug, the cash flow is positive—until other branded drugs (substitutes) enter the market, and eventually the patent expires and generics enter the market.

If price controls are imposed on a drug after it is approved by the FDA and marketed, the positive cash flow from the new drug is greatly diminished, as shown by the dotted line in Exhibit 28.3. To illustrate the financial effects of imposing price controls in the previous example, one would have to examine the present value of both the cash outlay and the positive cash return.

Money received in the future is worth less than the same amount of money received today. These money outflows (before the drug is sold) and inflows occur at different times. The cost of developing a new drug includes all the costs of bringing it to market, such as research expenditures, the cost of clinical trials, the cost of having the drug approved by the FDA, and marketing costs once it is approved. A company would calculate what it could

EXHIBIT 28.2

Life Cycle of a
New Drug

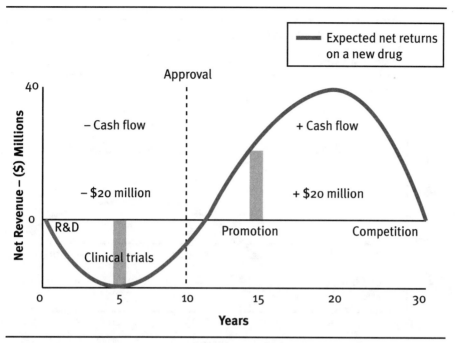

have earned on that investment if the funds were instead invested in a corporate bond and gained interest. For example, if $10 were invested today and earned 6 percent interest per year, in five years that initial investment would grow to $13.38. Thus, in calculating the cost of developing a new drug, the firm calculates both its cash outlay and what it could have earned on that money (the opportunity cost). Similarly, in calculating the return received from that new drug, which generates a positive cash flow in the future, it is necessary to discount (using the same interest rate) the positive cash flow and determine what money received in the future is worth in today's dollars (the present value).

Using the example shown in exhibits 28.2 and 28.3, if a firm invests $20 million in year 5, the present value of that investment equals $14.95 million. (In other words, $14.95 million invested today would be worth $20 million in five years.) If, after 15 years, a new drug earns $20 million, the present value of that return is only $8.35 million. Clearly, the $20 million spent and the $20 million earned are not equal. In this example, the drug firm would lose money on its investment—$6.6 million. Thus, the longer it takes to bring a drug to market, the longer the negative cash flow and the smaller the present value of the positive cash flow once the drug is marketed.

If price controls are imposed on a drug once it is marketed, as shown by the dotted line in Exhibit 28.3, both its positive cash flow and the present

EXHIBIT 28.3
**Effect of Price
Controls on
Drug Returns**

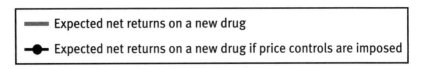

Expected net returns on a new drug

Expected net returns on a new drug if price controls are imposed

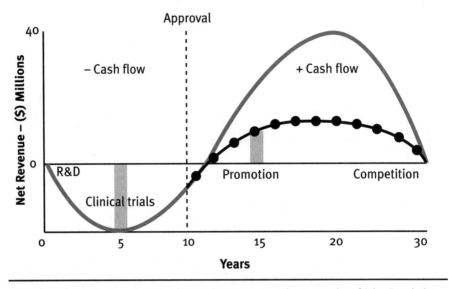

value of that reduced cash flow will be lower. Thus, if the firm earns only $10 million in year 15, the present value equals only $4.17 million. The present value of the cash outflow remains at $14.95 million (Helms 2004).

In the previous example of price controls reducing future returns, a drug firm would change its investment strategy: It would decrease its overall investment in R&D, invest in drugs with a quicker payoff, seek drugs with less-risky profitability outcomes, and invest in drugs whose market potential is very large and profitable, thereby abandoning research on drugs for diseases affecting fewer people.

Examples of Price Controls on US Prescription Drugs

The debate over President Clinton's health plan, introduced in the fall of 1993, provides an indication of the likely effect of price controls on prescription drugs. Included in the plan was the Advisory Council on Breakthrough Drugs, whose purpose was to review prices of new drugs. If the proposed council believed a new drug's price was excessive, it would try to have it reduced or, failing that, have the drug excluded from health insurance payment. The targeted drugs were those that were the most profitable and had high price markups—namely breakthrough drugs. The pharmaceutical industry was concerned that if the plan was enacted, price controls would be imposed on prescription drugs and the profitability of new drugs would be decreased. As a result, the annual rate of increase in R&D expenditures declined sharply, falling from 18.2 percent in 1992 to 5.6 percent by 1994, the smallest annual rate of increase in 30 years (see Exhibit 28.4). Once it became clear that the Clinton health plan would be defeated and price controls would not be imposed on new drugs, the annual rate of increase in pharmaceutical R&D spending rose again.

The next threat to the drug companies occurred in 2002, when the firms believed Congress was going to legalize reimportation of drugs from Canada and Europe (without the approval of the secretary of the Department of Health and Human Services). As a result, in 2002 R&D expenditures grew by only 4.2 percent, after having increased by 14.4 percent in 2001. Once there was no longer a threat of a more stringent form of reimportation, R&D expenditures again rose—to 11.1 percent in 2003.

In 2008 and 2009, the annual change in R&D expenditures sharply decreased over concerns that the newly elected Democratic president (Obama) and large Democratic majorities in Congress would adversely affect the industry by requiring reductions in Medicare and Medicaid prescription drug prices. In the fee-for-service part of Medicaid, drug firms pay a rebate to Medicaid for each drug the program purchases on behalf of its beneficiaries. President Obama's 2010 budget proposed to increase that rebate (ultimately lowering the price drug firms receive). Proposals were also made to require a rebate on drugs purchased by Medicare Part D beneficiaries. As the data indicate, R&D expenditures are sensitive to possible legislative changes that would reduce drug firms' profits (CBO 2009).

History does not offer much hope for drug manufacturers evading price controls. Governments in other countries have used various approaches to lower their drug expenditures. In a study of 19 OECD (Organisation for Economic Co-operation and Development) countries, Sood and colleagues (2008) found various forms of regulation that decreased pharmaceutical revenues. The types of controls used by these countries included fixing the price of drugs, delaying approval for expensive new drugs for several years, restricting the use of a drug once it has been approved, establishing global (country) budget caps, setting annual physician prescribing budget limits, applying profit controls, and setting the price of all drugs within a specific therapeutic category at the cost of the lowest-price drug. While a majority of the regulations decrease pharmaceutical revenues, direct price controls have the largest negative effect on revenues. If similar price controls were imposed in the United States, pharmaceutical revenues would fall as much as 20 percent. Further, the longer the regulations are in place, the greater their impact on revenues.

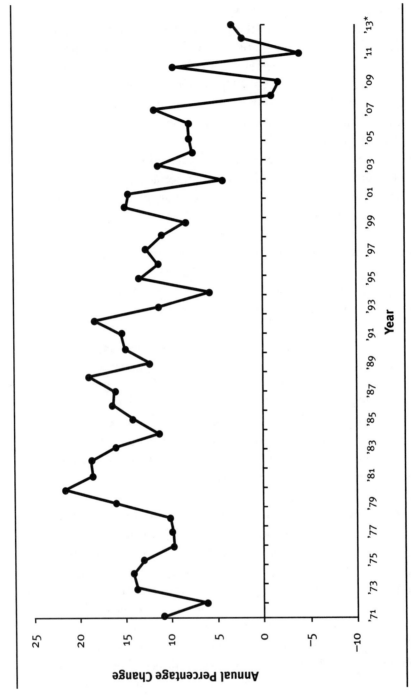

EXHIBIT 28.4
Annual
Percentage
Change in
US R&D,
Pharmaceutical
Companies,
1971–2013

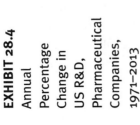

* Estimated for 2013
NOTE: Domestic US R&D includes expenditures within the United States by all PhRMA member companies. R&D abroad includes expenditures by US-owned PhRMA companies outside the United States and R&D conducted abroad by the US divisions of foreign-owned PhRMA member companies. R&D performed abroad by the foreign divisions of foreign-owned PhRMA member companies is excluded. Data for 1995 R&D affected by merger and acquisition activity.
SOURCE: Data from PhRMA (2014).

Several approaches have already been used in the United States to reduce government expenditures for prescription drugs (Vernon and Golec 2009). State Medicaid programs, because of their tight budgets, have more restrictive formularies than managed care plans do. Newer drugs that are more expensive but more effective are more likely to be excluded in favor of less-expensive generics. Further, Medicaid programs delay inclusion of expensive new innovative drugs in their formularies for several years. Studies have shown that the effect of limiting access to preferred drugs results in a shift to more costly settings, higher nursing home admissions, and greater risk of hospitalization among Medicaid populations (Soumerai 2004). Further, the savings in drug costs were offset by increases in the costs of hospitalization and emergency department care (Hsu et al. 2006).

A price-control approach used by the federal government requires the drug manufacturer to sell the drug to the government at its "best" price. In the 1980s, as a result of price competition among drug companies to have health maintenance organizations (HMOs) and group purchasing organizations (GPOs) include their drugs in HMO and GPO drug formularies, drug manufacturers gave large price discounts to certain HMOs and GPOs. In 1990, the federal government, in an attempt to reduce Medicaid expenditures, enacted a law that required drug manufacturers to give state Medicaid programs the same discounts they gave their best customers. Consequently, the drug companies gave smaller discounts to HMOs and GPOs. A study by the Congressional Budget Office (1996) found that the best (largest) price discount given to HMOs and GPOs declined in 1991 from 24 percent and 28 percent, respectively, and by 1994 to 14 percent and 15 percent, respectively, the minimum amount required by the government. The study concluded that drug companies were much less willing to give steep discounts to large purchasers when they had to give the same discounts to Medicaid. Drug prices and expenditures consequently increased for many private buyers.

Summary

Two important characteristics of the pharmaceutical industry are (1) the low costs of actually producing a drug pill and (2) the high cost of developing a new drug. The price at which a new drug is sold is determined not by its cost of production or the R&D investment in that drug but by its value to purchasers and whether any close substitutes to that drug are available. Valuable drugs that have no close substitutes (blockbuster drugs) will be priced high, relative to their costs of production. Lowering the price of these blockbuster drugs to make them more affordable will decrease pharmaceutical companies' incentive to invest hundreds of millions of dollars in drugs that may have great value to society. That is the public policy dilemma.

The pharmaceutical industry has been changing over time from large, vertically integrated organizations to an industry that still has large firms but also many small biotechnology firms (funded by venture capital) that are engaged in developing new blockbuster drugs. A great deal of private money is invested in these highly risky ventures in the hope of developing a valuable (and profitable) new drug.

The United States, compared with the rest of the world, has been a leader in developing important new drugs and is the country of first choice for introducing innovative new drugs. Government payment policies to reduce drug expenditures threaten both the US industry's leadership and patients' access to innovative drugs.

A growing concern is that federal government, which has become a large indirect purchaser of prescription drugs as a result of including Part D in Medicare, will attempt to lower its drug expenses by controlling the price of prescription drugs. Direct government negotiations with drug companies over the price of their drugs will be tantamount to the government fixing the price of drugs.

Implementing price controls will not have any immediate effect on the aged's access to drugs. However, over time, drug companies will invest less in R&D and redirect their R&D toward population groups and diseases where profitability is greater.

In coming years, enormous scientific progress is likely. The mapping of the human genome and advances in molecular biology are expected to lead to drug solutions for many diseases. Drug prices and expenditures would also likely be higher to reflect the increased willingness of people to pay for these new discoveries. It would be unfortunate if the desire to reduce the cost of drugs through price controls decreased the availability of breakthrough drugs.

Any public policy must deal with trade-offs: reducing the high price markup of breakthrough drugs versus maintaining incentives for investing in R&D. It is important to distinguish between the short- and long-term effects of public policy. Using price controls to lower drug prices results in a visible short-term benefit but comes at a less-visible longer-term cost of fewer breakthrough drugs. Future patients would be willing to pay for life-saving breakthrough drugs that were not developed because the government removed the incentives to do so. Given the trade-off between instituting regulation to reduce the cost of drugs or having innovative drugs to cure disease, reduce mortality, and lower the cost of medical treatment, society would likely choose the full benefits scientific discovery will offer.

Discussion Questions

1. How has the structure of the pharmaceutical industry changed over time?
2. What are alternative ways of judging whether the pharmaceutical industry is competitive?
3. Why are price controls on prescription drugs politically attractive?
4. Why would price controls not limit access to blockbuster drugs that are either currently on the market or have almost completed the FDA approval process?
5. What are the expected long-term consequences of price controls on R&D investments, quality of life, mortality rates, and the cost of medical care?

References

Cockburn, I., S. Stern, and J. Zausner. 2011. "Finding the Endless Frontier: Lessons from the Life Sciences Innovation System for Energy R&D." In *Accelerating Energy Innovation: Insights from Multiple Sectors,* edited by R. Henderson and R. Newell, 113–57. Chicago: University of Chicago Press.

Congressional Budget Office (CBO). 2009. "Pharmaceutical R&D and the Evolving Market for Prescription Drugs." *Economic and Budget Issue Brief,* October 26. www.cbo.gov/ftpdocs/106xx/doc10681/10-26-DrugR&D.pdf.

———. 1996. *CBO Papers: How the Medicaid Rebate on Prescription Drugs Affects Pricing in the Pharmaceutical Industry.* Washington, DC: US Government Printing Office.

Danzon, P., A. Epstein, and S. Nicholson. 2007. "Mergers and Acquisitions in the Pharmaceutical and Biotech Industries." *Managerial and Decision Economics* 28 (4–5): 307–28.

Golec, J., and J. A. Vernon. 2009. "Financial Risk of the Biotech Industry Versus the Pharmaceutical Industry." *Applied Health Economics and Policy* 7 (3): 155–65.

Grabowski, H., and Y. Wang. 2006. "The Quantity and Quality of Worldwide New Drug Introductions, 1982–2003." *Health Affairs* 25 (2): 452–60.

Helms, R. 2004. "The Economics of Price Regulation and Innovation." *Supplement to Managed Care* 13 (6): 10–12.

Hsu, J., M. Price, J. Huang, R. Brand, V. Fung, R. Hui, B. Fireman, J. Newhouse, and J. Selby. 2006. "Unintended Consequences of Caps on Medicare Drug Benefits." *New England Journal of Medicine* 354 (22): 2349–59.

IMS Health. 2014. "Top Companies by Non-Discounted Spending (U.S.)." Accessed April. www.imshealth.com/deployedfiles/imshealth/Global/

Content/Corporate/Press%20Room/2012_U.S/Top_Companies_by_Non-Discounted_Spending_U.S.pdf.

Lazonick, W., and O. Tulum. 2011. "US Biopharmaceutical Finance and the Sustainability of the Biotech Business Model." *Research Policy* 40 (9): 1170–87.

Light, D. 2009. "Global Drug Discovery: Europe Is Ahead." *Health Affairs* 28 (5): 969–77.

Pharmaceutical Research and Manufacturers of America (PhRMA). 2014. *2014 Biopharmaceutical Research Industry Profile*. Published April. www.phrma.org/sites/default/files/pdf/2014_PhRMA_PROFILE.pdf.

Sood, N., H. deVries, I. Gutierrez, D. Lakdawalla, and D. Goldman. 2008. "The Effect of Regulation on Pharmaceutical Revenues: Experience in Nineteen Countries." *Health Affairs* (web exclusive): W125–W135.

Soumerai, S. 2004. "Benefits and Risks of Increasing Restrictions on Access to Costly Drugs in Medicaid." *Health Affairs* 23 (1): 135–46.

Vernon, J., and J. Golec. 2009. *Pharmaceutical Price Regulation: Public Perceptions, Economic Realities, and Empirical Evidence*. Washington, DC: American Enterprise Institute Press.

Walker, J., and P. Loftus. 2013. "Merck to Cut Staff by 20% as Big Pharma Trims R&D." *Wall Street Journal*, October 2, pp. 1–2.

SHOULD KIDNEYS AND OTHER ORGANS BE BOUGHT AND SOLD?

29

B etween 1995 and 2013, 126,663 people on waiting lists for an organ died. During this period, the number of people waiting for a transplant rose 200 percent (from 43,937 to 132,019), while the number of organs donated increased by just 52 percent (from 23,255 in 1995 to 35,389 in 2013); see Exhibit 29.1. More than 80 percent of those waiting for organ transplants are waiting for kidneys; the remainder are waiting for a heart, liver, lung, intestine, or pancreas. The number of people who die each year while waiting for an organ transplant is increasing: In 2013, the number was 6,717, up from 3,722 in 1995.

Although the total number of transplants has increased (see Exhibit 29.2), the gap between those waiting for organ transplants and the supply of organs has also been growing rapidly as more patients are recommended for such transplants. Improved transplant techniques and the development of better immunosuppressive drugs to reduce the risk of rejection has greatly increased the success rate of organ transplants; success rates for kidney transplants have increased from approximately 60 percent in the late 1950s to 96 percent in 2013. Unfortunately, the number of organs is insufficient to keep up with the growing demand. Consequently, many of those waiting for a transplant die before an organ becomes available.[1]

Patients waiting for a kidney transplant must rely on kidney dialysis, which is costly. Kidney transplantation is a lower-cost form of treatment than dialysis. If all of the patients on dialysis who are waiting for a transplant could be given a kidney, the federal government—which pays for kidney dialysis and kidney transplants under Medicare—could save approximately $12.7 billion (in 2013 dollars) over a five-year period.[2] In addition to being higher cost, dialysis takes time—up to seven hours per day for several days a week. Kidney dialysis patients have a reduced quality of life as well as lower productivity.

Sources of Organs for Transplant

The two sources of supply for organ transplants are (1) living donors, such as family members who donate one of their kidneys, and (2) cadavers. Approximately 62 percent of kidneys—as well as other organs used for

EXHIBIT 29.1
Demand for
Organs and the
Total Number
of Organs
Donated, 1995–
2013

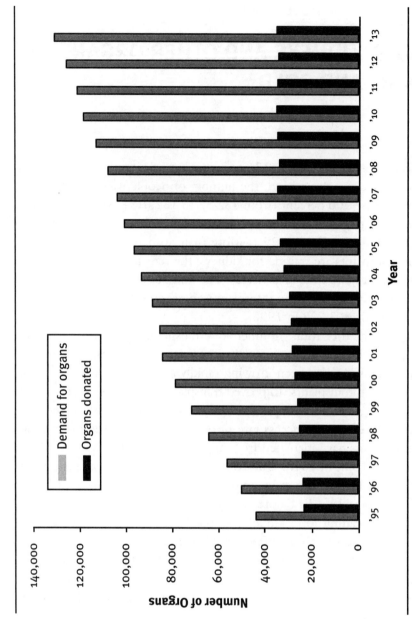

SOURCE: Data on the number of organs demanded are based on the waiting list of the Organ Procurement and Transplantation Network (OPTN) on the last day of each year. Data for the number of organs donated are from OPTN as of March 21, 2014 (see http://optn.transplant.hrsa.gov).

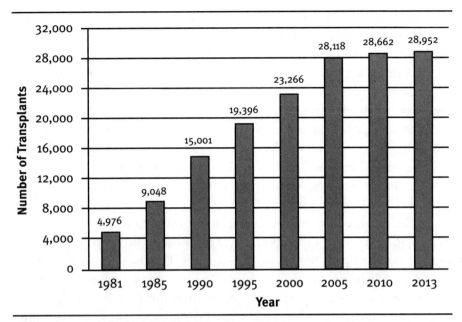

EXHIBIT 29.2
Number
of Organ
Transplants,
Selected Years,
1981–2013

SOURCE: Based on Organ Procurement and Transplantation Network data as of March 21, 2014 (see http://optn.transplant.hrsa.gov).

transplants (96 percent of livers, 99 percent of lungs, and 100 percent of pancreases and hearts)—come from victims who have just been killed in an accident. A total of 77 percent of all organs come from accident victims (OPTN n.d.).

The motivating force on which transplant patients have long depended is altruism. According to the National Organ Transplant Act of 1984, purchase or sale of human organs is illegal. Current efforts to increase the supply of organs rely on approaches to stimulate voluntary organ donations by the family members of those who die in accidents.

Currently, shortly after they have been notified of the death of their loved one, family members are asked by medical personnel to donate the deceased's organs. Physicians are often reluctant to make such a request to a grieving family, and the grieving family is reluctant to agree while still shocked by the death. For some families, the sorrow might be somewhat offset by the belief that another person's life might be saved. About 30 percent of families are still unwilling to give permission for their deceased family member's organs to be used for transplant patients (Goldberg, Halpern, and Reese 2013). For psychological reasons (such as the thought of dismemberment of a loved one) and religious reasons, families of the deceased are often unwilling to donate the deceased's organs. The period in which such a request can be made is short: Tissues may be recovered from donors up to 24 hours after the cessation of heartbeat; the organ will quickly deteriorate.

The family must be located, permission must be received, a recipient must be located through the national organ network, and a tissue match must be made between the recipient and the deceased.

Various approaches have been proposed to increase voluntary organ donations.[3] One is to use improved "marketing" techniques on how to approach (and who should talk to) grieving families, whose sorrow (as mentioned) may be lessened by the knowledge that they have saved another person's life by donating the deceased's organs. Another approach is to provide greater publicity and education to the public on registering to become a donor, which make a person's organs available to potential recipients. (Each US state has a donor registry and specific instructions for potential donors.)

Although education and publicity are likely to increase the number of people registering to become an organ donor (hence potential organ donations), the organ transplant community still seeks permission from the donor's family before harvesting organs. In some states, such as Texas, medical authorities have been legally granted permission to harvest organs from bodies if the family has not been identified within four hours. This authority, however, has rarely been used. Fear of lawsuits and unfavorable publicity and the desire to maintain the public's trust prevent physicians from immediately harvesting a deceased donor's organs.

Presumed consent laws have been proposed that would make the deceased's organs available unless the deceased or their family had previously opposed it. These laws, which are in force in many European countries, have increased organ donation rates about 25 percent to 30 percent over those in the United States; although in most countries with presumed consent laws, such as Spain, medical authorities do not authorize the removal of organs without an explicit family approval. Thus, while presumed consent would alleviate the organ shortage in the United States, it would not eliminate it (Abadie and Gay 2006).

Waiting for permission from the deceased's family often results in the organs being lost. Although about 20,000 people who die each year in the United States have organs suitable for harvesting, only 15 percent to 20 percent of those organs are actually donated. Under the current system of altruism, the supply of living and deceased donors has increased very slowly—from 5,909 in 1988 to 9,220 in 1996 to 14,010 in 2012.

Kidney exchanges have been established to increase the number of voluntary donations. A person who is willing to donate a kidney to his or her intended recipient may be unable to do so because of various types of donor (known as recipient incompatibility). Using a kidney exchange, however, two incompatible patient–donor pairs exchange kidneys with each patient receiving a compatible kidney from the other's donor (Roth, Sonmez, and Unver 2005).

Donor Compensation Proposals

The growing imbalance between supply and demand for organs has led some persons to advocate compensating donors to increase the supply of donated organs. Paying donors (or their families) is highly controversial and would require a change in current legislation prohibiting the purchase or sale of body organs. Organ payment proposals cover the spectrum from mild (paying family members for organs of their kin before or after death) to strong (paying a living donor for a kidney). The following discussion covers three such proposals.

Compensating Families After the Death of the Donor

One approach proposes that the burial costs of the deceased be paid if the family permits harvesting of the deceased's organs. Similarly, the family of the deceased could be paid an amount varying between $1,000 and $5,000. A potential problem with these proposals is that negotiating a financial transaction with a family traumatized by the death of a loved one may be awkward. Another possible problem is that organ purchases of the deceased, which would presumably be directed toward those with low income, might offend low-income minority families, who may feel that they are being exploited to benefit wealthy white people.

Compensating Donors Before Death

Allowing people to sell their organs in advance of their death has the advantage that family members would not be subject to the psychological and social pressure to make a quick decision at the time they suffer the loss of a loved one. Thus, a second approach is to allow people to sell the rights to their organs in return for reducing their health or auto insurance premiums. Health or automobile insurance companies might offer annually a choice of lower premiums to those who are willing to donate their organs if they die during the coming year. The insurance company would then have the right to harvest the deceased's organs during the period of the insurance contract. Each of the potential donors would be listed in a central computer registry, which a hospital would check when a patient died. Transplant recipients would also be listed in a national registry, and their health insurer or the government would reimburse the insurer a previously stated price for the organ.

For example, if the value of all of a deceased's organs is $100,000 at time of death and the probability of dying during the year is 10,000:1 (the current average chance of dying during a year), the annual premium reduction would be $10. If the value of all of the organs is greater than $100,000 or the probability of death is lower than 10,000:1, the premium reduction would be greater. Young drivers and motorcyclists, who are more likely to die in accidents, would presumably be offered larger automobile insurance reductions.

The price of organs could either be established competitively or by the government—for example, $10,000 for a kidney. These prices would be used by insurance companies, together with the probability that a subscriber would die during the next year, to establish the annual premium reduction for a potential donor. If too few insurance subscribers were willing to accept the premium reduction, the price of the organ (if established by the government) could be increased until the likely supply is large enough to satisfy the estimated demand for transplants. The greater the shortage of organs, the larger would be the reductions in insurance premiums for organ donors.

Compensating Living Kidney Donors

The most controversial approach is to pay living donors a sufficiently high price for them to part with one of their kidneys. Paying a market price to bring forth an increase in supply is already occurring in other highly sensitive areas of human behavior, such the use of sperm banks and surrogate mothers, who are willing to be impregnated with another couple's fertilized egg in return for a fee. Recently, it became legal to compensate bone marrow donors (Satel and Viard 2013). Previously, 2,000 to 3,000 people with cancer and blood diseases would die each year while waiting for a bone marrow transplant.[4]

Market transactions consist of a voluntary exchange of assets between two parties. People engage in voluntary exchange because they differ in their valuation of the asset and both parties expect to benefit from the transaction. If sales of kidneys were permitted, the person selling the kidney would receive a fee that she believes would compensate her for the loss of a kidney. The purchaser believes the kidney is worth at least what he is willing to pay for it. The purchaser is likely to be the government rather than an individual, as kidney transplants are covered under Medicare; in this case, paying for the kidney would be similar to paying the surgeon for the operation. No one is made worse off by voluntary trade. Thus, the first major advantage of legalizing the sale of kidneys is that both parties are likely better off with the voluntary exchange than when it is prohibited.

Permitting a commercial market for kidneys has other important advantages. Organs that would save the lives of all those waiting for a kidney could be purchased. No longer would they have to endure the suffering that occurs while waiting for a kidney donation, possibly dying before one becomes available. Further, the government would save a great deal of money by substituting kidney transplants for kidney dialysis, as a transplant is a lower-cost method of treatment than dialysis. Lastly, the quality of donated kidneys would increase, improving the success rate of transplants. Currently, donated kidneys that do not have good tissue matches are used because of the severe shortage of kidneys. Paying living donors for their kidneys would result in greater choice of donors, enabling tissue matches between recipient and donor to be made in advance.

Opposition to Using Financial Incentives

Opposition to using financial incentives to increase the supply of organs is based on several factors. First, some believe offering financial incentives would discourage voluntary organ donations, further reducing the supply of organs. Evidence that decreased supply may be the result of paying donors is demonstrated by what happened when financial incentives were used to augment the blood supply (Dunham 2008). Voluntary donations of blood went down, but the decline was more than offset by the growth of paid donations.

Second, some claim that paying living donors for their organs would exploit the poor to benefit the wealthy. The poor are likely to be the sellers of organs, whereas those with higher income are likely to be the beneficiaries. The poor, it is claimed, would be forced to sell their organs to provide for their families. However, the reason the poor have inadequate funds is that society is unwilling to provide them with sufficient subsidies or education so that they can raise their productivity and income. Prohibiting the poor from selling one of their assets would leave them worse off, and they would be prevented from doing something they believe will improve their situation. Although little risk is involved in selling one's kidney, a donor would be accepting a slightly higher risk of dying in return for greater financial rewards. Many people seek additional compensation by choosing to work in higher-risk occupations. Working in a coal mine, in a skyscraper, or on an offshore drilling platform carries occupational risks, yet society does not interfere with these voluntary transactions. Someone willing to make the trade-off between greater compensation and the loss of a kidney is not "forced" to sell her organs.

Third, some are concerned that those selling their kidneys might be subject to fraud and then regret selling their kidneys. Various protections could be included in legislation legalizing the sale of kidneys. A waiting period (such as six months) could be used in case the person decides to change his mind. The donor could be required to be of a minimum age. The donor could also be approved by a panel that includes a psychiatrist or social worker to assess the donor's ability to make rational choices.

When demand exceeds supply in a market, prices rise. When prices are not permitted to rise or sales are illegal, the potential for a black market exists. Although the sale of kidneys in the United States is illegal, a wealthy patient has access to an international black market, particularly from donors from less-developed countries, such as India and China. Demand for organs is lower when the activity is illegal than it would be if sales were legal. On the black market, the search for an organ donor is more expensive, purchasers are less certain of the organ's quality, no legal remedies are available if fraud occurs, and the purchaser has to pay the hospital's and surgeon's costs out of pocket. However, this option is available only to the wealthy. Therefore, prohibiting the sale of organs discriminates against the poor, who do not have access to the international black market in kidneys.

If a legal market in organs were permitted, would only the wealthy be able to afford kidney transplants once the price of a kidney is included in the already-high price of a transplant? The answer is no. Kidney transplants are currently paid for by the federal government; the higher cost would not be a deterrent to any recipient needing a transplant. Most of the costs for a transplant are for hospital and physician services, so including the price of the organ would not be a large addition to those costs. Currently, everyone associated with the transplant benefits—the recipient receives a new kidney, and the physician and hospital are paid for the transplantation surgery. Why should the donor not also benefit?

What if a low-income person desperate for money sells his kidney and subsequently suffers from kidney disease? Because the government currently pays for all kidney transplants as part of Medicare, that donor would become eligible for a free transplant. A new donor would be paid for a kidney to be used for the previous donor's transplant.

Would the opponents of a compensation system who are concerned with its effects on the poor be more positively inclined to using financial incentives if the poor—defined, for example, as those with income below the federal poverty level—were prohibited from selling their organs? Would the poor be better off if they were denied the right to sell one of their assets? A belief that society helps the poor when those with higher income limit their choices is paternalistic.

Additional Considerations

The poor and minority groups are placed at a disadvantage by the present altruistic system for securing and allocating organs. Many of those waiting for transplants have low income. Further, although African Americans are statistically more likely to suffer from kidney disease than whites, they are less likely to receive an organ transplant. In fact, while African Americans make up 13.1 percent of the population, they comprise 34 percent of the waiting list for kidney transplants. The relatively higher proportion of African Americans on the waiting list is due to three factors: (1) They need proportionately more kidneys than whites, (2) their tissue match rate with whites is low, and (3) they are not as likely to get donations from African-American families as from white families. (The refusal rate for organ donations among African-American families is 45 percent, compared with 23 percent for white families [Goldberg, Halpern, and Reese 2013].)

As Epstein (2006) wrote, "Only a bioethicist would prefer a world in which we have 1,000 altruists per annum and more than 6,500 excess deaths over one in which we have no altruists and no excess deaths." Markets and altruism are differing approaches for increasing the number of organ donations; they should be evaluated on the basis of which produces less loss of life.

Summary

The demand for transplantation will continue to grow as the incidence of obesity-driven diabetes and high blood pressure—the two main causes of end-stage kidney failure—rises, as the feasibility of transplants increases, and as more hospitals and physicians find status and profit in performing transplants. However, without any financial incentives for donors, the waiting lines for organ transplants will get longer and the shortage of organs will become more severe. As Cohen (2005) says, "If the benefits of an organs market are so clear, then why do we still...condemn people to death and suffering while the organs that could restore them to health are instead fed to worms?"

Perhaps the strongest objection to compensating donors for their organs is some people's ideological and moral beliefs. Financial incentives would replace altruism as a person's motivating force for donating her organs, an idea that is deeply offensive to many people. However, a trade-off must be considered. Although the thought of having people sell their organs is offensive, thousands of people die each year because they didn't receive the new organ they needed, and this number will rise. Which choice is more offensive—violating the strongly held beliefs of some people who think a market for human organs is repugnant or watching the suffering and subsequent loss of life of thousands of people needing an organ transplant?

Discussion Questions

1. Why have voluntary methods for increasing the supply of body organs been unsuccessful?

2. Evaluate the following proposal: People would be permitted to sell the rights to their organs (in the form of reduced health or auto insurance premiums) if they die in an accident in the coming year.

3. Would government expenditures for kidney disease (currently covered as part of Medicare for all persons) be higher or lower under a free-market system for kidneys?

4. Would the poor be disadvantaged to the benefit of the wealthy under a free-market system for selling kidneys?

5. Would it be equitable to prohibit the poor from selling their kidneys in a free market that otherwise permitted the sale of kidneys?

Notes

1. Under the current system, kidneys are distributed primarily to patients considered to be compatible for that kidney and those in the local area who have been waiting the longest. If there are no good matches for the kidney locally, then the search for a compatible patient expands regionally and then nationally.

2. The following is a rough calculation of Medicare's five-year savings: $93,200 is the annual cost of kidney dialysis, and $272,300 is the one-time cost of a kidney transplant (the annual cost of $18,900 for immunosuppressive drugs is included in the $272,300). According to the United Network for Organ Sharing, about 107,000 patients are currently waiting for kidney transplants. Assuming that these patients receive a kidney transplant this year, Medicare costs over a five-year period will equal ($272,300 × 107,000 + 4 × $18,900 × 107,000) = $37,225,300,000 (or $37.2 billion). However, if these patients use dialysis for the next five years, Medicare would spend 107,000 × $93,200 × 5 = $49,862,000,000 (or $ 49.9 billion). Therefore, if all of the patients on dialysis who are waiting for a transplant could receive a kidney, the federal government would save $49.9 billion – $37.2 billion = $12.7 billion over a five-year period. Data on the annual cost of kidney dialysis come from USRDS (2014), and data on the average cost of kidney transplants are from Bentley and Hanson (2011, Table 2). The 2011 annual cost estimates in these sources were updated to 2013 dollar costs.

3. Using an experimental game, a study found that giving priority on waiting lists to those who previously registered as organ donors (if they were to die) increased the numbers of registered donors (Kessler and Roth 2012).

4. Australia started a two-year experimental trial (to be reviewed in 2015) to compensate living kidney donors as a means of reducing the gap between the number of kidney donors and the number of recipients. Donors will be offered up to six weeks of paid leave.

Additional Readings

Becker, G., and J. Elias. 2007. "Introducing Incentives in the Market for Live and Cadaveric Organ Donations." *Journal of Economic Perspectives* 21 (3): 3–24.

Howard, D. 2007. "Producing Organ Donors." *Journal of Economic Perspectives* 21 (3): 25–36.

References

Abadie, A., and S. Gay. 2006. "The Impact of Presumed Consent Legislation on Cadaveric Organ Donation: A Cross-Country Study." *Journal of Health Economics* 25 (4): 599–620.

Bentley, T. S., and S. G. Hanson. 2011. *2011 U.S. Organ and Tissue Transplant Cost Estimate and Discussion*. Milliman Research Report. Published April. http://us.milliman.com/uploadedFiles/insight/research/health-rr/2011-us-organ-tissue.pdf.

Cohen, I. 2005. "Directions for the Disposition of My (and Your) Vital Organs." *Regulation* 28 (3): 32–38.

Dunham, C. 2008. "'Body Property': Challenging the Ethical Barriers in Organ Transplantation to Protect Individual Autonomy." *Annals of Health Law* 17 (1): 39–65.

Epstein, R. 2006. "Kidney Beancounters." *Wall Street Journal*, May 15, p. 15.

Goldberg, D., S. Halpern, and P. Reese. 2013. "Deceased Organ Donation Consent Rates Among Racial and Ethnic Minorities and Older Potential Donors." *Critical Care Medicine* 41 (2): 496–505.

Kessler, J., and A. Roth. 2012. "Organ Allocation Policy and the Decision to Donate." *American Economic Review* 102 (5): 2018–47.

Organ Procurement and Transplantation Network (OPTN). n.d. "Data Reports." Accessed March 2014. http://optn.transplant.hrsa.gov/latestData/viewDataReports.asp.

Roth, A., T. Sonmez, and M. Unver. 2005. "A Kidney Exchange Clearing House in New England." *American Economic Review* 95 (2): 376–80.

Satel, S., and A. Viard. 2013. "Don't Ban Compensation for Bone-Marrow Donors." American Enterprise Institute. Posted December 2. www.aei.org/

article/health/comment-on-rin-0906-ab02/?utm_source=today&utm_
medium=paramount&utm_campaign=120313.

United States Renal Data System (USRDS). 2014. "Costs of End Stage Renal
Disease." In *2013 USRDS Annual Data Report,* volume 2. www.usrds
.org/2013/pdf/v2_ch11_13.pdf.

THE ROLE OF GOVERNMENT IN MEDICAL CARE

30

Government intervention in the financing and delivery of medical services is pervasive. On the financing side, the Affordable Care Act (ACA) provides subsidies and tax credits to individuals, small businesses, and low-income employees, and employers are required to provide health insurance benefits to their employees. Further, hospital and physician services for the aged are subsidized (Medicare), and a separate payroll tax pays for those subsidies; Medicaid, a federal/state matching program, pays for medical services for the poor and near-poor; a large network of state and county hospitals is in place; health professional schools are subsidized; loan programs for students in the health professions are guaranteed by the government; employer-paid health insurance is excluded from taxable income; military members, retirees, and their families have access to a separate healthcare program called TRICARE; and medical research is subsidized. These programs and others make government a greater than 50 percent partner in total health expenditures.

In addition to these financing programs, extensive government regulations influence the financing and delivery of medical services. For example, state licensing boards determine the criteria for entry into the different professions, and practice regulations determine which tasks can be performed by various professional groups. In some states, hospital investment is subject to state review, hospital and physician prices under Medicare are regulated, health insurance companies are regulated by the states, and each state mandates what benefits (e.g., in Minnesota, hair transplants) and which providers (e.g., in Washington, naturopaths) should be included in health insurance sold in that state (Bunce 2013).

The role of government in the financing and delivery of medical services (and through federal and state regulations) is extensive. To understand the reasons for these different types of government intervention and at times seemingly contradictory policies, it is necessary to understand the two theories that underlie the government's objectives.

Public-Interest Theory of Government

The public-interest, or traditional, theory of government can be classified according to its policy objectives and the policy instruments used to achieve those objectives. The policy objectives of government in the healthcare field are twofold: (1) to redistribute medical resources to those least able to purchase medical services and (2) to improve the economic efficiency by which medical services are purchased and delivered. These traditional objectives of government—redistribution and economic efficiency (also referred to as *market failure*)—can be achieved by using one or more of the following policy instruments: expenditure, taxation, and regulation. (Government provision of services, such as Veterans Administration hospitals, is rarely proposed as a policy instrument in the United States.)

These policy instruments—expenditure, taxation, and regulation—can be applied to either the purchaser (demand) side or the supplier (provider) side of the market. For example, expenditure policies on the demand side are Medicare and Medicaid, and on the supply side are subsidies for hospital construction and health manpower training programs. Taxation policies on the demand side cover tax-exempt employer-paid health insurance and on the supply side are tax-exempt bonds for nonprofit hospitals. Regulation policies on the demand side contain the individual mandate to buy health insurance and on the supply side are licensing requirements, restrictions on the tasks different health professionals can perform, entry barriers to building a hospital or a new hospice in a region, and regulated provider prices for hospitals and physicians under Medicare.

These policy objectives and instruments—which can be used to classify each type of government health policy according to policy objectives, the type of policy instrument used, and whether the policy instrument is directed toward the demand or supply side of the market—are shown in Exhibit 30.1. According to the public-interest theory, each policy should easily be categorized as achieving one of the two government objectives.

Redistribution

Redistribution causes a change in wealth. According to the public-interest theory of government, society makes a value judgment that medical services should be provided to those with low income and should be financed by taxing those with high income. Redistributive programs typically lower the cost of services to a particular group by enabling members of that group to purchase those services at below-market prices. These benefits are financed by imposing a cost on some other group. Two large redistributive programs are Medicare for the aged and Medicaid for the medically indigent. The benefits

	Government Objectives	
Government Policy and Instruments	**Redistribution**	**Efficiency Improvement**
Expenditure { Demand side / Supply side		
Taxation (+/–) { Demand side / Supply side		
Regulation { Demand side / Supply side		

EXHIBIT 30.1
Health Policy Objectives and Interventions

and costs of any redistributive medical program, such as Medicaid, should have the effects shown in Exhibit 30.2.

Efficiency Improvement

The second traditional objective of government is to improve the efficiency with which society allocates resources. Inefficiency in resource allocation can occur, for example, when firms in a market have monopoly power or when externalities exist. A firm has monopoly power when it is able to charge a price that exceeds its cost by more than a normal profit. Monopoly is inefficient because it produces too small a level of service (output). The additional benefit to purchasers from consuming a service (as indicated by its price) is greater than the cost of producing that benefit; therefore, more resources should flow into that industry until the additional benefit equals the additional cost of producing it.

There exist several bases of monopoly power: (1) The market may have only one firm, as with a natural monopoly such as an electric company; (2) barriers to entry into a market may exist; (3) firms may collude on raising their prices; and (4) a lack of information may mean consumers are unable to judge the differences in price, quality, and service among suppliers. In each of these situations, the prices charged will exceed the costs of producing the product (which includes a normal profit). The appropriate

	Low Income	High Income
Benefits	x	
Costs		x

EXHIBIT 30.2
Determining the Redistributive Effects of Government Programs

government remedy for decreasing monopoly power is to eliminate barriers to entry into a market, prevent price collusion, and improve information among consumers.

The other situation in which the allocation of resources can be improved is when externalities occur—that is, when someone undertakes an action and in so doing affects others who are not part of that transaction. The effects on others could be positive or negative. For example, a utility company using high-sulfur coal to produce electricity also produces air pollution. As a result of the air pollution, residents in surrounding communities may have a higher-than-average incidence of respiratory illness. Resources are misallocated because the cost of producing electricity excludes the costs imposed on others. As a result, too much electricity is being generated. If the costs of electricity production also include the costs imposed on others, the price of electricity would be higher and its demand lower. The allocation of resources would be improved if the utility's costs include production and external costs. The appropriate role of government in such a situation is to determine the costs imposed on others and to tax the utility company an equivalent amount. (This subject is discussed more completely in Chapter 31.)

According to the public-interest theory, if a policy does not have redistribution as its objective then its goal should be to achieve greater economic efficiency.

Economic Theory of Regulation

Dissatisfaction with the public-interest theory occurred for several reasons. Instead of simply regulating natural monopolies, government has also regulated competitive industries (such as airlines, trucks, and taxicabs) as well as various professions. Further, unregulated firms always want to enter regulated markets. To prevent entry into regulated industries, the government establishes entry barriers. If the government supposedly reduces prices in regulated markets—hence the firm's profitability—why should firms seek to enter a regulated industry?

To reconcile these apparent contradictions with the public-interest theory of government, an alternative theory of government behavior—the economic theory of regulation—was developed (Stigler 1971). (For a more complete discussion of this theory and its applicability to the healthcare field see Feldstein [2006].) The basic assumption underlying the economic theory is that political markets are no different from economic markets; individuals and firms seek to further their self-interest. Firms undertake investments in private markets to achieve a high rate of return. Why would the same firms not invest in legislation if it also offered a high rate of return? Organized groups are willing to pay a price for legislative benefits. This price is political support, which brings together the suppliers and demanders of legislative benefits.

The Suppliers: Legislators

The suppliers of legislative benefits are legislators, and their assumed goal is to maximize their chances for reelection. As the late Senator Everett Dirksen said, "The first law of politics is to get elected; the second law is to be reelected." To be reelected requires political support, which consists of campaign contributions, votes, and volunteer time. Legislators are assumed to be rational—that is, to make cost–benefit calculations when faced with demands for legislation. However, the legislator's cost–benefit calculations are not the costs and benefits to society of enacting particular legislation. Instead, the benefits are the additional political support the legislator would receive from supporting the legislation, and the costs are the lost political support she would incur as a result of her actions. When the benefits to the legislators exceed their costs, they will support the legislation.

The Demanders: Those with a Concentrated Interest

Those who have a concentrated interest—that is, those on whose profitability the legislation will have a large effect by affecting their revenues or costs—are more likely to be successful in the legislative marketplace. It becomes worthwhile for the group to incur the costs to organize, represent its interests before legislators, and raise political support to achieve the profits favorable legislation can provide. For this reason, only those with a concentrated interest will demand legislative benefits.

Diffuse Costs

When legislative benefits are provided to one group, others must bear those costs. When only one group has a concentrated interest in the legislation, that group is more likely to be successful if the costs to finance those benefits are not obvious and can be spread over a large number of people. When this occurs, the costs are said to be diffuse. For example, assume there are ten firms in an industry, and if they can have legislation enacted that limits imports that compete with their products, they will be able to raise their prices and thereby receive $300 million in legislative benefits. These firms have a concentrated interest ($300 million) in trying to enact such legislation. The costs of these legislative benefits are financed by a small increase in the price of the product amounting to $1 per person.

Often, the fact that legislation raises their costs is not obvious to consumers. Further, even if consumers were aware of the legislation's effect, it would not be worthwhile for them to organize and represent their interests to forestall a price increase that will decrease their income by $1 a year. The costs of trying to prevent the cost increase would exceed their potential savings.

It is easier (less costly) for providers than for consumers to organize, provide political support, and impose a diffuse cost on others. For this reason, much legislation has affected entry into the health professions, which tasks are reserved to certain professions, how (and which) providers are paid under public medical programs, why subsidies for medical education are given to schools and not students (otherwise schools would have to compete for students), and so on. Most health issues have been relatively technical, such as the training of health professionals, certification of their quality, methods of payment, controls on hospital capital investment, and so on. The higher medical prices resulting from regulations that benefit physicians, for example, by successfully placing limits on nurses' scope of practice, have been diffuse and not visible to consumers.

Entry Barriers to Regulated Markets

The economic theory of regulation provides an explanation for these dissatisfactions with the public-interest theory. Firms in competitive markets seek regulation to earn higher profits than are available without regulation. Prices in regulated markets (such as interstate air travel) were always higher than in unregulated markets (such as intrastate air travel), enabling regulated firms to earn greater profits. These higher prices gave unregulated firms an incentive to try to enter regulated markets. Government, on behalf of the regulated industry, imposed entry barriers to keep out low-priced competitors. Otherwise, the regulated firms could not earn more than a competitive rate of return.

Through legislation, firms try to receive the monopoly profits they are unable to achieve through market competition.

Opposing Concentrated Interests

When only one group has a concentrated interest in the outcome of legislation and the costs are diffuse, legislators will respond to the political support the group is willing to pay to have favorable legislation enacted. When there are opposing groups, each with a concentrated interest in the outcome, legislators are likely to reach a compromise between the competing demanders of legislative benefits. Rather than balancing the gain in political support from one group against the loss from the other, legislators prefer to receive political support from both groups and impose diffuse costs on those offering little political support.

Visible Redistributive Effects

When the beneficiaries are specific population groups, such as the aged, the redistributive effects of legislation are meant to be very visible. An example of this is Medicare. By making clear which population groups will benefit, legislators hope to receive their political support. The costs (taxes) of financing such visible redistributive programs, however, are still designed to be diffuse so as not to generate political opposition from others.

A small, diffuse tax imposed on many people, such as a sales or a payroll tax, is the only way large sums of money to finance visible redistributive programs can be raised with little opposition. These taxes are regressive; the tax represents a greater portion of income from low-income employees and consumers. Economists have determined that payroll taxes, even when imposed on the employer, are borne mostly by the employee. (The employer is only interested in the total cost of an employee; thus, the employee eventually receives a lower wage than if those costs were not imposed.) By imposing part of the tax on the employer, however, employees appear to be paying a smaller portion of it than they really are. The remainder of the tax is shifted forward to consumers in the form of higher prices for the goods and services they purchase, which is also regressive.

Medicare: A Case Study of the Success of Concentrated Interests

The concentrated interests of medical providers and the subsequent diffuse (small) costs imposed on consumers explain much of the legislative history of the financing and delivery of medical services until the early 1960s. The enactment and design of Medicare illustrates the real purpose of visible redistribution policy: to redistribute wealth—that is, increase benefits to politically powerful groups without their paying the full costs of those benefits by shifting the costs to the less politically powerful.

Throughout the 1950s and early 1960s, the American Federation of Labor–Congress of Industrial Organizations (AFL–CIO) unions had a concentrated interest in their retirees' medical costs that placed them in opposition to the American Medical Association (AMA). Employers had not prefunded union retirees' medical costs but instead paid them as part of current labor expenses. If union retirees' medical expenses could be shifted away from the employer, those funds would be available to be paid as higher wages to union employees.

To ensure that their union retirees would be eligible for Medicare, AFL–CIO insisted that eligibility be based on those who had paid into the Social Security system while they were working and that the new Medicare program (hospital services) be financed by a separate Medicare payroll tax to be included as part of the Social Security tax. Although the current retirees had not contributed to the proposed Medicare program, they were to become immediately eligible because they had paid Social Security taxes. The use of the Social Security system to determine eligibility became the central issue in the debate over Medicare (Feldstein 2006).

The AMA was willing to have government assistance go to those unable to afford medical services, which would have increased the demand for physicians. Thus, the AMA favored a means-tested program funded by general tax revenues because it was concerned that including the non-poor in the new program would merely substitute government payment for private payment. The AMA believed such a program would cost too much, leading to controls on hospital and physician fees.

With the landslide victory of President Johnson in 1964, AFL–CIO achieved their objective. Once Social Security financing was used to determine eligibility for Medicare, Medicare Part B (physician services) was added, financed by general tax revenues. Although AFL–CIO won on the financing mechanism, Congress acceded to the demands of the AMA (as well as the American Hospital Association) on all other aspects of the legislation. The system of payment to hospitals and physicians promoted inefficiency (cost-plus payments to hospitals), and restrictions limiting competition were placed on alternative delivery systems.

This historic conflict between opposing concentrated interests in medical care left both sides victorious and illustrates how the power of government can be used to benefit politically important groups. As a result of Medicare, a massive redistribution of wealth occurred in society. The beneficiaries were the aged, union members, and medical providers, and the benefits were financed by a diffuse, regressive tax (the Medicare payroll tax) on a large group—the working population, who also paid higher prices for their medical services and more income taxes to finance Medicare Part B. Medicare was designed to be both inefficient and inequitable simply because it was in the economic interests of those with concentrated interests.

Medicaid and Medicare

Differences in the sources of political support are important for understanding the two main redistributive programs in the United States. Medicaid is a means-tested program for the poor funded from general tax revenues. Because the poor (who have low voting-participation rates) are unable to provide legislators with political support, the support for Medicaid comes from the middle class (who must agree to higher taxes to provide the poor with medical benefits). The inadequacy of Medicaid in every state, the conditions necessary for achieving Medicaid eligibility, the low levels of eligibility, and beneficiaries' lack of access to medical providers are related to the generosity (or lack thereof) of the middle class. The beneficiaries of Medicare, on the other hand, are the elderly (who generally have the highest voting-participation rate of any age group). The aged, together with their adult children, provide the political support for the program. As the cost of Medicare has risen, government has raised the Medicare payroll tax and lowered payments to providers rather than reduce benefits or beneficiaries from this politically powerful group.[1]

The political necessity of keeping costs diffuse explains why Medicare and producer regulation were financed using regressive taxes—either payroll taxes or higher prices for medical services. Spreading the costs over large populations keeps those costs diffuse, with the net effect that low-income people pay the costs and high-income people (such as physicians or well-to-do elderly) receive the benefits. Those receiving the benefits and those bearing the costs, according to the economic theory, are not based on income (see Exhibit 30.2) but rather on which groups are able to offer political support (the beneficiaries) and which groups are unable to do so (they bear the costs). Regressive taxes are typically used to finance producer regulation and to provide benefits to specific population groups.

Changes in Health Policies

Health policies change over time because groups who previously bore a diffuse cost develop a concentrated interest. Until the 1960s, medical societies were the main group with a concentrated interest in the financing and delivery of medical services. Thus, the delivery system was structured to benefit physicians. The physician-to-population ratio remained constant for 15 years (until the mid-1960s) at 141 per 100,000 (see Exhibit 4.1), state restrictions were imposed on health maintenance organizations (HMOs) to limit their development, advertising was prohibited, and restrictions were placed on other health professionals to limit their ability to compete with physicians. Financing mechanisms also benefited physicians; until the 1980s, capitation payment for HMOs was prohibited under Medicare and Medicaid, and competitors to physicians were excluded from reimbursement under public and private insurance systems.

As the costs of medical care continued to increase rapidly for government and employers, their previously diffuse costs became concentrated. Under Medicare, the government was faced with the choice of raising taxes or reducing benefits to the aged, both of which would have cost the presidential administration political support. Successive administrations developed a concentrated interest in lowering the rate of increase in medical expenditures. Similarly, large employers were concerned that rising medical costs were making them less competitive internationally. The pressures for cost containment increased as the costs of an inefficient delivery and payment system grew larger. Rising medical expenditures are no longer a diffuse cost to large purchasers of medical services.

Other professional organizations—such as the respective associations for psychologists, chiropractors, podiatrists, nurse practitioners, and nurse anesthetists—saw the potentially greater revenues their members could receive if they were better able to compete with physicians. These groups developed a concentrated interest in securing payment for their members under public and private insurance systems and expanding their scope of practice. The increase in opposing concentrated interests weakened the political influence of organized medicine.

Summary

The public-interest theory of government and economic theory of regulation provide opposing predictions of the redistributive and efficiency effects of government legislation, as shown in Exhibit 30.3. To determine which of these contrasting theories is a more accurate description of government, we must match the actual outcomes of legislation to each theory's predictions. Do the benefits of redistributive programs go to those with low income, and are they financed by taxes that impose a larger burden on those with higher income? Does the government try to improve the allocation of resources by reducing barriers to entry and, in markets where information is limited, by monitoring the quality of physicians and other medical services and making this information available?

EXHIBIT 30.3
Health Policy
Objectives
Under Different
Theories of
Government

Theories of Government	Objective of Government	
	Redistribution	**Efficiency Improvement**
Public-interest theory	Assist those with low income	Remove (and prevent) monopoly abuses and protect environment (externalities)
Economic theory of regulation	Provide benefits to those able to deliver political support and finance from those having little political support	Efficiency objective unimportant More likely to protect industries so as to provide them with redistributive benefits

The economic theory of regulation provides a better explanation (than other theories do) of why health policies are enacted and why they have changed over time. An indication of the inadequacy of the public-interest theory is the difficulty of placing demand-side and supply-side policies for each of the three policy instruments—expenditure, taxation, and regulation (described in Exhibit 30.1)—into a redistribution or efficiency improvement objective. The economic theory predicts that government is not concerned with efficiency issues. Redistribution is the main objective of government, but that objective is to redistribute wealth to those who are able to offer political support from those who are unable to do so. Thus, medical licensing boards are inadequately staffed, have never required reexamination for relicensure, and have failed to monitor practicing physicians because organized medicine has been opposed to any approaches for increasing quality that would adversely affect physicians' income. Regressive taxes are used to finance programs, such as Medicare and the ACA's employer mandate, not because legislators are unaware of their regressive nature but because the taxes are designed to be diffuse and not obvious to those with low income (who actually bear the burden of the benefits provided to those who have a concentrated interest).

The structure and financing of medical services is rational; the participants act according to their calculations of costs and benefits. Viewed in its entirety, however, health policy is uncoordinated and seemingly contradictory. Health policies are inequitable and inefficient; low-income persons end up subsidizing those with higher income. These results, however, are the consequences of a rational system. The outcomes were the result of policies intended by the legislators.

Discussion Questions

1. What were the dissatisfactions with the public-interest theory of government?
2. Contrast the benefit–cost calculations of legislators under the public-interest theory of government and the economic theory of regulation.
3. Why are concentrated interests and diffuse costs important in predicting legislative outcomes?
4. Contrast the predictions of the public-interest and economic theories regarding redistributive policies.
5. Evaluate the following policies according to the two differing theories:
   a. Medicare and Medicaid beneficiaries, taxation, and generosity of benefits
   b. The performance of state licensing boards in monitoring physician quality

Note

1. The political support offered by providers, such as hospitals and physicians, is important in determining how such redistributive legislation is designed. Providers benefit because such programs increase demand by those with low income. However, medical societies have opposed government coverage of entire population groups (such as the aged) regardless of income level because government payment would merely substitute for private payment for those who are not poor. Physicians were concerned that if government covered everyone or all of the aged, regardless of income, the cost of such programs would rise and the government would eventually control physician fees. This was the AMA's basic reason for opposing Medicare. To gain the political support of physicians, Congress acceded to physicians' preferences when Medicare was established by permitting physicians to decide whether or not to accept the government payment for treating Medicare patients. Medicaid was not controversial because it covered those with low income, and hospitals and physicians were paid according to their preferences. As the federal and state governments experienced large expenditure increases under each of these programs, government developed a concentrated interest in controlling hospital and medical spending.

References

Bunce, V. 2013. *Health Insurance Mandates in the States 2012.* Alexandria, VA: The Council for Affordable Health Insurance.

Feldstein, P. J. 2006. *The Politics of Health Legislation: An Economic Perspective,* 3rd ed. Chicago: Health Administration Press.

Stigler, G. J. 1971. "The Theory of Economic Regulation." *Bell Journal of Economics* 2 (1): 3–21.

MEDICAL RESEARCH, MEDICAL EDUCATION, ALCOHOL CONSUMPTION, AND POLLUTION: WHO SHOULD PAY?

A n important role of government is to improve the way markets allocate resources. When markets perform poorly, fewer goods and services are produced, and incomes are lower than they would be otherwise. The usual policy prescription for improving the performance of markets is for the government to eliminate barriers to entry and increase information. Competitive markets, in which no entry barriers are in place and purchasers and producers are fully informed, are likely to produce the correct (or optimal) rate of output. The correct rate occurs if individuals benefiting from the service pay the full cost of producing that service.

Resources are optimally allocated when the additional benefits from consuming the last unit equal the cost of producing that last unit. When still more units are consumed, the costs of those additional units exceed the benefits provided, and the resources would be better used to produce other goods and services whose benefits exceed their costs. As shown in Exhibit 31.1, when the costs are C_1 and benefits are B_1, the correct rate of output is Q_1.

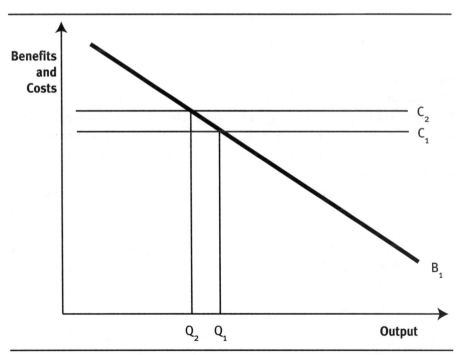

EXHIBIT 31.1
Optimal Rate of Output

The benefit curve is declining because the more one has of a good, the lower the value of an additional unit will be.

Under certain circumstances, however, even a competitive market may not allocate resources correctly. The optimal rate of output in a market occurs when *all* costs and benefits are included. Private decision makers consider only their *own* costs and benefits and exclude the costs or benefits imposed on others, if any. The effect may be that some services are underproduced, while others are overproduced.

The quantity of medical and health services may not be optimal because costs and benefits may be imposed on persons other than those who purchase and provide the service. What happens when costs or benefits are imposed on someone who is not a voluntary participant in that private transaction? Such external costs and benefits must be included; otherwise, either too much or too little of the service is produced and purchased. For example, when external costs are imposed on others, as shown by C_2 in Exhibit 31.1, the correct rate of output declines from Q_1 to Q_2, where both private (C_1) and external (C_2) costs equal the benefits (B_1) from consuming that good or service.

When such external costs or benefits exist, government should calculate their magnitude and use subsidies and taxes to achieve the "right" rate of output in the affected industry. Subsidies or taxes on the producers in that industry will change the costs of producing a service so that producers will adjust their levels of output. The difference between C_1 and C_2, the external cost, is also the size of the tax to be imposed on each unit of the product.

External Costs and Benefits

Pollution

One reason externalities, such as pollution, occur is that no one owns the resource being exploited. When a resource such as air or water is scarce and no one owns it, a firm may use it as though it were free; it does not become a cost of production as it would if the firm were charged a fee for its use. The lack of property rights over scarce resources is the basis for government intervention. For example, when a firm pollutes a stream in the process of producing its product, those who use the stream for recreational purposes are adversely affected; they bear a cost not included in the firm's calculation of its costs of producing the product. Because the firm has not had to include the external costs of production, it sells the product at a lower price, and the user pays less for that product than the product actually costs society. Because of its lower price, a greater quantity of the product is purchased and produced.

When no property rights over a scarce resource exist and that resource is used by large numbers of people and firms, negotiations among the parties over the use of that resource are likely to be difficult and costly. Government intervention is needed to calculate the external costs and, in the case of pollution, to impose a tax based on the proportional amount of pollution caused on each unit of the product sold. The product's higher price would include both the cost of production and the unit tax; therefore, less of the product would be sold. If all costs and benefits—both private and external—are part of the private decision-making process, the industry will produce the right rate of output.

A pollution tax could not be expected to eliminate all pollution, but it would reduce it to the correct level; the tax revenues received by the government would go toward cleaning up the pollution or compensating those who were adversely affected. If the government attempted to eliminate all of the pollution, it would have to stop production of that product completely. Eliminating all pollution could adversely affect a great many people if the total benefits derived from that product outweigh its costs, including the costs of pollution. Consider, for example, the effect of eliminating all air pollution originating from automobiles or electricity production. Clearly, people prefer some quantity of these products to zero air pollution, which means determining the correct amount of air pollution.

Imposing a tax on pollution has another important consequence. The producer of the product will attempt to lower the tax by devising methods to reduce pollution.[1] The firm may move to an area where the costs of pollution (hence the tax) are lower, or the firm may innovate in its production process to reduce pollution. The tax creates incentives for producers to lower their production costs, which include the tax.

Imposing a tax directly on pollution is preferable to such indirect methods of controlling pollution as allowing existing firms to continue polluting but not permitting others to enter the market or mandating that all firms use a particular production process to reduce pollution. Such indirect approaches eliminate incentives for producers to search for cheaper ways to reduce pollution.

Based on the example of the external costs of pollution, the role of government seems straightforward: When widespread external costs exist, the government should calculate the size of those costs and assess a tax on each unit of output produced. The purchasers and producers of that product will base their decisions about how much to purchase on all of the costs and benefits (external as well as private) of that product.

Medical Research

The analysis is similar when applied to external benefits. If a university medical researcher develops a new method of performing open-heart surgery that reduces the mortality rate of that procedure, other surgeons will copy the technique to benefit their own patients. An individual researcher/surgeon cannot declare ownership over all possible uses of that technique. However, if the university medical researcher were not compensated for all those who would eventually benefit, she would not find it feasible or worthwhile to invest time and resources to develop new medical techniques.

Similarly, if medical researchers were not properly compensated in some fashion, they would underproduce the discovery of basic scientific knowledge, because they presumably would not be able to charge all those who would eventually benefit from their research. Although it would be difficult, the government should attempt to calculate the potential benefits and subsidize medical research. Unless the external benefits are assessed and the costs are shared by potential beneficiaries, the costs of producing medical research will exceed the private benefits.

An alternative to offering a subsidy to private firms is to give them property rights or ownership over their discoveries in the form of patent protection. Drug companies need incentives to compensate them for the risks and investments made in research and development. Patent protection, however, is not possible for all basic research or for new surgical techniques. Unpatented medical research or new drug discoveries can be copied by others who then benefit from the discoveries.

Immunization

Another example of external benefits involves protection from contagious diseases. Individuals who decide to be immunized against contagious diseases primarily base their decisions on the costs and benefits to themselves of immunization. However, those who are not immunized also benefit by receiving a "free ride"; their chances of catching that disease are lowered. If immunization were solely a private decision, not enough individuals would be immunized. The costs incurred by those who chose to be immunized should be subsidized by imposing a small tax on those who are not immunized but who also benefit. In this manner, the "right" numbers of people become immunized. The immunization decision thus encompasses private benefits, external benefits, and the costs of immunization.

When transaction costs are high—that is, the administrative costs of monitoring, collecting taxes, and subsidizing individuals are substantial—it may be less costly to simply require everyone to be immunized against certain diseases.

Subsidies to the Medically Indigent

Externalities are also the rationale for providing subsidies to the medically indigent. If the only way the poor receive medical care were through voluntary contributions, many people who did not make such contributions would benefit by knowing that the poor were cared for through the contributions of others. Too little would be provided to the medically indigent because those who did not contribute receive a free ride; they would benefit without having to pay for that benefit. Government intervention would be appropriate to tax those who benefit by knowing the poor receive medical care.

Government Policies When Externalities Exist

In the examples described, the subsidies and taxes are related to the size of the external benefits and costs. Furthermore, the taxes imposed on products that pollute are to be spent for the benefit of those adversely affected. When external benefits exist, the subsidies are financed by taxes on those who receive the external benefit. Patents are an attempt to recover the external benefits of research. In each case, taxes and subsidies are matched according to external costs and benefits.

Recognizing how externalities affect the correct rate of output in an industry is useful for understanding which government policies would be appropriate in a number of additional areas. For example, when a motorcyclist has an accident and suffers a head injury as a result of not wearing a helmet, government (society) pays the medical expenses if the cyclist does not have insurance or sufficient personal funds. Fines for not wearing helmets are an attempt to make motorcyclists bear the responsibility for external costs that they would otherwise impose on others. At times, imposing requirements (e.g., helmet use, immunizations, grade school education) may be the least costly approach for achieving the correct output.

The same analogy can be used to describe those who can afford to buy health insurance but refuse to do so. When they incur catastrophic medical expenses they cannot pay for, they become a burden on society. Requiring everyone who can afford it to have catastrophic medical coverage is a way of preventing individuals from imposing external costs on others.[2]

Similarly, drunk drivers frequently impose costs on innocent victims. Penalties—such as jail terms, forfeiture of driver's licenses, fines, and higher alcohol taxes—have been used as attempts to shift the responsibility for these external costs back to those who drink and drive. One study concluded that federal and state alcohol taxes should be increased (from an average of 11 cents to 24 cents a drink) to compensate for the external costs imposed on others by excessive drinkers (Manning et al. 1989).

We should be aware, however, that some people might misapply the externalities argument to justify intervention by the government in all markets. For example, if you admire someone's garden, should you be taxed to subsidize the gardener? Should the student who asks a particularly clever question in class be subsidized by a tax on other students? These examples, although simple, illustrate several important points about externalities. First, when only a few individuals are involved, the parties concerned should be able to reach an accommodation among themselves without resorting to government intervention. Second, even when ownership to the property is clear, high transaction costs may make it too costly to charge for external benefits or costs. The owner of the garden can decide whether it is worthwhile to erect a fence and charge a viewing fee. Chances are the cost of doing so will exceed the amount others are willing to pay. Many may thus receive external benefits simply because excluding them or collecting from them is too costly. Only when the external benefits (or costs) become sufficiently large relative to their transaction costs does it pay for the provider of external benefits to either exclude others or charge them for their benefits.

Another point these examples illustrate concerns the relative size of private benefits compared with external benefits. Would the output of the gardener be too small if neighbors did not contribute? Although many goods and services provide external benefits to others, excluding these external benefits does not result in too small a rate of output. In markets in which the external benefits are sufficiently small relative to the total private benefits, excluding external benefits does not affect the optimal rate of output. This type of externality, referred to as an *inframarginal* externality, occurs within the market. Thus, gardeners may receive so much pleasure from their gardens that they put forth the same level of effort with or without their neighbors' financial contribution.

The concept of inframarginal benefit is important to understanding the issue of financing education for health professionals. We all benefit from knowing that we have access to physicians, dentists, and nurses if we become ill. However, if their educations were not subsidized, would too few physicians be available? The education of physicians is heavily subsidized. The average four-year subsidy for a medical education exceeds $500,000. One reason this cost is so high is that medical schools have little incentive for reducing those costs. Given the continual excess demand for a medical education, large subsidies that go to the school rather than directly to prospective medical students, and entry barriers established by the accrediting commission, nonprofit medical schools have little incentive to be efficient or innovative. This would change if medical schools had to compete for students who bore more of the cost themselves. For example, some medical educators claim that medical students could be admitted to medical school after two years of college, medical education could be reduced by at least one year, the residency period could be shortened, and innovations in teaching methods and curricula could reduce the cost still more.

Even if physicians had to pay their entire educational costs themselves, however, the economic return on the costs of becoming a physician has been estimated to be sufficiently attractive that we would have had no less than the current number of physicians. Over time, these economic returns on a medical (or dental) education have changed and varied according to specialty status; returns were higher in the 1950s to 1970s than they are currently. Thus, the concept of external benefits in the number of physicians is more likely a case of inframarginal benefits; sufficient private benefits to individuals from becoming a physician would ensure a sufficient supply of physicians even if no subsidies were provided.

A separate issue is whether low-income individuals could afford a medical education if subsidies were removed. Yet making medical and dental education affordable to all qualified individuals could be accomplished more efficiently by targeting subsidies and loan programs to those who need them than by equally subsidizing everyone who attends medical school regardless of income level. The rationale for large educational subsidies for a health professional education should be reexamined.

Divergence Between Theoretical and Actual Government Policy

Correcting for external costs and benefits creates winners and losers. Taxes and subsidies have redistributive effects; taxpayers have lower income, whereas subsidy recipients have higher income. Every group affected by external costs and benefits desires favorable treatment and has incentives to influence government policy. For example, an industry that pollutes the air and water has a concentrated interest in forestalling government policy that would increase its production costs. All who benefit from environmental protection must organize and provide legislators with political support if anything more than symbolic legislation is to be directed at imposing external costs on those who pollute. The growth of the environmental movement was an attempt to offset the imbalance between those with concentrated interests (polluters) and those bearing the diffuse costs (the public).

The Clean Air Act (1977 amendments) illustrates the divergence between the theoretical approach for resolving external costs and the real-world phenomenon of concentrated and diffuse interests. A greater amount of air pollution is caused when electric utilities burn high-sulfur coal rather than low-sulfur coal. Imposing a tax on the amount of sulfur dioxides (air pollution) emitted would shift the external costs of air pollution to the electric utilities, which would then have an incentive to search for ways to reduce this tax and consequently the amount of air pollution. One alternative would be for the utilities to switch to low-sulfur coal.

Low-sulfur coal, however, is produced only in the West (of the United States); furthermore, it is less expensive to mine low-sulfur coal than high-sulfur coal. Low-sulfur coal is therefore a competitive threat to the Eastern coal interests that produce high-sulfur coal. Faced with taxes based on the amount of air pollution emitted, Midwestern and Eastern utilities would find it less expensive to pay added transportation costs to have low-sulfur coal shipped from the West. However, the concentrated interests of the Eastern coal mines, their heavily unionized employees, and the Senate majority leader at that time (who was from West Virginia, which would have been adversely affected) were able to have legislation enacted that was directed toward the *process* of reducing pollution rather than the *amount* of pollution emitted.

Requiring utilities to merely use specified technology for reducing pollution eliminated the utilities' incentives to use low-sulfur coal. When specific technology is mandated, the utility loses its incentive to maintain that technology in good operating condition and to search for more efficient approaches to reducing pollution. Western utilities that used low-sulfur coal bore the higher costs of using mandated technology, although they could have achieved the desired outcomes by less expensive means (Feldstein 2006).

Summary

Even if medical care markets were competitive, the "right" quantity of output might not occur because of external costs and benefits. With regard to personal medical services, externalities are likely to exist related to medical services for the poor and for those who can afford catastrophic medical insurance but refuse to buy it. Why should medical and dental education be so heavily subsidized? Any external benefits are likely to be inframarginal, thereby not affecting the optimal number of health professionals. Imposing taxes on personal behaviors (or products), such as excessive alcohol consumption, that may result in external costs will also serve as an incentive to reduce these external costs. Most externalities in healthcare in the United States derive from medical research, medical services for the poor, lack of catastrophic insurance for those who can afford it, alcohol consumption, and pollution.

Implicit in discussions of externalities is the assumption that government regulation can correct these failures of competitive markets. Politicians, however, may at times be even less responsive to correcting external costs and benefits than producers and consumers. When externalities occur, a theoretical framework for determining appropriate government policy provides a basis for evaluating alternative policies. The divergence between theoretical and actual policies can often be explained by a comparison of the amounts of political support offered by those with concentrated and diffuse interests.

Discussion Questions

1. What is the economist's definition of the correct, or optimal, rate of output?
2. Why do externalities, such as air and water pollution, occur?
3. Why do economists believe there can be an optimal amount of pollution? What would occur if all pollution were eliminated?
4. Explain the rationale for requiring everyone who can afford it to purchase catastrophic health insurance.
5. The number of medical school spaces in this country is limited. Would fewer people become physicians if government subsidies for medical education were reduced?

Notes

1. Another approach to reducing pollution that also provides incentives for polluters to search for the most efficient method of reducing pollution is to establish a market for pollution rights. The 1990 Clean Air Act Amendments established the first large-scale use of the tradable permit approach to pollution control. A market for transferable sulfur dioxide emission allowances among electric utilities was established. Along with a cap on annual emissions, electric utilities had an opportunity to trade rights to emit sulfur dioxide. Firms facing high abatement costs had an opportunity to purchase the right to emit pollution from firms with lower costs.
2. The ACA includes an individual mandate. The penalty tax for not buying health insurance is small—$95 in 2014 and increasing to $695

by 2016 and beyond (indexed for inflation). The tax might alternatively be calculated as a percentage of income—0.1 percent in 2014 and up to 2.5 percent of income in 2016. The maximum tax will be $2,085 in 2016. Because the cost of health insurance for a single person is likely to be $3,000 to $5,000 (increased mandatory benefits, the excise tax on health insurers shifted to enrollees, and age rating provisions will increase the premiums for those who are young), it is likely that many individuals will find it less expensive to pay the tax rather than buy insurance. Should they become ill they could immediately buy insurance (no preexisting exclusion can apply) and then drop their insurance once they recover. Under these circumstances, the ACA's individual mandate will not shift back to the free riders the external cost that is imposed on the insured by those who can afford to buy insurance but do not do so.

Additional Readings

Goulder, L. 2013. "Markets for Pollution Allowances: What Are the (New) Lessons?" *Journal of Economic Perspectives* 27 (1): 87–102.

Joskow, P., R. Schmalensee, and E. Bailey. 1998. "The Market for Sulfur Dioxide Emissions." *American Economic Review* 88 (4): 669–85.

References

Feldstein, P. J. 2006. "The Control of Externalities: Medical Research, Epidemics, and the Environment." In *The Politics of Health Legislation: An Economic Perspective*, 3rd ed. Chicago: Health Administration Press.

Manning, W., E. Keeler, J. Newhouse, E. Sloss, and J. Wasserman. 1989. "The Taxes of Sin: Do Smokers and Drinkers Pay Their Way?" *JAMA* 261 (11): 1604–09.

THE CANADIAN HEALTHCARE SYSTEM

32

The Canadian healthcare system, a single-payer system, has been suggested as a model for the United States. Starting in the late 1960s, the Canadian government established the basic guidelines for the system, and each province was provided with federal funds contingent on its adherence to them. Under these guidelines, everyone has access to hospital and medical services, and no one has to pay any deductibles or copayments. Patients have free choice of physician and hospital. Unlike the single-payer system in Great Britain, it is not possible to buy out of the system; private health insurance is not permitted for these basic hospital and medical services.

The basic cost-control mechanism used in Canada is expenditure limits on health providers. Each province sets its own overall health budget and negotiates a total budget, which it cannot exceed, with each hospital. The province also negotiates with the medical association to establish uniform fees for all physicians, who are paid on a fee-for-service basis and must accept the province's fee as payment in full for their services.[1] In some provinces, physicians' income is also subject to controls; once physicians' revenues exceed a certain level, further billings are paid at 25 percent of their fee schedule.

These cost-containment measures have limited the increase in Canadian health expenditures, although providers complain about their budgets and occasionally physicians go on strike. Because each province finances its services through an income tax, receives federal funds, and pays all medical bills, the need for insurance companies is eliminated. The province controls the adoption and financing of high-technology equipment.

According to its proponents, the Canadian system offers higher life expectancy, universal coverage, comprehensive hospital and medical benefits, no out-of-pocket expenses for hospital and medical services,[2] and lower administrative costs, while devoting a smaller percentage of the gross domestic product (GDP) to healthcare and spending less per capita than the United States. Would the United States be better off if it adopted the Canadian single-payer health system?

Comparing the Canadian System with the US System

Life Expectancy and Lower Infant Mortality Rate

Proponents of the Canadian system claim that for less money they can achieve better health outcomes than the US healthcare system can. Life expectancy at birth for Canadians is about five years higher than for US and little more than one year higher at age 65. Canada also has a lower infant mortality rate per 1,000 live births.

Life expectancy and infant mortality rates, however, are inappropriate measures of the output of each country's medical care system. Many factors other than medical services affect these measures, such as lifestyle factors as diet, exercise, smoking, homicide, and so on. For example, the obesity rate among males and females is much greater in the United States than in Canada; the mortality rate among those younger than age 40 years due to accidents and homicides is also much higher in the United States than in Canada, as is the mortality rate for heart disease among those older than age 45 years (O'Neill and O'Neill 2008).

Treatment Outcomes and Prevention

More relevant to a comparison of each country's medical system are the treatments and outcomes of people who are ill. The United States has a greater percentage of total births that are low-birth-weight infants (under 1,500 grams) than does Canada (which is likely related to lifestyle factors); however, the United States has a lower mortality rate for those infants than does Canada (which is an effect of the medical system). Examining the percentage of those with a specific medical condition, such as high blood pressure or heart disease, who receive treatment shows that whites in the United States are more likely to be treated for their disease than are white Canadians. Similarly, rates of preventive screening for various types of cancer—such as mammograms for breast cancer, Pap smears for cervical cancer, PSA [prostate-specific antigen] tests for prostate cancer, and colonoscopies for colorectal cancer—are much higher in the United States than in Canada (O'Neill and O'Neill 2008; Preston and Ho 2010).

Another important indication of the performance of a country's medical system is the survival rate of those with cancer. (Relative survival is the ratio of survival noted in patients with cancer to patients subjected to normal mortality.) As shown in Exhibit 32.1, overall cancer survival rates are higher in California (with similar size population) than in Canada. In addition, California and US cancer survival rates are among the highest in the world. Although cancer survival rates vary among regions in the United States, the variation in survival rates is much greater in Europe and among Canadian provinces.

	Year of Diagnosis	Breast	Prostate	Colorectum	Lung
Canadian registries	1996–1998	86	91	60	16
	2006–2008	88	95	65	18
California registries	1996–1998	88.9	97.7	63.6	14.6
	2006–2008	91.5	99.7	67.1	17.9

EXHIBIT 32.1 Age-Standardized Five-Year Relative Survival Rates for Cancer in Canada and California, 1996–1998 and 2006–2008

NOTE: Updates on these data were not available at the time of this revision.
SOURCES: Data for Canada from Canadian Cancer Society (2007), Table 16, and Canadian Cancer Society (2013), Table 5.2. Data for California from Kwong (2013).

This discussion thus far is not meant to imply that the current US medical system does not need important reform changes to make it more equitable and efficient, just that, contrary to the beliefs of single-payer proponents, the Canadian system does not have better medical outcomes than the United States does.

Universal Coverage

According to its proponents, the Canadian system has two major advantages. The first is universal coverage. However, as adoption of the Canadian system is but one proposal for reform, it should be compared not to the current US system but to other healthcare reform proposals to achieve universal coverage (see Chapter 34). Thus, adopting the Canadian system solely to achieve universal coverage is not necessary. The second advantage is that, to many the Canadian system is based on its presumed ability to control the rising costs of healthcare.

Controlling Healthcare Costs in Canada

Proponents of the Canadian system point to two cost savings. The first is lower administrative costs, and the second is a slower rate of increase in healthcare costs. Each is discussed in the sections that follow.

Administrative Costs

Advocates of the Canadian system have claimed that if the United States adopted the Canadian system, it could greatly reduce its administrative costs, as health insurance companies would no longer be necessary; therefore, universal access could be financed at no additional cost (Woolhandler, Campbell, and Himmelstein 2003). Many agree that administrative costs in the United States could be somewhat lowered with standardization of claims processing and billing.

Simple comparisons of administrative expenses between the two countries, however, are misleading.[3] Administrative and marketing costs could be reduced if the United States eliminated choice of health plans and agreed to a standardized set of health benefits. The United States has a wide variety of health plans—such as health maintenance organizations (HMOs), point-of-service plans, and preferred provider organizations—that offer different benefits, cost-sharing levels, and access to providers. Competition among health plans offers consumers greater choice at different premiums.

Choice is costly. However, without choice, less innovation would occur in benefit design, patient satisfaction, and competition on health plan premiums. The diversity of insurance plans reflects differences in enrollees' preferences and how much they are willing to pay for those preferences.

Lower administrative costs are not synonymous with greater system efficiency. One can imagine very low administrative costs in a system in which physicians and hospitals send their bills to the government and the government simply pays them. These lower administrative costs cause higher healthcare expenditures because they do not detect or deter inappropriate use or overuse of services.

A trade-off occurs between lower administrative costs and higher health expenditures caused by insufficient monitoring of physician and hospital behavior. If higher administrative cost resulting from utilization management did not pay for itself by reducing medical expenses and over-utilization, managed care plans would not use these measures. For example, the US Medicare system, which has a similar design to the Canadian system, has much lower administrative costs than do private managed care plans. However, the US Government Accountability Office (1995) has in the past criticized Medicare for having administrative costs that are "too low," noting that billions of dollars could be saved "by adopting the healthcare management approach of private payers to Medicare's public payer role." Studies have shown that cost-containment approaches—such as preauthorization for hospital admissions, utilization review for hospitalized patients, catastrophic case management, and physician profiling for appropriateness of care—save money (e.g., NCSL 2011).

Due to its lack of controls and oversight, Medicare fraud and waste is widespread. The Centers for Medicare & Medicaid Services (CMS 2012) reported that Medicare had an overall payment error rate of 8.5 percent ($30 billion) and an error payment rate of 66 percent for improper or fake claims for durable medical equipment. Medicare's lack of scrutiny (it automatically pays 95 percent of all claims) results in lower overhead costs but makes the program highly vulnerable to fraud.

The health insurance industry in the United States is very competitive and would only increase administrative costs if the benefits from doing so exceeded their costs. Any savings in administrative costs by eliminating cost-containment techniques and patient cost sharing would be more than offset by the higher utilization that would occur. The Canadian system is forgoing substantial savings by not raising its administrative costs, investing more in cost-containment programs, and developing mechanisms to monitor physicians' practice patterns.

Rising Healthcare Costs

An oft-cited measure of the Canadian system's cost-containment success is that healthcare costs take up a smaller (than the US system's) percentage of the country's GDP. Although correct, this information can be misleading. At different times, GDP may increase faster in one country than in another, distorting any conclusion as to which country's healthcare costs are rising faster.

A more accurate indication of which country's healthcare costs have grown more slowly is the rise in per capita health expenditures. Again, one must be careful in making such comparisons, as 40 percent of US medical expenditures are by the government—for Medicare and Medicaid, which have limited cost controls. Some regions of the United States also have greater managed care penetration than others. The US medical system has evolved from one that, until the 1980s, provided limited if any incentives for efficiency to one in which the private sector (in some states more than others) emphasizes managed care delivery systems. Thus, the performance of the US system in the 1990s—particularly in states with a great portion of the population under managed care—is more relevant to compare with the Canadian system.

As shown in Exhibit 32.2, since the 1980s, per capita health expenditures (adjusted for inflation) have risen at a slower rate in Canada than in the United States. However, during some periods, Canada's rate has been higher to compensate for the serious lack of funding in previous years. The effect of managed care can be seen by the lower rate of increase in the United States during the mid-1990s than in prior years. (As a result of the backlash against managed care in the late 1990s, managed care's cost-containment methods were loosened and premiums rose more rapidly.) However, over the past decade—particularly between 2004 and 2012—Canada has had a *higher* average annual rate of increase in per capita health expenditures than the United States.

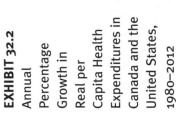

EXHIBIT 32.2
Annual
Percentage
Growth in
Real per
Capita Health
Expenditures in
Canada and the
United States,
1980–2012

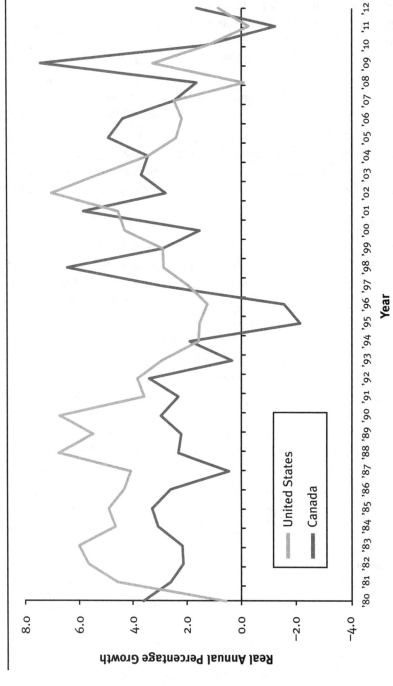

NOTE: Values adjusted for inflation using the consumer price index for each country.
SOURCE: Health expenditures per capita data from OECD (2013) and CMS (2014); consumer price index data from BLS (2014) and Statistics Canada (2013).

Does the Canadian healthcare system, compared with the US system, achieve lower per capita healthcare costs and consume a smaller percentage of its GDP because of greater efficiency?

Difference in Hospital Length of Stay

What were the reasons for the lower rate of increase in per capita healthcare spending in Canada? Is Canada more efficient than the United States in producing medical services? Although efficiency studies would have to control for many differences between the two countries—such as populations served, distribution of illnesses, outcomes of care, staffing patterns, wage rates, and so on—one simple, although partial, measure of efficiency is the difference in lengths of hospital stay.

Managed care systems in the United States have a financial incentive to use the least costly combination of medical services. Hospitals are the most expensive setting for providing care. Use of the hospital is subject to review; outpatient diagnostics and surgery are used whenever possible and catastrophic case management may involve renovating a patient's home to make it a lower-cost and more convenient setting in which to care for the patient.

The efficiency gains from managed care are evident in a comparison of utilization data between the United States and Canada. As shown in Exhibit 32.3, Canadian hospitals have a higher average length of stay than hospitals in the United States, but the difference is becoming smaller. In 1980, the length of stay in Canada was 10.2 days, compared with 7.6 days

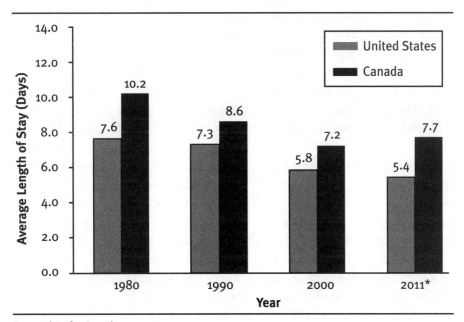

EXHIBIT 32.3
Average Length of Hospital Stay in Canada and the United States, 1980–2011

* 2010 data for Canada
SOURCE: Data from OECD (2013).

in the United States. In Canada (2010) and in the United States (2011), the most recent data available, the rate was 7.7 days and 5.4 days, respectively. In California, a state with high managed care penetration, it was 5.0 days (2011). The average length of stay for those aged 65 years and older is very high in Canada because few alternative arrangements are available. Canadian hospitals are used inappropriately; many services could be provided in an outpatient setting, the physician's office, or the patient's home.

Annual hospital budgets in Canada also provide administrators with an incentive to fill a portion of their beds with elderly patients who stay many days. If more surgical patients were admitted, hospitals would not receive additional funds to purchase the necessary supplies and nursing personnel to serve them. Thus, as inflation diminishes the real value of Canadian hospitals' budgets with which to purchase resources, they admit fewer acutely ill patients and prolong their stays.

If the lower rate of increase in Canada's health expenditures is not a result of greater efficiency, to what is it attributable?

Consequences of Strict Limits on Per Capita Costs

In the late 1980s, Canada was experiencing rising healthcare costs and a deep recession. As a result, the federal government reduced its financial commitment to the provinces from its initial 50 percent of each province's health spending to an average of about 18.6 percent (2012). As these federal cash and tax transfers fell, the growing cost of the Canadian health system placed a greater financial burden on each province.

The consequence of these costs for both the federal and provincial governments has been periods of reduced healthcare spending and then increased spending to compensate for the lack of access to care. As shown in Exhibit 32.2, the annual percentage increase in inflation-adjusted per capita health expenditures fell dramatically between 1994 and 1996. In contrast to the managed care revolution in the United States, this steep decline in Canada was attributable to cuts in government funding rather than new cost-containment approaches. In the past when such large decreases occurred (such as in the early and late 1970s), they were followed by sharp increases in following years. Consequently, over 2004 through 2010, Canada experienced a more rapid rate of growth in its per capita health expenditures to make up for the low and negative budgetary allocations in previous years. This pattern—years of slow growth in expenditures followed by years of high expenditures to make up for the previous reductions in access to care—repeats itself.

Government expenditure limits are the inevitable consequence of an unlimited demand for medical services. No government can fund all of the medical care that is demanded at zero price. Because expenditure limits result in less care being provided than is demanded at zero price, choices must be made as to how scarce healthcare resources are to be allocated. Many trade-offs must be made—for example, between preventive care, acute care, access to new technology, and patient waiting times to receive treatment. With limited dollars, providing more of one choice means less money is available to fulfill other choices.

The inevitable consequences of tight per capita expenditure limits, as have occurred in Canada, are more shortages in medical services and less access to new technology. Further, because the beneficial effects of preventive care occur in the future, existing resources are allocated to acute services for patients whose needs are immediate.

Access to Technology

One of the distinguishing features of the US medical system is the rapid diffusion of technologic innovation. Major advances in diagnostic and treatment procedures have occurred. Imaging equipment has improved diagnostic accuracy and minimized the need for exploratory surgery. New technology has resulted in less invasive procedures, quicker recovery times, and better treatment outcomes. Technologic advances have increased the survival rate of low-birth-weight babies and permitted a growing number and type of organ transplants. Any comparison of the Canadian and US health systems should consider the rate at which new technology is diffused and made available to patients.

Managed care, which is characteristic of the private US healthcare system, uses different criteria (from those used in Canada) for adopting and diffusing new technology. Two types of technologic advances occur. The first type, and simplest to evaluate under managed care, is when new technology reduces costs and improves patient satisfaction. A competitive managed care system invests the necessary capital to bring about these technologic savings. The second type is when new technology improves medical outcomes but is much more costly than existing treatment. Particularly troublesome is new technology that may have only a low probability of success—for example, 10 percent to 20 percent. In such cases, the patient would like access to the expensive treatment, while the insurer may believe it is not worth the expenditure given the low success rate.

Technology that is clearly believed to be beneficial is highly likely to be adopted. If one health plan decided not to adopt the technology when its competitors did, it would lose enrollees. Competition among health plans forces the adoption of highly beneficial technology. The costs of such technology are eventually passed on to enrollees in the form of higher premiums.

New technology that offers small beneficial effects (e.g., a new method of conducting Pap smears that increases cancer detection by 5 percent or experimental breast cancer treatments for late-stage cancer patients) has caused problems for managed care firms. Several health plans that have denied such treatments suffered penalties of up to $100 million as a result of lawsuits. To reduce their liability, more health plans have delegated such decisions to outside firms made up of ethicists and physicians who have no financial stake in the decision.

In Canada, the availability of capital to invest in cost-saving and benefit-increasing technology is determined by the government, not the hospital. Given its budget constraints and reluctance to raise taxes, the government is less likely to provide capital for new technology and for as many units than are firms that compete for enrollees. Outpatient diagnostic and surgical services are less available in Canada, denying patients the benefits (and society, the cost savings) of such technologic improvements. Costly benefit-increasing technology, such as transplants and experimental treatments, is also less available to Canadians.

A competitive managed care system may adopt technology too soon and have excess technologic capacity. Excess capacity, however, means faster access and lower patient risks. Enrollees may be willing to pay higher premiums to have that excess capacity available. If so, excess technologic capacity is appropriate; the benefits to enrollees of that excess capacity are at least equal to their willingness to pay for it. The adoption of new technology under managed care competition is different from what a government (or quasi-governmental agency) would use, as the government would be concerned with losing political support if it had to raise taxes or incur large budget deficits to increase access to new technology.

Examples of differences in availability of technology between Canada and the United States are shown in Exhibit 32.4. Twice as many gamma cameras per person are available in the United States than in Canada, four times as many MRI (magnetic resonance imaging) units and PET (positron emission tomography) scanners, and almost three times as many CT (computed tomography) scanners. Clearly, the likelihood of a patient in the United States receiving any of the services shown in Exhibit 32.4 is much greater than that of a patient in Canada with equal or similar needs. (How successful would an HMO be in the United States if it used access criteria similar to those used in Canada?)

The Technological Change in Healthcare (TECH) Research Network is an international group of researchers who examine differences in technologic change across countries in the treatment, resource costs, and health outcomes for common health problems (Bech et al. 2009; TECH Research Network 2001). Because knowledge of heart attack treatment has

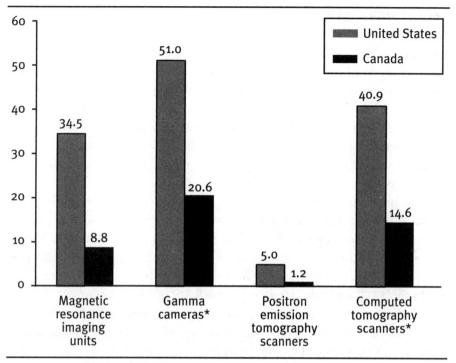

EXHIBIT 32.4
Indicators of Medical Technology per Million People, 2011 and 2012

NOTE: 2011 data for United States, 2012 data for Canada
SOURCE: Data from OECD (2013).

greatly changed in recent years and data from various studies have shown that improvements in outcomes may be the result of differences in medical practices, variations in adopting technology for inpatient care of heart attacks are likely to occur between countries.

The researchers found different patterns of technologic change between countries in adopting more intensive cardiac procedures. The United States adopted an "early start and fast growth" pattern, which resulted in relatively high treatment rates in the overall population as well as in the elderly population. Conversely, in Canada the adoption of new technology starts later, its diffusion is slower (as well as lower than in the United States), and both the elderly and general populations have lower treatment rates. The TECH Research Network (2001, 37) attributed these differences in the adoption and diffusion of beneficial technology for care of heart attack patients to differences in funding and decision making, "such as global budgets for hospitals and central planning of the availability of intensive services" in Canada. The researchers further stated that "it is clear that if high-quality care requires rapid innovation and diffusion of valuable high-cost as well as low-cost treatments, quality of care may differ greatly around the world, and national health policy may influence quality in important ways" (TECH Research Network 2001, 38).

Patient Waiting Times

As demand for services exceeds available supply, waiting time is used to ration nonemergency care. For some types of care, the quantity demanded increases because patients have no copayments. Facing a zero price, patients demand a high volume of physician visits. Consequently, to see more patients, physicians spend less time per visit. The physician then asks the patient to return for multiple short visits rather than provide all the needed services during one visit. Patient time costs are, therefore, high under a "free" system with tight fee controls because each visit requires the same patient travel and waiting time regardless of the length of the visit.[4]

Expenditure limits invariably result in high time costs being imposed on patients. However, not all care rationed by waiting time is of low value to the patient. According to a Fraser Institute report on the Canadian healthcare system, in 2013 Canadian patients had to wait, on average, 8.3 weeks for an MRI (the range was 5 to 16 weeks, depending on the province), 3.6 weeks for a CT scan (the range was 3 to 5.3 weeks), and almost 3.8 weeks for an ultrasound (the range was 2 to 6.5 weeks) (Barua and Esmail 2013). The long waits for first-time mammograms, which can vary from several weeks to a year within the same province, virtually eliminate this screening mechanism as a preventive method (CBC News 2009). Acknowledging these long waits and their adverse effects on patients, several Canadian provinces pay for heart surgery and radiation oncology treatment in the United States, which is Canada's safety valve. Ontario has contracted with hospitals in Buffalo (New York) and Detroit for MRI services. Quebec has sent hundreds of cancer patients to the United States for treatment, because they waited more than eight weeks for radiation or chemotherapy (more than four weeks of waiting time is considered medically risky) (Anstett 2009).

The Fraser Institute performs annual surveys on waiting times from referral by the general practitioner to an appointment with a specialist and on the waiting time from appointment with a specialist to treatment. These surveys are done by medical specialty for each Canadian province. Exhibit 32.5 describes the waiting time for treatment by specialty. For example, for orthopedic surgery (e.g., hips and knees) a person would have to wait, on average, 39.6 weeks to receive treatment; in some provinces, however, the wait to have the surgery performed may be as short as 26.6 weeks or as long as 75.5 weeks. (In 1991, aged patients in some provinces had to wait up to four years for a hip or knee replacement.) Ophthalmology (e.g., cataract removal) requires an average wait of 19.4 weeks, but this can vary by province from 14.4 to 62 weeks. For neurosurgery, the average waiting time is 24.7 weeks, but it varies by province between 13.1 and 54.9 weeks.

The Fraser Institute also asks specialists how long a patient *should* wait before he receives the recommended treatment. For example, in Nova Scotia the

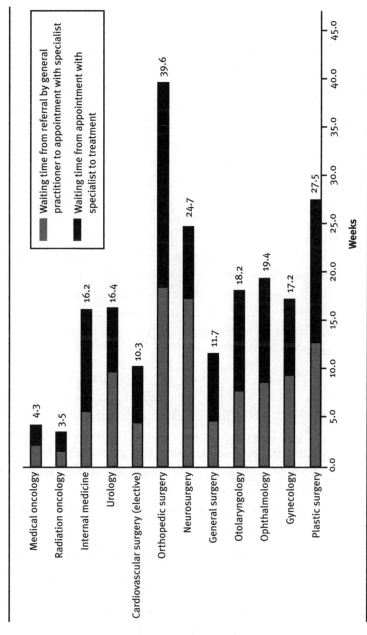

EXHIBIT 32.5
Canadian
Hospital
Waiting Lists:
Total Expected
Waiting Time
from Referral
by General
Practitioner to
Treatment, by
Specialty, 2013

Legend:
- Waiting time from referral by general practitioner to appointment with specialist
- Waiting time from appointment with specialist to treatment

Specialty	Total (weeks)
Medical oncology	4.3
Radiation oncology	3.5
Internal medicine	16.2
Urology	16.4
Cardiovascular surgery (elective)	10.3
Orthopedic surgery	39.6
Neurosurgery	24.7
General surgery	11.7
Otolaryngology	18.2
Ophthalmology	19.4
Gynecology	17.2
Plastic surgery	27.5

Weeks

SOURCE: Data from Barua and Esmail (2013).

actual waiting time for urgent cardiovascular surgery after a patient had seen a specialist is more than four weeks, whereas specialists believe the reasonable waiting time should not exceed one week; for elective cardiovascular surgery, the actual waiting time is much longer. There have been reports of patients dying while waiting for heart surgery. Clearly, access to care depends on the province in which one lives. Furthermore, in a province the waiting time is not the same for every procedure.

Canada does not have an egalitarian system. Access to care depends not only on the province in which one lives but also on whether a person can afford to pay for her care in the United States. The failure to consider the higher patient time costs in the Canadian system *understates* health expenditures in that country. As demand for services exceeds the available supply, many people would be willing to pay more rather than incur the cost of multiple trips, waiting, or doing without. Unfortunately, the Canadian system prohibits the purchase of private health insurance for hospital and medical services. Thus, people are legally prohibited from insuring themselves against the risks of not receiving timely care when they require it.

An important consequence of these long waits for medical service is that patients (GAO 1991, 59)

> experience pain and discomfort, and some may develop psychological problems.... The condition of some patients may worsen, making surgery more risky...because of the long queue for lithotripsy treatment, many doctors perform surgery to remove kidney stones (also resulting in higher costs), putting the patient at higher risk than with a lithotripsy procedure.... Often patients experience a financial setback, such as decreased income or loss of a job (while waiting in queues).... Patients are unable to work because they are physically immobile while they wait for a hip or other joint replacement.

Those who are wealthy can afford to skip the queues and purchase medical services in the United States, as did the then-premier of Newfoundland and Labrador. When he learned that he needed heart surgery in 2010, instead of waiting his turn, at his own expense he went to the United States for his operation (CBC News 2010). Similarly, the politically powerful are able to jump to the head of the queue, as occurred with Canada's health minister, who was able to have his surgery after being diagnosed with prostate cancer in 2001. Other prostate cancer patients were angered by his quick surgery after they had to wait much longer—some as long as a year between diagnosis and surgery (Rupert 2001).

Is Canada Abandoning Its Single-Payer System?

A Quebec patient, forced to wait a year for a hip replacement and prohibited from paying privately for his operation, brought a lawsuit against the Quebec government to the Canadian Supreme Court. In a surprise ruling, the Supreme Court concluded that the wait for medical services had become so long that the health system and its ban on private practice violated patients' "life and personal security, inviolability and freedom," which are part of Quebec's Charter of Rights and Freedoms. Further, "The evidence in this case shows that delays in the public healthcare system are widespread, and that, in some serious cases, patients die as a result of waiting lists for public healthcare.... In sum, the prohibition on obtaining private health insurance is not constitutional where the public system fails to deliver reasonable services." Although the ruling applied to Quebec, it has affected all of Canada's provinces (Krauss 2005). As a consequence of this ruling, private diagnostic and special surgery clinics have rapidly expanded.

The amount of private care that is now available across Canada varies widely from province to province. Privately funded primary and surgical care in British Columbia and Quebec have seen rapid growth but remains unavailable in other parts of the country, such as in New Brunswick, although patients can travel to British Columbia or Quebec. Private healthcare firms—such as Medisys, Medcan, Preventous, and Copeman—are expanding their services, and several provinces contract with and pay for treatments in privately operated surgical clinics. As in the United States, Canadian physicians have also started concierge practices for those willing to pay for better access. According to Shimo (2006), "...the spreading dissatisfaction with Canada's publicly funded system has begun to break down Canadians' traditional hostility toward for-profit health. Private health care in Canada is about more than increased choice for the very rich. It's about providing options to people on wait lists who are suffering in pain and have had to put their lives on hold. For some, it's about gaining access to life-saving drugs or cutting-edge treatments that aren't funded by the public system."

In addition, a new industry consisting of medical travel agents has been created to assist Canadian patients seeking medical treatment in other countries. These agents, such as MedSolution, specialize in out-of-country hospital care to places like France, Turkey, and India. Other medical travel agents, such as Vancouver-based Timely Medical Alternatives, offer package deals on hotels and operations at US clinics not more than a two-hour drive from the border. Private health insurance in Canada, however, has not expanded and is still not permitted in many provinces. However, court actions in British Columbia, Alberta, and Ontario are challenging the government's monopoly. These legal challenges should be decided in the next several years (Esmail 2013).

Supporters of the single-payer system are opposed to a two-tier medical system, believing the private sector will draw physicians and nurses away from the public system, where a severe physician shortage already exists, making waiting times even longer. The dam has already broken, however. As of 2009, 130 for-profit clinics are in operation across Canada, offering surgeries, MRIs, and access to physician services (Canadian Health Coalition 2009). Patients must pay with cash, but the wait time is short.[5] Stopping the trend toward privatization and a two-tier medical system, which already exist in other countries, will be difficult.

Should the United States Adopt the Canadian System?

Canada has been the only Westernized country with a single-payer system. Other countries that started with a single-payer system, such as Great Britain, moved to a two-tier system that permitted private medical markets. Canada is also moving in the same direction. Governments find that it eventually becomes too expensive to fund all the new technology and medical services its population demands when they do not have to pay any out-of-pocket costs. Inequities develop in a single-payer system; the wealthy can reduce their waiting by traveling to another country, and the politically powerful are able to jump the queue. A two-tier medical system recognizes that there are people willing to spend more of their money in return for quicker access to medical services and the latest medical technology.

Alternative approaches exist to achieve the objectives claimed for a single-payer system. With regard to the equity criterion—namely how to provide for the uninsured—the Canadian system should be compared not with the current US system but with a system in which the goal is universal coverage. This goal can be achieved in alternative ways, such as by providing income-related subsidies to those with low income (see Chapter 34). A single-payer system, as evidenced by the Canadian system, does not provide everyone with equal access to medical care. It should be acknowledged that every health system has multiple tiers; those who can afford it will be able to purchase more medical services or have quicker access to care. Unequal access to care exists in Canada depending on the province in which people live or whether they can afford to pay for their care in the United States.

Arbitrarily limiting the growth in medical expenditures, the cost-containment method used in single-payer systems, will not increase efficiency. Efficiency incentives on the part of patients or medical providers are not used in the Canadian system. Efficiency incentives are important because they affect the cost of any national health insurance plan and the willingness of the public to provide subsidies to those less fortunate than themselves. To whom are government decision makers accountable? What information do they have to make decisions? In a competitive market, people can leave a health plan when they are dissatisfied with that plan; in a monopolized system (single payer), they have no similar way in which to express their dissatisfaction with the system. In a single-payer system, information on waiting times and access problems is either unavailable or dated, making it difficult for decision makers to make adjustments based on changes in demand or supply conditions. Also important to which national health insurance plan is adopted are the criteria used for access to and investment in new medical technology. Efficiency, innovation, and capital investment are determined by incentives; a government bureaucracy is highly unlikely to outperform competitive markets in this regard.[6]

Political versus private decision making will result in differences in access to care, technology adoption, efficiency, equity, and even health outcomes. Before the United States places its healthcare system (which accounts for almost one-sixth of its economy) under complete government control, single-payer advocates should provide evidence (more than just opinion) showing why a single-payer system will not suffer the same fate experienced by other countries that have tried and subsequently abandoned their own single-payer systems. Further, why would the problems of a single-payer system differ from the problems experienced by the two single-payer systems that currently exist in the United States—namely Medicare (which has a $34 trillion deficit and will have to be reformed to avoid bankruptcy; see Chapter 8) and Medicaid (which offers poor access to care; see Chapter 9)?

Summary

Proposals for further healthcare reform of the US healthcare system should not be evaluated against the Canadian single-payer system but against other national health insurance proposals aiming to achieve universal coverage and to limit rising healthcare expenditures. Further, single-payer advocates should not dismiss the flaws of the Canadian system by claiming that the United States would be able to devote more money to a single-payer system. Given growing medical costs, advancements in medical technology, and no limits on patients' access to care, evidence based on the experience of every country that has tried a single-payer system suggests that a single-payer system in the United States would eventually suffer the same fate as the Canadian system.

Before the United States selects another country's medical system to emulate, it should know all the facts—good and bad—about the performance of that country's medical system and the criteria by which a system should be evaluated. Controlling the percentage of GDP devoted to medical care or the rise in per capita expenditures should not be the overriding objectives of a medical system; if they were, the United States could use Great Britain's National Health Service, which performs better than the Canadian system on these criteria but is clearly unacceptable on other grounds.

Patient preferences differ regarding how much they are willing to spend for faster access to care and for the latest advances in medical science. Single-payer systems disregard such differences in preferences. The appropriate rate of growth in medical expenditures should be based on how much people are willing to pay (directly and through taxes). There are legitimate reasons for increased medical expenditures—such as an aging population, more chronic illness, new technology that saves and improves the quality of life, new diseases, shortages of personnel (thereby requiring wage increases), and so on. Arbitrary expenditure limits would result in reduced access to medical services and technology.

Discussion Questions

1. Describe the Canadian healthcare system and the methods used to control costs.
2. What are the consequences of making medical services free to everyone?
3. Why is the size of administrative expenses (as a percentage of total medical expenditures) a poor indication of a healthcare system's efficiency?
4. What are the costs (negative effects) of expenditure limits?
5. Contrast the criteria used in Canada with those used in competitive managed care systems for deciding whether an investment should be made in new technology.

Notes

1. Hutchison and Glazier (2013) discuss recent changes in primary care payment to physicians in Ontario using fee-for-service, capitation, and pay for performance.
2. As of 2013, provincial governments pay, on average, only about 70 percent of total medical expenses—mainly for hospital and physician

services. Canadian patients pay the remaining 30 percent, which include outpatient prescription drugs, dental care, vision care, and other hospital and professional services. Despite first-dollar public coverage for hospital and physician services, Canadians spend more privately on healthcare than citizens of most European countries (Canadian Institute for Health Information 2013).

3. The administrative savings of moving to a Canadian system are believed to be grossly overstated. For example, in calculating administrative savings, the expense of administering self-insured employer plans was included in the expense ratio of insurers. However, the claims payments made on behalf of self-insured employers were not included as part of the insurers' premiums, falsely inflating the expense ratio. Further, included as part of insurers' overhead are premium taxes (a transfer payment to state governments), investment income (essentially a return to employers for advance payment of premiums), and a return on capital (which would also have to be calculated for a public insurer); see Danzon (1992). (Chapter 7 also discusses problems inherent in comparisons of administrative costs.)

4. The value to the patient of additional physician visits when there are no out-of-pocket payments is low. Generally, the approaches used to limit use of services whose value is worth less than their costs of production are cost-containment techniques and requiring patients to wait longer. Cost containment is included as an explicit administrative expense, whereas implicit patient waiting cost is not.

5. One physician who has opened private medical clinics said, "This is a country in which dogs can get a hip replacement in under a week and in which humans can wait two to three years" (Krauss 2006). Dogs have also had preferential treatment with regard to diagnostic tests. The government provides funding for hospitals to operate its MRIs only eight hours a day. In 1998, a Canadian hospital offered MRIs to pets in the middle of the night in an effort to make money. After an outcry from angry humans, who at that time were waiting up to a year for nonurgent scans, the hospital was forced to stop this practice (Walkom 2002).

6. For a brief critique of single-payer plans, see Emanuel (2008).

References

Anstett, P., 2009. "Canadians Visit U.S. to Get Health Care." *Michigan Business*, August 20. www.freep.com/article/20090820/ BUSINESS06/908200420/Canadians-visit-U.S.-to-get-health-care.

Barua, B., and N. Esmail. 2013. *Waiting Your Turn: Wait Times for Health Care in Canada, 2013 Report.* The Fraser Institute. Published October. www .fraserinstitute.org/uploadedFiles/fraser-ca/Content/research-news/ research/publications/waiting-your-turn-2013.pdf.

Bech, M., T. Christiansen, K. Dunham, J. Lauridsen, C. H. Lyttkens, K. McDonald, A. McGuire, and TECH Investigators. 2009. "The Influence of Economic Incentives and Regulatory Factors on the Adoption of Treatment Technologies: A Case Study of Technologies Used to Treat Heart Attacks." *Health Economics* 18 (10): 1114–32.

Bureau of Labor Statistics (BLS). 2014. "Consumer Price Index." Accessed January. www.bls.gov/cpi/home.htm.

Canadian Cancer Society, National Cancer Institute of Canada, Statistics Canada, Provincial/Territorial Cancer Registries, and Public Health Agency of Canada. 2013. *Canadian Cancer Statistics*, 2013. Published May. www .cancer.ca/~/media/cancer.ca/CW/cancer%20information/cancer%20101/ Canadian%20cancer%20statistics/canadian-cancer-statistics-2013-EN.pdf.

———. 2007. *Canadian Cancer Statistics*, 2007. Published April. www.cancer .ca/~/media/cancer.ca/CW/cancer%20information/cancer%20101/ Canadian%20cancer%20statistics/%20Canadian-Cancer-Statistics-2007- EN.pdf.

Canadian Health Coalition. 2009. "Private, For-Profit Clinics." Published March. http://medicare.ca/wp-content/uploads/2009/05/factsheet1-20091.pdf.

Canadian Institute for Health Information. 2013. *National Health Expenditure Trends, 1975 to 2013.* Published October 29. www.cihi.ca/CIHI-ext-portal/ internet/en/document/spending+and+health+workforce/spending/ release_29oct13_infogra1pg.

CBC News. 2010. "Danny Williams Going to US for Heart Surgery." Posted February 1. www.cbc.ca/news/canada/newfoundland-labrador/danny- williams-going-to-u-s-for-heart-surgery-1.878492.

———. 2009. "Digital Mammography Cuts Wait Times in Moncton." Posted September 29. www.cbc.ca/news/canada/new-brunswick/digital- mammography-cuts-wait-times-in-moncton-1.835426.

Centers for Medicare & Medicaid Services (CMS). 2014. "Historical." Accessed January. www.cms.gov/Research-Statistics-Data-and- Systems/Statistics-Trends-and-Reports/NationalHealthExpendData/ NationalHealthAccountsHistorical.html.

———. 2012. "Fiscal Year 2012 Improper Payment Rates for CMS Programs." Accessed January 2014. www.cms.gov/apps/media/press/factsheet.asp? Counter=4484.

Danzon, P. M. 1992. "Hidden Overhead Costs: Is Canada's System Really Less Expensive?" *Health Affairs* 11 (1): 21–43.

Emanuel, E. J. 2008. "The Problem with Single-Payer Plans." *Hastings Center Report* 38: 38–41.

Esmail, N. 2013. Personal correspondence with the author, June 5.

Hutchison, B., and R. Glazier. 2013. "Ontario's Primary Care Reforms Have Transformed the Local Landscape, But a Plan Is Needed for Ongoing Improvement." *Health Affairs* 32 (4): 695–703.

Krauss, C. 2006. "Canada's Private Clinics Surge as Public System Falters." *New York Times,* February 28, p. A3.

———. 2005. "In Blow to Canada's Health System, Quebec Law Is Voided." *New York Times,* June 10, p. A3.

Kwong, S. 2013. Personal correspondence with the author, December 23.

National Conference of State Legislatures (NCSL). 2011. *Health Cost Containments and Efficiencies.* Washington, DC: NCSL.

O'Neill, J. E., and D. M. O'Neill. 2008. "Health Status, Health Care and Inequality: Canada vs. the U.S." *Forum for Health Economics & Policy* 10 (1): 1558–9544.

Organisation for Economic Co-operation and Development (OECD). 2013. *2013 OECD Health Data.* Paris: OECD.

Preston, S., and J. Ho. 2010. "Low Life Expectancy in the United States: Is the Health Care System at Fault." In *International Differences in Mortality at Older Ages: Dimensions and Sources,* edited by E. Crimmins, S. Preston, and B. Cohen, 268–308. Washington, DC: National Academies Press.

Rupert, J. 2001. "Man Protests Rock's Speedy Surgery." *Ottawa Citizen,* February 17, p. D3.

Shimo, A. 2006. "The Rise of Private Care in Canada: All the Health Services Money Can Buy." Published April 25. www.macleans.ca/article.jsp?cont ent=20060501_125881_125881.

Statistics Canada. 2013. "Consumer Price Index, Historical Summary." Accessed December. www.statcan.gc.ca/tables-tableaux/sum-som/l01/cst01/ econ46a-eng.htm.

Technological Change in Health Care (TECH) Research Network. 2001. "Technological Change Around the World: Evidence from Heart Attack Care." *Health Affairs* 20 (3): 25–42.

US Government Accountability Office (GAO). 1995. *Medicare: Rapid Spending Growth Calls for More Prudent Purchasing.* GAO/T-HEHS-95-193. Washington, DC: US Government Printing Office.

———. 1991. *Canadian Health Insurance.* GAO/HRD-91-90. Washington, DC: US Government Printing Office.

Walkom, T. 2002. "No Pets Ahead of People." *Toronto Star,* January 11, p. A6.

Woolhandler, S., T. Campbell, and D. Himmelstein. 2003. "Costs of Health Care Administration in the United States and Canada." *New England Journal of Medicine* 349 (8): 768–75.

EMPLOYER-MANDATED NATIONAL HEALTH INSURANCE

An employer mandate for health insurance has had a great deal of political support. President Nixon proposed it, as did President Clinton; Hawaii and Massachusetts instituted it; and it was included as part of President Obama's 2010 Affordable Care Act (ACA). Starting in 2014, employers are required to provide health insurance to their employees and dependents or pay a tax per employee.

In 2012, approximately 57 million people under age 65 years were uninsured. About 88 percent of the uninsured were either employed (full-time or part-time) or in a family with an employed member. Therefore, mandating employers to provide their employees with health insurance covers a large percentage of the uninsured at small cost to the government. According to the ACA, if employers (with 50 or more employees working 30 or more hours a week) choose not to provide health insurance to their employees, they have to pay a new payroll tax of $2,000 per employee—hence the name "play-or-pay" national health insurance.

Several variations on the basic approach have previously been proposed. Mandated employer proposals have generally required the employer to pay 80 percent and the employee 20 percent of the cost of the insurance. And instead of a fixed tax per employee, President Clinton proposed requiring employers to spend a fixed percentage of wages for health insurance. Play-or-pay proposals generally exclude firms with fewer than 50 employees realizing that, although small firms have a high rate of uninsured workers, the additional cost to such firms would represent a financial hardship. Firms with fewer employees are provided with tax credits to offset the higher costs.

Before analyzing the economic consequences of mandating employers to provide health insurance to the working uninsured, we must examine who the uninsured are and why they do not have insurance.

The Uninsured

In 2012, of the 266 million persons who were under age 65 years (at which Medicare eligibility begins), 22 percent (or 57 million) were without health insurance (AHRQ 2013, Table 1).[1] Medicaid covers about 12 percent (or

22 million) low-income nonelderly (18 to 64 years old). As part of the ACA, the federal government will pay 100 percent of the costs between 2014 and 2016 and 90 percent thereafter to encourage states to expand Medicaid eligibility from 100 to 133 percent of the federal poverty level. Many states, however, have decided not to participate in this Medicaid expansion because they believe the additional cost to the state after 2016 will still be significant and because they are unsure whether the federal government (with its large deficits) will continue paying 90 percent of the cost.

The age group with the highest percentage of uninsured employees comprises 25- to 34-year-olds; 22 percent of them do not have insurance. About 5.6 percent of those under 18 years old who work are uninsured (see Exhibit 33.1). These young, employed age groups are generally single adults who are not eligible for their parent's health insurance. (As part of the ACA, young adults can join or remain on a parent's health insurance policy until they reach age 26, as long as they are not eligible for coverage under their own employer's policy. Premiums have increased as a result of families adding adult children to their policies.) The percentage of uninsured workers declines with each higher age group.

When uninsured workers in each age group are examined as a percentage of all uninsured workers, those aged 25 to 34 years represent the greatest portion of all uninsured workers—at 30.0 percent. The second highest are those aged 45 to 64 years—at 29.8 percent. The distribution of uninsured workers in the remaining age groups—aged 19 to 24 and 35 to 44 years—are 15.8 and 23.5 percent, respectively, of the total number of uninsured workers.

When one examines the percentage distribution of the total uninsured population, about 11 percent of the uninsured are children. This number has decreased since the 1997 enactment of the Children's Health Insurance Program (CHIP), which covers low-income children.

EXHIBIT 33.1
Uninsured Workers, by Age Group, 2011

Age in Years	Working Population in Thousands	% Distribution of Workers	% Uninsured Within Each Age Group	% Distribution of All Uninsured
16–18	3,601	2.3	5.6	0.8
19–24	18,722	12.1	21.4	15.8
25–34	35,152	22.8	21.6	30.0
35–44	33,827	21.9	17.6	23.5
45–64	62,975	40.8	12.0	29.8

SOURCE: Data from Rhoades (2013).

Whites represent 48 percent of the total number of uninsured, although only 14 percent of all whites are uninsured. Twenty-two percent of all African Americans are uninsured, and Hispanics have the highest uninsured percentage at 33 percent. Regionally, most of the uninsured (44 percent) are in the South, the West is second with 26 percent, the Midwest has 16 percent, and the Northeast has the fewest with 15 percent (AHRQ 2013, Table 1).

The first important characteristic of the employed uninsured is the size of the firm in which they work. The fewer the number of employees, the greater is the likelihood that the employer does not provide health insurance (see Exhibit 33.2). Twenty-five percent of employees in small firms (defined as those with fewer than ten employees) are uninsured, compared with only 4.6 percent in large firms (those with more than 500 employees). Of all the employed uninsured (including self-employed workers), 69.3 percent are in firms with fewer than 25 employees and 9.9 percent are in firms with 25 to 49 employees. Thus, 79.2 percent of the total employed uninsured are in firms with fewer than 50 employees. If self-employed workers are excluded, 47.4 percent of uninsured workers are in firms with fewer than 25 employees and 9.9 percent are in firms with 25 to 49 employees.

Characteristic	Working Population in Thousands[a]	% Distribution of Workers	% Uninsured Within Each Group	% Distribution of All Uninsured
Self-employed	16,470	11.6	30.3	21.9
Fewer than 10 workers	25,265	17.8	24.9	27.6
10–24 workers	22,365	15.8	20.1	19.8
25–49 workers	14,839	10.5	15.2	9.9
50–99 workers	16,768	11.8	10.5	7.7
100–499 workers	25,934	18.3	8.0	9.2
500 or more workers	19,987	14.1	4.6	4.0

EXHIBIT 33.2 Uninsured Workers, by Size of Firm, 2011

[a] Excludes persons with unknown self-employment status and size of establishment
SOURCE: Data from Rhoades (2013).

The second important characteristic of the employed uninsured is their low wages. As shown in Exhibit 33.3, as of 2011, 45.4 percent of the employed uninsured earned less than $10 an hour, and another 31.6 percent earned between $10 and $15 per hour. Thus, 77 percent earned less than $15 per hour. With respect to part-time work, 23.5 percent of uninsured workers work fewer than 30 hours per week.

With all these traits considered, the general picture of the uninsured that emerges is of young people who work in small firms and earn low wages.

Why the Uninsured Do Not Have Health Insurance

The employed uninsured have not had health insurance for two important reasons.

First, the price of insurance is high for those who are employed in small firms. Small firms are unable to take advantage of economies in administering and marketing health insurance, which results in higher insurance costs per employee. Insurance companies also previously charged small firms higher premiums to make allowance for adverse selection, believing many employees would join just to take advantage of health benefits. For example,

EXHIBIT 33.3
Percentage Distribution of Uninsured Workers, by Wage Rate and Hours Worked, 2011

Characteristic	Working Population in Thousands[a]	% Distribution of Workers	% Uninsured Within Each Group	% Distribution of All Uninsured
Hours of Work				
Fewer than 20	12,247	8.2	17.4	8.8
20–29	14,790	9.9	24.0	14.7
30 or more	122,987	82.0	15.0	76.4
Hourly Wage				
Less than $5.00	2,029	1.5	26.1	2.7
$5.00–$9.99	27,005	19.9	30.9	42.7
$10.00–$14.99	32,375	23.9	19.0	31.6
$15.00–$19.99	23,311	17.2	10.3	12.3
$20.00 or more	50,733	37.5	4.1	10.8

[a] Excludes persons with unknown hours of work and unknown hourly wages
SOURCE: Data from Rhoades (2013).

an owner might hire a sick relative so that her medical costs can be paid. In large firms with lower turnover rates, employment is less likely for the primary purpose of receiving health benefits. Finally, many states have mandated various benefits, such as in vitro fertilization and hair transplants, that must be included in any health insurance plan sold in their state. Once included in the insurance policy, employees use these services, increasing the insurance premium. Large firms, however, are able to self-insure, making them exempt from the costs of these additional mandates. Small firms are too small to self-insure and therefore have to pay the higher premium, which lessens their demand for health insurance.

Second, the demand for health insurance is low among employees in small firms because of their low income. Because 77 percent of the employed uninsured earn less than $15 per hour, health insurance premiums would result in a major reduction in their funds available for other necessities. For example, most uninsured workers (45.4 percent) earn $10 per hour or less, or roughly $20,000 a year. Requiring them to purchase health insurance would reduce their income by 30 percent; in 2013, insurance cost an average of $5,884 per person per year and $16,351 per year for a family of four (Kaiser Family Foundation and HRET 2013). Instead, when these low-wage employees or their families become ill, they are likely to become eligible for Medicaid, which does not cost them anything. For low-wage workers and their families, Medicaid is their health insurance plan.

Consequences of Employer-Mandated Health Insurance

Failure to Achieve Universal Coverage

Employer-mandated health insurance by itself cannot achieve universal coverage. Even if all working uninsured were covered by an employer mandate, those employed part-time and those not employed, together with their dependents, would still not have insurance coverage. This would leave approximately one-third of the uninsured without coverage. To achieve universal coverage, an employer mandate must be combined with an individual mandate, together with insurance subsidies for these other population groups. Unless everyone is required to have health insurance (with subsidies for those unable to afford insurance), universal coverage will not occur. It is for this reason the ACA has both an employer and an individual mandate.

Inequitable Method of Financing

Advocates of an employer mandate have proposed that small firms be given tax credits or subsidies to induce them to offer health insurance to their employees. This approach, however, will likely be inequitable. Although many low-wage employees work in small firms, not everyone employed by small firms earns a low income; consider those who work for small legal firms or physician groups, for example. To rectify this inequity, the subsidy could be limited to those small firms with low average income. However, some low-wage employees in large firms would not receive subsidies. To eliminate these inequities, tax subsidies should be targeted to those in need (i.e., they should be income related) regardless of the size of the employer. (This issue is discussed below as one of the concerns with the ACA.)

Who Pays for Employer Mandates?

Proposals for an employer mandate have always required the employer to pay a significant part (such as 80 percent) and the employee to pay for a small part (such as 20 percent) of the cost of health insurance. The ACA requires employers (with 50 or more employees) to buy their employees health insurance or pay a $2,000 tax for each employee without health insurance (excluding the first 30 employees). Thus, most of the cost would appear to be borne by the firm. However, whether the employer or the employee actually bears the burden of the tax does not depend on whom the tax is imposed. In competitive industries, firms do not make excess profits; otherwise, other firms (including foreign firms) would enter that industry until excess profits ceased to exist. When employers are earning a competitive rate of return, they are unable to bear the burden of an additional tax themselves—or they eventually go out of business. Instead, faced with a new employee tax, within a short period employers shift the cost of that tax to others by increasing their prices, decreasing the cash wages paid to their employees, or both.

Imposing a per employee tax on the employer is likely to result in one of two possible outcomes (Blumberg 1999). Exactly which combination occurs depends on the particular labor and product markets in which the firm competes, because the nature of these markets determines how much of the higher labor cost is shifted back to the employee and how much is shifted forward in the form of higher consumer prices.

First, to the extent that employees are flexible about the relative portions of their total compensation that go to cash wages and fringe benefits (including health insurance), the cost of labor to the employer is unchanged. A greater employer tax to pay for employees' insurance would result in lower wages, consequently not increasing the cost of labor to the firm.[2] Although employees receive more health insurance, they clearly value the health insurance less than the cash wages it takes to purchase it, because they could have purchased the insurance previously but chose not to. Thus, the first effect of a per employee tax is to make uninsured low-wage employees worse off by forcing a change in how they spend their limited income.

Second, the cost of labor to the firm will be raised because the mix between wages and health insurance is not perfectly flexible, particularly right away. With higher labor costs, the firm will have to increase the prices of its goods and services. These prices in turn will lead consumers to purchase fewer goods and services. To the extent that labor costs are increased, part of the employee tax is shifted forward in the form of higher consumer prices. This second effect of the tax results in a regressive form of consumer taxation because all consumers, regardless of their income, pay higher prices. Those higher prices represent a greater portion of the income of low-income consumers than of high-income consumers. Such a tax is an inequitable method of financing universal health insurance.

Employers Reducing the Number of Employees and Work Hours

One of the major concerns with an employer mandate is its effect on firms' demand for labor. When part of the cost of labor is passed on to consumers in the form of higher prices, the demand for the firm's output decreases; with less demand for its output, the firm will need fewer employees. Further, employers not offering their employees health insurance are required to pay a $2,000 penalty tax. Many employees near the minimum wage whose wages cannot be reduced to offset the employer tax will likely be let go. The Congressional Budget Office (CBO 2012) estimated that the ACA employer mandate will result in employment decreases of approximately one-half of 1 percent. This is equivalent to about 700,000 people losing their jobs. Those at the greatest risk of job loss are low-income workers.

Employers not offering insurance and having fewer than 50 employees are exempt from paying a per employee penalty of $2,000. Anecdotal evidence suggests that many employers have refused to hire more than 49 employees.[3] Firms may also decrease their use of full-time employees and increase their use of part-time employees because, under the ACA, the employer does not have to buy insurance for employees working fewer than 30 hours a week. Thus, another effect of a health insurance tax per employee is that fewer full-time workers may be employed, firms may be reluctant to increase hiring above 49 employees, and more part-time employees are likely to be hired.

Employers Dropping Health Coverage

Many employers will decide that paying an employee tax is less costly than providing their employees with health insurance. During the ACA debate, the CBO estimated that only about 20 million people would take advantage of subsidies in the exchanges. The remainder of those eligible would continue to obtain coverage at work or through the newly expanded Medicaid program. Several economists, however, estimated that the number of people taking advantage of the exchange subsidies may be as high as 50 million. Shifting more employees into the subsidized state health insurance exchanges greatly increases the federal government's cost of providing exchange subsidies.

To meet the employer mandate requirement, the employer has several choices. Employers with fewer than 50 employees that do not offer insurance are exempt from paying a per employee penalty of $2,000 (after the first 30 employees). Employers with 50 or more employees can provide their employees with the mandated coverage and not incur a penalty. Alternatively, the employer could decide to pay the penalty and not provide health insurance to their employees. If the employer chooses not to provide coverage, the employees are then eligible to buy subsidized insurance from state health insurance exchanges. (The state insurance exchanges are also available to others, such as the self-employed.)

The percentage of the premium families without access to an employer-provided plan have to pay on the exchange increases the higher the family's income; families earning 133 percent of the federal poverty level ($31,721 for a family of four in 2014) will pay no more than 3 percent of their income, while a family earning 400 percent of the poverty level ($95,400) will pay no more than 9.5 percent of their income in premiums.

Both employers and their low-wage employees would be better off if employers dropped employee health coverage. Economists generally agree that employee costs, such as payroll taxes and health insurance, are paid for by reduced employee wages. Higher employee costs result in lower wages. The advantage of having the employer pay for the employee's health insurance is that it is bought with pretax dollars. Exchange subsidies are worth much more to lower-wage workers than the federal tax subsidy associated with employer-paid insurance premiums. The CBO (2012, 15, Table 1) has estimated that, in 2016, a family of four with a household income of $50,000 would be better off by more than $11,000 if they got their insurance through a state exchange instead of from an employer. For example, the tax subsidy received by a low-wage worker from an employer-paid $15,000 insurance plan is only about $3,000. However, a worker earning $30,000 a year would have to have her cash wages reduced by $15,000 for an employer-paid policy. Clearly, such a worker would be opposed to substituting a $15,000 plan for an equivalent reduction of cash wages.

If the employer does not offer insurance, the worker becomes eligible to join the exchange and buy a $15,000 plan, which would only cost 3 percent, or about $1,000, of a low-income employee's wages. Low-wage employees, then, would prefer to have the employer deduct the $2,000 penalty from their wages and buy a subsidized $15,000 plan on the exchange that would only cost 3 percent of their income. Thus, two low-income employees—both with the same income, but one works for a firm that provides health insurance and the other does not—have cash wages that are largely different. The employee working for an employer that provides insurance is much worse off. Large firms with many low-wage employees likely will decide not to offer health insurance, otherwise their employees likely will shift to an employer that does not offer health insurance. It is inequitable policy to treat two workers with the same income so differently.

High-income, exchange-eligible employees have to pay 9.5 percent of their income when buying a plan on the exchange. High-income employees (e.g., those earning 400 percent of the federal poverty level) would prefer to have their employer continue purchasing their insurance because the tax subsidy of employer-paid health insurance is worth more to them than the government subsidy (plan premium minus 9.5 percent of their income plus the $2,000 employer penalty they would have to pay) if they bought insurance on the exchange.

The point at which the benefits of the tax subsidy exceed the exchange subsidy occurs at 350 percent of the federal poverty level ($82,425 a year in 2013) for a household of four people with one worker. (This "crossover" point depends on family size and number of workers per household (Pauly and Leive 2013).

Financing national health insurance through an employer mandate relies on a hidden and inequitable method of financing health insurance for the uninsured. Imposing the tax on the employer makes it appear as though the employer bears the cost of the tax. The tax, however, would be shifted to both consumers and employees. In both cases, the tax would be regressive. If the tax were borne by labor in the form of lower cash wages, low-income employees would have to pay a higher percentage of their income for health insurance than high-wage employees would. This hidden tax on consumers and employees also understates its budgetary effects on the government. Federal and state governments lose tax revenues.

State Health Insurance Exchanges

The ACA created state health insurance exchanges to serve as marketplaces where individuals and small businesses can compare and buy subsidized private health insurance meeting federal and state standards, including mandated benefits likely costing between $15,000 and $20,000 for family coverage in 2016. Insurers competing on the exchanges offer four types of standardized plans so that purchasers can more easily compare price and service. Bronze plans cover about 60 percent of the costs of medical services; Silver, Gold, and Platinum plans cover 70, 80, and 90 percent, respectively, with the balance paid by the family. All plans cover the same ten essential benefits, including preventive services, hospitalizations, mental health, and prescription drugs. Premiums are lowest for the Bronze plans, although their deductibles and copayments are the highest.

Federal exchange subsidies are only available to individuals and families with income from 133 percent to 400 percent of the federal poverty level who do not have access to an employer health plan. Employees who have access to an employer health plan are ineligible to buy insurance on the exchange. (Families whose income is below 133 percent of the federal poverty level are eligible for Medicaid.) The benchmark federal subsidy is based on the Silver plan, and those choosing a more expensive plan pay more of the additional premium; similarly, for those choosing the Bronze plan, the subsidy pays more of the premium.

It is inequitable to treat households having the same income very differently, depending on whether their employer provides insurance or they buy insurance on the exchange. *Horizontal equity* is violated when low income households receiving exchange subsidies receive greater benefits than similar households unable to access the exchange subsidies.

The number of people eligible to buy insurance on the exchange will grow over time. Starting in 2016, exchanges will have to offer insurance to businesses with 51 to 100 employees and, in 2017, large employers will be allowed to buy insurance on the exchanges. States also have the authority, although many states have not yet exercised it, to prohibit insurers from selling insurance to individuals and small businesses outside the exchange (or require insurers to sell the same plans inside and outside the exchange) so that insurers cannot engage in preferred risk selection, enrolling good risks outside the exchange and having sicker individuals enroll on the exchange.

Age-Rated Premiums

Several important concerns have arisen with regard to the exchanges. The first concerns the premiums charged on the exchanges. Age-related premiums cannot vary by more than 3:1. Thus, those who are aged 50 to 60 years and incur, on average, six times more medical costs than 21-year-olds will pay a lower premium than they would otherwise, while 21-year-olds will pay a higher premium than one based on their expected medical costs. Further increasing the premiums for younger age groups are the additional mandated benefits included in the offered plans. These higher premiums will discourage many young people from buying health insurance on the exchange. The penalty under the individual mandate—$95 or 1 percent of income in 2014 and going up to $695 or 2.5 percent of income per adult in 2016—for not buying insurance is much less costly than paying a premium, even though the premium is subsidized. (If a serious illness occurs, the individual can then buy insurance, because insurers can no longer exclude people with preexisting conditions).

Those who are older have an incentive to buy insurance on the exchange because they receive two subsidies—a federal subsidy based on income and one subsidized by those who are younger and based on a lower age-rated premium. Young people generally have a higher uninsurance rate than older adults because they have lower income and believe they are less likely to need health insurance. However, because premiums are age rated at 3:1 rather than 6:1, fewer young people will buy insurance, causing average premiums to increase. Insurers are concerned that adverse selection will occur under an age-rated premium of 3:1 as the purchase of insurance by high-risk groups will not be offset by the low-risk groups.

Offering very narrow networks of providers that patients can see is an approach being used by insurers to limit the costs of adverse selection. By excluding costly major medical centers and specialists and negotiating lower rates with providers included in a limited network, the medical costs (and access to care) of enrollees with serious illnesses will be reduced.

Political Consequences of Employer-Mandated Health Insurance

Advantages

Given the inequities and inefficiencies associated with an employer mandate, why has it received so much political support? The political advantages received by various interest groups outweigh the inequities and inefficiencies that an employer mandate imposes on others. The employer mandate is attractive to government because it would appear that government would not have to raise a large amount of tax revenues for an employer-mandated national health insurance plan; such a plan could even reduce Medicaid expenditures by shifting the cost of low-wage labor off Medicaid to the employees and their employers. Thus, national health insurance offers the illusion that federal expenditures are little affected. States, whose Medicaid expenditures are increasing faster than any other expenditure, are reluctant to raise taxes. If the states are able to shift the medical costs of low-wage employees and their dependents from Medicaid to the employees and their employers, the states' own fiscal problems would be alleviated.

However, an employer mandate is more costly to the government than it appears. First, because employer-paid health insurance is not considered to be taxable income, the change in compensation from cash wages to health insurance decreases Social Security taxes as well as state and federal income taxes. Second, government welfare expenditures will be higher as a result of the increase in unemployment that results from layoffs of those with low wages and the reduction of employee income as more are shifted from full-time to part-time work. Third, additional federal subsidies and taxes are necessary to finance care for approximately one-third of the uninsured who are not employed or are dependents of an employee if this approach is to achieve universal coverage.

Hospital and physician organizations favor an employer mandate because it would provide insurance to those previously without it, increasing the demand for hospital and physician services. Payment levels to health providers would be higher than Medicaid payment levels. Health insurance companies would similarly benefit because the demand for their services would grow. Health insurers favored the ACA's employer mandate but opposed the final bill when the individual mandate penalty for not buying insurance was weakened. With the elimination of the preexisting condition exclusion and a small penalty for not having insurance, insurers were concerned that adverse selection would occur.

Large employers and their unions—which thought they would be unaffected because they already provide health benefits in excess of the mandated minimum—believed they would benefit competitively from employer-mandated insurance because the labor costs of their low-wage competitors would increase, making those competitors less price competitive. More than two decades ago, Robert Crandall, the chair of American Airlines, stated that as a result of the difference between the medical costs of American employees and those of Continental Airlines employees, "Continental's unit cost advantage vs. American's is enormous—and worse yet, is growing! ... which is why we're supporting ... legislation mandating minimum [health] benefit levels for all employees" (*Wall Street Journal* 1987).

Opposition

The major political opposition to an employer mandate has come from small businesses. These firms are aware of the consequences of an employee tax on the prices they would have to charge, on demand for their goods and services, and on their demand for labor. Opposition by small businesses was an important reason the Clinton Administration's legislation failed. In an attempt to buy off the political opposition of the powerful small business lobby, the Obama Administration treated small businesses (those with fewer than 50 employees) differently: They would be provided with subsidies to offset their higher costs. These promised subsidies did not overcome the skepticism of small businesses, however.

Summary

An employer-mandated national health insurance plan has numerous political advantages. Although an employer mandate statutorily imposes most of the cost on employers, in reality a large portion of the cost is shifted to the employee in the form of lower wages (or other fringe benefits). An employer mandate is not equitable because it disproportionately affects less-skilled workers and treats employees with the same income differently, depending on whether their employers provide health insurance. The mandate increases the cost to employers of low-wage workers and imposes a financial burden on those least able to afford it. An important reason for low-wage employees' lack of insurance is that they have more pressing needs for their limited income, and Medicaid is available to them as a substitute to buying private health insurance.

An employer mandate does not achieve universal coverage because not all of the uninsured are employed. (Thus, an individual mandate was added to an employer mandate to achieve universal coverage, together with the ACA's provision for state health insurance exchanges and income-related federal subsidies.) Further, likely unintended consequences of the ACA's employer mandate are decreases in demand for low-wage labor and a reduction in employee work hours so that employers can avoid the tax imposed for having employees without health insurance. Alternative approaches for achieving national health insurance need to be examined to avoid these labor market distortions.

Discussion Questions

1. What are the characteristics of the uninsured?
2. Would it be equitable to provide all employees in small firms with a subsidy to purchase health insurance?
3. What is the likely effect of employer-mandated health insurance on the employer's demand for labor?
4. Does an employer-mandated health insurance tax have a regressive, proportional, or progressive effect on the income of employees and consumers?
5. Which groups favor and which groups oppose an employer mandate for achieving national health insurance? Why?
6. Why did the ACA include an individual mandate with the employer mandate?

Notes

1. The Medical Expenditure Panel Survey–Household Component produces estimates of the uninsured for three different periods within a year: any time during the year, throughout the first half of the year, and the entire year. In 2011—the latest year for which all three measures are available—25.2 percent of the population younger than age 65 years (nonelderly) were uninsured at some point during the year, 21.1 percent were uninsured throughout the first half of the year, and 14.5 percent were uninsured the entire year (Chu 2013).

2. Kolstad and Kowalski (2012) estimated that the employer mandate instituted in Massachusetts decreased wages by an average of $6,058 annually, which was only slightly smaller than the average cost of the mandate to employers.

3. If an employer hires a 50th employee, the ACA's employer mandate creates a huge tax on that additional employee. The employer would have to pay a penalty of $2,000 per employee, minus the first 30 employees; thus, the additional cost of the 50th employee, excluding her wages, is $40,000 (50 − 30 = 20 employees × $2,000). This high marginal tax on a 50th employee is a disincentive for the employer to hire that additional employee.

Additional Reading

Krueger, A., and U. Reinhardt. 1994. "Economics of Employer Versus Individual Mandates." *Health Affairs* 13 (2, Part II): 34–53.

References

Agency for Healthcare Research and Quality (AHRQ). 2013. *Health Insurance Coverage of the Civilian Noninstitutionalized Population: Percent by Type of Coverage and Selected Population Characteristics, United States, First Half of 2012.* Accessed March 2014. http://meps.ahrq.gov/mepsweb/data_stats/ summ_tables/hc/hlth_insr/2012/alltables.pdf.

Blumberg, L. 1999. "Who Pays for Employer-Sponsored Health Insurance?" *Health Affairs* 18 (6): 58–61.

Chu, M. C. 2013. "The Uninsured in America, 1996–2012: Estimates for the U.S. Civilian Noninstitutionalized Population Under Age 65." *Statistical Brief* No. 420, August. http://meps.ahrq.gov/data_files/publications/st420/ stat420.shtml.

Congressional Budget Office (CBO). 2012. "CBO and JCT's Estimates of the Effects of the Affordable Care Act on the Number of People Obtaining Employment-Based Health Insurance." Posted March. http://cbo.gov/sites/default/files/cbofiles/attachments/03-15-ACA_and_Insurance_2.pdf.

Kaiser Family Foundation and the Health Research and Educational Trust (HRET). 2013. "Employer Health Benefits: 2013 Annual Survey." Published August 20. http://kaiserfamilyfoundation.files.wordpress.com/2013/08/8465-employer-health-benefits-20132.pdf.

Kolstad, J., and A. Kowalski. 2012. *Mandate-Based Health Reform and the Labor Market: Evidence from the Massachusetts Reform. NBER Working Paper* No. 17933. Cambridge, MA: National Bureau of Economic Research.

Pauly, M., and A. Leive. 2013. "The Unintended Consequences of Postponing the Employer Mandate." *New England Journal of Medicine* 369: 691–93.

Rhoades, J. 2013. Personal correspondence with the author, December 4.

Wall Street Journal. 1987. "Notable and Quotable." *Wall Street Journal* August 8, p. 16.

CHAPTER

NATIONAL HEALTH INSURANCE: WHICH APPROACH AND WHY?

34

Ntional health insurance is an idea whose time has often come and then gone. However, in 2010 President Obama with the Democrats controlling both Houses of Congress enacted the Affordable Care Act (ACA), over the opposition of all House and Senate Republicans. The legislation was intended to provide medical coverage for 95 percent of the population by covering an additional 32 million. The legislation is complex; it expands coverage by increasing eligibility for Medicaid, by providing insurance subsidies on government insurance exchanges, and by requiring everyone to have insurance (individual mandate). Also included are financial penalties if people are not insured, a series of different types of taxes, and reductions in Medicare provider reimbursement to pay for the program. Regulations were imposed on the insurance industry, and state-based insurance exchanges are to be established. Most of the legislation's benefits were phased in at the beginning of 2014, with the last ones implemented in 2019. (See the Appendix for a brief description of different elements of the legislation.)

The ACA is not the end of the quest for national health insurance; instead, it is a beginning. It is likely that many aspects will be revised as regulations are written regarding its implementation; the long-term care program (CLASS Act) has already been repealed as being unworkable; the dramatic payment reductions to hospitals (productivity adjustments) will need to be changed; and the ACA's financing will have to be revisited so that it does not contribute to an already enormous federal deficit.[1] Thus, many of the plan's features will change, evolve over time, and return to the political agenda.

To have a basis by which the new legislation can be evaluated, we examine in this chapter different proposals for national health insurance. The current system is a mixture of private and public financing with elements of market competition and regulation; the ACA continues this mix of public and private aspects. In contrast, general national health insurance proposals rely more on one approach to financing and delivery.

A variety of national health insurance plans have been proposed—from replicating the Canadian (single-payer) system to expanding existing public programs for the poor to mandating employers to provide coverage for their employees to providing tax credits for the purchase of health insurance. The proponents of each approach claim different virtues for their plans—one plan is more likely to limit the growth of medical expenditures, one will require a small tax increase to implement, another will allow individuals greater choice, and still another may be more politically acceptable. Unless some commonly accepted criteria are established on what national health insurance should accomplish, evaluating and choosing among these plans will be difficult.

Criteria for National Health Insurance

Economists are concerned with two issues: efficiency and equity. Efficiency has two parts: production efficiency and consumption efficiency. The equity criterion is concerned with equitable redistribution.

Production Efficiency

Production efficiency, as the first criterion, determines whether the services (for a given level of quality) are produced at the lowest cost. Efficiency in production not only includes whether the hospital portion of a treatment is produced at the lowest cost but also whether the treatment itself is produced at the minimum cost. Unless the treatment is provided in the lowest cost mix of settings—such as hospitals, outpatient care, and home care—the overall cost of providing the treatment will not be as low as possible.

Ensuring that each component of the treatment (such as hospital services), as well as the entire medical treatment, is produced efficiently requires appropriate financial incentives. These incentives are usually placed on the providers of medical services; however, they could also be placed on consumers, as would occur when enrollees choose among competing health plans and pay out of pocket the additional cost of more expensive plans (or under a health savings account approach). On whom to place the incentives is a controversial issue, but whether the plan includes appropriate incentives for efficiency in production is not.

Consumption Efficiency

Consumption efficiency is controversial. In other sectors of the economy, consumers make choices regarding the amount of income to allocate to different goods and services. Consumers have incentives to consider the costs and benefits of their choices. Spending their funds on one good or service means forgoing the benefits of another good or service. When consumers allocate their funds in this manner, resources are directed to their highest-valued uses as perceived by consumers.

Some are opposed to having consumers decide how much should be spent on medical services. They would prefer to have the government decide how much is allocated to medical care, as in the Canadian healthcare system. Yet Canadians are unable to purchase additional private health insurance to forgo waits for open-heart surgery, hip replacements, or treatment of other illnesses. Inherent in the concept of consumption efficiency is that the purpose of national health insurance is to benefit the consumer and that the consumer will be free to purchase more medical services than the minimum level offered in any health insurance plan.

Even if one accepts the concept of consumer decision making, concern has arisen that the costs of consumers' choices may be distorted. If the cost of one choice is subsidized and other choices are not, consumers will demand more of the subsidized choice than if they had to pay its full costs, resulting in consumption inefficiency. For example, the government does not consider employer-purchased health insurance to be taxable income to the employee. Consumers purchase more health insurance because health insurance is paid with before-tax dollars, whereas other choices (such as education and housing) must be paid for with after-tax dollars. The tax-free status of employer-paid health insurance, therefore, is a cause of inefficiency. Thus, this second criterion for national health insurance plans is whether consumers are able to decide how much of their income they want to spend on medical services and whether any subsidies distort the costs of their choices.

When production and consumption efficiency are achieved through the use of appropriate incentives, *the rate of increase in medical expenditures is considered to be appropriate.* Having a national health insurance objective of limiting the rate of increase in medical expenditures to, for example, a specified percent increase in growth domestic product (GDP) per capita, would be inappropriate if achieving this objective meant sacrificing the goals of consumption and production efficiency.

Equitable Redistribution

Presumably, an important (and some would say the only) objective of national health insurance is to provide additional medical services to the poor. When national health insurance plans are evaluated on how those with low income are to be subsidized, one must examine which population groups benefit (or are subsidized) and which population groups bear the costs (or pay higher taxes). For *equitable redistribution* to occur, those with higher income are expected to incur net costs (their taxes are in excess of their benefits), whereas those with low income should receive net benefits (benefits in excess of costs). When an individual's costs are not equal to the benefits he receives, redistribution occurs. Thus, if redistribution is the goal, high-income groups should subsidize the care of those with low income; whether equitable redistribution occurs is the third criterion for evaluating alternative national health insurance plans.

Crucial for determining whether redistribution goes from high- to low-income groups is the definition of beneficiaries and how the plan is financed. Ideally, those with the lowest income should receive the largest subsidy (which would decline as income rises), and the subsidy should be financed by a tax that is either proportional or progressive to income. If the tax is proportional to income (e.g., a flat tax of 5 percent regardless of income), those with the lowest income will receive a net benefit because the subsidy they receive (sufficient to purchase a minimum benefit package) will exceed the taxes they pay. When a progressive tax such as an income tax (with a rate that increases as income level increases) is used to finance benefits to those with low income, the redistribution from those with high income to those with low income is even greater.

An income tax is the most equitable method of financing a redistributive program because it is either a proportional tax or a progressive tax and would place the greater cost burden on those with high income. The disadvantages of an income tax are that it is highly visible and therefore likely to generate political opposition from middle- and high-income groups. Further, while income tax financing is generally regarded as being more equitable, it is a tax on work effort and may therefore cause a decrease in the supply of such effort.

Payroll taxes are imposed on the employer and their employees. A regressive payroll tax (a certain dollar amount per employee or a percent of the employee's income up to a certain amount of income), such as Social Security tax or a sales tax, takes a higher portion of income from those who have low income than from those with high income (because a greater portion of the the latter group's income is above the threshold for taxation). Because regressive taxes require low-income employees to pay a higher percentage of their income than required of high-income employees, such taxes are a less desirable method of financing redistributive programs. A sales tax—particularly if it does not exclude such expenditures as food—could be regressive in that those with low income pay a higher percentage of their income than do those with high income. A small increase in a sales tax typically generates a great deal of tax revenue and is not as visible a tax as income or property taxes; property taxes are paid in a lump sum, making their magnitude very visible to voters. "Sin" taxes—taxes on alcohol and cigarettes, for example—are also regressive but are economically efficient when the beneficiaries of such goods are required to pay the full costs of their consumption.

In fact, when a regressive tax is used, the tax paid by many low-income persons may exceed the value of the benefits they receive. For example, if everyone is eligible to receive the same set of benefits but those with high income use more medical services—perhaps because they are located closer to medical providers or their attitudes toward seeking care are different from those with less education (who also may have low income)—the taxes paid by those with low income may exceed the benefits they receive. Perversely, those with low income may end up subsidizing the care received by those with high income. (This also occurs when low-income nonelderly workers subsidize the health benefits of high-income elderly.)

A user tax occurs when those receiving the benefits incur the full cost of those benefits. An example is a tax on cigarettes, which is used to pay the additional medical costs incurred by smokers. An individual mandate—whereby everyone must purchase a minimum or a defined health insurance policy (discussed later in the chapter)—may also be considered similar to a user fee; everyone would pay for their expected medical costs.

Deficit financing—whereby the government borrows the money to subsidize different population groups—shifts the cost burden to future generations. Therein lie both its political advantage and its inequity. Deficit financing from a legislator's perspective is ideal; future generations do not vote on current policies, thereby politicians can provide benefits without imposing any costs on current voters. Deficit financing is regressive in that current populations, including those with high income, are subsidized by future generations, including those with low income (depending on the type of tax used for financing the deficit). As the federal deficit becomes too large, however, macroeconomic effects may occur, and the public is likely to view a presidential administration that greatly increases the deficit as being too reckless.

An examination of the size of the benefits received by income level in relation to the amount of tax paid is important. Income tax financing is the preferred way to achieve redistribution because it results in greater net benefits to those with low income.

The different types of taxes that have been used in financing Medicaid, Medicare, and the ACA, as well as additional types of taxes that might be used, are shown in Exhibit 34.1. Included with each type of tax is its visibility and equitability.

Based on our discussion of efficiency and equitable redistribution thus far, a national health insurance plan should provide incentives for efficiency in production; should enable consumers to decide how much of their income they want to spend on medical care; and should be redistributive—those with low income should receive net benefits, whereas those with high income should bear costs in excess of their benefits. All national health insurance proposals should be judged by how well they fulfill these criteria.

An important reason national health insurance plans fail to meet these efficiency and equitable redistribution criteria is that national health insurance proposals have objectives other than improving efficiency or equitable redistribution. These other objectives become obvious when the explicit efficiency and redistributive criteria are used.

National Health Insurance Proposals

Many different types of national health insurance plans have been proposed. Some proposals are incremental in that they build on the current system and do not propose changes in the delivery of medical services. Others are more radical, and dramatic changes are proposed in the financing and delivery of medical services. In general, however, the types of national health insurance plans proposed can be classified into three broad categories: (1) a single-payer (Canadian) system, (2) employer-mandated health insurance with an individual mandate, and (3) income-related tax credits. Although separate chapters are devoted to the Canadian approach and an employer mandate, we present a brief description of each, together with an evaluation of how well they achieve the three criteria.

Single-Payer System

Under a single-payer system the entire population is covered; benefits are uniform for all; no out-of-pocket expenses are incurred for basic medical services; and, most important, private insurance for hospital and medical services is not permitted (one cannot opt out of the single-payer system). The method of financing may be a combination of income taxes and other sources

EXHIBIT 34.1
Taxes for
Financing
Redistributive
Healthcare
Programs

Type of Tax	Visibility	Equitability	Medicaid	Medicare	ACA
Income tax	High	Progressive		Parts B & D	
Sales tax	Low	Regressive			Insurer, medical devices, etc.
Sin tax	Low	Regressive			Premiums on smokers
Payroll tax	Low	Regressive (becoming progressive)		Part A, ACA	Employer mandate
User fee	High	B = C			Individual mandate
Deficit financing	Low	Regressive B = current generation C = future generation	Federal Medicaid	Parts B & D, ACA	

NOTE: Property taxes are not considered as a source for financing healthcare services.
B = Benefits
C = Costs

of funds, such as payroll taxes on the employer and employee, Medicare and Medicaid payments, "sin" taxes (on alcohol and tobacco), or even a sales tax.

The major advantage of a single-payer system is its apparent simplicity in achieving universal coverage. Access to care by those with low income and the uninsured is likely to be improved. Single-payer proponents also claim that less would be spent per capita on medical services and total medical expenses would account for a smaller percentage of GDP.

The major disadvantages of a single-payer approach concern consumption and production efficiency (see Chapter 32). Global budget caps are used to limit total medical expenditures. Fixed budgets are imposed on hospitals, their capital outlays are controlled by a central authority, and annual limits are placed on the amount each physician can earn. These arbitrarily determined budget levels limit the amount consumers can spend on medical services, forcing them to wait for services or do without. Those with higher income are able to skip the queue by traveling outside the country for their medical services. The result is consumer inefficiency. Further, incentives to achieve production efficiency are lacking in a single-payer system, as are incentives for prevention and innovation.

Expansion of Public Programs

Somewhat similar to a single-payer system is the proposal to expand existing public programs, such as Medicaid, by increasing the income limits to allow greater numbers of those with low income and the uninsured to become eligible.[2] Medicaid is funded by general income taxes, and its beneficiaries are those with low income; thus, the equitable redistribution goal would be appropriate. Advocates of expanding public programs claim that no major changes in the financing or delivery system are required; only changes in the eligibility criteria are needed. Similarly, more uninsured children could be covered by the Children's Health Insurance Program (CHIP) simply by expanding its eligibility levels, which was done in the 2010 renewal of CHIP.

Some have also proposed that uninsured adults aged 55 to 65 years be allowed to buy into Medicare. Expanding Medicare to include those younger than age 65 years and increasing Medicaid and CHIP eligibility to include those with higher income would eventually bring more people into a single-payer-type system (often the goal of such proponents). Although differences between Medicare and Medicaid exist, both programs have the same characteristics as a single-payer system. Beneficiaries of these programs pay little if anything for use of medical services (particularly when the Medicare patient has Medigap supplementary coverage) and have free choice of provider (except for those enrolled in a Medicaid HMO), providers are paid fee-for-service, and the government controls expenditures by limiting provider fees. These programs have none of the cost-containment and quality programs—such as utilization management and care coordination—used by the private sector, nor do they have any incentives for provider efficiency.[3]

Some advocates of expanding public programs view "Medicare for All" as an approach to achieving a single-payer system in the United States. As private health insurance premiums and out-of-pocket expenses increase and as private health plans limit their provider networks and restrict referrals, many privately insured would prefer becoming part of traditional Medicare with its unlimited access to providers, ability to self-refer to any provider, and heavily subsidized costs. However, expanding Medicare to include all those younger than 65 years old would merely hasten the time before the inefficient Medicare system goes bankrupt, the federal deficit for Medicare soars beyond its current deficit of $43 trillion (Boards of Trustees 2013, tables V.G2, V.G4, and V.G6), and payroll and income taxes would have to increase along with premiums and cost sharing. Eventually, price controls are placed on providers, severely limiting patient's access to care, as occurs under the Canadian system and Medicaid.[4]

The problem with expanding Medicaid to care for a greater portion of the uninsured (up to 133 percent of the federal poverty level, as proposed by the ACA) is that many states cannot afford their share of the matching funds required to include more of the uninsured. Particularly in times of recession, states lack the funds and are reluctant to increase taxes to expand eligibility limits. In fact, many states have been reducing enrollment in CHIP as their tax revenues have fallen and they face budget deficits. Medicaid and CHIP do not have a stable source of funding, and many states are reluctant to commit themselves to expanding these programs.

Employer-Mandated Health Insurance

An employer mandate requires employers to either purchase health insurance for their employees or pay a specified amount (tax) per employee. Although the financial burden for purchasing health insurance is placed on the employer, studies have found that the burden is shifted back to the employee in the form of lower wages. In effect, a tax is imposed on low-wage workers (who are typically without health insurance), requiring them to buy health insurance. Under the ACA, the employer tax for not providing health insurance to their employees is $2,000 per employee, which is shifted back to the employee in the form of lower wages (or slower raises). Many employees earning near the minimum wage whose wages cannot be reduced to offset the employer tax will likely be let go.

The ACA requires that private health insurance cover the 10 Essential Health Benefits.[5] These mandated benefits that individuals and employees are required to purchase are more than most low-wage and other workers are willing or able to pay. Thus, consumption efficiency is difficult to achieve. (If the employer does not buy insurance for their employees, then their low-wage employees are eligible for subsidies when buying insurance on the exchange.)

Production efficiency can be achieved under an employer mandate by having health plans compete for employees. However, the inability to achieve equitable redistribution (the employer tax is shifted to low-wage employees) is the biggest disadvantage of the employer mandate.

Individual Mandate

An employer mandate will not, by itself, achieve universal coverage. To achieve universal coverage, the government must ensure that the two groups without health insurance—those who can afford insurance but refuse to purchase it and those who cannot afford insurance—have coverage. It is for this reason the ACA has imposed an individual mandate; everyone above a minimum level of income is required to have health insurance, the remainder (except for the undocumented) become eligible for Medicaid. Many uninsured are financially able to purchase a high-deductible health insurance plan but choose not to do so. If someone who can afford insurance does not have catastrophic coverage and suffers a large medical expense that has to be subsidized by the community, the person is shifting the risk—hence the cost of catastrophic coverage—to the rest of the community.[6] Thus, for an employer mandate to achieve universal coverage, it must be combined with an individual mandate. The ACA continues and expands Medicaid for low-wage employees and the unemployed whose income is below 133 percent of the federal poverty level.

Under the ACA, proof of insurance must be included on the person's federal income tax form. Lack of such evidence would result in the government collecting the appropriate penalty.[7] Thus, those who could afford health insurance would not become a burden to others if they suffered a serious illness or accident.

Income-Related Tax Credits

Various income-related tax credit approaches have been proposed over the years. The following proposal attempts to achieve universal coverage in an equitable manner while providing incentives for efficiency in the use and delivery of medical services.

Refundable Tax Credits

A refundable tax credit would replace the current, inequitable system whereby the employer purchases health insurance for their employees and the employers' contribution is not considered to be taxable income to the employee. As shown in exhibits 6.2 and 6.3, high-wage employees benefit more (than low-wage workers do) from tax-exempt, employer-paid health insurance because they are in a higher tax bracket. An additional inequity is that employees whose employer does not buy health insurance and those who are self-employed are not eligible for the same tax-free benefit when they buy insurance.

As part of the refundable tax credit proposal, the current exclusion of employer-purchased health insurance from an employee's taxable income would be removed as the tax credit is substituted in its place. The lost revenues from this open-ended subsidy would be an important revenue source to be made available for a refundable tax credit (in 2013 dollars, this amounted to an annual loss of federal, state, and Social Security taxes of $248 billion) (CBO 2013).[8]

A refundable tax credit of $5,000 would be provided to individuals and $10,000 would be provided to families. Everyone would receive a refundable tax credit for the purchase of health insurance. Taxpayers would be allowed to subtract the tax credit to purchase health insurance from their income taxes. Individuals whose tax credit exceeds their tax liabilities would receive a refund for the difference. Thus, if a person's income is too low to pay taxes, the full amount of the credit would be used to provide her with a voucher for a managed care plan. As a person's income increases to the point where she has an income tax liability, the tax credit would offset part of the liability, leaving her with part of the tax credit to be used toward purchasing a health insurance voucher. The tax credit would have to be refundable, or the benefits would go only to those who pay taxes, excluding those with low income.

The full tax-credit subsidy would be equal to the premium of a managed care plan. (These refundable tax credits essentially would be vouchers for a health plan for persons with little or no tax liability.) The tax credit could be an equal dollar amount for all families, such as $10,000, or could be lower for those with higher income. Under a refundable tax credit that declines with higher income, the subsidy would go to those with the lowest income. However, providing a tax credit of an absolute dollar amount would be more politically acceptable in that those earning middle and high income would also receive some benefit.

The value of the voucher could be determined in several ways. First, the government may take bids from managed care plans, as occurs under Medicare Advantage. Second, the voucher could equal the premium of the lowest (or second-lowest) cost managed care plan in the market; this approach is used by more and more employers. In this manner, the preferences of the non-poor for what they want to purchase from a managed care plan would determine the benefits to be offered to those with low income.

(Those receiving a full or partial voucher could choose a more expensive health plan by paying the additional cost themselves.)

To achieve universal coverage, a refundable tax credit could also be combined with an individual mandate. For those opposed to an individual mandate, the tax credit would be an incentive to purchase insurance, which would slowly decline in value the longer the person delays purchasing insurance. (A similar approach is used in encouraging seniors to enroll in Medicare Parts B and D by increasing their premiums the longer they delay enrolling).

The refundable tax credit would also replace the current Medicaid program, using Medicaid expenditures to partially offset the cost of the refundable credit. Currently, eligible Medicaid adults and children would receive the same refundable tax credit as others and have greater choice in their selection of health plans. Eventually, as Medicare must be restructured to become financially viable, Medicare could also be included in a refundable tax credit plan. There is little reason to have different financing systems for different population groups—those who work, those who are retired, and those who are uninsured because of their low income.

Consumption efficiency would be achieved by permitting individuals to purchase greater coverage or policies with fewer restrictions on access to providers by paying the additional premium for such plans. Production efficiency would presumably occur as health plans compete for enrollees based on price, quality of services, and access to care. By providing a refundable tax credit, financed from general income taxes, redistributive equity would be achieved.

Health Savings Accounts

A proposal that places greater responsibility for medical expenses on the individual is the use of a health savings account (HSA) in conjunction with a high-deductible, catastrophic health insurance policy. HSAs could be an option under the employer mandate and the refundable tax credit proposals.

The basic idea behind an HSA is to combine an inexpensive high-deductible insurance policy with a tax-free savings account. An HSA plan works as follows: A person (or his employer acting on his behalf) purchases a high-deductible health plan and then annually contributes a specified tax-free amount into the HSA. (A high-deductible catastrophic policy has a much lower premium than a comprehensive health insurance policy has.) In 2014, the maximum that can be contributed each year to an HSA account is $3,300 for an individual and $6,550 for a family—or the amount of the deductible of the high-deductible health plan, whichever is lower. The maximum out-of-pocket expenses for which the person is liable can be as high as $6,350 a year for an individual or $12,700 for a family. A person would be at risk for the difference between the out-of-pocket maximum ($6,350) and his annual contribution to his HSA ($3,300), which is $3,050.[9]

HSA proponents claim that an HSA reduces the monthly insurance premium and provides individuals with a financial incentive to be concerned with the prices they pay for medical services and think carefully about which services they really need. (Most high-deductible health plans also include several preventive visits.) Proponents believe that if consumers have a greater financial incentive, medical expenditures will increase at a lower rate. The funds in the HSA account can be invested, grow tax free, and be used later for long-term care expenses (or any other uses, as the funds belong to the individual).

Opponents of HSAs claim that any savings would be relatively small because once the out-of-pocket maximum is reached; the patient has no incentive to spend less. Critics also claim that the adoption and availability of new technology, which is typically used in an inpatient setting, determine expenditure increases, not spending for outpatient services. HSA critics further claim that HSAs would split the insurance risk pools; healthier, lower-risk persons would choose HSAs (thereby gaining financially), and higher-risk persons would remain in more comprehensive plans. HSA proponents disagree, arguing that higher-risk persons would also benefit from and choose HSAs because their total medical out-of-pocket expenses, including prescription drugs, would be subject to a limit. Under Medicare, for example, out-of-pocket expenses are *not* limited.

HSAs include financial incentives for consumption efficiency to occur. (If consumers are to become informed purchasers, however, more information on provider performance and prices is needed.) Presumably, production efficiency would result as providers compete on price and as managed care plans become responsible for providing catastrophic services. Government subsidies would be needed to enable those with low income to establish HSAs.

Health Insurance Exchanges

With a refundable tax credit, the health insurance would belong to the individual. If the individual changes jobs, she would not have to worry about what type of coverage the new employer offered or whether she would have a waiting period for a preexisting medical condition. Further, employers—particularly small employers—would not have to be concerned with administering or bearing any health insurance costs if they hire low-wage employees; *health insurance would no longer be connected to the workplace.* Previously, employers purchased their employees' health insurance because employer-paid health insurance was tax-exempt. In place of the employer, everyone could use state health insurance exchanges. Everyone would be able to choose among competing insurers offering different benefit coverage. (State health insurance exchanges were included in the ACA, although many states declined to start an exchange and the ACA's regulations are more restrictive than many would prefer; for example, insurers must offer more costly benefit coverage, modified community rating, and gender rating.) State health insurance exchanges—which existed before the ACA in a number of states, including Massachusetts and Utah—make for a more competitive health insurance market.

Under the refundable tax credit proposal, people buying insurance on the exchange would be classified into risk categories by age and family status. The current cross-subsidies that exist as part of the ACA, such as young adults subsidizing older persons, would be eliminated; each risk group's premium would reflect its actuarial cost, thereby lowering the cost of insurance for those who are young and have lower income.

Preexisting condition exclusions have long been a concern of those unable to purchase health insurance. In the past, many states established high-risk pools to provide subsidized insurance for those with a preexisting condition. The ACA prohibits insurers from excluding those with preexisting conditions, assuming that the individual mandate will provide insurers with a sufficiently large insurance pool to negate any effects of adverse selection. Unfortunately, the ACA's penalty for not having insurance is so low that many people who decide to remain uninsured will not be deterred by it. A stronger penalty should be adopted, or as with a tax credit proposal, individuals would receive a declining value of the tax credit the longer they refuse to buy insurance.

Eliminating State Mandates

State health mandates require private health insurance to cover specific health providers, such as chiropractors, acupuncturists, marriage therapists, and athletic trainers; specific insurance benefits, such as hair transplants, in vitro fertilization, and massage therapy; and specific populations, such as non-custodial children and terminated workers. There are 2,271 state mandates across the 50 states (as of 2012). Many states also have regulations requiring *any willing provider* (AWP) laws, which restrict a health plan's ability to exclude hospitals and physicians from its provider networks.

These state mandates increase the cost of health insurance, making it too expensive for those with low income. Depending on where one lives, mandates can increase the cost of a policy by between 10 percent and 50 percent (Bunce 2013). The high cost of state mandates (as high as several thousand dollars in insurance premiums per person per year) directly affects the number of insured (and uninsured) in a state.

These state regulations would not be needed under this proposal, and eliminating them would reduce the cost of health insurance. If individuals wish to purchase these services—such as hair transplants and fertility treatments—on their own with after-tax dollars, they would be free to do so.

Advantages of Income-Related Tax Credits

The income-related voucher meets the efficiency and equitable redistribution criteria in the following ways:

Everyone is obligated to have a minimum set of health insurance benefits. Those with the lowest income would be assured of adequate health insurance and would receive the largest net benefits under the proposed plan.

The size of the subsidy would decline as income grows. Employer-purchased health insurance would no longer be tax exempt, and the employee's taxable income would increase. The higher tax revenues, together with funds from the income tax system and Medicaid, would then provide the funding for the income-related subsidies. Thus, the financing source is based on progressive taxation.

Requiring universal coverage through an individual mandate means that cost shifting by those who do not purchase insurance to those who do would no longer occur.

The mandate to have insurance is on the *individual,* not the employer; thus, the individual would be able to change jobs without fear of losing insurance or being denied coverage because of a preexisting condition. Because everyone would be required to have insurance, an employer should be willing to hire someone who is older, is less healthy, or has a preexisting condition because no additional health insurance cost would be incurred by the employer or other employees.

Employees would have incentives to make cost-conscious choices, and a competitive health insurance market would help achieve efficiency and quality. The greater out-of-pocket liability for employees purchasing more expensive health plans would increase their price sensitivity to different managed care plans. Price (premium) sensitivity by employees (and employers acting on their behalf) would provide price incentives for managed care plans and providers, such as hospitals and physicians, to be as efficient as possible. Unless health plans were responsive to consumers at a premium the consumer was willing to pay, the health plans would not be able to compete in a price-competitive market.

A brief description and comparison of the three national health insurance proposals is presented in Exhibit 34.2.

EXHIBIT 34.2
A Comparison
of Three
National Health
Insurance
Proposals

Feature	Employer Mandate	Single-Payer System	Refundable Tax Credit (With or Without an Individual Mandate)
How does it work?	Requires all employers to buy health insurance for their employees or pay into a pool	Provides comprehensive coverage with no out-of-pocket payments; private insurance not permitted	Everyone is provided with a refundable tax credit to purchase health insurance; those with low income receive a voucher
Does it provide universal coverage?	Excludes those who work part-time and those who are not working; achieves universal coverage when an individual mandate is included	Achieves universal coverage	Achieves universal coverage when an individual mandate is included; the insurance belongs to the individual and not tied to the workplace
Is there consumption efficiency?	Partially: minimum mandated benefits are greater than low-income workers prefer, and employer may not provide choice of health plans	No: persons are not permitted to buy medical services or private insurance for services covered by the basic health plan	Yes: participants can choose among different health plans and can purchase additional medical services and insurance above minimum required catastrophic insurance
Is there production efficiency?	Plan relies on market-based competition to achieve production efficiency	No consumer or provider incentives are included to encourage efficiency, to minimize the cost of a treatment, or to provide preventive care	Plan includes consumer and provider incentives for efficiency; it relies on market-based competition to achieve production efficiency
Is it equitably financed?	Regressive: the plan retains tax-exempt employer coverage and a tax is imposed on employers and employees, including low-income employees without insurance	Partially regressive: there is pooling of funds from employers, Medicare, Medicaid, and increased payroll taxes	Progressive: tax-exempt employer-paid insurance is replaced with a refundable tax credit to everyone; those with low income receive income-related subsidies
What are the administrative costs?	High costs: because of multiple health plans, monitoring and enforcement of mandate	Low costs: too low to detect fraud and abuse or to institute disease management and other types of programs	High costs: because of multiple health plans, monitoring and enforcement of mandate
How are healthcare costs controlled?	Plan relies on the market to achieve appropriate rate of increase in costs	Plan relies on arbitrary budget caps and regulated fees	Plan relies on market to achieve appropriate rate of increase in costs

Fundamental Differences in Perspectives Regarding Government's Health Policy Role

The reason it is so difficult to achieve compromise when discussing health policy is that fundamental differences exist regarding the role of government and the private sector. These differences are ideological and reflect differences in constituent interests. For example, there are those who distrust the profit motive in healthcare and of individuals' ability to make appropriate healthcare choices. Others disagree, placing greater trust in market competition than government to achieve efficiency and ability to respond to consumer preferences.

These differences in belief in the role of government and the private sector also reflect the economic interests of important constituencies. Unions would like to shift their members' healthcare costs to the government (the taxpayer), thereby resulting in higher take-home wages for their members. Unions believe a single-payer system would achieve this goal, as they were able to shift their retirees' healthcare costs by having these retirees enroll in Medicare. Hospitals, physicians, insurers, and pharmaceutical companies believe they would be more profitable under a private system where the government's main role is to subsidize those with low income to enable them to buy healthcare in a privately operated system.

Exhibit 34.3 describes these differences in values, cost-containment approaches, and types of health plan preferred by each of these opposing ideologies/constituent interests.

Summary

National health insurance proposals should be judged according to their production efficiency, consumption efficiency, and equitable redistribution (whether those with low income receive a net benefit). A market-based system, in contrast to a single-payer system, has demonstrated its ability to achieve the goals of production efficiency and consumption efficiency. Subsidies to those with low income, such as through a refundable tax credit, are a direct method of improving equity and can provide greater choices and result in production efficiency when provided through a market-based system.

An important role of government under national health insurance would be to monitor quality and access to care received by those with low income. Government has not performed this function well for Medicaid patients. However, Medicaid can be eliminated by providing everyone with a refundable tax credit. Allowing those with low income to enroll in managed care plans that also serve other population groups and buying

Ideology	Values	Cost Containment	Redistribution
Left	• Trust in government as regulator • Distrust of profit motive • Distrust of consumers' ability to make choices	• Fee and price controls IPAB (hospitals, MDs) • Government negotiation with pharmaceutical companies • Comparative/cost-effectiveness	• Expand existing public programs • Expand eligibility for Medicare (age 55+) • Expand eligibility for Medicaid (by income and age) • Maintain employer-paid system • Single-payer program (by combining above programs)
Right	• Trust in market competition • Belief in necessity of financial incentives • Values consumer sovereignty and choices	• Markets and competition • FEHB for Medicare • Individual choice (HSAs) • Eliminate state mandates	• Income-related refundable tax credits • Medicare a fixed contribution program (premium support) • Income-related public programs • Cap amount of health insurance premiums that are tax exempt

EXHIBIT 34.3
Constituent/
Ideological
Differences on
Health Policy

FEHB: federal employees health benefits; HSA: health savings account; IPAB: independent payment advisory board

health insurance in state insurance exchanges would provide consumers with greater choice of health plans and achieve greater competition among insurers. Information on health plans, their prices, and the quality and access they provide would be important in achieving a competitive market. In addition to states providing information on each plan's performance, other organizations and websites likely would develop and offer information to assist consumers in making informed choices. These reporting and monitoring activities would benefit all enrollees, including those subsidized by the government.

Under a market-based national health insurance system, the rate of increase in medical expenditures would be based on what consumers, balancing cost and use of services, decide is appropriate. The government would not need to set arbitrary limits on total medical expenditures as occurs in a single-payer system and the ACA. Instead, the rate of increase in medical expenditures would be the "correct" rate because consumers, through their choices, would make the trade-off between access to care and premiums to pay for that level of access.

Discussion Questions

1. Discuss the criteria that should be used for evaluating alternative national health insurance proposals.
2. Evaluate the desirability of the following types of taxes for financing national health insurance: payroll, sales, and income tax.
3. What is the justification for requiring everyone (all those who can afford it) to purchase a minimum level of health insurance?
4. Outline (and justify) a proposal for national health insurance. As part of your proposal, discuss the benefits package, beneficiaries, method of financing, delivery of services, and role of government. How well does your proposal meet the criteria discussed in the chapter?
5. What are alternative ways for treating Medicare under national health insurance?

Notes

1. One stated objective of the administration in designing the new legislation was that it would not contribute to the federal deficit over a ten-year period. To achieve this goal, the new taxes and the reductions in Medicare expenditures used to finance the new benefits start at the beginning of the ten-year period, while the benefits (expenditures) become effective in only the last six of the ten years.
2. Proponents of the ACA claimed that the number of uninsured will decrease by 32 million; expanded Medicaid eligibility is intended to cover 16 million of those uninsured.
3. Medicaid production efficiency would be improved if the state were to offer Medicaid recipients a choice of competing health plans. Proposals for Medicare reform have similarly proposed providing all the aged with a subsidy to cover the cost of a basic health plan and allowing the aged to choose among different competing health plans, paying out-of-pocket the additional cost of a more expensive health plan, such as traditional Medicare. Such Medicare reform proposals would improve consumption efficiency and production efficiency.

4. Allowing just the uninsured to buy into Medicare would result in adverse selection; sicker individuals—those without employment-based health insurance—would pay a premium that is below their expected costs.

5. The ACA requires insurers to cover a broad range of mandated "essential" benefits, the scope of which is greater than typical individual policies previously sold. Insurers are required to permit parents to include their children, up to age 26 years, on their insurance policies and not be charged any more than for coverage of younger children. Mandated benefits include preventive services with no copayments, behavioral health, contraceptives, maternity care (even for single men and women past child-bearing age), outpatient prescription drugs, and pediatric dental and vision; annual lifetime limits on health benefits are prohibited. The more comprehensive and generous the insurance, the more expensive it is.

6. The ACA permits those younger than age 30 years to buy a catastrophic health plan.

7. Two serious problems with the individual mandate as enacted in the ACA are that the penalty for not buying insurance is low and that, effective in 2014, all insurers must accept anyone who wants to buy insurance, even if they have a preexisting medical condition. Thus, it is expected that many will pay the annual penalty and then, when they become ill, buy health insurance. Once they are better, they will drop their insurance. This form of adverse selection, unless changed, can destroy the health insurance market.

8. The ACA imposes a 40 percent tax on health coverage that exceeds $10,200 for individuals and $27,500 for families, thereafter indexed for inflation, starting in 2018.

9. Additional information on HSAs may be found at www.treasury.gov/resource-center/faqs/Taxes/Pages/Health-Savings-Accounts.aspx.

Additional Readings

Fuchs, V. 2009. "The Proposed Government Health Insurance Company: No Substitute for Real Reform." *New England Journal of Medicine* 360 (22): 2273–75.

Furman, J. 2008. "Health Reform Through Tax Reform: A Primer." *Health Affairs* 27 (3): 622–32.

References

Boards of Trustees of the Federal Hospital Insurance and Federal Supplementary Medical Insurance Trust Funds. 2013. *2013 Annual Report*. Published May. www.cms.gov/Research-Statistics-Data-and-Systems/Statistics-Trends-and-Reports/ReportsTrustFunds/Downloads/TR2013.pdf.

Bunce, V. C. 2013. *Health Insurance Mandates in the States 2012*. Executive Summary. The Council for Affordable Health Insurance. Published April. www.cahi.org/cahi_contents/resources/pdf/Mandatesinthestates2012Execsumm.pdf.

Congressional Budget Office (CBO). 2013. *The Distribution of Major Tax Expenditures in the Individual Income Tax System*. Published May. www.cbo.gov/sites/default/files/cbofiles/attachments/43768_DistributionTaxExpenditures.pdf.

FINANCING LONG-TERM CARE

Spending for long-term care services is expected to increase sharply over the next several decades. For the elderly (and their families), long-term care (LTC) expenditures represent a large uninsured financial risk; only a small percentage of the elderly protect themselves against possibly catastrophic LTC expenses by buying private LTC insurance. Federal and state governments also face huge financial pressures for paying for the LTC needs of the growing number of elderly. Medicaid, the primary government insurance program for LTC, pays for the majority of all LTC services (Calmus 2013).

How federal and state governments can limit their financial burden for paying for LTC for the aged, while ensuring that the elderly are protected from possibly catastrophic LTC expenditures, is a major public policy dilemma. More generally, how should LTC services should be financed, and by whom?[1]

The population is aging, as shown in Exhibit 35.1. The number of seniors are expected to increase from 37.3 million in 2012 (13.7 percent of the population) to 63.8 million in 2030 (20.3 percent of the population) to 65.8 million in 2050 (20.9 percent of the population). An aging population that is living longer increases the number at risk for needing LTC services. The fastest-growing group of the aged comprises those aged 85 years or older. This older group is expected to grow from 13.7 percent of all aged in 2012 (the oldest of the baby boomers started to retire in 2011) to 20.9 percent in 2050. As the impaired aged demand more services to assist them in activities necessary for daily living, the cost of providing those services is rising at a faster rate than is general inflation.

The Nature of Long-Term Care

LTC consists of a range of services for those who are unable to function independently, including services that can be provided in the person's home, such as shopping, preparing meals, and housekeeping; in community-based facilities, such as adult day care; and in nursing homes for those who are unable to perform most of the activities of daily living, such as bathing, toileting,

EXHIBIT 35.1

Percentage of US Population Aged 65 Years and Older, 1980–2050

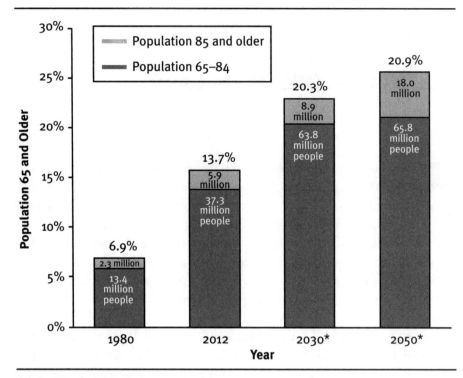

* Projected
SOURCE: Data from Census Bureau (2012).

and dressing. A nursing home is but the end of a spectrum for those with the most physical and mental impairments.

The need for LTC increases with age. As shown in exhibits 35.2 and 35.3, the group needing LTC the most comprises 50 percent of those aged 85 years and older. The need for nursing home care also increases with age. At any point in time (as of 2012), approximately 2.8 percent of the aged (about 1.2 million) are in a nursing home. An estimated 1 percent of those aged 65 to 74 years are in nursing homes, compared with 3 percent of those aged 75 to 84 years and 10 percent of those aged 85 years and older (AoA 2013). The main reasons for nursing home use are severe functional deficiencies, mental disabilities (such as Alzheimer's), and lack of a family member to provide services in the elderly's own home. As shown in Exhibit 35.3, the number of functional limitations increases with age.

Most LTC occurs in the home rather than in an institutional setting. Informal caregivers are predominantly family members or close relatives. Older men with a disability are more likely to have a surviving spouse to provide them with LTC than are older women. However, as those requiring LTC age, it becomes increasingly difficult for their spouse to provide the care or services they need. In 2004 (latest data available), wives provided 19.3 percent of husbands' LTC needs; husbands (because there were fewer

	Adult Day Services Center	Home Health Agency	Hospice	Nursing Home	Residential Care Community
Number of users (including under age 65)	273,200	4,742,500	1,244,500	1,383,700	713,300
Age	**Percentage of Users**				
Under 65	36.5	17.6	5.5	14.9	6.7
65 and over	63.5	82.4	94.5	85.1	93.3
65–74	19.4	24.6	16.4	14.9	10.4
75–84	27.2	32.2	31.3	27.9	32.4
85+	16.9	25.5	46.8	42.3	50.5

EXHIBIT 35.2
Users of Long-Term Care Services, by Provider Type and User Age, 2012

SOURCE: Data from Harris-Kojetin and colleagues (2013), Table 4.

	All Medicare Beneficiaries				
	Total	< 65	65–74	75–84	85+
Beneficiaries (in thousands)	50,186	8,382	22,321	13,089	6,394
Functional Limitation	**Beneficiaries as a Percentage of Column Total**				
None	49.3	21.5	65.8	51.0	24.8
IADL only	14.1	23.4	10.4	13.4	16.4
One to two ADLs	22.4	31.7	16.6	23.3	28.7
Three to six ADLs	14.2	23.5	7.2	12.4	30.1

EXHIBIT 35.3
Medicare Beneficiaries, by Age and Disability Level, 2011

ADL: activity of daily living; IADL: instrumental activity of daily living
SOURCE: Data from CMS (2011), Table 2.1.

husbands) provided 14.7 percent of wives' LTC needs. Daughters provided 43.2 percent, and sons provided 22.8 percent (Houser, Gibson, and Redfoot 2010, 54, Table A6).

Children bear a great portion of the informal care needs of their parents. Women more often than men provide this uncompensated care. When the impaired aged is a woman, typically a widow, children and relatives are the most frequent caregivers. These services by family members, although uncompensated, are costly to the caregivers in terms of added strain and reduced hours at work.

Current State of Long-Term Care Financing

LTC is expensive and represents a significant financial risk to the elderly. In 2014, the national average annual cost for a private room in a nursing home was $87,600 (Genworth Financial Inc. 2014, 18), and this figure is expected to almost triple by 2025 (MetLife Mature Market Institute 2012). A person turning 65 years old in 2000 had a 44 percent chance of entering a nursing home at some point in his life. Most of the aged who enter a nursing home will do so for a short period, but 19 percent will stay longer than five years and incur 89 percent of all nursing home costs. Because women have a longer life expectancy, a 65-year-old woman has a 51 percent chance of entering a nursing home during her lifetime and, upon entering, has an expected average stay of two years. In-home care is also expensive; the average cost for a home health aide is $21 per hour (MetLife Mature Market Institute 2012). Thus, LTC services in a nursing home or from an aide who comes to the home are too costly for most elderly on a fixed income and with limited assets. The uneven expenditures for LTC services and the very large financial risk for about 20 percent of the elderly indicate that insurance against such large possible losses would give rise to a large demand for private LTC insurance. And yet this has not occurred.

Many aged mistakenly believe Medicare will pay for their LTC needs; in fact, Medicare pays for certain, limited LTC expenses. Included as part of Medicare are home health care for those aged who need part-time skilled nursing care or therapy services and are under the care of a physician. A limited number of post-acute care days (100) in a skilled nursing home are covered for those discharged from a hospital. Medicare spending on these services accounted for about 29.7 percent of total LTC spending in 2012 (about $68.2 billion). Medicare does not cover the services needed when an aged person has decreased ability to care for himself because of chronic illness, a disability, or normal aging.

In 2012, spending from all public and private sources for LTC (for all ages) was $229.4 billion, which represented about 8.2 percent of total healthcare expenditures. The largest component of LTC services is for nursing homes, which represents 66 percent of such expenditures; home care represents 34 percent. The major sources of LTC financing are public programs—primarily Medicaid and Medicare—at 66.7 percent. Individuals provide about 25.5 percent of the costs out of pocket, and the remainder (about 7.7 percent) is covered by private LTC insurance. These percentages differ according to whether the LTC is provided in a nursing home or in the patient's home. LTC insurance covers 7.9 percent of nursing home costs and 7.2 percent of home health care. Private LTC insurance is beginning to become prevalent, but very few of the aged have such insurance. See Exhibit 35.4.

On average, 34 percent of all nursing home care costs, a significant financial burden for many, are paid out of pocket. Although the aged and their families pay about 9.4 percent of home health costs, these costs do not include the substantial nonfinancial burden imposed on families and relatives

Payment Source	Nursing Home Care	Home Health Care	Total
	Billions of Dollars		
Total	$151.6	$77.8	$229.4
Medicare	34.4	33.8	68.2
Medicaid	46.3	28.9	75.2
Other federal	4.4	1.0	5.4
Other state and local	3.1	1.1	4.2
Private insurance	12.0	5.6	17.6
Out-of-pocket and other sources	51.3	7.3	58.6
	Percentage of Total		
Total	100.0	100.0	100.0
Medicare	22.7	43.4	29.7
Medicaid	30.5	37.1	32.8
Other federal	2.9	1.3	2.4
Other state and local	2.0	1.4	1.8
Private insurance	7.9	7.2	7.7
Out-of-pocket and other sources	33.8	9.4	25.5

EXHIBIT 35.4
Estimated Spending on Long-Term Care Services, by Type of Service and Payment Source, 2012

SOURCE: Data from CMS (2014d).

who are unpaid caregivers. The Congressional Budget Office (2013) estimated that the economic value of family caregiving in 2011 for those aged 65 years and older was $234 billion. Lynn Feinberg and colleagues (2011) estimated that the economic value of family caregiving for people of all ages in 2009 was $450 billion.

Medicaid LTC Expenditures

Medicaid is a joint federal–state financing program for those with low income. Total Medicaid expenditures were $409 billion in 2012, of which 30.5 percent was for payment of LTC services; the remainder was for acute care services (CMS 2014a). States vary greatly in their per capita (per person within the state) annual expenditures for LTC—ranging from $1,189 in New York to $171 in Utah (CMS 2014e).

Medicaid is the major payer for nursing home care (30.5 percent) and pays for a limited amount of in-home coverage (37.1 percent). Medicaid is the payer of last resort, covering LTC expenses only after the impaired aged have exhausted their own financial resources. To qualify for Medicaid, an individual must first spend down his assets and is allowed to keep only $2,000. Current law permits a spouse to retain half of the couple's financial assets up to a maximum of $117,240 (inflation adjusted) in addition to a private home of any value if it is the principal residence (CMS 2014b).

To limit their Medicaid expenditures, states have restricted the availability of nursing home beds, paid nursing homes low rates, and provided limited in-home services to those eligible for Medicaid. The consequence of these policies has been a continual excess demand for nursing home beds by the impaired aged. Because demand exceeds supply and states set low payment rates, the quality of services provided is often poor. Few states pay nursing homes according to the level of care needed by the patient; thus, nursing homes have an incentive to admit Medicaid patients who have lower care needs and are less costly to care for. When a private-pay patient seeks nursing home care, he will be admitted before the Medicaid patient because his payment exceeds Medicaid reimbursement. As nursing home demand by private patients rises, the excess demand by Medicaid patients will become greater in those states that continue to limit the number of nursing home beds.

The risk of a person entering a nursing home as a private patient and having to spend down her assets was only 6.3 percent in 1985 (latest available data). (The probabilities vary by race and gender.) Most of the aged (59.2 percent) entering a nursing home were private patients; the remainder were those already eligible for Medicaid (17.3 percent) and Medicare or other payers (23.5 percent). Of those private-pay patients who used fewer than three months of nursing home care, 2.7 percent had to spend down their assets to qualify for Medicaid eligibility. For a stay up to six months, a total of 10.5

percent of the aged had to spend down. As the stay increased up to two years, 18.2 percent had to spend down (Spillman and Kemper 1995).

The probability of entering a nursing home for 65-year-old men is 27 percent and for 65-year-old women is 44 percent. Of those who do, 12 percent of men and 22 percent of women will spend more than five years there (Brown and Finkelstein 2008). Nursing homes cost nearly $90,000 per year. Although the lifetime risk of a person entering a nursing home and having to spend down her assets is relatively low, the fear of incurring this financial burden is the basis of the demand for LTC insurance and government subsidies.

Home care expenditures have become a growing share of Medicaid LTC expenditures. From 2000 to 2012, Medicaid spending on home care rose from $6.8 billion to $29 billion, an average annual rate of 27 percent, compared with 4 percent on nursing homes (CMS 2014c). States have also attempted to reduce their nursing home spending by substituting it with less costly in-home and community-based LTC services.[2]

Why Do So Few Aged Buy Private LTC Insurance?

When people are at risk for a large unexpected expense but only a few will actually incur such catastrophic costs, private insurance is a solution—for those who can afford it. A private insurance market enables people to reduce their financial risk in exchange for a premium. Given the growing number of aged at such risk, the potential market for LTC insurance is huge. Dependence on Medicaid and government LTC subsidies would diminish if more of the elderly purchase LTC coverage, yet fewer than 15 percent of the elderly have done so.

Why has private LTC insurance not grown more rapidly? How feasible is it to expect this insurance to alleviate the middle-class elderly's concerns that their LTC needs will be provided and paid for without burdening their family caregivers or spending down their estates?

Characteristics of LTC Insurance Policies

About 80 percent of LTC insurance is sold to individuals, in contrast to medical insurance, which is mainly sold to groups. This is so, even though group LTC insurance is eligible for the same tax subsidy as employer-purchased health insurance is. Given the predominance of individual LTC coverage, our discussion focuses on this market. Most LTC insurance policies cover all forms of LTC needs, including nursing homes, home care, and assisted-living facilities. Case management services, medical equipment in the home, and training of caregivers may also be included. Most plans also have a deductible in the form of days of care the individual must pay (30 to 100 days) before the policy is effective. These deductible provisions ensure that the policy is for a chronic condition and does not cover acute medical or rehabilitative services, which are the responsibility of Medicare or private medical insurance.

LTC plans also contain benefit maximum. Policies may limit lifetime benefits to five years in a nursing home. In addition, most policies contain a maximum daily payment for care in a nursing home or for reimbursement for care in the home. These maximum daily benefits are either fixed over time or (for an additional premium) increased by an annual percentage amount. Further, to qualify for LTC benefits, the individual must meet certain criteria, such as requiring substantial assistance to perform specific activities of daily living for an extended period, such as 90 days.

Premiums of LTC insurance reflect the cost of providing the services and the risk that the person will need the services as he ages. In 2014, the average annual premium (with 5 percent inflation protection) was $2,853 at age 65 years, $4,715 at age 75 years, and $9,150 at age 85 years. If a policy is purchased at age 30 years, the premium is only $770 per year; this rate reflects both the lower risk of the young enrollee and the assumption that the person would be paying the premium over a greater number of years than someone who purchased the coverage when he was older (FLTCIP n.d.).

The type of benefits included in an LTC policy greatly affects the premiums charged. For example, the premium on a policy sold in 2014 to a 70-year-old will vary from a low of about $1,377 to a high of $4,892 per year, depending on the benefits included.

Premiums are also higher if the purchaser wishes to protect herself against inflation in LTC costs. Because most policies provide specified cash benefits in the event that the purchaser requires LTC, a policy that pays $100 per day for care in a nursing home is not sufficient if nursing home costs increase at the previous annual growth rate of 6.7 percent; over 20 years, the cost per day will be $366. Protection against these additional financial risks raises the premium.

LTC policies are guaranteed renewable, and premiums vary by age and risk class, of which there are usually three: preferred, standard, and extra risk. Once a person has purchased a plan, she is not charged an additional amount as her age or health condition changes (RMM n.d.).

Possible explanations for why less than 15 percent of the elderly have LTC insurance can be classified according to (1) the factors that limit the demand for LTC insurance and (2) the possible market imperfections in the supply of LTC insurance.

Factors Limiting the Demand for LTC Insurance

The aged's income and ability to pay for insurance vary. The oldest old—those most in need of LTC services—generally have lower income than do the younger seniors and are in a high-risk group, which makes their insurance premiums much higher.

A great deal of misinformation exists among the aged. Many believe Medicare and Medigap insurance (private insurance that pays Medicare's deductibles and copayments) cover LTC, but they do not. Additionally, the elderly may be unaware of their potential LTC risks and the financial consequences of those risks. Further, the number and types of policies available, with their differing copayments and benefits, may be confusing to some elderly people.

The availability of Medicaid also contributes to the reasons many elderly do not buy (or are less likely to buy) private LTC insurance. They (and perhaps their family members) view Medicaid as a low-cost substitute to LTC insurance. If the older aged need to enter a nursing home, they have to rely on Medicaid. To those elderly, however, who wish to bequeath their assets to their children or loved ones, Medicaid is a poor substitute to purchased private insurance because they need to spend most of their assets first before they can qualify for Medicaid to pay their LTC expenses. In effect, Medicaid imposes a high implicit tax on the assets of the aged.

Expectations of the elderly that their family members will provide financial and nonfinancial support to them if they require LTC affects their demand for insurance as well. Publicly funded or family-provided LTC decreases the demand for private insurance (Brown, Goda, and McGarry 2012).

Possible Market Imperfections in the Supply of LTC Insurance

Supply-side concerns relate to whether LTC plans are priced significantly above their actuarial fair value (their pure premium), in which case the premiums would greatly exceed the policy's expected benefits. The greater the difference between the premium and expected benefits (referred to as the *loading charge*), the lower the demand for such insurance.

Premiums for LTC plans may be much higher than the expected benefits for several reasons. When LTC insurance policies are sold to individuals, the marketing and administrative costs are much higher than if it were sold to large employer groups. The loading charges for individually sold LTC insurance are estimated to be 32 percent to 50 percent, but loading charges for group purchasers are only 10 percent (Brown and Finkelstein 2011).

Also increasing the loading charge is insurers' concern about adverse selection.[3] Individual LTC insurance is bought on a voluntary basis, whereas employer-paid health insurance includes everyone in a group, which eliminates the chance that only sick employees will buy the insurance. Because insurance premiums are based on the average expected claims experience (use rate multiplied by the price of the service) of a particular age group, insurers are concerned that a higher proportion of the impaired aged will purchase

LTC insurance. If the premium is based on an expected high-risk group than exists among the general population of elderly desiring to buy insurance, those elderly of an average risk level will find the premium greatly in excess of their expected benefits. (Delay-of-benefits provisions, indemnity coverage with a large deductible, and copayments are usually included in policies to discourage adverse selection.)

Insurers are also concerned that as insurance becomes available to pay for in-home LTC services, the demand for such services will sharply increase beyond the amount believed necessary. To the extent that such moral hazard occurs and is not controlled by the insurer, the premium will reflect these higher use rates and greatly exceed the expected benefits for those seniors who would not increase their use of services once their insurance starts paying for those services.[4]

Conclusions About the Small Market for Private LTC Insurance

The size of the loading charge does not seem to be the determining factor causing the small demand for LTC insurance.[5] Such policies charge the same premiums for men and women of the same age. Brown and Finkelstein (2008) estimated the loading charge for a 65-year-old man to be 44 percent—that is, he would expect to receive $56 worth of benefits in return for paying a $100 premium. However, because premiums are the same regardless of sex, the loading charge for a 65-year-old woman was estimated to be negative—that is, her expected benefits are greater than the premium paid: $104 in expected benefits in return for a $100 premium. Despite the favorable pricing for women, still only about 10 percent of elderly women purchase LTC policies, which is no different from the percentage of men purchasing such policies. These findings suggest that market-supply imperfections, reflected by the loading charge, are insufficient to understanding the limited demand for LTC insurance.

Demand factors are, therefore, more likely explanations for the limited insurance demand. Brown and Finkelstein (2011) believed that the availability of Medicaid is critical in explaining the small demand, as Medicaid crowds out the demand. For an elderly person with median wealth, most of the premiums for a private LTC policy pay for the same benefits that are covered by Medicaid. Further, women are more likely than men to end up on Medicaid—regardless of whether they have private LTC insurance—because of their much greater expected lifetime utilization of LTC services. Thus, women, even though they might be able to buy a policy with a zero loading charge, would still not buy it because of the availability of Medicaid. As long as Medicaid exists in its present form, expanding the demand for private LTC insurance will be difficult.

In their survey to learn more about the factors affecting this demand, Brown, Goda, and McGarry (2012) concluded that if the demand is to be increased, public policy should address multiple factors, such as the high cost of insurance, the availability of Medicaid and unpaid care from family members, the existence of a person's savings to pay for his care, and the limited knowledge of the risk of needing such care.

Approaches to Financing Long-Term Care

The LTC needs of the older aged, the aged's fear of having to spend down their assets, and the high cost of private LTC insurance form the basis of the demand for government LTC subsidies. Providing the aged with a range of services—from in-home services to nursing home care—without financially burdening the aged or their children requires huge government subsidies. Given the rapid increase in the number and proportion of aged, federal and state subsidies for LTC would be a very large financial burden on the non-elderly, who already face the financial burden of paying for the enormous federal deficit.

Federal spending on programs benefiting the aged—Medicare, Medicaid, and Social Security—consumed 9.8 percent of gross domestic product (GDP) in 2014. By 2039, inflation-adjusted expenditures on these programs will rise to 14.3 percent of GDP (CBO 2014, Table 1-1). Federal spending on the elderly will absorb a larger and ultimately unsustainable share of the federal budget and economic resources. Thanks in part to medical advances, people are living longer and spending more time in retirement, which places greater demands on these three federal programs. The aged are a growing portion of the total population, the oldest baby boomers have already started to retire, and the number of workers per aged to finance the costs of Medicaid, Medicare, and Social Security is declining. These demographic, technologic, and economic pressures have profound implications for the US economy and the continued funding of these entitlement programs.

Medicaid is the fastest-growing and second-largest program in state spending. About 67 percent of Medicaid expenditures are on behalf of the aged and those with disabilities. The growing number of aged will place a greater burden on state budgets in coming years. Expanding public subsidies for LTC would not only exacerbate federal and state fiscal pressures but also serve as a disincentive to the purchase of private LTC insurance.

Given these trends in both the number and percentage of aged and the likely inability of government to continue financing these benefits, subsidies for LTC are likely to be curtailed rather than expanded. The public policy dilemma concerns the role of government in financing LTC.

Stimulating the Demand for Private LTC Insurance

Increasing the demand for private LTC insurance would, over time, decrease the demand for Medicaid subsidies for LTC services. To stimulate the insurance demand, it is necessary to make Medicaid a less attractive substitute. Government subsidies for buying private LTC insurance could offset the low-cost advantage of Medicaid (once the spend-down requirement is met) if an individual requires LTC.

One type of government subsidy is a tax subsidy that is similar to tax-exempt employer-paid health insurance. Since 1996, employees do not have to pay income taxes on their employer's contributions toward their LTC insurance premiums; however, most private LTC insurance is sold on the individual market, where the premiums are not tax exempt. Even if the law were changed to make such premiums tax exempt, the benefits would primarily accrue to those in high marginal tax brackets, who otherwise are not eligible for Medicaid.

Under the 2010 Affordable Care Act (ACA), a voluntary federal insurance program for LTC was established—the Community Living Assistance Services and Supports (CLASS) Act. With this program, the federal government would serve as the insurer and would sell private LTC insurance directly to the public. As an insurer, the government—rather than private insurers—would bear the liability if premiums fell short of the program's outlays. Those purchasing the insurance would have to wait a minimum of five years before they became eligible to collect benefits. Once eligible, if a person had two or more functional limitations—that is, unable to perform certain activities of daily living (such as eating or bathing) and are certified by a healthcare practitioner to continue to suffer these limitations for more than 90 days—the person would receive a cash benefit of not less than $75 per day (adjusted for inflation) for the rest of his life, assuming his limitations continue. These funds could be used to purchase nonmedical services and supports necessary to maintain a community residence, such as hiring an aide (or a family member) to bathe the person or prepare meals at his home. Proponents of the CLASS Act claimed that the new program, which was to be privately financed by premiums, would reduce Medicaid expenditures because care in the home is less costly than residency in a nursing home.

In 2011, the government claimed the program could not be implemented because it would be fiscally unsustainable. In addition to permitting those below the federal poverty level to enroll at below actuarial rates, there was the problem of adverse selection. Enrollment in the CLASS Act was voluntary, and after only a short period an enrollee could become eligible for benefits. A voluntary program was more likely to attract those who expect to benefit from the program, particularly because the premiums were adjusted for age but not for health status. As more high-risk people enrolled, the premiums would increase and those with low risk would either not enroll or would drop out. As proportionately more high-risk people enrolled, benefit payouts would exceed premiums. As the unfunded deficit for this program increased over time, premiums would have to be raised and, possibly, everyone would have been required to enroll to increase the size of the risk pool (to include more healthy enrollees).

The Government as a Safety Net

Given the fiscal pressures on the federal and state governments, government policy is likely to be (1) a safety net for low-income aged and (2) a method to improve the effectiveness of how those subsidies are spent. When government acts as a safety net, primary responsibility for paying LTC expenses is placed on the individual and the family. The government fills the gap between the needs of the elderly and what their families and financial resources can provide. Availability of government assistance, such as Medicaid, is based on an elderly person's income and assets and is financed from general taxes; those with high income bear the financial burden of subsidizing those with low income. Because states differ in their generosity and financial capacity, the availability of LTC services (access to nursing homes and in-home care) varies greatly among state Medicaid programs.

Most states now have provisions that prevent people from qualifying for Medicaid within three years of voluntarily impoverishing themselves through bequests of their assets to family members. (States are going after middle- and high-income persons who have adopted estate-planning strategies that permit them to qualify for Medicaid by transferring their assets just before they need nursing home care.) Further, because some assets are excluded for purposes of determining Medicaid eligibility—such as having a house, spending assets on home improvements, having an automobile, and placing assets in certain types of trusts—tightening Medicaid requirements would further reduce eligibility and increase public subsidies for those most in need.

Lengthening the period for asset transfers from three to five years (which is opposed by the AARP), limiting excludable assets, and enforcing these requirements would reduce Medicaid expenditures; make Medicaid a less desirable substitute to insurance for middle- and high-income elderly; and, consequently, increase the demand for private LTC plans. Even if all these actions were undertaken, however, a majority of the elderly would still be unlikely to buy private LTC coverage.

Given that Medicaid will continue to be the major source of LTC funding for a majority of aged needing such services and that government expenditures for LTC are expected to significantly rise in coming years, how can Medicaid be made more effective?

Improving the Effectiveness of Government LTC Programs

Several states have developed innovative LTC programs with the expectation that Medicaid's LTC expenditures will decrease. These states also hope to improve patient satisfaction with the care they receive. Several states use consumer-directed "cash and counseling" programs, for example. Under this approach, Medicaid beneficiaries living in the community are provided with funds to purchase LTC services rather than rely on Medicaid-provided services. Beneficiaries are given more choice in the type and providers of LTC services. Medicaid beneficiaries currently have no financial incentive to use LTC efficiently. Cash and counseling programs give beneficiaries an incentive to shop for lower-priced services and get more care for their budgets. Preliminary evidence from these demonstration projects indicates that participants are more satisfied with the care received and have fewer unmet needs than beneficiaries in traditional Medicaid (Doty, Mahoney, and Sciegaj 2010).

Other innovative programs integrate acute and long-term care. Social health maintenance organizations (S/HMOs) receive a monthly premium in return for providing acute and LTC services to their enrollees. The S/HMO is at financial risk for the cost of all the medical and LTC services its enrollees require. Both healthy and impaired aged are able to enroll in the S/HMO, which has an incentive to improve the efficiency of the care received by its enrollees by coordinating care and reducing unnecessary services.

The Program of All-Inclusive Care for the Elderly (PACE) model is directed toward Medicare- and Medicaid-eligible beneficiaries who are eligible for nursing home care but want to continue living at home. PACE organizations receive a monthly capitation payment; use a multidisciplinary team of providers, such as physicians, nurses, and case managers; and provide services to enrollees in adult day care centers. Preliminary evaluations indicate that PACE enrollees use less nursing home and hospital care. These results may be biased, however, by favorable selection; PACE enrollees may be less impaired than nursing home patients, which is their comparison group.

Public subsidies affect the demand for private LTC insurance. The lower the aged's responsibility for their LTC expenses, the lower is their likelihood of buying insurance. Appropriate public policy should do two things: (1) encourage those who can afford it to purchase private LTC insurance, and (2) stipulate that limited public funds be used for those unable to afford LTC insurance.

Summary

Fewer than 40 percent of the aged are likely able to afford private LTC insurance. Although this percentage indicates that the private insurance market can greatly grow, it also indicates that a sizable number—mainly comprising the older aged—will be unable to purchase insurance for the LTC services they need, forcing them to rely on Medicaid.

A fundamental issue here concerns the extent to which the government should provide LTC subsidies to the aged. LTC policy requires making choices. The elderly have greater needs for care, do not wish to be a burden on family members, do not want to spend down their hard-earned assets, and would like to be assured of a high-quality nursing home (should they require one). Yet given the projected number of aged, government subsidies would be very costly. Such subsidies would require large tax hikes at a time when Medicare taxes will also be increased to keep it from going bankrupt. These tax increases would represent a huge financial burden on workers because the number of workers per aged person is declining.

Subsidies also reduce the incentive for many aged to rely on their children or to purchase private LTC insurance. To reduce the cost of LTC subsidies, subsidies should be targeted to those with the lowest income. Estate-planning strategies that enable middle- and high-income aged to transfer their assets shortly before qualifying for Medicaid are inequitable in that they shift their costs to others. To the extent that Medicaid rules are enforced and Medicaid becomes a less desirable substitute to private insurance, the demand for LTC insurance will grow. Greater growth in demand will reduce Medicaid LTC expenditures. Educating both workers and the aged about the need to protect themselves against catastrophic LTC costs is also important.

Discussion Questions

1. Describe the demographic and economic trends affecting the outlook for LTC.
2. What should be the objectives of an LTC policy? How do these objectives differ from the long-term care goals of the middle class?
3. Why has the market for LTC insurance grown so slowly?
4. How can Medicaid be changed so it is not a low-cost substitute for private LTC insurance for the middle-income aged?
5. Why does private LTC insurance, when sold to the aged, have such a high loading charge relative to the pure premium?
6. Why did the government decide not to implement the CLASS Act?

Notes

1. Although many nonelderly have disabilities requiring LTC services, the expected large growth in the number of elderly (particularly the

oldest old, who are much greater users of LTC services) and the financing of their care have been the main concern of LTC policy.

2. States cover nonmedical and social support services to allow people to remain in the community. These services include personal care, home-maker assistance, adult day care, chore assistance, and other services shown to be cost-effective and necessary to avoid nursing home insti-tutionalization. To control costs, however, states limit eligibility and the scope of services covered.

3. Since the late 1980s, insurers have marketed LTC insurance to large employee groups. Group policies have lower loading charges because of their lower administrative and marketing costs. Adverse selection is also less of a concern when everyone in a group participates, particu-larly when they are at low risk for LTC. Further, because employees would not be at risk for many years, group policies could be sold at very low premiums. Employer-sponsored policies are a more useful financing source for future than for current aged.

4. To lower the cost of providing LTC, insurers provide comprehensive services—both in-home assistance and nursing home care. In-home services are less expensive (and are preferred by the impaired aged) when they reduce use of the more expensive nursing home. Case managers would ideally be used to evaluate the elderly's needs and determine the mix of services to be provided. In-home services could be substituted for nursing home care, and the discretionary use of in-home assistance could be minimized. Controlling adverse selec-tion and discretionary use of services is essential to keeping private LTC insurance premiums low. Currently, greater reliance is placed on financial incentives (deductibles and copayments) than on the use of case managers to control costs.

5. The importance of price on the demand for LTC insurance has been estimated to be between –0.23 and –0.87; that is, if the price of insurance were to decrease by 1 percent, demand would increase by less than 1 percent (Stevenson, Frank, and Tau 2009).

References

Administration on Aging (AoA). 2013. *A Profile of Older Americans: 2013.* Accessed September 2014. www.aoa.gov/Aging_Statistics/Profile/2013/docs/2013_Profile.pdf.

Brown, J., and A. Finkelstein. 2011. "Insuring Long Term Care in the United States." *Journal of Economic Perspectives* 25 (4): 119–42.

———. 2008. "The Interaction of Public and Private Insurance: Medicaid and the Long Term Insurance Market." *American Economic Review* 98 (3): 1083–102.

Brown, J., R. G. Goda, and K. McGarry. 2012. "Long-Term Care Insurance Demand Limited by Beliefs About Needs, Concerns About Insurers, and Care Available from Family." *Health Affairs* 31 (6): 1294–302.

Calmus, D. 2013. "The Long-Term Care Financing Crisis." Center for Policy Innovation Discussion Paper No. 7 on Health Care, February 6. www.heritage.org/research/reports/2013/02/the-long-term-care-financing-crisis.

Centers for Medicare & Medicaid Services (CMS). 2014a. "CMS-64 Quarterly Expense Report." Accessed February. http://medicaid.gov/Medicaid-CHIP-Program-Information/By-Topics/Data-and-Systems/MBES/CMS-64-Quarterly-Expense-Report.html.

———. 2014b. "2014 SSI and Spousal Impoverishment Standards." Accessed February. www.medicaid.gov/Medicaid-CHIP-Program-Information/By-Topics/Eligibility/Downloads/Spousal-Impoverishment-2014.pdf.

———. 2014c. "National Health Expenditures Tables." Accessed January. http://cms.gov/Research-Statistics-Data-and-Systems/Statistics-Trends-and-Reports/NationalHealthExpendData/Downloads/tables.pdf.

———. 2014d. "National Health Expenditure Data." Last modified May 5. cms.gov/Research-Statistics-Data-and-Systems/Statistics-Trends-and-Reports/NationalHealthExpendData/index.html.

———. 2014e. "Medicaid Expenditures for Long Term Services and Supports in FFY 2012." Accessed September. www.medicaid.gov/Medicaid-CHIP-Program-Information/By-Topics/Long-Term-Services-and-Supports/Downloads/LTSS-Expenditures-2012.pdf.

———. 2011. "2011 Characteristics and Perceptions of the Medicare Population." Accessed February 2014. www.cms.gov/Research-Statistics-Data-and-Systems/Research/MCBS/Data-Tables-Items/2011CharAndPerc.html.

Congressional Budget Office (CBO). 2014. *The 2014 Long-Term Budget Outlook.* Published July. www.cbo.gov/sites/default/files/cbofiles/attachments/45471-Long-TermBudgetOutlook_7-29.pdf.

———. 2013. *Rising Demand for Long-Term Services and Supports for Elderly People.* Published June. www.cbo.gov/sites/default/files/cbofiles/attachments/44363-LTC.pdf.

Doty, P., K. Mahoney, and M. Sciegaj. 2010. "New State Strategies to Meet Long-Term Care Needs." *Health Affairs* 29 (1): 49–56.

The Federal Long Term Care Insurance Program (FLTCIP). n.d. "Monthly Premium Rates." Accessed February 2014. www.ltcfeds.com/programdetails/monthlyrateschart.html.

Feinberg, L., S. C. Reinhard, A. Houser, and R. Choula. 2011. "Valuing the Invaluable: 2011 Update. The Growing Contributions and Costs of Family Caregiving." *Insight on the Issues* 51, June. AARP Public Policy Institute. http://assets.aarp.org/rgcenter/ppi/ltc/i51-caregiving.pdf.

Genworth Financial Inc. 2014. *Genworth 2014 Cost of Care Survey,* 11th ed. Published March. www.genworth.com/dam/Americas/US/PDFs/ Consumer/corporate/130568_032514_CostofCare_FINAL_nonsecure.pdf.

Harris-Kojetin, L., M. Sengupta, E. Park-Lee, and R. Valverde. 2013. *Long-Term Care Services in the United States: 2013 Overview.* Accessed February 2014. www.cdc.gov/nchs/data/nsltcp/long_term_care_services_2013.pdf.

Houser, A., M. Gibson, and D. Redfoot. 2010. *Trends in Family Caregiving and Paid Home Care for Older People with Disabilities in the Community: Data from the National Long-Term Care Survey.* AARP Public Policy Institute. Published September. http://assets.aarp.org/rgcenter/ppi/ltc/2010-09-caregiving.pdf.

MetLife Mature Market Institute. 2012. *Market Survey of Long-Term Care Costs: The 2012 MetLife Market Survey of Nursing Home, Assisted Living, Adult Day Services, and Home Care Costs.* Published November. www.metlife .com/assets/cao/mmi/publications/studies/2012/studies/mmi-2012-market-survey-long-term-care-costs.pdf.

RMM Inc. n.d. "What Senior Citizens Need to Know About Private Long Term Care Insurance." Accessed February 2014. www.rmminc.net/articles-ltc_ ins/need_to_know.shtml#Premium%20Increases.

Spillman, B., and P. Kemper. 1995. "Lifetime Patterns of Payment for Nursing Home Care." *Medical Care* 33 (3): 288–96.

Stevenson, D., R. Frank, and J. Tau. 2009. "Private Long-Term Care Insurance and State Tax Incentives." *Inquiry* 46 (3): 305–21.

US Census Bureau. 2012. *2012 National Population Projections.* Accessed January 2014. www.census.gov/population/projections/data/national/2012/ downloadablefiles.html.

THE POLITICS OF HEALTHCARE REFORM

I n 2010, the Affordable Care Act (ACA) was enacted. The legislation was several thousand pages long. Many legislators never read or fully understood the legislation. Its provisions were controversial, and it was passed with only Democratic support. Not one Republican senator or representative voted for the final bill. The bill's major provisions did not become effective until 2014—and some as late as 2018 and 2020. (See the Appendix for a brief summary of the legislation.)

Although dissatisfaction with the US health system exists, the ACA continues to be unpopular. The Obama Administration believed that Democrats would receive political support from the public for enacting the ACA, whose goals include extending health coverage to an additional 32 million people (and making that expansion be budget neutral so that it would not increase the federal deficit), eliminating the middle class' fear of losing their health insurance in case of illness, and slowing down the rise of insurance premiums and the US health expenditures. When campaigning during the 2010 congressional midterm elections, however, many legislators who voted for the ACA were reluctant to publicize their vote in TV ads. More significantly, the dissatisfaction with the ACA led to the rise of the Tea Party and the Democrats' loss of the majority in the House of Representatives.

To understand the difficulties of enacting healthcare reform and the relative unpopularity of the ACA, we must examine the goals of different political constituencies, how the Obama Administration attempted to satisfy these constituencies, and what the Obama Administration's own objectives were in designing the ACA. In doing so, it becomes obvious that healthcare reform and national health insurance mean different things to different groups. Further, the process and outcome of the legislation were a cause for dissatisfaction among many members of the middle class, including the aged.

Differing Goals of Healthcare Reform

Benefiting the Poor

Many assume that the main purpose of healthcare reform and national health insurance is to increase the availability of medical services to those with low income. Certainly, many individuals support more and better services to the poor, but this is not and has never been the driving force behind national health insurance. Medicaid is national health insurance for the poor. To use the power of government to achieve one's objectives requires political power. The inadequate structure and funding of Medicaid is indicative of the limited political power of the poor and their advocates. These inadequacies are not attributable to the actions of a few miserly bureaucrats or legislators but instead are reflective of the resources that society—mainly the middle class—is willing to devote to the poor. States vary in their generosity and in the criteria used for determining Medicaid eligibility. Few states provide Medicaid eligibility for all those at the federal poverty level, and some states provide benefits only to people whose income is 16 percent of the federal poverty level (Kaiser Family Foundation 2014, Table 3). How much the non-poor are willing to tax themselves for charity depends on how much the non-poor themselves have, how culturally similar the poor and non-poor are, and how much providing for the poor costs.

Because the non-poor have the political power to determine the allocation of resources to the poor, one must assume that the inadequacies of Medicaid are reflections of insufficient interest among the non-poor in improving Medicaid and increasing funding for the poor. If society is unwilling to improve Medicaid, why would it tax itself to enact national health insurance for the poor?

Benefiting Politically Powerful Groups

If national health insurance is not primarily for the poor, its broader purpose must be to use the power of government to benefit politically powerful groups. Important groups must receive benefits in excess of their costs, if visible redistributive legislation affecting everyone's health coverage is to be enacted. These groups are the middle class and the aged (who determine the outcome of elections) as well as healthcare providers, businesses, and labor groups (who have a concentrated interest in the legislation's provisions and are able to provide legislators with financial support). Healthcare providers and other interest groups are relatively easy to accommodate in the short run. The problem with enacting healthcare reform or national health insurance has always been the middle class. If the middle class is to receive net benefits, which group will have to bear the costs of financing those benefits? Whichever group has to pay more will oppose legislators who vote to raise their taxes. The major difficulty in healthcare reform has been finding groups that can be taxed to provide net benefits to politically powerful constituencies.

In the past, politically important groups received visible redistributive benefits that less politically powerful groups were taxed to provide. Regressive taxation was typically used to finance universal redistributive legislation, such as Social Security and Medicare Part A.[1] Over time, these regressive taxes became more progressive as the cost of the programs exceeded projections. To lessen the opposition of those being taxed, the tax was hidden. Splitting the Social Security tax and the Medicare payroll tax between the employer and the employee makes it appear that the employee bears only half of the tax. In reality, economists believe that most of the employer share is shifted back to the employee in the form of lower wages, while the rest is shifted forward to consumers in the form of higher prices for goods and services.

Politically influential groups have a concentrated interest in a particular issue and are able to organize themselves to provide political support to legislators by means of campaign contributions, votes, and volunteer time. A group is said to have a concentrated interest if specific regulation or legislation will have a sufficiently large effect to make it worthwhile for the group to invest its resources either to forestall or to promote that effect. The potential legislative benefits must exceed the group's costs of organizing and providing political support.

This discussion of concentrated interests assumes that legislators will respond to political support because their objective is to be reelected. Legislators are assumed to be similar to other participants in the policy process and to rationally undertake cost–benefit calculations of their actions. However, they weigh the political support gained and lost by their legislative actions and not by the legislation's effect on society.

Initially, physicians and hospitals were the major groups with a concentrated interest in health legislation. Physician and hospital associations represented (successfully) their concentrated interests before both state and federal legislatures and in so doing were able to affect the financing and delivery of medical services. These legislative actions by physician and hospital associations were neither very obvious nor initially very costly to the consumers of medical services. Medical prices rose faster than they would have otherwise, and alternatives to the fee-for-service system, such as managed care, were delayed for many years. These costs to consumers were not sufficiently large to make it worthwhile for them to organize, represent their interests before legislatures, and offer political support to legislators who were favorable to their interests.

Over time, growing medical costs resulted in the rise of other groups, such as unions and employers, with a concentrated interest in limiting medical cost increases. Groups with opposing concentrated interests—such as physicians and hospitals (who wanted increased medical spending) and unions and employers and their insurers (who wanted to limit medical spending)—made political compromise more difficult. Healthcare reform had to attempt to receive support from such opposing groups.

The Need for Visible Benefits to the Middle Class and Aged

In 2009, the first year of the Obama Administration, the United States was in a severe recession; unemployment was high and the number of uninsured was rising; and, because insurance was tied to their jobs, the middle class were concerned with losing their health insurance. The administration believed that with the country's economic stress the public would be amenable to government programs that provided greater healthcare security. Given the public concern with the huge federal deficit, the administration realized that a new healthcare reform program had to be financed without visibly further adding to the federal deficit. In addition, while expanding health coverage to 32 million people, the administration had to gain the political support of the middle class and the aged.

The middle class and the aged are two important voting constituencies who determine the outcome of elections. The middle class (those in the middle-income group) has a disproportionate amount of political power because they are the median voters. It is difficult to form a majority of voters without those in the middle. The aged have the highest voting rate of any age group (see Exhibit 36.1), and the near-aged have the next highest voting participation rate. Those aged 18 to 24 years have the lowest voting

EXHIBIT 36.1
Voting Participation Rates in Presidential Elections, by Age, 1984–2012

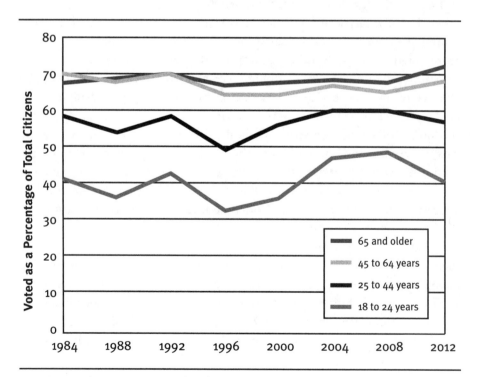

SOURCE: Data from Census Bureau (2013).

participation rates, and future generations who do not currently vote offer the least amount of political support to legislators. Thus, the cost of providing current benefits is shifted to those who are less important politically. To enact highly visible redistributive legislation, such as healthcare reform, legislators attempt to provide the middle class and the aged with benefits at no additional cost so as to gain their political support for reelection.

The Middle Class

As medical costs and insurance premiums continued their rapid increase, middle-class dissatisfaction with the current system grew. Their out-of-pocket medical expenses had gone up as their employers began shifting a greater portion of their healthcare costs back to them, asking them to pay more of their health insurance premiums and to pay higher copayments and deductibles. The middle class were also concerned that if they lost or changed their jobs, they would lose their health insurance. They wanted unrestricted access to specialists (traditional fee-for-service insurance), low out-of-pocket copayments, limited monthly health insurance premiums, and the security of having health insurance.

The problem with coming to grips with serious reform is not with special-interest groups but with the middle class. They are unwilling to have the government raise their taxes to pay for health insurance for the uninsured. Further, they are unwilling to recognize that they must make a trade-off between the higher cost of unlimited access to medical services and the amount they are willing to pay.

The difficulty in enacting healthcare reform is that legislators are unable to provide the middle class with more benefits at no additional cost. Which population group can be made to bear the cost of subsidizing the middle class?

To receive the political support of the middle class, the Obama Administration emphasized "health insurance" reform rather than "healthcare" reform. Because the middle class has health insurance, they do not want to lose it or pay more in premiums. Thus, President Obama promised the following: "if you are happy with your health plan, you can keep it," insurance premiums will *decrease* by $2,500 per year because the legislation will "bend the cost curve down," the legislation will not "add a dime to the deficit," and "it will be fully paid for." Further, the middle class would not have to pay higher taxes; only those whose family income is greater than $250,000 would pay increased taxes. To expand coverage to the uninsured, the administration assured the middle class that healthcare reform would not cost them anything, and in fact, they would also receive additional benefits. It was to be a "free lunch."

The Aged

The second politically powerful group is the aged (and near-aged). The aged have their own national health insurance—Medicare. The near-aged want to ensure that Medicare is available for them when they retire. The children of the aged and near-aged also want to ensure that Medicare is maintained because they do not want the financial responsibility of caring for their parents' health needs. In addition to their desire to maintain Medicare, the aged want to reduce their out-of-pocket expenses—particularly for Medicare Part D—and limit the premium increases for Medicare Parts B and D. Both political parties compete for the political support of the aged; in December 2003, this led to a new prescription drug benefit—Medicare Part D (Feldstein 2006). To reduce the cost of the drug benefit, Congress created a "donut hole" (a large deductible), which became a financial burden for seniors with high drug costs.

The ACA phases out the donut hole. Further, because this benefit will not be immediately visible to the aged, the administration sent $250 checks to millions of middle-class seniors who fell into the donut hole to secure their political support for the ACA before the 2010 midterm elections. (Seniors with low income and high drug costs were already enrolled in Medicaid.)

The ACA reduced the premiums of the near-aged—those aged younger than 65 years, who will be buying insurance through the new health insurance exchanges—by requiring health insurers to only allow age-related premiums to vary by a difference of 3:1 rather than a 6:1 ratio, which reflects the much higher medical costs of older adults. The effect of lowering premiums for older adults by narrowing age-related premiums was higher premiums for young adults, who happen to have lower voting participation rates. Young adults, who have lower income, are to subsidize older adults.

Groups with a Concentrated Interest in Healthcare Reform

Many groups have a concentrated interest in health legislation. To understand the conflicting forces that affected the design of the ACA, we have to examine the objectives of several important groups.

At the time the ACA was being drafted, President Obama had a high approval rating and the Democrats controlled a large majority in the House of Representatives as well as a filibuster-proof margin (60) in the Senate. (Senator Arlen Specter switched from the Republicans to the Democrats, and a contested Minnesota Senate election was decided in favor of the Democrats, giving them the 60 votes needed for cloture.) It appeared that healthcare reform was inevitable, so provider organizations thought they had to negotiate the best possible deal with the administration, which promised them a better deal than if their fate was left to Congress, which was anxious to impose severe payment reductions. The saying was "you're either at the table or on the menu." Consequently, the Obama Administration was able to induce almost all of the major groups with a concentrated interest in healthcare reform (pharmaceutical firms, the American Medical Association, the American Hospital Association, unions, AARP, employers, and health insurers) into supporting the ACA. Industry groups were also promised a pool of millions of additional patients, funded in full or in part by the government.

Pharmaceutical Research and Manufacturers of America

Pharmaceutical firms have an interest in expanding their market of paying patients and retaining their ability to price their drugs according to what the market will bear. Yet the Pharmaceutical Research and Manufacturers of America (PhRMA), the trade association for the pharmaceutical industry, agreed to cut drug prices by $80 billion over ten years (the time frame for calculating the revenues and costs of the ACA). The Obama Administration used this reduction estimate in its budget calculations to minimize the overall cost of the ACA. In addition, PhRMA agreed to spend $100 million in TV advertising to endorse the legislation. In return, the administration agreed that the ACA would not include price controls on any Medicare prescription drugs, a major concern of the drug firms, and that Congress would not enact legislation allowing Americans to import low-cost prescription drugs from overseas. The drug firms also received protection for their high-tech biological medicines against early competition from low-cost generics.

The American Medical Association

The American Medical Association (AMA) has had a long history of opposing federal intervention in healthcare, opposing President Truman's proposed national health insurance bill in 1946, Medicare in 1965, and President Clinton's healthcare proposal in 1993. The AMA's endorsement of the ACA was important to the Obama Administration because it did not want physicians claiming that not enough physicians are available to care for an additional 32 million people; if that were to happen, the middle class and aged would become concerned about their decreased access to care. It is difficult to know the AMA's rationale for endorsing the bill, given that the association received no assurance that its two important objectives—both of which concern money—would be achieved through the ACA and thus benefit physicians.

The first AMA objective was to have Congress change Medicare's physician payment system, which relies on the sustainable growth rate (SGR) for determining annual fee updates. According to the SGR formula, physicians were scheduled for a 21 percent decrease in Medicare fees. However, each year Congress overrules the proposed decrease. Achieving a permanent fix would have required adding to the federal deficit $280 billion over the next ten years. Surprisingly, the AMA's support for the ACA was not contingent on having Congress enact a permanent payment fix; the Democratic Congress subsequently did not include a permanent fix as part of the ACA.

The second AMA legislative priority was tort reform. While the ACA includes a section establishing an incentive program for states to adopt and implement alternatives to medical liability litigation, tort reform is essentially negated by another provision in the ACA: A state is not eligible for the incentive payments if that state enacts a law that limits attorney's fees or imposes caps on damages. Limits on attorney's fees and damage caps were two tort-reform priorities of the AMA. Given the significant financial support provided by trial lawyers to Democrats, the trial lawyers' income was protected from any harm.

Critics claim the AMA had a different reason for endorsing the ACA. The AMA has a trademark monopoly, created by the federal government, on the medical coding system known as current procedural terminology (CPT) (Geiger 2009; Roy 2011). Each medical and surgical procedure and diagnostic service used by hospitals and healthcare professionals is assigned a CPT code, and insurers pay the AMA a fee when using the CPT codes to reimburse healthcare providers. Annual income generated by this monopoly provides the AMA with about $70 million in 2010, more than they received from membership dues ($38 million). ACA critics believed the administration threatened the AMA with the loss of its CPT monopoly (and revenues). These revenues are extremely important to the AMA because its membership has declined from 75 percent of all physicians in the 1970s to almost 27 percent (224,503 physicians) in 2012 (Vincent 2013). When the AMA receives twice as much money from the government than from its members, its interests lie more with the government than with its members. The AMA's management had a conflict of interest with its membership.

If the AMA's support was based on increasing the association's revenues (maintaining CPT revenues), then the AMA was not acting in its members' economic interests. (Several state associations and many members denounced the AMA's ACA endorsement.) If the AMA's support was based on including a permanent fix to the SGR system or establishing meaningful tort reform, then the AMA would have demanded that both be incorporated into the final legislation (which did not happen). In any case, it appears the AMA gave its support either because of its own economic interest (maintaining or increasing CPT revenues) or because of the expectation (but not assurance) that the SGR system would be changed and tort reform legislation would be developed.

American Hospital Association

Hospitals derive a significant portion of their revenues from Medicare and Medicaid, a fact that places hospitals in direct conflict with state and federal efforts to reduce publicly financed hospital expenditures. The American Hospital Association's (AHA) healthcare reform objective has been to grow hospital reimbursement.

Given the political environment, the AHA agreed (on behalf of hospitals) to a $155 billion payment reduction from the federal government over ten years to help pay for healthcare reform. In return, under the new law hospitals would receive an increase in the number of funded patients. Previously, hospitals treated many uninsured patients and incurred a large amount of bad debts. The additional revenues hospitals stand to gain from the great influx of patients—whose care is funded either by the federal government or government-subsidized private insurance—are expected to more than offset the payment reductions AHA agreed to. In addition, in exchange for agreeing to payment reductions, hospitals would be exempt for ten years from any other payment cuts that may be recommended by ACA's newly established Independent Payment Advisory Board. Another benefit is that hospitals forestalled threatened changes in nonprofit hospitals' tax-exempt status and were able to eliminate competition from physician-owned specialty hospitals by making the development of new physician-owned facilities illegal.

Unions

Unions were among the strongest supporters of healthcare reform and spent a great deal of money in support of it. The unions publicly argued that the healthcare system performs poorly, and they strongly favored the government-run public option, which they believed would lead to a single-payer system. The public option was to be a government-run insurance plan offered on the state exchanges. The unions believed that the government plan would be able to reduce the rates it pays providers, as it does under Medicare, thereby lowering its premiums, and drive the private plans from the market. Eventually, everyone would join the public option and a single-payer system would evolve.

The unions had several self-interest motives for favoring a government-run health plan. First, the economic interests of the major unions, such as the United Auto Workers (UAW), have not changed since the enactment of Medicare. At that time, they were successful in shifting part of their retirees' medical costs onto the general working population through the Medicare payroll tax. Since then, the unions' legislative objective has been to maintain their benefits without having to pay the required cost. Large private-sector unions, such as the UAW, have generous medical benefits, which are among the most expensive of any employee benefits. As the cost of medical care has risen, these unions have had to accept smaller wage increases to maintain their comprehensive medical benefits. These private-sector unions prefer a single-payer system so that their members' healthcare costs can be shifted to the taxpayer. Because employers are only interested in the total cost of labor—and not in how the compensation is divided between wages and benefits—the unions could increase their members' wages by the cost of health benefits shifted to the taxpayer.

Second, unions wanted to expand the number of unionized employees. Unions have been more successful in organizing public-sector employees than private-sector employees. The percentage of unionized private-sector employees is declining and was only 6.7 percent in 2013. In contrast, 35.3 percent of government employees are unionized (Bureau of Labor Statistics 2014). The Canadian single-payer system has a much higher rate of unionization than exists in the US healthcare system. Unions in the United States believe that, under a government health system, they could increase their membership by millions of employees, who would then pay billions of dollars in union dues.

Third, unions have far more power in a single-payer system to increase their wages and benefits. A powerful public-sector union bargaining with a public-sector health monopoly will do better than if it were bargaining against competing private-sector providers. Examples of union success in bargaining with public entities are the higher wages, pensions, and health benefits of union members who work for cities, counties, and states compared to workers in the private sector.

Unions benefited from ACA in additional ways. The legislation included $5 billion to pay for medical costs for millions of unionized autoworkers, steelworkers, schoolteachers, and other early retirees in underfunded retiree health benefit plans. Company, municipal, and union-sponsored plans that meet certain eligibility criteria were reimbursed up to 80 percent for early retirees' (ages 55 to 64 years) medical costs.

To help fund the legislation, Senator Max Baucus (D-MT), chair of the Senate finance committee, proposed taxing health insurance plans, a proposal favored by many economists to provide enrollees with an incentive to choose less costly health plans. Unions strongly opposed this tax on "Cadillac" health plans. Many unionized state employees, such as teacher unions, receive generous health benefits for which they would have been taxed. To assuage the unions, the premium threshold for the tax was increased and the implementation date delayed until 2018.

AARP

AARP is supposed to represent the economic interests of the aged, particularly those on Medicare. The ACA includes almost $600 billion in cuts to the Medicare program over ten years, leading the Medicare Actuary to claim that the ACA cuts in Medicare hospital payments are so severe that 15 percent of hospitals will have to stop admitting Medicare patients. Payments to Medicare Advantage plans, which enroll about 25 percent of Medicare beneficiaries, will be reduced by about $150 billion, resulting in higher premiums and/or reduced benefits and causing an estimated 4 million elderly to shift away from such plans. Further, the ACA did not forestall the scheduled 21 percent reductions in Medicare physician fees scheduled to occur (thereby reducing seniors' access to physicians).

Yet AARP strongly endorsed the ACA. AARP claimed that it did not oppose the almost $600 billion in Medicare cuts because reducing fraud and waste will make Medicare stronger over time. Is it possible that AARP's interests and those of the seniors it purports to represent are not aligned? An alternative hypothesis is that AARP has a conflict of interest between representing seniors and increasing its own revenues. AARP receives a majority of its revenues—hundreds of millions of dollars each year—from health insurers and others that use its endorsement in selling their products (including insurance, restaurant discounts, and credit cards). The largest share of these royalty revenues comes from insurers that sell Medigap policies (supplemental insurance to cover Medicare's deductibles and copayments). (AARP receives a 4.95 percent royalty each time someone buys a Medigap policy with the AARP brand name). If more seniors leave Medicare Advantage plans and return to traditional Medicare and buy Medigap policies, AARP makes more money.

Medicare Advantage plans are strong competitors to Medigap plans. Medicare Advantage plans received about 12 percent to 14 percent more funding per enrollee than does traditional Medicare and were able to provide additional benefits to their enrollees. Reducing payments to Medicare Advantage plans by about $150 billion forces these plans to reduce benefits while increasing copayments and premiums; consequently, many of these plan's enrollees will switch and buy Medigap plans, thereby increasing AARP's royalties.[2]

Employers

Many employers believe they bear part of the cost of their employees' health insurance premiums, and when premiums increase employers believe this causes them to increase their prices. Consequently, employers favor reform that lowers rising healthcare costs or enables those costs to be shifted to others. The business community was divided on the employer mandate, which requires employers either to provide their employees with health insurance that meets federal standards or to pay a tax. The highest percentage of uninsured employees work for small businesses. The National Federation of

Independent Business (NFIB)—the trade association for small business—opposed ACA because small business owners would increase their labor costs, thereby forcing them to raise their prices and hire fewer workers. The NFIB also opposed the income tax increase imposed on those with high income to help fund the legislation, because it would affect many small business owners. Several large businesses, such as Walmart (the nation's largest private employer), favored the bill because they currently provide health insurance to their employees and wanted to increase the cost to competitors who do not. Walmart also felt that if the employer provision were enacted, more onerous provisions affecting lower-wage employers would be less likely to be passed.

Health Insurers

Insurers have a concentrated interest in healthcare reform—namely, to have access to a greater number of potential enrollees and not be displaced by a government plan. Health insurers were initially in favor of healthcare reform because they believed that, because health insurance in the employer market was decreasing, the only way for them to increase enrollment was through government subsidies to the uninsured. They were strongly opposed, however, to the government-run public option, which they saw as a subsidized competitor, crowding out private insurance by forcing hospitals and physicians to accept low rates (as is done in Medicare) and, together with unlimited federal subsidies, undercutting the premiums charged by private insurers. With lower premiums in the government plan, private enrollees would shift to the public plan.

The public option was viewed by insurers (and others) as a forerunner to a single-payer system. In 2003 President Obama stated, "I happen to be a proponent of a single-payer universal healthcare program... But as all of you know, we may not get there immediately." Further, Barney Frank (D-MA), commenting on why the Democrats were not backing a single-payer system, said, "We don't have the votes for it. I wish we did. I think if we had a good public option it would lead to single-payer" (*Wall Street Journal* 2009).

Once the Senate removed the public option (to secure the 60th Senate vote needed for cloture) and competition from a government plan was eliminated, insurers favored the individual mandate requiring everyone to buy insurance because it would provide them with more enrollees. However, the small penalty included in the individual mandate for not buying insurance, together with the elimination of the preexisting condition exclusion, led insurers to oppose the ACA. Insurers believed that they would be subject to adverse selection; people would wait until they were sick to buy insurance. Insurers were also opposed to many aspects of insurance reform included in the bill, such as mandated minimum medical loss ratios, government-standardized generous benefit coverage, limits on out-of-pocket spending, and review of their premium increases—all of which would adversely affect their business. Insurers claimed that various insurance requirements—such as elimination of caps on lifetime benefits and adding children up to age 26 on family policies—would result in higher costs and hence higher premiums, which would then subject them to rate review. The insurance industry was criticized as "villains" by the Obama Administration.

The Legislative Process

The Obama approach to healthcare reform appeared to follow what Tom Daschle (who was nominated to become secretary of the Department of Health and Human Services [HHS] but withdrew over income tax problems) wrote in his book outlining his proposal for healthcare reform (Daschle, Greenberger, and Lambrew 2008). Daschle, a former Democratic Senate majority leader, advised the Obama Administration to move fast before there could be public debate and to write as vague a bill as possible. The bill would delegate to the HHS secretary the authority to write many regulations governing the financing and delivery of medical services. President Obama accepted the advice and wanted the bill to be quickly enacted before the summer 2009 legislative recess.

The 2008 elections gave Democrats an overwhelming majority in the House of Representatives and a filibuster-proof majority (60) in the Senate. Liberal House Democrats enacted their version of healthcare reform because they saw little reason to negotiate a compromise healthcare reform bill with House Republicans given the large Democratic majority.

The Ideological Divide

Ideological differences on healthcare reform between the two parties—which reflected differing economic interests, such as unions and trial lawyers versus health insurers, healthcare providers, and pharmaceutical firms—had previously been an impediment to healthcare reform. In the latter half of the 1990s, huge federal budget surpluses were projected far into the future. The middle class would not have been required to tax themselves to provide for the uninsured. It was an opportune time to cover the uninsured without seeming to impose a financial burden on anyone. And yet the ideological divisions between the political parties made it impossible for Congress to enact universal healthcare.

Since the 1990s, Congress had not been able to agree on how the uninsured should be assisted. Republicans favored providing the uninsured with refundable tax credits to buy insurance.[3] Their objective was to strengthen the private health insurance system and to allow the insured to have greater choice of health plans. They also favored placing greater fiscal responsibility on the insured for their healthcare choices and relying on health plan competition to reduce rising medical costs.

Conversely, the Democrats supported making the uninsured eligible for existing public programs, such as Medicaid. President Clinton proposed expanding Medicare by allowing those between the ages of 55 and 65 to buy into Medicare. The Democrats also favored expanding Medicaid eligibility of children (up to age 18 years) and childless adults. Expanding the number of people in public programs (Medicare and Medicaid) makes it easier to convert these programs into a single-payer system like the Canadian healthcare system. The next step would have been to include in the single-payer system employer health insurance premiums on behalf of their employees. Accumulating all these funds would not necessitate a huge tax increase.

Proponents of a single-payer system oppose proposals such as refundable tax credits and competitive health plans, including Medicare Advantage plans, in which plans compete to enroll seniors. Providing incentives for the aged and others to choose less costly health plans would strengthen a competitive private healthcare system. Democrats prefer the traditional Medicare approach, which resembles a single-payer system. Proposals allowing greater choice of health plans move the medical care system away from the direction single-payer proponents favor. Instead, single-payer proponents favor increasing the cost of private health insurers (such as by imposing additional regulations) to raise their premiums, which will cause the public to demand an alternative system—namely a publicly financed system, such as "Medicare for All." This ideological dispute between proponents of strengthening the private system and those favoring an expanded public (eventually single-payer) system limited opportunities for reaching a compromise on healthcare reform.

The Public Option

Democrats in the House of Representatives included in their version of ACA a public option. The initial design of the public option would have had the government establish a single national health plan, set provider payment equal to Medicare rates, and allow anyone to join the public option plan. Proponents of the public option claimed insufficient competition existed among health insurers. They claimed that a public option plan would provide more choice and compete against the private health insurance industry, driving down premiums and reducing healthcare costs because the government plan's bargaining power would be able to negotiate lower prices directly with healthcare providers.[4]

In markets with few competitors, the dominant insurer is typically a nonprofit Blue Cross plan. Nonprofit insurers—such as Blue Cross and Blue

Shield plans—currently compete in the health insurance market, and it is not obvious how the objectives and performance of a public option would differ from these nonprofit plans. It is not clear that a public plan would have lower costs (and thus the ability to charge a lower price than what health insurers charged) unless it was subsidized and subject to a different set of rules. The public plan's administrative costs would be higher than Medicare's because it would have to incur marketing costs to compete for enrollees, profile physicians and other providers as it forms provider networks in different markets, offer different benefit plans, perform utilization management to reduce fraud and waste, and bill and collect premiums from enrollees. None of these tasks is currently performed by Medicare (Conover and Miller 2010).

If too few insurers are available because they have monopolized the market (no evidence of which was presented) the appropriate remedy would be to use the antitrust laws, as is done in every other industry. If barriers to entry exist in health insurance, those barriers should be eliminated. Concern over monopoly behavior with Microsoft, among hospitals, or in other industries has not led to proposals for the federal government to go into the software business to compete with Microsoft or have the government build its own hospitals.

Instead, the real purpose of a public plan was quite different than its stated purpose; it was not to increase competition but to decrease it. A subsidized government insurer using its regulatory powers would result in decreased private insurer enrollment, leading to the government becoming the dominant health insurer and making the transition to single payer more inevitable.[5]

Growing Opposition by the Middle Class and Aged to Healthcare Reform

The House and Senate missed the Obama Administration's summer deadline for passing healthcare reform. The delay in passing the bill provided the opposition with the opportunity to disparage the bill and weaken political support for it. When legislators returned home for the summer recess and held town hall meetings, they were met with a great deal of public anger. The unexpected anger was driven by both accurate and inaccurate media discussions of various provisions being considered as part of the healthcare legislation, such as paying doctors to provide end-of-life counseling to Medicare patients; talk of government-run "death panels" frightened the aged. Included in the legislation were funds for comparative effectiveness research, which opponents claimed would go beyond simply providing information on the effectiveness of different treatments and eventually be used by the government for deciding which treatments would be reimbursed.

Distrust of the proposed bill grew. Coverage was to be expanded to an additional 32 million people, Medicare expenditures were to be reduced by almost $600 billion over ten years, payments to Medicare Advantage plans would be decreased, access to care would be less for seniors if they had to compete with more newly insured amid a growing shortage of primary care physicians, out-of-pocket payments and premiums would be increased, and growing doubt emerged that the legislation would "bend the cost curve down." Instead, more people became concerned that the plan would increase the deficit, contrary to the projections of the administration and the Congressional Budget Office. (To be fully paid for over ten years, the legislation delayed the start of the costly benefit increases for four years, but the taxes, excise fees, and provider payment reductions were to start at the beginning of the ten-year period.)

The administration failed to convince the middle class or Medicare seniors that they would benefit from reform, and it and Congress both were surprised by the intense opposition. The protests were not from the healthcare industry, which came out in favor of reform, but from grassroots segments of the public—some of whom were members of the newly formed but loosely organized Tea Party. Initially, these angry protests and the Tea Party were derided by most of the media, but they proved to be an early indication of the public's dissatisfaction with the proposed healthcare bill and with the growing role of government. The public also became concerned about the increasing federal deficit and the government's involvement into different sectors of the economy, such as with the bailouts of the auto companies and the banks, the large amount spent on the stimulus bill, and the government "takeover" of the health sector. The public also feared that the new reform bill would not be completely paid for. There was a great deal of confusion concerning various provisions and what they meant, and many legislators admitted to not having read the complex 2,600-page draft of the legislation.

During this period, congressional Republicans and other opponents of the legislation proposed going slower on healthcare reform, doing more to lower healthcare costs before greatly expanding public and private coverage, and working to reduce the federal deficit. Because the bill was being crafted without Republican support, it was in the Republicans' political interest to criticize the bill as the public turned against it.

Enactment of the ACA

As polls showed the legislation was losing public support, the Obama Administration believed that Democrats had more to lose politically by abandoning the health bill than by pushing it through. It was argued that, in 1994, as a result of failing to pass the Clinton healthcare bill, the Democrats lost control of Congress. The administration believed that, by the 2010 midterm election, the public would favor the bill.

The House of Representatives finally enacted their reform bill in November 2009, but with a surprisingly close vote—220 to 215. Democratic legislators had become fearful of their reelection prospects after the public's anger during the summer. The next step was the Senate. Attempts by the Senate finance committee chair to devise a compromise bill delayed the Senate's vote until the end of 2009. Liberal senators were reluctant to make many concessions to achieve a broad bipartisan bill because the Democrats had a filibuster-proof majority.

To secure the 60 votes needed to withstand a Republican filibuster, it was necessary that all Senate Democrats vote in favor of the legislation. Consequently, each Democratic senator had market power; many Democratic senators were able to negotiate special deals for their constituents, several of which became publicized and derided. For example, a senator from Nebraska engineered the "Cornhusker Kickback," which stipulates that the federal government will pay 100 percent of Nebraska's Medicaid expansions in perpetuity.[6] Media publicity on some of these special deals angered the public. The Senate passed its bill in late December 2009.

The outcome of the bill, which received 60 Senate votes, had more to do with special deals than good public policy: $100 million for a particular but unnamed hospital in Connecticut, ethanol subsidies, exemption from a new insurance tax for Blue Cross Blue Shield in Michigan, increased payments for hospitals in Nevada, and so on. (All the hundreds of special deals and exemptions from taxes negotiated on behalf of groups with a concentrated interest illustrate how budget and allocation decisions are made when the government enacts a broad redistributive program and how such future decisions are likely to be influenced.)

Because the Senate bill differed in substantial ways from the House bill, the normal process would have been for the two bills to be reconciled in a House and Senate conference committee and then for the Senate and House to vote on the new compromise bill. An unexpected event derailed the normal process of using the conference committee. In a major upset, a Republican won the January special Senate election to fill the late Senator Edward Kennedy's (D-MA) seat. Senator Scott Brown (R-MA) vowed to vote against the healthcare bill. A conference committee bill could not be sent back to the Senate, where the Republicans gained their forty-first seat, sufficient to filibuster the bill. Thus, the previously passed Senate bill became the basis for the legislation. To make some changes in the Senate bill desired by House leaders, a budget reconciliation bill was agreed upon between the House and Senate, which only required a simple Senate majority to pass. ACA was enacted in March 2010.

The administration believed it could enact near universal coverage by convincing the middle class and the aged that not only would it not cost them anything but that they would benefit from the legislation—a necessary condition for a far-reaching, expensive, visible redistributive program. By the time Congress voted on the legislation, many of the middle class and aged concluded they would be better off without it.

The Obama Administration's Objective for Healthcare Reform: A Hypothesis

The healthcare reform legislation had conflicting objectives.

- Insurance coverage was to be expanded (through increased Medicaid eligibility and state exchange premium subsidies) to an additional 32 million—yet the administration claimed it would also reduce the federal deficit.
- More costly, comprehensive insurance benefits were mandated, although the administration said the ACA would lower the typical family's premiums by $2,500 a year.
- The president stated, "if you are happy with your health plan, you can keep it." However, if the employer makes changes to employees' health benefits, their plan is no longer grandfathered, and they can't keep their plan. Additionally, payments to Medicare Advantage plans would be decreased, causing many seniors to switch back to traditional Medicare or remain in Medicare Advantage plans and pay higher premiums or receive fewer benefits.
- Healthcare reform was supposed to add health plan choices, yet fewer health plan choices (Bronze, Silver, Gold, and Platinum) were to become available, and insurance regulations (such as minimum medical loss ratios) would force many plans to exit state exchanges.
- Over the next ten years, the rate of increase in Medicare expenditures would be reduced by almost $600 billion (to fund subsidies on the exchanges), but the administration stated that access and quality of care for Medicare patients would not be affected.
- Lastly, healthcare reform was going to "bend the cost curve down." Yet no consumer or provider incentives were changed that would reduce healthcare spending.[7]

To drastically change the healthcare system, it is necessary to have political support from the middle class and the aged. Thus, the administration had to promise them that they would benefit from the change.

These conflicting objectives and statements, however, do not clarify the administration's goal in proposing such a vast undertaking. If the administration just wanted to cover the uninsured, it could have done so with less change to the entire system and without a complicated bill that few legislators who voted for it even read.

One can only hypothesize what the administration's underlying objective was for healthcare reform. Coverage was to be expanded to an additional 32 million people and insurance benefits for the middle class and the aged were to be increased—at no additional cost, which would be expected to greatly increase demand for medical services. During this period of high demand, the supply of medical services (such as physicians and other medical personnel) could not be similarly expanded. Medical prices and expenditures would be expected to sharply rise.[8] However, the administration claimed that broad tax hikes would not be needed to pay for the additional coverage or benefits nor would the federal deficit be affected. Because the legislation does not change consumer and provider incentives to spend less money, the only way this conflicting scenario can be achieved is by imposing stringent government controls over medical prices and expenditures.[9]

Medicare expenditures have been rising at an unsustainable rate and are a major unfunded liability for the federal government. These expenditures make up a growing portion of the federal budget (leaving less money available for other federal programs) and are projected to greatly explode the federal deficit (Exhibit 2.1). Estimates are that Medicare benefits for current and future participants, discounted to their present value, will add $27.5 trillion to the deficit (Part A: $5.9 trillion, Part B: $ 14.8 trillion, and Part D: $6.8 trillion) (Department of the Treasury 2013, 46–47). In addition, the federal government is responsible for its share of Medicaid expenditures, which were $251 billion in 2012 and are projected to increase to $391 billion in 2018, or a total of $2.261 trillion over the period 2012 to 2018. The federal government will be unable to fund these programs without limiting access to care and/or raising taxes.

If Medicare expenditures were to be reduced by paying physicians and other providers less, providers would reallocate their time to where they can make more money; they would serve fewer Medicare patients and care for more privately insured patients, as occurs with Medicaid. Less access by Medicare patients would become a significant political problem. The government would have to reduce providers' incentives to serve fewer Medicare patients. To do so, providers would have to receive the same fees for serving Medicare and private patients.

Thus, a proposed solution to Medicare and Medicaid's unsustainable increases in the federal deficit while preventing providers from reducing access to Medicare patients is a Canadian type single-payer system. Everyone would have the same benefits and would be in the same system. The government would establish provider payments and control total expenditures. The aged would continue to have the same benefits (as would everyone) and no less access than anyone else.

The government-run public option plan was meant to evolve into a single-payer system. A heavily subsidized government plan available to everyone, together with stringent regulations on private insurers, would eventually drive most insurers out of the market. Medicare, Medicaid, and the public option plan would then encompass most of the population. Remaining employer health plans would eventually be included in the single-payer system at no visible cost to the employee; the government would collect the funds from the employer.

Orzag and Emanuel (2010), two administration architects of the ACA, explained how regulation would be used to control rising medical costs:

> The most important institutional change in the ACA, however, is likely to be the establishment of the Independent Payment Advisory Board (IPAB), an independent panel of medical experts tasked with devising changes to Medicare's payment system. Beginning in January 2014, each year that Medicare's per capita costs exceed a certain threshold, the IPAB will develop and propose policies for reducing this inflation. The secretary of HHS must institute the policies unless Congress enacts alternative policies leading to equivalent savings. The threshold is a bit complex; initially, it is a combination of general and medical inflation, but in 2018 and thereafter, the cap is set at general inflation plus 1%.

The ACA, however, prohibited the IPAB from proposing to control expenditure growth rates by changing Medicare benefits or eligibility or from increasing beneficiary cost sharing or premium percentage. The only alternative cost-control measures left to the IPAB are to cut provider payments and/or the price of certain costly treatments, making them less available.

Limiting cost growth to a level below medical inflation is difficult to achieve. The fact that legislators regularly ignore Medicare physician payment reductions indicated by the SGR is cited by some as proof that Congress cannot cut Medicare costs. The reason for the establishment of the IPAB and for the difficulty Congress faced to simply override IPAB recommendations is that legislators would be unable, politically, to reduce benefits or provider payments. If the IPAB is able to decrease Medicare's payment rates but not private payers' rates, the gap between Medicare rates and private rates will increase and providers will be less likely to serve Medicare patients. To prevent physicians from abandoning Medicare patients, prices in the private market would have to be similarly controlled; a public option plan would have enabled this to occur, similar to the adoption of a single-payer system.

Implementation of the ACA

The implementation of the ACA sign-up in 2013 was disastrous. The federal exchange website (substituting for 27 states that refused to initiate their own exchanges) functioned very poorly. (Websites for states having their own exchanges performed better.) It became frustrating for the millions of people who wanted to sign up during the open enrollment period. A great deal of unfavorable media publicity occurred. Adding to the bad publicity, Republicans in the House of Representatives held hearings on why, after more than three years of preparation, the federal website was not operable.

During this period, most of those enrolled in the individual insurance market (about 5 percent, or 8 million, of the privately insured population) began receiving cancellation notices from their insurer. Their previous coverage did not meet the higher benefit coverage mandated by the ACA; they had to enroll on the federal and state websites to buy insurance. However, many were unable to sign up through the federal exchange because the website was not working. Those who were ill and under the care of a physician were very upset; they were afraid that they would be without insurance after the first of the year.

President Obama's earlier claim, repeated over and over—"if you are happy with your health plan, you can keep it"—turned out not to be true. Those who believed in the ACA and then received a cancellation notice were very upset. The president apologized but because of his broken promise, his poll ratings dropped. He had been previously aware that many would lose their insurance, yet he continued to make his claim. Belief in the president's "trustworthiness" fell sharply. Other claims made to sell the ACA to the middle class also fell by the wayside. Instead of seeing their premiums decrease by $2,500, people found the new plans on the exchange were quite expensive and had large deductibles (even after receiving premium subsidies), particularly for the young whose premiums were subsidizing those who were older. The new plans also included mandated additional benefits, which raised the cost of the plans. Fewer young people enrolled in the exchanges, and insurers were concerned that they would have more costly, sicker, enrollees. To control what they believed would be adverse selection, insurer plans used very narrow networks of hospitals and physicians. Another claim that "you can keep your doctor" was also no longer accurate.

In addition to all the bad media publicity surrounding the failed website and the millions of cancellations, the unions—staunch backers of the ACA—came out in opposition to the ACA. Unions representing workers in industries with small employers have what are referred to as multiemployer health insurance plans. Unions and employers contribute to the cost of the insurance. About 20 million workers—from high-wage construction workers to low-wage restaurant workers—are enrolled in these plans. Access to union-negotiated health insurance benefits by workers employed in these industries have been an important reason they joined unions. Under the ACA, small employers can drop their employer-sponsored coverage and send their employees to the exchanges, once their current collective bargaining agreements end. The employees can then buy subsidized coverage on the exchanges and would have less incentive to pay dues to join a union.

Unions want their members, who already have employer-sponsored insurance, to receive the same subsidies as are available on the exchanges. According to the ACA, employees with employer-sponsored insurance are not eligible for exchange subsidies. The unions have threatened the administration that they would work to repeal the law if their members do not also receive subsidies. It is surprising that the unions did not foresee such a crucial aspect of the legislation.

Democrats who voted for the ACA and who were up for reelection in 2014 began distancing themselves from the ACA. The Republicans, however, were intent on reminding the voters—particularly in states carried by Romney in the 2012 election—which Democrats voted for the law.

Many millions of people who work for small businesses were due to receive their cancellation notices in fall 2014. Health insurance, access to healthcare, and the patient–physician relationship are very personal issues. As a political issue, the ACA will continue to remain in the headlines and influence election outcomes.

The Years Ahead

The purpose of visible redistributive legislation is to be able to provide politically powerful groups with benefits in excess of their costs. The only way this can be achieved is if the government legislates it. The Obama Administration was able to receive the political support for its healthcare reform legislation from most groups with a concentrated interest, such as the PhRMA, AMA, AHA, unions, AARP, and employers. The administration tried to convince the middle class and aged that they can keep what they have, their costs would be lower, and their access to care would not decrease. For broad visible redistribution to occur, general agreement is needed from the middle class and the aged; if not, it will eventually be changed. This is what occurred with the Medicare Catastrophic Act of 1988, which was repealed the following year.

Healthcare reform has to impose increased cost (such as higher taxes or reduced access) on some population groups if greater benefits are to be provided to others (such as the uninsured and those with low income).

Expanding access to an additional 32 million (mandating comprehensive benefits to everyone) without changing consumer or provider incentives, while claiming costs will be lower, is irreconcilable.

Four years after the passage of the ACA, the law remains deeply unpopular; more than 60 percent of those polled (as of 2014) favor major changes or repeal. The unions, who were important backers of the law, are now strongly opposed to certain provisions. Many states have decided against forming insurance exchanges and a number of states have refused to expand their Medicaid eligibility levels. It is uncertain whether sufficient numbers of younger people will enroll in the exchanges, causing significantly higher premiums for older groups. The ACA is also causing changes to the labor market as employers are cutting the hours of work for their least-skilled and lowest-income employees so as not to provide their employees with insurance or to pay a penalty. Many large employers and their employees may decide it is in both their interests for employees to buy subsidized insurance on the exchanges, thereby greatly expanding the number of enrollees on the exchanges. Lastly, the cost of the ACA is highly likely to exceed its estimated costs, placing greater pressure on the federal deficit, resulting in political fights over ACA subsidies and other federal entitlements.

The next several elections are likely to decide the future of the ACA. If dissatisfaction with the ACA among the middle class, aged, and unions continues, the law is likely to be drastically changed. These changes may move the healthcare system toward greater price and insurer regulation (and possibly a single-payer system, such as "Medicare for All") or toward a different direction—such as greater reliance on patient and provider incentives to reduce costs and greater choice of health plans—within a more competitive medical marketplace. It is too early to judge how healthcare reform will evolve.

Discussion Questions

1. What are alternative hypotheses regarding what national health insurance should achieve?
2. Why are groups that have a concentrated interest in a particular legislation likely to be more influential in the policy process than groups that have a diffuse interest in the legislation's outcome?
3. What are the conflicting objectives of healthcare reform?
4. How did President Obama try to convince the middle class that they would benefit from healthcare reform at no additional cost?
5. What benefits did the ACA provide for the aged?
6. Why were many aged opposed to the ACA?
7. What aspects of the public option plan concerned health insurers?

8. Why are health insurers concerned that even without the public option being explicitly included in the legislation, a government-run health plan may still occur?

Notes

1. Regressive taxation occurs when the tax represents a greater percentage of income for low-income groups than for high-income groups. A payroll tax of a flat dollar amount or a percentage of income up to a certain level of income results in high-wage earners paying a smaller percentage than low-wage earners.

2. Another example of AARP's possible conflict of interest was the Medicare Catastrophic Act of 1988, which provided seniors with a prescription drug benefit and financed it by increasing taxes on high-income aged. The AARP's endorsement convinced legislators that seniors would be pleased by their efforts. The AARP offered drug plans and stood to make a great deal of money from the increase in demand for such plans. Many seniors, however, were so upset with the financing provisions that Congress repealed the law the following year.

3. Persons whose tax credit exceeds their tax liabilities would receive a refund for the difference. For those with little or no tax liability, the tax credit is essentially a voucher for a health plan.

4. Although advocates claimed that the public option would create needed competition to insurers, various provisions in the bill were expected to reduce the number of competing insurers and choice of coverage, suggesting that its advocates were really opposed to increasing competitive forces in healthcare. The successful competition among private firms to deliver the Medicare Part D drug benefit, which reduced premiums, was to be limited by requiring competing firms to offer only one, rather than multiple, drug plans. Regulations imposed on insurers—such as specifying minimum loss ratios, standard benefit plans, and review of premium increases—all belie the notion that greater competition was truly desired by the bill's proponents.

5. One study estimated that about 140 million would switch to the public option (Halpin and Harbage 2010).

6. When Republicans complained about special deals being included in the bill, Senate majority leader Harry Reid (D-NV) replied, "There's a hundred senators here, and I don't know if there is a senator that

doesn't have something in this bill that was important to them. If they don't have something in it important to them, then it doesn't speak well of them. That's what this legislation is all about. It's the art of compromise" (Pear 2010).

7. President Obama claimed that the ACA has helped slow the growth in healthcare prices and spending. However, the Centers for Medicare & Medicaid Services, the Congressional Budget Office, and various researchers attributed the slow growth to the depth and severity of the recession, greater cost sharing in private plans, and a slower rate of introduction of new technology—all of which started before President Obama was elected (Chandra, Holmes, and Skinner 2013; also see Kaiser Family Foundation 2013 and Exhibit 1.3).

8. A study by the Office of the Actuary claims that medical expenditures will be greater, not less, under healthcare reform (Cuckler et al. 2013).

9. Included in the new law are various approaches to control medical costs, such as eliminating fraud and waste (which has been proposed by various administrations); greater use of electronic medical records; and new pilot programs, such as developing accountable care organizations, bundled payments, and comparative effectiveness research. Although these programs may be promising, there has been no evidence that they can control costs (Goldsmith 2013).

References

Bureau of Labor Statistics. 2014. "Union Members Summary." *Economic News Release*. Posted January 24. www.bls.gov/news.release/union2.nr0.htm.

Chandra, A., J. Holmes, and J. Skinner. 2013. "Is This Time Different? The Slowdown in Healthcare Spending." *Brookings Panel on Economic Activity*. September 19–20. www.brookings.edu/~/media/Projects/BPEA/Fall%20 2013/2013b%20chandra%20healthcare%20spending.pdf.

Conover, C., and T. Miller. 2010. "Why a Public Option Is Unnecessary to Stimulate Competition." *AEI Working Paper* No. 162, January. www.aei .org/paper/100077.

Cuckler, G., A. Sisko, S. Keehan, S. Smith, A. Madison, J. Poisal, C. Wolfe, J. Lizonitz, and D. Stone. 2013. "National Health Expenditure Projections, 2012–22: Slow Growth Until Coverage Expands and Economy Improves." *Health Affairs* 32 (10): 1820–31. http://content.healthaffairs.org/ content/32/10/1820.abstract?etoc.

Daschle, T., S. Greenberger, and J. Lambrew. 2008. *Critical: What We Can Do About the Health-Care Crisis*. New York: Thomas Dunne Publisher.

Feldstein, P. 2006. "The Medicare Modernization Act, 2003." In *The Politics of Health Legislation: An Economic Perspective*, 3rd ed. Chicago: Health Administration Press.

Geiger, K. 2009. "Medical Billing Code Monopoly Explains American Medical Association's Support for Health Plan, Critics Say." *Chicagotribune.com*, December 27. www.chicago tribune.com/health/chi-sun-health-ama-1227dec27,0,4125322.story.

Goldsmith, J. 2013. "Pioneer ACOs' Disappointing First Year." *Health Affairs* blog. Posted August 13. http://healthaffairs.org/blog/2013/08/15/pioneer-acos-disappointing-first-year/.

Halpin, H., and P. Harbage. 2010. "The Origins and Demise of the Public Option." *Health Affairs* 29 (6): 1117–123.

Kaiser Family Foundation. 2014. "Where Are States Today? Medicaid and CHIP Eligibility Levels for Children and Non-Disabled Adults as of January 1, 2014." Posted January 13. http://kaiserfamilyfoundation.files.wordpress.com/2014/01/7993-04-tables-where-are-states-today-medicaid-and-chip-eligibility-levels.pdf).

———. 2013. "Assessing the Effects of the Economy on the Recent Slowdown in Health Spending." Published April 22. http://kff.org/health-costs/issue-brief/assessing-the-effects-of-the-economy-on-the-recent-slowdown-in-health-spending-2/.

Orzag, P., and E. Emanuel. 2010. "Health Care Reform and Cost Control." *NEMJ.org Postings*. Posted June 16. http://healthcare reform.nejm.org/?p=3564&query=home.

Pear, R. 2010. "In Health Bill for Everyone, Provisions for a Few." *New York Times*, January 4. www.nytimes.com/2010/01/04/health/policy/04health.html?pagewanted=print.

Roy, A. 2011. "Why the American Medical Association Had 72 Million Reasons to Shrink Doctors' Pay." *Forbes*, November 11. www.forbes.com/sites/theapothecary/2011/11/28/why-the-american-medical-association-had-72-million-reasons-to-help-shrink-doctors-pay/.

US Census Bureau. 2013. *2013 Current Population Reports. Population Characteristics, P20 Series*. Various editions. Accessed September 2014. www.census.gov/hhes/www/socdemo/voting/publications/p20/.

US Department of the Treasury. 2013. *Citizen's Guide to the 2012 Financial Report of the United States Government*. Accessed February 2014. www.fms.treas.gov/fr/12frusg/12frusg.pdf.

Vincent, H. 2013. *Demographic Characteristics of the House of Delegates and AMA Leadership.* CLRPD Report 2-A-13. American Medical Association. Accessed February 2014. www.ama-assn.org/resources/doc/clrpd/2013-demographic-report.pdf.

Wall Street Journal. 2009. "The Public Option Goes Over." Editorial. *Wall Street Journal,* August 18, p. A16.

APPENDIX: A BRIEF SUMMARY OF THE PATIENT PROTECTION AND AFFORDABLE CARE ACT OF 2010

In 2010, President Obama and large Democratic majorities in the House and Senate, without any support from House or Senate Republicans, enacted healthcare legislation that has been described as the most far-reaching health legislation since Medicare and Medicaid were enacted in 1965. This law—the Patient Protection and Affordable Care Act (ACA)—is very complex and will affect everyone in one way or another.[1] The law applies to US citizens and legal immigrants. Many aspects of the law continued to be defined through an extensive number of administrative regulations. The Obama Administration has delayed implementing several provisions of the law.

The following describes the basic elements of the ACA, much of which did not take effect until 2014 and will not be completely phased in until 2019.

Coverage

Medicaid Expansions

States are permitted to expand their Medicaid programs by covering individuals and families up to 133 percent of the federal poverty level (FPL), effective 2014. (For individuals 133 percent of the FPL is $15,521 and $31,720 for a family of four in 2014). (Contrary to the ACA, which required states to expand their Medicaid eligibility, the US Supreme Court ruled that Medicaid expansion is optional.) The federal government will pay 100 percent of the cost of Medicaid expansion in 2014–2016; thereafter, the federal share will decline to 90 percent in 2020 and beyond.

An Individual Mandate

Individuals must obtain minimum "essential" coverage for themselves and their families, effective 2014. Failure to do so results in a tax of $95 in 2014, increasing to $695 by 2016 and beyond (indexed for inflation). The tax might alternatively be a percentage of income—0.1 percent in 2014 up to 2.5 percent of taxable income in 2016. (The maximum tax will be $2,085 in 2016). Individuals who qualify on hardship grounds are exempt from the tax.

An Employer Mandate

Employers with *more than 50 employees* must offer qualified coverage to their employees. If an employer does not offer qualified coverage and has at least one employee receiving a premium tax credit, the employer is fined $2,000 per full-time employee (excluding the first 30 employees).[2] Employers with *50 or fewer full-time employees* are exempt from any of these penalties.

Individual Tax Credits

Individuals and families with incomes between 133 percent and 400 percent of the FPL who purchase their insurance on an insurance exchange will receive premium credits and cost-sharing subsidies on a sliding scale and as a percentage of income. (For individuals, 133 percent of the FPL is $15,521 and $31,720 for a family of four in 2014; 400 percent of the FPL is $46,680 for individuals and $95,400 for a family of four). For example, a family with income at 400 percent of the FPL will pay 9.5 percent of its income, or $9,063.

Small Business Tax Credits

Small firms can receive tax credits equal to 50 percent of the amount paid for their employees' health coverage if they have 25 or fewer employees with average annual wages below $50,000.

Medicare Prescription Drug Benefit (Part D)

The "donut hole"—where seniors pay 100 percent of the costs of drugs—will be reduced by 50 percent in 2011, and by 2020 that gap will be eliminated. Seniors that reached the donut hole in 2010 received a $250 rebate.

Medicare Preventive Services

The ACA waives cost sharing for preventive services, such as prostate, colon, and breast cancer screenings, and seniors will have access to a comprehensive health-risk assessment.

Public Health and Workforce Issues

The federal government will finance various grant, loan, and funding programs for healthcare professionals. Also included is funding for community health centers ($11 billion).

Health Insurance Changes

Dependent Coverage

Insurers that offer dependent coverage must allow uninsured children to remain on or join their parent's coverage until age 26 years, regardless of whether the child has a preexisting condition. Insurers can increase the premium for adding the dependent child.

Preventive Services

Insurers must offer preventive services and immunizations, without cost sharing.

Guaranteed Issue, Lifetime Limits, and Rescinding Coverage

Insurers will be barred from rejecting applicants based on health status, medical condition or history, or genetic information. (Elimination of preexisting condition exclusion). Individual and group health plans are prohibited from placing lifetime limits on the dollar value of coverage, and insurers are prohibited from rescinding coverage except in cases of fraud.

High-Risk Pools

Until the health insurance exchanges became available in 2013, a temporary high-risk insurance pool was available for uninsured people who have been denied coverage by insurers because of a preexisting medical condition.

Medical Loss Ratio (MLR)

Group plans must have an MLR not less than 85 percent and individual plans not less than 80 percent.

Insurance Rating (Pricing)

Differential prices cannot be based on health or gender. Insurance premiums can only vary by a ratio of 1.5:1 for tobacco users, 3:1 according to age, and according to family composition and geography.

Insurer Rate Review

Insurers will be required to submit justifications for premium increases. Plans with "excessive" rate increases will be prohibited from participating in the health insurance exchanges.

Health Insurance Exchanges

States had the option to establish an insurance exchange by 2014 that will facilitate the purchase of "qualified" health plans. The exchange can only be a government agency or a nonprofit organization. The federal government established an exchange for those states declining to participate.

Health insurance plans in the individual and small group market must provide the "essential" benefits package effective 2014. Four benefit categories of plans are offered on the exchange. All plans offered on the exchange must include basic medical services and will be one of four types—Bronze, Silver, Gold, and Platinum—based on their coverage. The Bronze plan would cover 60 percent of the benefit costs of the plan, Silver 70 percent, Gold 80 percent, and Platinum 90 percent.

People in their 20s have the option of buying a catastrophic plan ($6,000 out-of-pocket expenses before coverage begins) that has lower premiums. Three primary care visits and preventive care are to be included in the plan with no cost sharing.

Small employers (100 or fewer employees) are eligible to use the exchange and, with state permission, so are employers with more than 100 employees. Qualified individuals are also eligible to use the exchange.

Essential Benefits Package

All qualified health benefits plans—including those offered through the exchanges and those offered in the individual and small group markets outside the exchanges (except grandfathered individual and employer-sponsored plans)—are required to offer at least the essential health benefits package.

Long-Term Care

A new voluntary long-term care program was established for the purpose of purchasing community living assistance services and supports (CLASS Act). After a five-year vesting period, the program was supposed to provide individuals with functional limitations a cash benefit of not less than $50 per day to purchase nonmedical services and supports necessary to maintain a community residence. The Obama Administration claimed the CLASS Act was unworkable, and it was subsequently repealed by Congress.

How the Health Benefits and Coverage Are Financed

The higher government expenditures called for in the ACA were estimated to be paid for by increased taxes on individuals and different segments of the health industry and $500 billion in Medicare payment reductions to different providers. Demonstration programs were established in the expectation that they would eventually be able to reduce rising healthcare costs, but no specific estimate of their potential savings was included.

Individual Income Taxes

The Medicare payroll tax is increased 0.9 percent—from 1.45 percent to 2.35 percent—on individuals earning more than $200,000 and families earning more than $250,000. In addition, a 3.8 percent Medicare tax is imposed on all unearned income, such as investment income, dividends, royalties, and capital gains, for individuals earning more than $200,000 and families earning more than $250,000. These income amounts are not adjusted for inflation.

Reduced Medicare Healthcare Provider Payments

All Medicare providers will have their annual provider payment updates reduced, either as a result of changes in their market basket updates or by an assumed productivity increase, which would reduce annual update payments, effective 2011. Physicians are provided with a financial incentive to participate in a quality reporting system and are penalized if they do not participate by 2015.

Medicare Advantage Plans

Medicare Advantage plans had been receiving payments in excess of the costs of treating comparable (risk-adjusted) Medicare beneficiaries in traditional (fee-for-service) Medicare; these additional payments will be reduced.

Excise Tax on High Cost Health Plans ("Cadillac" Plans)

A 40 percent tax will be imposed on health coverage that exceeds $10,200 for individuals and $27,500 for families (thereafter indexed for inflation), effective 2018. Stand-alone dental and vision plans are not subject to the tax.

Health Insurance Industry User Fee

An annual fee will be imposed on the health insurance industry of $8 billion in 2014, rising to $14.3 billion in 2018 and increasing by the rate of growth in premiums thereafter. Nonprofit insurers are subject to a smaller tax.

Medical Device Industry Excise Tax

A 2.3 percent excise tax is imposed on gross revenues of all medical devices sold in the United States.

Pharmaceutical Industry User Fee

An annual fee is imposed on manufacturers of brand name prescription drugs of $2.5 billion in 2011, increasing to $4.1 billion in 2018 and then to $2.8 billion in 2019 and beyond.

Medical Expense Deduction

The medical expense deduction threshold for claiming the itemized deduction for medical expenses is increased from 7.5 percent to 10 percent.

Employer Tax Deduction for Medicare Part D Expenses

The tax deduction for employers who receive Medicare Part D drug subsidy payments is eliminated.

Health Savings Accounts (HSAs)

A 20 percent tax is imposed on funds from HSA accounts that are not used for medical expenses.

Flexible Spending Accounts (FSAs)

FSA contributions are limited to $2,500 a year adjusted for inflation.

Independent Medicare Payment Advisory Board

An Independent Payment Advisory Board is established to develop and submit proposals to Congress aimed at extending the solvency of Medicare, slowing growth in costs, improving quality of care, and reducing national health expenditures. Congress constrained the board's options in that the board cannot include recommendations to ration healthcare, raise revenues under premiums, increase beneficiary cost sharing, or restrict benefits. Options available to the board to reduce Medicare expenditures may include decreasing provider payments, changing the age of eligibility, or making a change to the benefits offered. The board's proposals will be automatically implemented unless Congress opposes them. Proposals to modify Medicare payments will be effective starting in 2015 (2020 for hospitals). To date, no board members have been appointed.

Comparative Effectiveness Research

The Patient-Centered Outcomes Research Institute is established to identify national priorities for comparative clinical effectiveness research. The institute is prohibited from mandating coverage or reimbursement policies based on the institute's research.

Other Legislative Initiatives

Accountable Care Organizations (ACOs)

Medicare will establish a shared savings program to promote accountability and coordination of Medicare Parts A and B. Groups of providers who meet certain criteria will be recognized as ACOs and become eligible to share in the cost savings achieved by Medicare.

Medicare Payment Innovations

This establishes a new Center for Medicare and Medicaid Innovation to test, evaluate, and expand different payment structures and methodologies. The government will develop a national, voluntary, bundled payment pilot program to provide incentives for providers to coordinate care. The Independent Medicare Advisory Board will test medical home models.

Specialty Hospitals

New or expanded physician-owned specialty hospitals are prohibited; existing physician-owned specialty hospitals are grandfathered in.

Medicare Quality and Transparency Initiatives

Several approaches are proposed to increase quality reporting and transparency.

Notes

1. The Kaiser Family Foundation website has a detailed summary of the ACA; see http://kaiserfamilyfoundation.files.wordpress .com/2011/04/8061-021.pdf.
2. Low-wage employees whose employer does not offer health insurance are able to receive almost fully subsidized insurance in a state health insurance exchange. The same employee, however, who is required to buy insurance at work does not receive a similar subsidy.

GLOSSARY

accountable care organization—Network of hospitals, physicians, and other providers receiving payment incentives from Medicare for coordinating care for a defined group of Medicare patients.

actual versus list price—Actual prices are the fees collected or paid for a particular good or service. The differences between actual and list prices are provider discounts, which vary by type of payer.

actuarially fair insurance—Expected insurance payments (benefits) are equivalent to premiums paid by beneficiaries (plus a competitive loading charge).

adverse selection—Occurs when high-risk individuals have more information on their health status than the insurer and are thus able to buy insurance at a premium based on a lower-risk group.

all-payer system—Each payer pays the same charges for hospital and medical services.

American Medical Association (AMA)—A national organization established in 1897 to represent the collective interests of physicians.

antitrust laws—A body of legislation that promotes competition in the US economy.

any willing provider (AWP) laws—These laws lessen price competition in that they permit any physician to have access to a health plan's enrollees at the negotiated price. Because physicians cannot be assured of having a greater number of enrollees in return for discounting their prices, physicians have no incentive to compete on price to be included in the health plan's network.

assignment/participation—An agreement whereby the provider accepts the approved fee from the third-party payer and is not permitted to charge the patient more, except for the appropriate copayment fees.

balance billing—When the physician collects from the patient the difference between the third-party payer's approved fee and the physician's fee.

barriers to entry—Barriers, which may be legal (e.g., licensing laws and patents) or economic (e.g., economies of scale), that limit entry into an industry.

benefit–premium ratio—The percentage of the total premium paid out in benefits to each insured group divided by the price of insurance. (Also referred to as the medical loss ratio.)

budget neutral—Total payments to providers under the current payment system are set equal to what was spent under the previous payment system.

Canadian-type health system—A form of national health insurance in which medical services are free to everyone and providers are paid by the government. Expenditure limits are used to restrict the growth in medical use and costs.

capitation incentive—When the provider is capitated, he becomes concerned with the coordination of all medical services, providing care in the least costly manner, monitoring the cost of enrollees' hospital use, increasing physician productivity, prescribing less costly drugs, and being innovative in the delivery of medical services. Conversely, the provider has an incentive to reduce use of services and decrease patient access.

capitation payment—A risk-sharing arrangement in which the provider group receives a predetermined fixed payment per member per month in return for providing all of the contracted services.

case-mix index—A measure of the relative complexity of the patient mix treated in a given medical care setting.

certificate-of-need (CON) laws—State laws requiring healthcare providers to receive prior approval from a state agency for capital expenditures exceeding predetermined levels. CON laws are an entry barrier.

coinsurance—A fixed percentage of the medical provider's fee paid by the insurance beneficiary at the point of service.

community rating—The insurance premium is the same to all of the insured, regardless of their claims experience or risk group.

competitive market—The interaction between a large number of buyers and suppliers, where no single seller or buyer can influence the market price.

concentrated interest—When some regulation or legislation has a sufficiently large effect on a group to make it worthwhile for that group to invest resources to either forestall or promote that effect.

consumer-driven healthcare (CDHC)—Consumers purchase high-deductible health insurance and bear greater responsibility for their use of medical services and the prices they pay healthcare providers.

consumer sovereignty—Consumers, rather than health professionals or the government, choose the goods and services they can purchase with their income.

copayment—A specific dollar amount paid by the patient at the point of service.

cost-containment program—Approaches used to reduce healthcare costs, such as utilization review and patient cost sharing.

cost shifting—The belief that providers charge a higher price to privately insured patients because some payers, such as Medicaid or the uninsured, do not pay their full costs.

declining marginal productivity of health inputs—The additional contribution to output of a health input declines as more of that input is used.

deductible—Consumers pay a flat dollar amount for a medical service before their insurance picks up all or part of the remainder of the price of that service.

diagnosis-related group (DRG)—A method of reimbursement established under Medicare to pay hospitals based on a fixed price per admission according to the diagnosis for which the patient is admitted.

diffuse cost—When the burden of a tax or program is spread over a large population and is relatively small per person so that the per person cost of opposing such a burden exceeds the actual size of the burden on the person.

economic theory of regulation—A theory of legislative and regulatory outcomes that assumes political markets are no different from economic markets in that organized groups seek to further their self-interests.

economies of scale—The relationship between cost per unit and size of firm. As firm size increases, cost per unit falls, reaches a minimum, and eventually rises. In a competitive market, each firm operates at the size that has the lowest per unit costs. For a given size market, the larger the firm size required to achieve the minimum costs of production, the fewer the number of firms that will be able to compete.

economies of scope—Occur when it is less costly for a firm to produce certain services (or products) jointly than if separate firms produced each of the same services independently.

employer-mandated health insurance—Starting in 2014, employers are required to provide health insurance to their employees and dependents or pay a tax per employee.

experience rating—Insurance premiums are based on the claims experience or risk level, such as age, of each insured group.

externality—Occurs when an action undertaken by an individual (or firm) has secondary effects on others, and these effects are not taken into account by the normal operations of the price system.

fee-for-service payment—A method of payment for medical care services in which payment is made for each unit of service provided.

free choice of provider—This was included in the original Medicare and Medicaid legislation and specified that all beneficiaries had to have access to all providers. This precluded closed provider panels and capitated HMOs. Economists consider the provision to be anticompetitive in that it limits competition; beneficiaries could not choose a closed provider panel in return for lower prices or increased benefits.

gatekeeper—In many HMOs, the primary care physician or gatekeeper is responsible for the administration of the patient's treatment and must coordinate and authorize all medical services, laboratory studies, specialty referrals, and hospitalizations.

geographic market definition—Used in antitrust analysis to determine the relevant market in which a healthcare provider competes. The broader the geographic market, the greater the number of substitutes available to the purchaser and hence the smaller the market share of merging firms.

guaranteed issue—Health insurers have to offer health insurance to those willing to purchase it.

guaranteed renewal—Requires health insurers to renew all health insurance policies, as long as premiums are paid, regardless of changes in the health of the insured. Any premium changes must be for the entire class of policyholders.

health maintenance organization (HMO)—A type of managed care plan that offers prepaid comprehensive healthcare coverage for hospital and physician services, relying on its medical providers to minimize the cost of providing medical services. HMOs contract with or directly employ participating healthcare providers. Enrollees must pay the full cost of receiving services from non-network providers.

health savings account (HSA)—Enacted as part of the Medicare Modernization Act, individuals are permitted to have a high-deductible insurance plan together with a savings account to use toward healthcare expenses. The unused portion of the savings account can accumulate over time.

horizontal merger—When two or more firms from the same market merge to form one firm.

income elasticity—The percentage change in quantity that occurs with a given percentage change in income. When the percentage change in quantity exceeds the percentage change in income, the service is income "elastic."

indemnity insurance—Medical insurance that pays the provider or the patient a predetermined amount for the medical service provided.

independent practice association (IPA)—A physician-owned and physician-controlled contracting organization comprising solo and small groups of physicians (on a nonexclusive basis) that enables physicians to contract with payers on a unified basis.

individual mandate—Under the ACA, everyone is required to have health insurance or pay a penalty. Subsidies to purchase insurance are to be provided to those with low income.

insurance premium—Consists of two parts: the expected medical expense of the insured group and the loading charge, which includes administrative expenses and profit.

integrated delivery system (IDS)—A healthcare delivery system that includes or contracts with all of the healthcare providers to provide coordinated medical services to the patient. An IDS also views itself as being responsible for the health status of its enrolled population.

law of demand—A decrease in price will result in an increase in quantity demanded, other factors affecting demand held constant.

managed care organization (MCO)—An organization that controls medical care costs and quality through provider price discounts, utilization management, drug formularies, and profiling participating providers according to their appropriate use of medical services.

mandated benefits—According to state insurance laws, specific medical services, providers, or population groups must be included in health insurance policies.

marginal benefit—The change in total benefits from purchasing one additional unit.

marginal contribution of medical care to health—The increase in health status resulting from an additional increment of medical services.

marginal cost—The change in total costs from producing one additional unit.

Medicaid—A health insurance program financed by federal and state governments and administered by the states for qualifying segments of the low-income population.

Medicaid risk contract—A Medicaid managed care program in which an HMO contracts to provide medical services in return for a capitation premium.

medical care price index—Calculated by the Bureau of Labor Statistics and included as part of the Consumer Price Index, it is used as a measure of the rate of inflation in medical care prices.

medical group—A group of physicians who coordinate their activities in one or more group facilities and share common overhead expenses; medical records; and professional, technical, and administrative staffs.

medical loss ratio—See *benefit–premium ratio.*

Medicare—A federally sponsored and supervised health insurance plan for the elderly. Part A provides hospital insurance for inpatient care, home health agency visits, hospice, and skilled nursing facilities. The aged are responsible for a deductible but do not have to pay an annual premium. Part B provides payments for physician services, physician-ordered supplies and services, and outpatient hospital services. Part B is voluntary, and the aged pay an annual premium that is 25 percent of the cost of the program in addition to a deductible and copayment. Part C permits private health plans to compete for serving the aged. Part D is a prescription drug benefit that includes deductibles and copayments and requires a monthly premium.

Medicare Advantage plans—Enacted as part of the Medicare Modernization Act, private health plans receive a monthly capitation payment from Medicare and accept full financial risk for the cost of all medical benefits (Part A, Part B, and Part D services) to which their enrollees are entitled. Enrollees using nonparticipating providers are responsible for the full charges of such providers. Previously referred to as Medicare+Choice plans.

Medicare risk contract—See *Medicare Advantage plans.*

Medigap insurance policy—Insurance policy privately purchased by the elderly to supplement Medicare coverage by covering deductibles and copayments.

monopoly—A market structure in which there is a single seller of a product that has no close substitutes.

moral hazard—Occurs when patients can affect the size of their loss, as when patients increase their use of medical services when the price of those services is reduced.

multihospital system—A system in which a corporation owns, leases, or manages two or more acute care hospitals.

multipayer system—A system in which reimbursement for medical services is made by multiple third-party payers.

network HMO—A type of HMO that signs contracts with a number of group practices to provide medical services.

nonprice hospital competition—Hospitals compete on the basis of their facilities and services and the latest technology rather than on price.

not-for-profit—An institution that cannot distribute profits to shareholders and is tax exempt.

nurse participation rate—The percentage of trained nurses who are employed.

opportunity cost—Relevant costs for economic decision making; they include explicit and implicit costs. For example, the opportunity costs of a medical education include the forgone income the student could have earned had she not gone to medical school.

out-of-pocket price—The amount that the beneficiary must pay after all other payments have been considered by the health plan.

over-the-counter drug—A drug that is available for public purchase and self-directed use without a prescription.

patient dumping—A situation in which high-cost patients are not admitted to or are discharged early from a hospital because the patient has no insurance or the amount reimbursed by the third-party payer will be less than the cost of caring for that patient.

Patient Protection and Affordable Care Act of 2010—Better known as the ACA, contentious legislation that expands coverage to an additional 30 million people by increasing Medicaid eligibility and providing federal subsidies to those enrolled in state and federal health insurance exchanges.

pay for performance—Higher payments are made to those healthcare providers who demonstrate that they provide higher-quality services.

per diem payment—A method of payment to institutional providers that is based on a fixed daily amount and does not differ according to the level of service provided.

pharmacy benefit manager (PBM)—Firm that provides administrative services and processes outpatient prescription drug claims for health insurers' prescription drug plans.

physician agency relationship—The physician acts on behalf of the patient. Agency relationships may be perfect or imperfect, and the method of physician payment (fee-for-service or capitation) produces different behavioral responses among imperfect physician agents.

physician–hospital organization (PHO)—An organization in which hospitals and their medical staffs develop new types of group practice arrangements that will allow the hospitals to seek contracts from HMOs and other carriers on behalf of the physicians and hospitals together.

play or pay—Employers are required to provide medical insurance to their employees (play) or pay a certain amount of tax per employee.

point-of-service plan—A plan that allows the beneficiary to select from participating providers (the health plan) or use nonparticipating providers and pay a high copayment.

portability—Included as part of health insurance reform that enables the insured to change jobs without losing their insurance.

preexisting exclusion—To protect themselves against adverse selection by new enrollees, insurers used a preexisting exclusion clause that excluded treatment for any or specified illnesses diagnosed within the previous (usually 12) months. Under the ACA, preexisting-condition exclusion can no longer be used to deny health insurance to those willing to buy insurance.

preferred provider organization (PPO)—An arrangement between a panel of healthcare providers and purchasers of healthcare services in which a closed panel of providers agrees to supply services to a defined group of patients on a discounted fee-for-service basis. This type of plan offers its members a limited number of physicians and hospitals, negotiated fee schedules, utilization review, and consumer incentives to use PPO-participating providers.

preferred risk selection—Occurs when insurers receive the same premium for everyone in an insured group and try to attract only those with lower risks, whose expected medical costs would be less than the group's average premium.

prescription drug—A drug that can be obtained only with a physician's order. It includes the following:

- **breakthrough (or innovator) drug**—The first brand-name drug to use a particular therapeutic mechanism (that is, a particular method of treating a given disease).
- **generic drug**—A copy of a breakthrough drug that the Food and Drug Administration judges to be comparable in terms of such factors as strength, quality, and therapeutic effectiveness. Generic drugs are sold after the patent on a brand-name drug has expired and generally under their chemical names.
- **"me-too" drug**—A brand-name drug that uses the same therapeutic mechanism as a breakthrough drug and thus directly competes with it.
- **multiple-source drug**—A drug available in both brand-name and generic versions from a variety of manufacturers.
- **single-source drug**—A brand-name drug that is still under patent and thus is usually available from only one manufacturer.

price discrimination—An indication of monopoly power by a provider. The provider is able to charge different purchasers different prices according to the purchaser's elasticity of demand (willingness to pay) for the same or a similar service.

price elasticity—The percentage change in quantity divided by the percentage change in price. When the percentage change in quantity exceeds the percentage change in price, the service is price "elastic."

primary care physician—A physician who coordinates all of the routine medical care needs of an individual. Typically, this type of physician specializes in family practice, internal medicine, pediatrics, or obstetrics/gynecology.

process measures of quality—A type of quality assessment that evaluates process of care by measuring the specific way in which care is provided or, with respect to health manpower, the educational requirements.

product market definition—Used in antitrust cases to determine whether the product or service in question has close substitutes, which depends on the willingness of purchasers to use other services if the relative prices change. The closer the substitutes, the smaller is the market share of the product being examined.

prospective payment system (PPS)—A method of payment for medical services in which providers are paid a predetermined rate for the services rendered regardless of the actual costs of care incurred. Medicare uses a PPS for hospital care based on a fixed price per hospital admission (by diagnosis).

public-interest theory of government—Assumes that legislation is enacted to serve the public interest. According to this theory, the two basic objectives of government are to improve market efficiency and, based on a societal value judgment, redistribute income.

pure premium—The expected claims experience for an insured group, exclusive of the loading charge. The pure premium for an individual is calculated by multiplying the size of the loss by the probability the loss will occur.

redistribution—When, as a result of public policy, the benefits and costs to a person are not equal, redistribution occurs. For example, based on a societal value judgment that those with higher income should be taxed to provide for those with lower income, the benefits and costs are not equal for either of the groups affected.

reference pricing—An employer (or insurer) determines the maximum price it will pay the provider for an employee's medical treatment, such as a hip replacement. The reference price is usually based on the treatment price at high-quality hospitals. If the employee goes to other hospitals for treatment, the employee pays the difference between the reference price and the hospital's price.

refundable tax credit—A proposal for national health insurance under which individuals are given a tax credit to purchase health insurance. The tax credit may be income related (i.e., declining at higher levels of income). Persons whose tax credit exceeds their tax liabilities would receive a refund for the difference. For those with little or no tax liability the tax credit is essentially a voucher for a health plan.

regressive tax—When those with lower income pay a higher portion of their income for a given tax than do those with higher income.

report card—Standardized data representing process and outcome measures of quality that are collected by independent organizations to enable purchasers to make more informed choices of health plans and their participating providers.

resource-based relative value scale (RBRVS)—The current Medicare fee-for-service payment system for physicians, initiated in 1992, under which each physician service is assigned a relative value based on the presumed resource costs of performing that service. The relative value for each service is then multiplied by a conversion factor (in dollars) to arrive at the physician's fee.

risk-adjusted premium—The employer adjusts the insurance premium to reflect the risk levels of the employees enrolled with different insurers.

risk pool—Represents a population group that is defined by its expected claim experience.

risk selection—Occurs when insurers attempt to attract a more favorable risk group than the average risk group, which was the basis for the group's premium (preferred risk selection). Similarly, enrollees may seek to join a health plan at a premium that reflects a lower level of risk than their own (adverse selection).

rule of reason—Used in antitrust cases to determine whether the anticompetitive harm caused by a particular activity (e.g., merger) exceeds the procompetitive benefits of not permitting the particular activity.

second opinion—A utilization-review approach in which decisions to initiate a medical intervention are typically reviewed by two physicians.

self-funding self-insurance—A healthcare program in which employers fund benefit plans from their own resources without purchasing insurance. Self-funded plans may be self-administered, or the employer may contract with an outside administrator for an administrative-service-only arrangement. Employers who self-fund can limit their liability via stop-loss insurance.

single payer—A form of national health insurance in which a single third-party payer (usually the government) pays healthcare providers and the entire population has free choice of all providers at zero (or little) out-of-pocket expense.

skilled nursing facility—A long-term care facility that provides inpatient skilled nursing care and rehabilitation services.

specialty PPO—A type of PPO that offers one or more limited healthcare services or benefits, such as anesthesia, vision, and dental services.

staff-model HMO—A type of HMO that hires salaried physicians to provide healthcare services on an exclusive basis to the HMO's enrollees.

stop-loss insurance—Insurance coverage providing protection from losses resulting from claims greater than a specific dollar amount (equivalent to a large deductible).

supplier-induced demand—When physicians modify their diagnosis and treatment to favorably affect their own economic well-being.

sustainable growth rate (SGR)—Medicare's expenditure limit on physician payments consists of four elements: the percentage increase in real GDP per capita, a medical inflation rate of physician fee increases, the annual percentage increase in Part B enrollees, and the percentage change in spending for physicians' services resulting from changes in laws and regulations (e.g., expanded Medicare coverage for preventive services).

target income hypothesis—A model of supplier-induced demand that assumes physicians will induce demand only to the extent they will achieve a target income, which is determined by the local income distribution, particularly with respect to the relative income of other physicians and professionals in the area.

tax-exempt employer-paid health insurance—Health insurance purchased by the employer on behalf of its employees is not considered to be taxable income to the employee. By lowering the price of insurance the quantity demanded is increased (as is its comprehensiveness). The major beneficiaries are those in higher income-tax brackets.

tertiary care—This type of care includes the most complex services (such as transplantation, open-heart surgery, and burn treatment) provided in inpatient hospital settings.

third-party administrator (TPA)—An independent entity that provides administrative services, such as claims processing, to a company that self-insures. A third-party administrator does not underwrite the risk.

third-party payer—An organization (such as an HMO, an insurance company, or a government agency) that pays for all or part of the insured's medical services.

triple-option health plan—A type of health plan in which employees may choose from an HMO, a PPO, or an indemnity plan depending on how much they are willing to contribute.

unbundling—Occurs when a provider charges separately for each of the services previously provided together as part of a treatment.

uncompensated care—Services rendered by the provider without reimbursement, as in the case of charity care and bad debts.

universal coverage—When the entire population is eligible for medical services or health insurance.

upcoding—Occurs when the provider bills for a higher-priced diagnosis or service rather than the lower-cost service actually provided.

usual, customary, and reasonable fee—A method of reimbursement in which the fee is "usual" in that physician's office, "customary" in that community, and "reasonable" in terms of the distribution of all physician charges for that service in the community.

vacancy rate—The percentage of a hospital's budgeted RN positions that are unfilled.

vertical integration—The organization of a delivery system that provides an entire range of services to include inpatient care, ambulatory care clinics, outpatient surgery, and home care.

vertical merger—A merger between two firms that have a supplier–buyer relationship.

virtual integration—The organization of a delivery system that relies on contractual relationships rather than complete ownership to provide all medical services required by the patient.

voluntary performance standard—An expenditure target adopted by the Medicare program in 1992 to limit the rate of increase in its expenditures for physicians' services. This was replaced by the SGR formula as part of the Balanced Budget Act of 1997.

INDEX

A

Abortion, 35, 36

ACA. *See* Patient Protection and Affordable Care Act (PPACA)

Access, to healthcare
equity in, 31
limitations to, 28

Accountable care organizations (ACOs), 105–106, 260, 319, 320
financial incentives for, 106, 198
financial risk of, 266
opposition to, 319
provider payment strategies of, 194

Administrative costs, in healthcare
of health insurance, 22, 70, 73–74
of Medicare, 510–511
US–Canada comparison of, 507, 509–511, 525n

Admissions. *See* Hospital admissions

Adverse selection, 82–85
under Affordable Care Act, 89–90
insurers' protection against, 83–85
in long-term care insurance, 573–574, 580n

Advertising, in healthcare
AMA's restrictions on, 10, 331
of prescription drugs, 314, 414, 418n

Affordable Care Act (ACA). *See* Patient Protection and Affordable Care Act (PPACA)

AFL-CIO (American Federation of Labor-Congress of Industrial Organizations), 491–492

Age factors. *See also* Children; Elderly population
in mortality causes, 37, 38

Agency relationship, between physicians and patients, 43–49
imperfect agent model of, 44, 46–49
perfect agent model of, 43–44, 48–49

Aid to Families with Dependent Children (AFDC), 125, 126

Alcohol tax, 502, 504–505, 548, 550

Ambulatory surgery centers, 238, 240

American Academy of Family Physicians, 180

American Association of Retired Persons (AARP), 91, 577, 592–593

American Federation of Labor-Congress of Industrial Organizations (AFL-CIO), 491–492

American Hospital Association (AHA), 195, 591

American Medical Association (AMA)
Affordable Care Act endorsement from, 589–593
antitrust lawsuits against, 10, 331
Current Procedural Terminology (CPT) trademark monopoly of, 590
position on managed care, 315
position on Medicare, 491, 492, 496n
survey of time requirements for medical procedures, 156–157, 288–289
survey on physician practice settings, 186–187, 188

Antitrust laws, 247
applied to nurses' wages, 386
effect on medical marketplace, 10–11
purpose of, 333

Antitrust lawsuits
against American Medical Association, 10, 331
against hospital mergers, 253, 333

Any willing provider (AWP) laws, 315, 334, 557

Automobile industry
employee healthcare costs of, 359, 368n–369n
labor costs of, 361
retiree health insurance coverage in, 364–365
United Auto Workers (UAW), 364–365, 591–592

B

Baby boom generation, 113–114, 155, 156, 257, 258, 565, 575

Balance-billing payment method, 145, 152

Balanced Budget Act of 1997, 127, 150

Baucus, Max, 592

Biologics. *See* Biotechnology drugs

Biotechnology companies, 458–459, 460

Biotechnology drugs, 409–410, 460–461

Block grants, 137–139

ABOUT THE AUTHOR

Paul J. Feldstein, PhD, has been a professor and the Robert Gumbiner Chair in Health Care Management at the Paul Merage School of Business, University of California, Irvine, since 1987. His previous position was at the University of Michigan as a professor in both the Department of Economics and the School of Public Health. Before that, he was the director of the Division of Research at the American Hospital Association. Professor Feldstein received his PhD from the University of Chicago.

Professor Feldstein has written eight books and more than 70 articles on healthcare. His book *Health Care Economics* is one of the most widely used texts on health economics. His book *The Politics of Health Legislation: An Economic Perspective* uses economic analysis to explain the outcome of health legislation in terms of the interest groups affected.

During leaves from the university, Professor Feldstein worked at the Office of Management and Budget, the Social Security Administration, and the World Health Organization. He has been a consultant to many government and private health agencies; has served as an expert witness on health antitrust issues; and was a board member of Sutter Health (a large not-for-profit healthcare organization serving Northern California), Province Healthcare (a hospital company serving nonurban populations), and Odyssey Healthcare (a hospice company).